The Massachusetts General Hospital Handbook of Pain Management

Second Edition

The Massachusetts General Hospital Handbook of Pain Management

Second Edition

Editor

Jane Ballantyne, M.D., FRCA
Director, MGH Pain Center
Department of Anesthesia and Critical Care
Massachusetts General Hospital
Assistant Professor of Anesthesia
Harvard Medical School
Boston, Massachusetts

Associate Editors

Scott M. Fishman, M.D.
Chief, Division of Pain Medicine
Associate Professor of Anesthesiology
University of California, Davis
Davis, California

Salahadin Abdi, M.D., PH.D.
Director, Pain Fellowship Program
Department of Anesthesia and Critical Care
Massachusetts General Hospital
Assistant Professor of Anesthesiology
Harvard Medical School
Boston, Massachusetts

Foreword by
Howard L. Fields, M.D., PH.D.

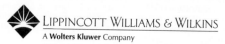
LIPPINCOTT WILLIAMS & WILKINS
A **Wolters Kluwer** Company
Philadelphia · Baltimore · New York · London
Buenos Aires · Hong Kong · Sydney · Tokyo

Acquisitions Editor: Craig Percy
Developmental Editor: Lisa Consoli
Production Editor: Jeffrey Somers
Manufacturing Manager: Colin Warnock
Compositor: Circle Graphics
Printer: R.R. Donnelley–Crawfordsville

© 2002 by Department of Anesthesia and Critical Care, Massachusetts General Hospital.
Published by LIPPINCOTT WILLIAMS & WILKINS
530 Walnut Street
Philadelphia, PA 19106 USA
LWW.com

Printed in the USA

Library of Congress Cataloging-in-Publication Data

The Massachusetts General Hospital handbook of pain management / edited by Jane Ballantyne ; associate editors, Scott Fishman, Salahadin Abdi ; foreword by Howard L. Fields.—2nd ed.
    p. ; cm.
  Includes bibliographical references and index.
  ISBN 0-7817-2377-9 (alk. paper)
    1. Pain—Treatment—Handbooks, manuals, etc. 2. Analgesia—Handbooks, manuals, etc. I. Title: Handbook of pain management. II. Ballantyne, Jane, 1948– III. Fishman, Scott, 1959– IV. Salahadin, Abdi. V. Massachusetts General Hospital
  [DNLM: 1. Pain—therapy—Handbooks. WL 39 M414 2002]
  RB127.M389 2002
  616'.0472—dc21
                                                                    2001041286

10 9 8 7 6 5

Contents

IV.   Therapeutic Options:
Nonpharmacologic Approaches

V.   Acute Pain

VI.   Chronic Pain

VII. Pain Due to Cancer

VIII. Special Situations

Appendices

Contributing Authors

Salahadin Abdi, M.D., Ph.D. *Assistant Professor of Anesthesiology, Harvard Medical School; Massachusetts General Hospital, Department of Anesthesia and Critical Care, Boston, Massachusetts*

Martin A. Acquadro, M.D., D.M.D. *Assistant Clinical Professor, Anaesthesia, Harvard Medical School; Associate Anesthetist, Massachusetts General Hospital, Boston, Massachusetts*

David K. Ahern, Ph.D. *Assistant Professor of Psychology, Department of Psychiatry, Massachusetts General Hospital, Boston, Massachusetts*

Shihab U. Ahmed, M.D. *Instructor in Anesthesia, Harvard Medical School; Department of Anesthesia and Critical Care, Massachusetts General Hospital, Boston, Massachusetts*

Joseph F. Audette, M.D. *Instructor, Harvard Medical School, Department of Physical Medicine and Rehabilitation; Director, Outpatient Pain Services, Spaulding Rehabilitation Hospital, Medford, Massachusetts*

Jane Ballantyne, M.D., FRCA *Director, MGH Pain Center; Assistant Professor of Anesthesia, Harvard Medical School; Department of Anesthesia and Critical Care, Massachusetts General Hospital, Boston, Massachusetts*

Pramit Bhasin, M.D. *Clinical Fellow, Harvard Medical School, Partners Headache Center, Massachusetts General Hospital / The Brigham and Women's Hospital, Boston, Massachusetts*

J. Andrew Billings, M.D. *Director, MGH Palliative Care; Co-Director, Center for Palliative Care; Assistant Clinical Professor, Harvard Medical School; Department of Palliative Care, Massachusetts General Hospital, Boston, Massachusetts*

Gary J. Brenner, M.D. *Instructor in Anesthesia, Harvard Medical School; Department of Anesthesia and Critical Care, Massachusetts General Hospital, Boston, Massachusetts*

Onassis A. Caneris, M.D. *Director, Comprehensive Pain Management, Northeast Rehabilitation Hospital, Salem, New Hampshire*

Paul J. Christo, M.D. *Postdoctoral Fellow, The Johns Hopkins University School of Medicine; Clinical Fellow in Pain Medicine, The Johns Hopkins Hospital, Baltimore, Maryland*

Robert S. Cluff, M.D. *Director of Neurology Section, Spine Care Pain Management Center, Seton Hospital, Daly City, California*

Steven P. Cohen, M.D. *Assistant Professor, Department of Anesthesia, Uniformed Services, University of the Health Sciences; Attending Physician, Pain Management Center, Walter Reed Army Medical Center, Massapequa, New York*

G. Rees Cosgrove, M.D., F.R.C.S.(C) *Associate Professor of Surgery, Harvard Medical School; Department of Neurosurgery, Massachusetts General Hospital, Boston, Massachusetts*

F. Michael Cutrer, M.D. *Director, Partners Headache Center; Assistant Professor of Neurology, Harvard Medical School; Department of Neurology, Massachusetts General Hospital, Boston, Massachusetts*

Isabelle Decosterd, M.D. *Centre Hospitalier Universitaire Vaudois, Anesthesiologie, Pav. 4, 1011 Lausanne, Suisse*

Thomas F. Delaney, M.D. *Lecturer in Radiation Oncology, Associate Professor of Radiation Oncology, Harvard Medical School; Department of Radiation Oncology, Massachusetts General Hospital, Boston, Massachusetts*

William T. Denman, M.D. *Director, Department of Pediatric Anesthesia, Associate Professor of Anesthesia, Tufts University Medical School, Tufts New England Medical Center, Boston, Massachusetts*

Brian W. Dubois, M.D., Ph.D. *Instructor in Anesthesia, Harvard Medical School; Department of Anesthesia and Critical Care, Massachusetts General Hospital, Boston, Massachusetts*

Annabel D. Edwards, R.N., M.S.N., A.N.P. *Clinical Nurse Specialist, Cancer Pain Service, Department of Anesthesia and Critical Care, Massachusetts General Hospital, Boston, Massachusetts*

Emad Eskandar, M.D. *Instructor in Neurosurgery, Instructor in Neurobiology, Harvard Medical School; Department of Neurosurgery, Massachusetts General Hospital, Boston, Massachusetts*

Scott M. Fishman, M.D. *Chief, Division of Pain Medicine, Associate Professor of Anesthesiology, Department of Anesthesiology and Pain Medicine, University of California, Davis; Davis, California*

Katharine H. Fleischmann, M.D. *Department of Anesthesia & Critical Care, Massachusetts General Hospital; Instructor in Anesthesia, Harvard Medical School, Boston, Massachusetts*

Jatinder S. Gill, M.D. *Department of Anesthesia and Critical Care, Massachusetts General Hospital; Instructor in Anesthesia, Harvard Medical School, Boston, Massachusetts*

Asteghik Hacobian, M.D.   *Clinical Associate, Department of Anesthesia and Critical Care, Massachusetts General Hospital, Boston, Massachusetts; Northeast Medical Consultants, Somersworth, New Hampshire*

Penelope Herbert, P.T., M.S.   *Program Director of Musculoskeletal Services, Spaulding Rehabilitation Hospital, Boston, Massachusetts*

Alyssa A. LeBel, M.D.   *Assistant Professor in Anesthesia and Neurology, Department of Anesthesia & Critical Care & Neurology, Children's Hospital of Philadelphia, Philadelphia, Pennsylvania*

Elizabeth Loder, M.D.   *Director, Pain and Headache Management Programs, Assistant Professor of Medicine, Harvard Medical School, Spaulding Rehabilitation Hospital, Boston, Massachusetts*

Edward Lubin, M.D., Ph.D.   *Clinical Fellow, The Yale School of Medicine; Attending Anesthesiologist, Yale-New Haven Hospital, West Haven, Connecticut*

Avine M. Lydon, F.F.A.R.C.S.I.   *Clinical Fellow in Anesthesia, Department of Anesthesia & Critical Care, Massachusetts General Hospital, Boston, Massachusetts*

Jianren Mao, M.D., Ph.D.   *Assistant Professor in Anesthesia, Harvard Medical School; Department of Anesthesia and Critical Care, Massachusetts General Hospital, Boston, Massachusetts*

John D. Markman, M.D.   *Clinical Fellow, Arnold Pain Management Center; Department of Anesthesia, Harvard Medical School, Beth Israel Deaconess Medical Center, Boston, Massachusetts*

Patricia McAlary, R.N., Ed.D.   *Program Director, Pain Management Program, Spaulding Rehabilitation Hospital, Boston, Massachusetts*

Bucknam J. McPeek, M.D.   *Associate Professor in Anesthesia, Harvard Medical School; Department of Anesthesiology & Critical Care, Massachusetts General Hospital, Boston, Massachusetts*

Theresa Hoskins Michel, P.T., M.S.   *Clinical Associate Professor, Massachusetts General Hospital Institute of Health Professions, Massachusetts General Hospital, Boston, Massachusetts*

Jeffrey A. Norton, M.D.   *Staff, Northeast Rehabilitation Hospital Pain Management Clinic, New England Neurological Associates, North Sutton, Massachusetts*

Anne Louise Oaklander, M.D., Ph.D. *Assistant Professor of Anesthesiology and Neurology, Harvard Medical School; Department of Anesthesia and Critical Care, Massachusetts General Hospital, Boston, Massachusetts*

May C. M. Pian-Smith, M.D., M.S. *Co-Chief, Division of Obstetric Anesthesia, Instructor in Anesthesia, Harvard Medical School; Department of Anesthesia and Critical Care, Massachusetts General Hospital, Boston, Massachusetts*

Andrew T. Putnam, M.D. *Clinical Fellow, Palliative Care Services, Massachusetts General Hospital, Boston, Massachusetts*

Daniel M. Rockers, Ph.D. *Psychologist, Division of Pain Medicine, Department of Anesthesiology and Pain Medicine, University of California, Davis Medical Center, University of California, Davis, Davis, California*

Elizabeth Ryder, R.N., M.S.N. *Clinical Nurse Specialist, Department of Anesthesia and Critical Care, Massachusetts General Hospital, Boston, Massachusetts*

Christine N. Sang, M.D., M.P.H. *Assistant Professor in Anesthesia, Harvard Medical School; Department of Anesthesia and Critical Care, Massachusetts General Hospital, Boston, Massachusetts*

Jan Slezak, M.D. *Clinical Associate, Department of Anesthesia & Critical Care, Massachusetts General Hospital, Boston, Massachusetts; Medical Director, Northeast Pain Research Center, Associate, Northeast Pain Consultants, Rochester, New Hampshire*

Milan Stojanovic, M.D. *Director, Interventional Pain Program, Instructor in Anesthesia, Department of Anesthesia and Critical Care, Massachusetts General Hospital, Boston, Massachusetts*

Jeffrey Uppington, M.D. *Department of Anesthesiology and Critical Care, Massachusetts General Hospital; Assistant Professor, Harvard Medical School, Boston, Massachusetts*

Barth L. Wilsey, M.D. *Associate Professor of Anesthesiology, Department of Anesthesiology and Pain Medicine, University of California, Davis, Davis, Massachusetts*

Harriet M. Wittink, Ph.D., PT, MS *Clinical Specialist, Assistant Professor, Tufts Medical School; Pain Management Program, Tufts New England Medical Center, Boston, Massachusetts*

Clifford J. Woolf, M.D., Ph.D. *Professor of Anesthesia Research, Harvard Medical School; Director, Neural Plasticity Research Group, Massachusetts General Hospital, Boston, Massachusetts*

YiLi Zhou, M.D., Ph.D. *Clinical Fellow, Harvard Medical School; Department of Anesthesia and Critical Care, Massachusetts General Hospital, Boston, Massachusetts*

Foreword

After three decades of progress in mapping the neural mechanisms of pain, a revolution is underway in the clinical practice of pain management: increasing numbers of physicians are taking responsibility for the relief of their patients' pain. *The Massachusetts General Hospital Handbook of Pain Management* provides an integrated and useful overview of the knowledge base required for effective treatment of pain. This timely new edition is much improved and mastering its contents will provide a sound basis for pain management.

Several factors have contributed to the revolution in pain management. Perhaps the most important is the evolution of attitude in individuals who are no longer willing to suffer pain in silence. Pain has moved progressively from the realm of the moral to that of the medical. Scientific discoveries that explain some of the most puzzling features of pain have facilitated this change in attitude. Dramatic advances have been made in understanding the neural basis of pain. For example, several critical transducer molecules have been discovered that convert chemical signals of tissue damage and intense thermal stimuli to coded electrochemical messages in the peripheral and central nerve cells that confer pain sensitivity; these are described in Chapter 2. In addition, the central nervous system pathways that transmit the information to higher centers have been described and, remarkably, we can now visualize the metabolic trace of neural activity produced in the brain of awake human subjects by painful stimuli. Beyond transduction and the transmission pathways, there are well-described brain circuits through which psychological factors can selectively amplify or suppress pain signals (see Chapter 1.) This is a discovery that has done much to explain the tremendous variability of pain severity reported by different patients with similar injuries. The public at large is familiar with the idea that endogenous opioid substances (endorphins) in the brain can produce bliss and pain relief. The objective description of pathways and mechanisms helps remove pain from the realm of the purely personal, making it less of a burden that one is expected to bear with resignation, like fear of death, and more of a sign of disease, like fever or bleeding. Clearly, the latter are matters of shared concern for both patient and physician.

This growth in our knowledge of neural mechanisms has been paralleled by increased interest on the part of physicians in actively treating pain. Although relief of suffering is accepted as a major goal for physicians, many doctors traditionally assume that pain relief per se is a simple task for which no special training is required. In fact, although acute pain is generally managed in an adequate manner, many health care professionals continue to manage acute and cancer pain inadequately, and chronic pain remains a major challenge. Fortunately, there has been increasing recognition among physicians that persistent pain is a serious and complex problem that often requires the skills of a variety of health care professionals for optimal assessment and treatment. Multidisciplinary pain clinics, a concept originated by the late John J. Bonica at the University of Washington, have now spread around the world, and it is unusual to find an academic medical center that does not have a pain management service. Appendix III of this handbook provides a useful list of resources, including reference to a list of pain centers across the country.

Despite the challenge presented by the complexity of pain, it is imperative that all physicians be experienced in its assessment and treatment. There are some simple guidelines, but the most important is to ask the patient how severe his or her pain is and what things make it worse. It is also essential to quickly establish the efficacy (or lack of efficacy) of the treatment given. In chronic pain, psychosocial factors loom large and must be assessed in the initial clinical encounter. This aspect of pain management is described in Chapter 15 of this handbook. The bottom line is that current practice standards make it unacceptable to allow a patient to suffer unnecessary pain.

This second edition of *The Massachusetts General Hospital Handbook of Pain Management* both reflects and supports the revolution in pain management by providing a broad introduction to the diagnostic complexities, assessment tools, and multiple treatment modalities that are now available. Master its contents and you will have gone far toward the goal of optimal care for pain patients.

Howard L. Fields, M.D., Ph.D.
Professor of Neurology and Physiology
UCSF School of Medicine
San Francisco, California

Preface

This book is dedicated to Donald P. Todd who instituted pain services at Massachusetts General Hospital in 1948, and who died after a short illness in 1998 while still active in the MGH Pain Center. Don was a kind and gentle physician who had enormous empathy for patients experiencing unrelenting pain. He was sure there was a way to help them. He spent many hours poring over anatomy texts and X-rays, with neurosurgeons and radiologists, devising safe and effective ways to block nerves. Over the years he taught generations of MGH fellows and residents the techniques he had mastered. He taught us, and we continue to teach our fellows and residents his techniques. Pain management has come a long way since the days when Don Todd and others were working out how to block nerves to provide pain relief, but they founded our specialty, and their role in our development will not be forgotten.

Our thanks go to David Borsook (editor and author) and to many other authors involved in the first edition of this handbook: Zahid Bajwa, Andreas Dauber, John DiCapua, Elon Eisenberg, Roberto Feliz, David Frim, Janet Hsieh, Keith Kettelberger, Suzanne LaCross, Khyati Mohamed, Shaffin Mohamed, Robert Ong, Terry Rabinowitz, Sharona Soumekh, Seth Waldman, Ursula Wesselmann, Nicolas Wieder, Melissa Wolff and Tina Wolter. This second edition of *The Massachusetts General Hospital Handbook of Pain Management* is based on their work. We owe them a debt, especially David Borsook, for formulating the concept of a pocket book on pain management to help residents, fellows, primary care practitioners, nurse practitioners, and others manage pain patients on the fly, and for contributing much of the text in the present edition.

We are also indebted to Tina Toland for her help with organizing the materials for this book, and researching the missing pieces. Last but not least, we thank our chairman, Warren Zapol, for his unbending support of this project.

Jane Ballantyne
Salahadin Abdi
Scott M. Fishman

Definitions and Abbreviations

Addiction   a disorder characterized by compulsive use of a drug resulting in physical, psychologic, and/or social dysfunction to the user and continued use despite that dysfunction

Allodynia   pain due to a stimulus such as light touch that does not normally provoke pain

Analgesia   absence of pain; commonly used to mean pain relief

Anesthesia   absence of sensation

Arthralgia   pain in a joint

Breakthrough pain   pain that breaks through the analgesia achieved by long-acting medications

Causalgia   see **CRPS II**

CNS Central nervous system

Central pain   pain that originates in the central nervous system, usually the spinothalamocortical pathway

Central sensitization   a long-term potentiation of pain signals associated with NMDA activation and with the induction of specific genes; a CNS response to prolonged painful stimulation

Chronic pain   pain that persists a month beyond the usual course of an acute injury or disease; this definition varies by treating clinician

CNMP   Chronic Non-Malignant Pain

Complex Regional Pain Syndrome (CRPS)   a chronic neuropathic pain syndrome characterized by its association at some point with evidence of edema, changes in skin blood flow, abnormal sudomotor activity in the region of pain, allodynia, hyperalgesia, or hyperpathia

CRPS I   (formerly known as **reflex sympathetic dystrophy [RSD]**); a painful condition that is associated with a continuous burning pain and sympathetic over-activity in an extremity after trauma but without major nerve injury; is not limited to the distribution of a single peripheral nerve, and is apparently disproportional to the inciting event

CRPS II   (formerly known as **causalgia**); burning pain, allodynia, and hyperpathia, often accompanied by vasomotor, sudomotor, and late trophic changes, occurring after partial injury of a nerve (or one of its major branches) in part of a limb (usually hand or foot) innervated by the damaged nerve

CSF   Cerebrospinal fluid

DEA   Drug Enforcement Agency

Deafferentation pain   pain resulting from loss of sensory input to the CNS; may arise in the periphery (e.g. peripheral nerve avulsion), or in the CNS itself (e.g. spinal cord lesions, multiple sclerosis)

Dysesthesia   an abnormal sensation, spontaneous or evoked, that is considered unpleasant

Drug dependence   (also known as physical dependence); this relates to the expression of a withdrawal syndrome upon sudden drug cessation; it occurs with the use of both addictive and nonaddictive drugs (e.g. opioids, local anesthetics, clonidine)

Drug tolerance   this occurs when a fixed dose of a drug produces a decreasing effect, so that a dose increase is required to maintain a stable effect; occurs particularly with opioids

FDA   Federal Drug Agency

Fibromyalgia   a pain syndrome that is diffuse through the body and characterized by predictable tender areas within muscles

Hypalgesia   same as **hypoalgesia**; an increased pain threshold (a decreased sensitivity to noxious stimulation)

Hypesthesia   an increased detection threshold (a decreased sensitivity to stimulation); definition excludes the special senses

Hyperalgesia   a decreased pain threshold (an exaggerated painful response to a pain-provoking stimulus)

Hyperesthesia   a decreased detection threshold (an increased sensitivity to stimulation); definition excludes the special senses

Hyperpathia   increased pain either after repetitive stimulation or due to decreased pain threshold

IASP   International Association for the Study of Pain

Meralgia paresthetica   a dysesthesia in an area of lateral femoral cutaneous nerve innervation

Myofascial pain   muscle pain stemming from muscles

Neuralgia   nerve pain along a specific anatomically distinct nerve or nerves

Neuraxis   the spinal cord and brain; the term "neuraxial" drug delivery is commonly used to encompass intrathecal and/or epidural delivery, although strictly the term should include intraventricular delivery

Neuritis   inflammation of a nerve or nerves

Neuropathy   a disturbance of function or pathologic change in individual nerves or groups of nerves; *mononeuropathy* involves a single nerve, *mononeuropathy multiplex* involves several nerves, *polyneuropathy* involves several nerves bilaterally or symmetrically

Neuropathic pain   pain caused by nerve injury or disease, or by involvement of nerves in other disease processes such as tumor or inflammation; may occur in the periphery or the CNS

NMDA   N-methyl-D-aspartate;   an important neurotransmitter associated with its own receptor, involved in the wind-up phenomenon, central sensitization, and the development of opioid tolerance

Nocebo   the noxious effects of a placebo; includes undesirable side effects (e.g. nausea), and increased pain

Nociceptive pain   pain arising from activation of nociceptors

Nociceptor   a receptor that is preferentially sensitive to noxious stimuli or to stimuli that become noxious if prolonged; a term that may also be used to refer to the entire nociceptive primary afferent from receptor through dorsal root ganglion to dorsal horn

NSAID   Nonsteroidal anti-inflammatory drug

Opiate   an opioid drug

Opioid   a substance active at endogenous opioid receptors; includes opiates (drugs) and endogenous opioids (e.g. endorphins and enkephalins)

Pain   an unpleasant sensory and emotional experience associated with actual or potential tissue damage, or described in terms of damage

Pain threshold   the lowest intensity of stimulus at which a subject experiences pain

Pain tolerance level   the greatest level of pain that a subject is able to tolerate

Paresthesia   an abnormal sensation, spontaneous or evoked, that is not considered unpleasant; the term dysesthesia should be used for an unpleasant abnormal sensation

PCA   patient-controlled analgesia

Peripheral neuropathy   neuropathic pain due to generalized or focal disease of peripheral nerves; characteristically this is constant or intermittent burning, aching or lancinating limb pain

Phantom pain   pain felt in an anatomical structure that has been surgically or traumatically removed

Physical dependence   see drug dependence

Placebo   a drug or therapy that simulates medical treatment but has no specific action on the condition being treated

Preemptive analgesia   analgesic treatment provided before and during painful stimulation that aims to modify the initial and subsequent pain responses

Pseudoaddiction   a phenomenon of drug-seeking behavior that results from undertreatment with a drug; resolves when the dose of the drug the patient seeks is increased appropriately; should be distinguished from true addiction, where drug-seeking behavior continues despite adequate and appropriate dosing

Psychogenic pain   pain inconsistent with the likely anatomic distribution of the presumed generator, or pain existing with no apparent organic pathology despite extensive evaluation

Radicular pain   pain that is evoked by stimulation of nociceptive afferent fibers in spinal nerves, their roots or ganglia, or by other neuropathic mechanisms; the symptom is caused by ectopic impulse generation; distinct from radiculopathy, but the two may arise together

Radiculopathy   a pathological condition of the nerve root (or multiple nerve roots) that results in conduction blockade and produces sensory and motor changes as well as pain in the area of its distribution; distinct from radicular pain, but the two may arise together

Referred pain   pain perceived as arising in a n area remote from its source; occurs because the nerve supply to both areas (i.e., the area pain is perceived, and the area pain is produced) is connected proximally

Reflex sympathetic dystrophy (RSD)   see **CRPS I**

Somatic pain   pain that arises from stimulation of nerves in the skin and musculoskeletal system, including bone, ligament, joint, and muscle

TCA   Tricyclic antidepressant

Tic douloureaux   a condition that produces sharp pain in the face due to abnormal firing of the trigeminal nerve; also know as trigeminal neuralgia

Tolerance   see drug tolerance

Trigger point   an area within a muscle or connective tissue that transmits pain to a distant area

VAS   Visual or verbal analogue scale;   pain assessment tools utilizing analogues (either a measured line [visual] or a numeric scale [verbal]) to represent pain

Visceral pain   pain due to stimulation of nerve endings in viscera; these nerves characteristically respond to stretch more than to other changes (e.g. cutting, inflammation, crushing); pain is usually referred to other areas (e.g. flank, skin, perineum, legs, shoulders)

WHO   World Health Organization

Wind-up   a short-term potentiation of pain signals associated with repeated high frequency (C-fiber) stimulation and with NMDA activation; ceases as soon as the stimuli cease

SELECTED READINGS

Mersky, H: Classification of chronic pain. Description of chronic pain syndromes and definition of pain terms. *Pain* (suppl 3):S1, 1986

Merskey N, Bogduk N (eds); *Classification of chronic pain, IASP Task Force on Taxonomy, 2nd ed*. IASP Press, Seattle, 1994, pp. 209–214.

Portenoy RK, Kanner RM: Definition and assessment of pain. In: Portenoy RK, Kanner RM (eds): *Pain Management: Theory and Practice*. Philadelphia, F.A. Davis, 1996, pp. 3–18.

General Considerations

General Considerations

Neural Basis of Pain

Gary J. Brenner

> Severe pain is world destroying.
> —*Elaine Scarry from The Body in Pain*

One of the most important functions of the nervous system is to provide information about potential bodily injury. Pain is defined by the International Association for Study of Pain (IASP) as "an unpleasant sensory and emotional experience associated with actual or potential tissue damage." The body's perception of pain is termed **nociception**. The pain system may be grossly divided into the following components:

1. **Nociceptors** are the specialized receptors in the peripheral nervous system that detect noxious stimuli. **Primary nociceptive afferent fibers**, normally A-delta (Aδ) and C fibers, transmit information regarding noxious stimuli to the **dorsal horn** of the spinal cord.
2. **Ascending nociceptive tracts**, for example the spinothalamic and spinohypothalamic tracts, convey nociceptive stimuli from the dorsal horn of the spinal cord to higher centers in the central nervous system (CNS).
3. **Higher centers in the CNS** are involved in pain discrimination, including affective components of pain,

3

memory components of pain, and motor control related
to the immediate aversive response to painful stimuli.
4. **Descending systems** allow higher centers of the CNS
to modify nociceptive information at multiple levels.

I. NOCICEPTORS

1. Definitions

Although it is somewhat confusing, the term *nociceptor* is used
to refer to the free nerve terminals of primary afferent fibers that
respond to painful, potentially injurious stimuli, as well as to the
entire apparatus (sensory neuron including free terminals) capable of transducing *and* transmitting information regarding noxious
stimuli. In this chapter, the term *nociceptor* will be used to refer to
the entire nociceptive primary afferent.

Free nerve terminals contain receptors capable of transducing
chemical, mechanical, and thermal signals. Recently, for example,
a membrane receptor that responds to heat has been discovered,
and, interestingly, this receptor is also stimulated by capsaicin, the
molecule responsible for the "hot" sensation associated with hot
peppers. Nociceptive terminals innervate a wide variety of tissues
and are present in both somatic and visceral structures including
the cornea, tooth pulp, muscles, joints, the respiratory system, the
cardiovascular system, the digestive system, the urogenital system, and the meninges, as well as the skin.

Nociceptors may be divided according to three criteria: degree of
myelination, type(s) of stimulation that evokes a response, and response characteristics. Using the criterion of degree of myelination
(which is related to conduction velocity), nociceptors can be divided
into two classes: Aδ fibers are thinly myelinated and conduct at a
velocity of 2 to 30 meters per second. C fibers are unmyelinated and
conduct at less than 2 m/sec (Table 1).

Aδ and C nociceptors can be further divided according to the
stimuli that they sense. They may respond to mechanical, chemical, or thermal (heat and cold) stimuli, or to a combination of these
(polymodal). For example, C-fiber mechano-heat receptors respond
to noxious mechanical stimuli and intermediate heat stimuli (41°
to 49°C), have a slow conduction velocity, and constitute the majority of nociceptive afferent fibers. Aδ-fiber mechano-heat receptors can be divided into two subtypes. Type I receptors have a high
heat threshold (>53°C) and conduct at relatively fast velocities
(30 to 55 m/sec). These receptors detect pain sensation during
high-intensity heat responses. Type II receptors have a lower heat
threshold and conduct at a slower velocity (15 m/sec). Some receptors respond to both warmth and thermal pain. There are also both
C and Aδ fibers that are mechanically insensitive but respond to
heat, cold, and a variety of chemicals, such as bradykinin, hydrogen
ions, serotonin, histamine, arachidonic acid, and prostacyclin.

2. Primary afferent fibers

The neural impulses originating from the free endings of nociceptors are transmitted via primary afferent nerves to the spinal
cord, or via cranial nerves to the brainstem if they come from the
head or neck. Most primary afferent fibers innervating tissues
below the level of the head have cell bodies located in the **dorsal
root ganglion** (DRG) of spinal nerves. Primary afferent fibers of

Table 1. Classification of fibers in peripheral nerves

Fiber group	Innervation	Mean diameter (µm)	Mean conduction velocity (m/sec)
A-alpha	Primary muscle spindle motor to skeletal muscle	15	100
A-beta	Cutaneous touch and pressure afferent fibers	8	50
A-gamma	Motor to muscle spindle	6	20
A-delta	Mechanoreceptors, **nociceptors,** thermoreceptors	<3	15
B	Sympathetic preganglionic	3	7
C	Mechanoreceptors, **nociceptors,** thermoreceptors, sympathetic postganglionic	1	1

Source: From JJ Bonica. Anatomic and physiologic basis of nociception and pain. In: JJ Bonica, ed. *The management of pain,* 2nd ed. Philadelphia: Lea & Febiger, 1990:31.

cranial nerves V, VII, IX, and X (the sensory cranial nerves) have cell bodies in their respective sensory ganglia.

The majority of nociceptors are C fibers, and 80% to 90% of C fibers respond to nociceptive input. The differences in conduction velocities and response characteristics of Aδ and C fibers may explain the typical subjective pain experience associated with a noxious stimulus: a first pain (called epicritic pain) that is rapid, well localized, and pricking in character (Aδ), followed by a second pain (called protopathic pain) that is burning and diffuse (C). Visceral afferent nociceptive fibers (Aδ and C) travel with sympathetic and parasympathetic fibers; their cell bodies are also found in the DRG. Muscle is also innervated by both Aδ and C fibers and, interestingly, muscle pain appears to be limited in quality to that of a cramp.

3. Dorsal horn synapses and biochemical mediators

Primary afferent nociceptors enter the spinal cord via Lissauer's tract and synapse on neurons in the dorsal horn (Fig. 1). Lissauer's tract is a bundle of predominately (80%) primary afferent fibers, consisting mainly of Aδ and C fibers that penetrate the spinal cord en route to the dorsal horn. After entering the spinal cord, Aδ and

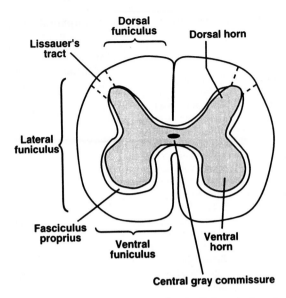

Figure 1. Diagrammatic cross section of the spinal cord.

C fibers run up or down one or two segments before synapsing with second-order neurons in the dorsal horn.

The dorsal horn synapse is an important site of further processing and integration of the incoming nociceptive information. The dorsal horn may be a point at which nociceptive information is conducted to higher centers, or it may be a point at which nociceptive information is inhibited by descending systems. The responsiveness of dorsal horn neurons may change in response to prior noxious afferent input, particularly repetitive input (central sensitization).

Biochemical mediators

Numerous neurotransmitters and other biochemical mediators are released in the dorsal horn. These substances are derived from three main sources:

a. Primary afferent fibers
b. Interneurons
c. Descending fiber systems

The neurochemistry of the dorsal horn is complicated and there are qualitative differences between the pharmacology of acute pain and that of the facilitated pain states associated with chronic noxious stimulation. Some of the neurochemical mediators can be categorized as excitatory or inhibitory, although many serve complex and mixed functions. For example, the endogenous opioid dynorphin may be inhibitory or excitatory depending on the state of the nervous system. The following are examples of excitatory and inhibitory substances active in the dorsal horn.

Excitatory neuromediators:
- Excitatory amino acids—glutamate and aspartate
- Neuropeptides—substance P (SP) and calcitonin gene-related peptide (CGRP)
- Growth factor—brain-derived neurotrophic factor (BDNF)

Inhibitory neuromediators:
- Endogenous opioids, such as enkephalin and β-endorphin
- Gamma-aminobutyric acid (GABA)
- Glycine

Cells of the dorsal horn possess specific receptors for the substances just listed, as well as receptors for a multitude of other neurochemicals (some probably undiscovered). Of particular note is one of the glutamate receptors, the *N*-**methyl**-D-**aspartate** (NMDA) receptor, which is widely distributed in the dorsal horn. Extensive experimental data now implicate the NMDA receptor in the generation and maintenance of facilitated pain states.

4. Peripheral sensitization

Prolonged noxious stimulation can sensitize nociceptors. *Sensitization* refers to a decreased threshold as well as to an increased response to suprathreshold stimulation. It is observed following direct nerve injury and inflammation, and it is the result of a complex set of transcriptional and post-translational changes in the primary nociceptive afferents. Sensitization of the entire nociceptive pathway can arise secondary to changes in the CNS (central sensitization) or the periphery (peripheral sensitization). Once sensitization is established, it may be impossible to separate central contributions from peripheral contributions to the process of sensitization. The related topics of hyperalgesia, allodynia, inflammation, and nerve injury are briefly discussed next.

Hyperalgesia

Tissue damage results in activation of nociceptors, and if the damage is prolonged and intense it can generate a state in which there is a lowered threshold to painful stimuli. This state is known as **hyperalgesia**. In areas of hyperalgesia it is also possible to observe an increased response to noxious stimuli. There are alterations in both the subjective and the neurophysiologic responses to stimuli. The subjective response is characterized by a lowered pain threshold and an increase in pain response, while nociceptors demonstrate a corresponding decreased threshold and increased response. **Primary hyperalgesia** is hyperalgesia at the site of injury, and **secondary hyperalgesia** refers to hyperalgesia in the surrounding skin. Neural changes producing hyperalgesia can also occur in the CNS (central sensitization).

Allodynia

In addition to the development of a lowered threshold for noxious stimuli following tissue damage (hyperalgesia), it is possible to observe a post-injury state in which normally innocuous stimuli are perceived as painful. This phenomenon is termed **allodynia**. For example, very light touch in the area of a burn or associated with post-herpetic neuralgia can generate excruciating pain. Like hyperalgesia, allodynia is most likely caused by plastic changes in both primary sensory fibers and spinal cord neurons.

Inflammation

Inflammation, the characteristic reaction to injury, results in **rubor, calor, dolor, tumor, and functio laesa** (i.e., redness, heat, pain, swelling, and loss of function). During an inflammatory response, activation of nociceptive pathways can lead to sensitization resulting clinically in spontaneous and increased stimulation-induced pain (i.e., hyperalgesia and allodynia). Release of prostaglandins, cytokines, growth factors, and other mediators by inflammatory cells can directly stimulate nociceptors. The precise nature of this interaction between the immune and nervous systems and the manner in which this can lead to pathologic pain states, however, remains to be clarified. The critical observation is that inflammation is an important cause of both acute and chronic alterations in pain processing and sensation.

Nerve injury

Direct neural trauma can also lead to pathologic pain states characterized by **spontaneous pain** (i.e., pain occurring in the absence of any stimulus), hyperalgesia, and allodynia. Such **neuropathic pain** can arise following injury to peripheral or central elements of the pain system. A clinical example of this is complex regional pain syndrome type I (CRPS-I), formerly called reflex sympathetic dystrophy (RSD), in which an apparently minor injury can lead to sensitization of pain processing in a region including but not limited to that involved in the injury.

II. ASCENDING NOCICEPTIVE PATHWAYS

1. Topographical arrangement of the dorsal horn (rexed laminae)

The gray matter of the spinal cord can be divided into 10 laminae (the Rexed laminae I through X) on the basis of the histologic organization of the numerous types of cell bodies and dendrites. The dorsal horn is composed of laminae I through VI (Fig. 2). The majority of nociceptive input converges on lamina I (the marginal zone), lamina II (the substantia gelatinosa), and lamina V in the dorsal horn. However, some primary visceral and somatic nociceptive afferent fibers synapse in other laminae. Cutaneous mechanoreceptor Aδ afferent fibers synapse in laminae I, II, and V; visceral mechanoreceptor Aδ fibers synapse in laminae I and V; cutaneous nociceptor C fibers synapse in laminae I and II; and visceral nociceptive C fibers synapse in many laminae including I, II, IV, V, and X. The ascending spinal pathways involved with nociceptive transmission arise mainly from laminae I, II, and V (Fig. 3). These pathways include the spinothalamic tract, the spinohypothalamic tract, the spinoreticular tract, and the spinopontoamygdala tract.

2. Dorsal horn projection neurons

The **second-order neurons** in the pain pathway are the dorsal horn projection neurons (or their equivalent in cranial pathways). Their cell bodies are in the spinal cord (or in cranial nerve nuclei in

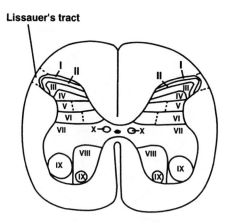

Figure 2.   Rexed laminae I through X of the spinal cord.

the head and neck), and they are classified according to their response characteristics. High-threshold [HT; also called nociceptive-specific (NS)] cells respond exclusively to noxious stimuli; these cells receive input only from nociceptors (i.e., Aδ and C fibers). Their receptive fields are small and organized somatotopically, being most abundant in lamina I.

Other cells, called wide dynamic range (WDR) cells, respond to a range of stimuli from innocuous to noxious. They integrate information from A-beta (Aβ; transmitters of information about non-noxious stimuli), Aδ, and C fibers. These cells have larger receptive fields, are the most prevalent cells in the dorsal horn, and are found in all laminae, with a concentration in lamina V. The convergence of sensory information onto a single dorsal horn neuron is critical for the coding of stimulus intensity in terms of output frequency by these second-order neurons.

3. Spinothalamic tract

The spinothalamic tract (STT) (Fig. 3) is the most important of the ascending pathways for the transmission of nociceptive stimuli. It is located in the anterolateral quadrant of the spinal cord. The cell bodies of STT neurons reside in the dorsal horn; most of their axons cross at the midline in the ventral white commissure of the spinal cord and ascend in the opposite anterolateral quadrant, although some do remain ipsilateral. Neurons from more distal regions of the body (e.g., the sacral region) are found more laterally, and neurons from more proximal regions (e.g., the cervical region) are found more medially within the spinothalamic tract as it ascends. STT neurons segregate into medial and lateral projections to the thalamus (see Limbic System, later).

Neurons that project to the **lateral thalamus** arise from laminae I, II, and V, and from there they synapse with fibers that project to the somatosensory cortex. The fibers are thought to be involved in sensory and discriminative aspects of pain.

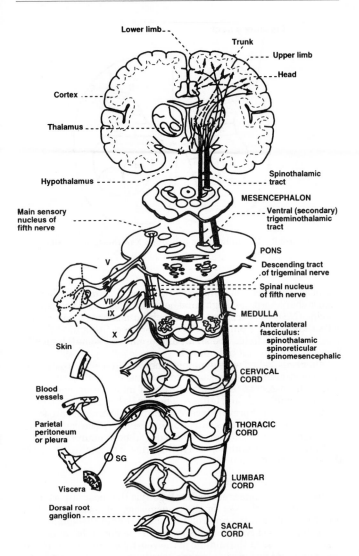

Figure 3.   Ascending pain pathways. (Reproduced with permission from Bonica JJ, ed. *The Management of Pain*, vol. 1. Philadelphia: Lea and Febiger, 1990:29.)

Neurons that project to the **medial thalamus** originate from the deeper laminae VI and IX. The neurons send collateral projections to the reticular formation of the brainstem and midbrain, the periaqueductal gray matter (PAG), and the hypothalamus, or directly to other areas of the basal forebrain and somatosensory cortex. They are thought to be involved with autonomic reflex responses, state of arousal, and emotional aspects of pain.

4. Spinohypothalamic tract

Nociceptive and non-nociceptive information from neurons within the dorsal horn is conveyed directly to diencephalic structures, such as the hypothalamus, by a recently discovered pathway—the **spinohypothalamic tract**. This pathway projects to the region of the brain (the hypothalamus) that is involved in autonomic functions such as sleep, appetite, temperature regulation, and stress response. In fact, the majority (60%) of SHT neurons project to the contralateral medial or lateral hypothalamus and, therefore, are presumed to have a significant role in autonomic and neuroendocrine responses to painful stimuli. Thus, the SHT appears to form the anatomic substrate that coordinates reflex autonomic reactions to painful stimuli. Some of its connections (e.g., to the suprachiasmatic nucleus, which partly controls the sleep/wake pattern) may account for behaviors such as difficulty in sleeping with painful conditions, particularly chronic pain. The majority of SHT neurons respond preferentially to mechanical nociceptive stimulation, and a smaller number respond to noxious thermal stimulation. The fibers of the SHT cross midline in the supraoptic decussation. The spinoreticular tract (SRT) and the spinopontoamygdala tract are also probably involved with state of arousal and emotional aspects of pain.

5. Cranial nerves

The transmission of pain in the head and neck has many of the same characteristics as the nociceptive system, which has first-order synapses in the dorsal horn of the spinal cord. The face and oral cavity are richly innervated with nociceptors. The primary nociceptive afferent fibers for the head originate mainly from cranial nerve V but also from cranial nerves VII, IX, and X, and from the upper cervical spinal nerves. The primary afferent fibers of the cranial nerves project mainly to nuclei of the trigeminal system, whereas the upper cervical nerves project to second-order neurons in the dorsal horn of the spinal cord. From there, projections continue to the supraspinal systems.

Trigeminal System

The trigeminal system (V) receives afferent input from the three divisions of the trigeminal nerve (ophthalmic, maxillary, and mandibular), which serve the entire face as well as the dura and the vessels from a large portion of the anterior two thirds of the brain. The trigeminal has three sensory nuclei, all of which receive projections from cells that have cell bodies located within the trigeminal ganglion, a structure similar to the DRG. The three nuclei are the mesencephalic, the main sensory, and the spinal trigeminal. The latter is further divided into the subnucleus oralis, the subnucleus interpolaris, and the subnucleus caudalis. The subnucleus caudalis (also known as the medullary dorsal horn) extends caudally from the medulla to the level of the upper cervical segments of the spinal cord (C3 to C4).

The trigeminal nuclei give rise to several ascending pathways. The axons of cell bodies in the main sensory nucleus and the subnucleus oralis project either ipsilaterally, forming the dorsal trigeminothalamic tract, or contralaterally, in the ventral trigeminothalamic tract. Both tracts terminate in the thalamus. The subnucleus caudalis contributes as well to the trigeminothalamic tracts, but it also has direct projections to the thalamus, the reticular formation, and the hypothalamus.

Glossopharyngeal nerve

The glossopharyngeal nerve (IX) conveys impulses associated with tactile sense, thermal sense, and pain from the mucous membranes of the posterior third of the tongue, tonsil, posterior pharyngeal wall, and eustachian tubes.

Vagus nerve

The vagus nerve (X) conveys impulses associated with tactile sense from the posterior auricular skin and external auditory meatus, and those associated with visceral sensation from the pharynx, larynx, trachea, esophagus, and thoracic and abdominal viscera, via the spinal trigeminal tract and the fasciculus solitarius (the sensory tract of VII, IX, and X).

6. Central Sensitization

Just as prolonged noxious stimulation of nociceptors can result in altered pain states (peripheral sensitization), so repetitive stimulation of second-order (and higher-order) neurons can alter pain processing (**central sensitization**). Hyperalgesia and allodynia are manifestations of central as well as peripheral sensitization (see Peripheral Sensitization, earlier). The ability of the neural tissue to change in response to various incoming stimuli is a key function of the nervous system, and it is termed **neural plasticity**. Presumably, this function has some evolutionary or protective advantage, although in clinical pain practice, a disadvantage is often seen—the development of chronic pain. Both short-term and long-term plastic changes occur in the dorsal horn. **Wind-up** is an increase in the ratio of outgoing to incoming action potentials of a dorsal horn neuron with each successive nociceptive stimulus. It occurs in response to repetitive C-fiber stimulation, and it is reversed as soon as the stimulation ceases. This is an example of a short-term plastic change. Central sensitization (including wind-up) is associated with NMDA receptor activation. In the case of long-term sensitization, various mechanisms produce the changes and there may be associated new gene expression (e.g., C-*fos*).

III. SUPRASPINAL SYSTEMS: INTEGRATION AND HIGHER PROCESSING

Integration of pain in higher centers is complex and poorly understood. At a basic level, the integration and processing of painful stimuli may fall into the following broad categories:

Discriminative component: This somatotopically specific component involves the primary (SI) and secondary (SII) sensory cortex. The level of integration allows the brain to define the location of the painful stimulus. Integration of somatic pain, as opposed to visceral pain, takes place at this level. The primary and secondary cortices receive input predominantly from the ventrobasal complex of the thalamus, which is also somatotopically organized.

Affective component: The integration of the affective component of pain is very complex and involves various limbic structures. In particular, the cingulate cortex is involved in the affective components of pain (it receives input from the parafascicular thalamic nuclei and projects to various limbic regions). The amygdala is also involved in the integration of noxious stimuli.

Memory components of pain: Recent evidence has demonstrated that painful stimuli activate CNS regions such as the anterior insula.

Motor control and pain: The supplemental motor area is thought to be involved in the integration of the motor response to pain.

1. Thalamus

The thalamus is a complex structure that acts as the relaying center for incoming nociceptive stimuli, and it has two important divisions that receive nociceptive input. First is the **lateral division**, formed by the ventrobasal complex in which nociceptive specific input from NS and WDR neurons synapses. It is somatotopically organized and projects to the somatosensory cortex. Second is the **medial division**, which consists of the posterior nucleus and the centrolateral nucleus. It is thought that these nuclei project to limbic structures involved in the affective component of pain, because there is no nociceptive-specific information conveyed by them to higher cortical regions.

The **medial and intralaminar nuclei** receive input from many ascending tracts, in particular the STT, and the reticular formation. There is little evidence of somatotopic organization of these nuclei. The **ventrobasal thalamus** is organized somatotopically and can be further subdivided into (a) the **ventral posterior lateral nucleus**, which receives input mainly from the STT but also from the dorsal column system and the somatosensory cortex, to which it projects, and (b) the ventral **posterior medial nucleus**, which receives input from the face via the trigeminothalamic tract and projects to the somatosensory cortical regions of the face. Input to the **posterior thalamus** comes mainly from the STT, the spinocortical tract, and the dorsal column nuclei. The receptive fields are large and bilateral and lack somatotopic organization. The posterior nuclei project to the somatosensory cortex and appear to have a role in the sensory experience of pain. The STT also sends projections to the **centrolateral nucleus**, which is involved in motor activity (e.g., the cerebellar and cerebral cortex).

2. Hypothalamus

The hypothalamus receives innocuous and noxious stimuli from all over the body, including deep tissues such as the viscera (see Spinohypothalamic Tract, earlier). The hypothalamic neurons are not somatotopically organized and therefore do not provide discriminatory aspects and localization of pain. Some hypothalamic nuclei send projections to the pituitary gland via the hypophyseal stalk, the brainstem, and the spinal cord. The gland regulates both the autonomic nervous system and neuroendocrine response to stress, including pain.

3. Limbic system

The limbic system consists of subcortical regions of the telencephalon, mesencephalon, and diencephalon. It receives input from the STT, the thalamus, and the reticular formation, and it projects to various parts of the cerebral cortex, particularly the frontal and temporal cortex. It is involved in the motivational and emotional aspects of pain, including mood and experience.

4. Cerebral cortex

The somatosensory cortex and the cingulate cortex are involved in pain. The somatosensory cortex is the most important area for nociception. It is located posterior to the central sulcus of the brain, and it receives input from the various nuclei of the thalamus, particularly the ventral posterior lateral and medial nuclei and the posterior thalamus. The somatosensory cortex is cytoarchitecturally organized and therefore has an important role in the discriminatory aspect and localization of pain. Efferent fibers from the somatosensory cortex travel back to the thalamus and contribute to the descending nociceptive system.

5. Cingulate cortex

The cingulate cortex is a component of the limbic system. The limbic system receives sensory and cortical impulses and activates visceral and somatic effectors; it contributes to the physiologic expression of behavior and emotion. The limbic system includes the subcallosal, cingulate, and parahippocampal gyri and hippocampal formation as well as the following subcortical nuclei: the amygdala, the septal nuclei, the hypothalamus, the anterior thalamic nuclei, and the nuclei in the basal ganglia. Recent work has demonstrated that the cingulate gyrus is activated in humans by painful stimuli. Cingulate cortex lesions have been used in an attempt to alleviate pain and suffering.

IV. PAIN MODULATION

Figure 4 and 5 illustrate pathways involved in the modulation of nociceptive information. The evidence for descending controls came from two basic observations. The first observation, in the late 1960s, was that neurons in the dorsal horn of decerebrate animals are more responsive to painful stimuli with spinal cord blockade. The second observation, in the late 1980s, was that electrical stimulation of the PAG profoundly relieved pain in animals. So great was the stimulation-produced analgesia that surgery could be performed on these animals without apparent pain. Furthermore, the animals behaved normally in every other way and there was no observed effect on other sensory modalities. These studies were pivotal in demonstrating an anatomic basis for the "natural equivalent" of **stimulation-produced analgesia**. Furthermore, subsequent studies demonstrated that small concentrations of morphine, when injected into regions such as the PAG, produced significant analgesia. Interestingly, both stress-induced analgesia and stimulation-induced analgesia can be reversed by

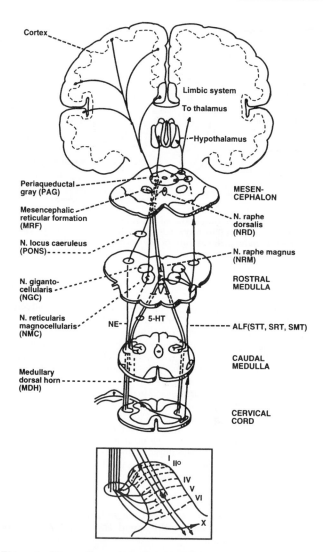

Figure 4.   Descending pain pathways. 5-HT, serotonin; NE, noradrenergic input; ALF, anterolateral fasciculus; STT, spinothalamic tract; SRT, spinoreticular tract; SMT, spinomesencephalic tract. (Reproduced with permission from Bonica JJ, ed. *The Management of Pain*, vol. 1. Philadelphia: Lea and Febiger, 1990:108.)

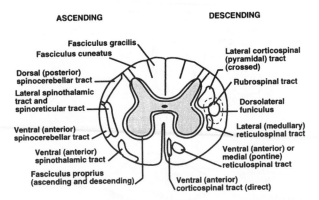

ASCENDING   **DESCENDING**

Fasciculus gracilis
Fasciculus cuneatus

Dorsal (posterior)
spinocerebellar tract
Lateral spinothalamic
tract and
spinoreticular tract

Ventral (anterior)
spinocerebellar tract

Ventral (anterior)
spinothalamic tract

Fasciculus proprius
(ascending and descending)

Lateral corticospinal
(pyramidal) tract
(crossed)

Rubrospinal tract

Dorsolateral
funiculus

Lateral (medullary)
reticulospinal tract

Ventral (anterior) or
medial (pontine)
reticulospinal tract

Ventral (anterior)
corticospinal tract (direct)

Figure 5.   Cross section of the spinal cord showing the location of the ascending pain pathways (e.g., the spinothalamic tract). The descending pain pathways are in the dorsolateral funiculus (not shown) of the spinal cord.

opioid antagonists. A number of brain centers are involved in the intrinsic modulation of noxious stimuli. These include the somatosensory cortex, the hypothalamus (paraventricular nucleus, lateral hypothalamus), the midbrain PAG, areas in the pons including the lateral tegmental area, and the raphe magnus. Electrical stimulation of these regions in humans (in some cases) and in animals produces analgesia.

Fibers from these central structures descend directly or indirectly (e.g., PAG to raphe magnus) via the dorsolateral funiculus to the spinal cord and send projections to laminae I and V. Activation of the descending analgesic system has a direct effect on the integration and passage of nociceptive information at the level of the dorsal horn. Blockade of the dorsolateral funiculus (with cold or sectioning) increases the response of nociceptive second-order neurons following activation by painful stimuli.

1. Descending systems

The descending system appears to have three major functionally interrelated components: the opioid, the noradrenergic, and the serotonergic systems.

Opioid system

The opioid system is involved in descending analgesia. Opioid precursors (pro-opiomelanocortin, proenkephalin, and prodynorphin) and their respective peptides (beta-endorphin, met- and leu-enkephalin, and dynorphin) are present in the amygdala, the hypothalamus, the PAG, the raphe magnus, and the dorsal horn. With the recent advent of opioid receptor cloning, knowledge is steadily increasing about the action sites of the various opioids (i.e., on mu, delta, and kappa receptors).

Noradrenergic System

Noradrenergic neurons project from the locus caeruleus and other noradrenergic cell groups in the medulla and pons. These projections are found in the dorsolateral funiculus. Stimulation of these areas produces analgesia, as does the administration (direct or intrathecal) of an alpha-2-receptor agonist such as clonidine.

Serotonergic System

Many neurons in the raphe magnus are known to contain serotonin [5-hydroxytryptamine (5-HT)], and they send projections to the spinal cord via the dorsolateral funiculus. Pharmacologic blockade, or lesioning, of the raphe magnus can reduce the effects of morphine, and administration of 5-HT to the spinal cord produces analgesia.

2. "On" and "off" cells: a component of descending analgesia

Nociceptive cells in the dorsal horn can be activated or inhibited following stimulation of the PAG. Therefore, it is reasonable to posit the existence of brain centers that provide both excitatory and inhibitory descending output. The raphe magnus, and other brain regions known to be involved in descending modulation (e.g., the PAG), appears to generate such output. Several types of neurons involved in the control of nociceptive information reside in the raphe magnus: in particular, there are neurons named "on" cells and "off" cells based on apparent function.

"On" cells are active prior to a nocifensive withdrawal reflex (e.g., tailflick). These cells are stimulated by nociceptive input; they are excited by stimulation and are inhibited by morphine. "On" cells facilitate nociceptive transmission in the dorsal horn. "Off" cells shut off prior to a nocifensive withdrawal reflex. These cells are inhibited by noxious stimuli, whereas they are excited by electrical stimulation and by morphine. It has been postulated that opioids act to inhibit inhibitory interneurons (GABAergic) that act on "off" cells and that, in this way, they produce a net excitatory effect on these cells. "Off" cells inhibit nociceptive transmission in the dorsal horn.

3. Projections to the dorsal horn

The nerve fibers that originate in nuclei that are involved in pain modulation terminate in the dorsal horn predominately in laminae I and II but also in other laminae, including IV, V, VI, and X. Thus there is a circuitry of projecting neurons acting directly or indirectly via interneurons on afferent fibers as well as projecting neurons such as the spinothalamic tract neurons.

V. CONCLUSION

The neuroanatomy and neurochemistry of the pain system is extremely complex. Neuroanatomic techniques have taught us a great deal about the "connectivity" of the system. Newer techniques have enabled the study of individual cells and specific cell populations in an attempt to elucidate roles in both ascending and descending systems. Sophisticated imaging—for example, functional magnetic resonance imaging and positron emission tomography—have allowed investigation of *in vivo* brain activity in the presence of acute and chronic pain. Thus, the nociceptive system continues to be investigated using reductionistic and holistic approaches to better understand its resting and pathologic states.

SELECTED READING

1. Fields HL. *Pain.* New York: McGraw-Hill, 1999.
2. Kruger L, ed. *Pain and touch.* San Diego: Academic Press, 1996.
3. Scarry E. *The body in pain: The making and unmaking of the world.* Oxford: Oxford University Press, 1985.
4. Simone DA. Peripheral mechanisms of pain perception. In: Abram SE, ed. *The atlas of anesthesia: Pain management.* Philadelphia: Churchill-Livingstone, 1998:1.1–1.11.
5. Waldman SD, Winnie AP, eds. Part I. Anatomy and physiology of pain: Clinical correlates. In: *Interventional pain management*, 4th ed. Philadelphia: WB Saunders, 1996:1–72.
6. Wall PD, Melzack R, eds. *Textbook of pain*, 4th ed. Philadelphia: Churchill-Livingstone, 1999.

Pain Mechanisms and Their Importance in Clinical Practice and Research

Isabelle Decosterd and Clifford J. Woolf

After great pain, a formal feeling comes
The Nerves sit ceremonious, like Tombs
The stiff Heart questions was it He, that bore,
And Yesterday, or Centuries before?
—*Emily Dickinson, 1830–1886*

It has become increasingly clear from animal models and from preclinical and clinical studies that multiple mechanisms operating at different sites and with different temporal profiles induce chronic pain syndromes. The identification of these mechanisms may provide the best lead to effective pain treatment, especially in the case of novel treatments. Whereas primary disease factors initiate pain mechanisms, it is the pain mechanisms, not the disease factors, that produce chronic pain. Identifying the causes of diseases is important, but it is also essential to differentiate them from pain mechanisms. Because a particular disease may activate several different pain mechanisms, a disease-based classification is useful primarily for disease-modifying therapy, but less for pain therapy. Similarly, symptoms are not equivalent to mechanisms, although they may reflect them. The same symptom may be produced by different mechanisms and a single mechanism may elicit different symptoms.

In this chapter, we propose a new way of analyzing pain, based on the current understanding of pain mechanisms, and we show the implications of this for assessing pain in individual patients and for evaluating new forms of diagnosis and therapy.

I. FUNDAMENTAL PAIN MECHANISMS

1. Response to acute painful stimuli

Acute pain is initiated by a subset of highly specialized primary neurons, the high-threshold nociceptors, innervating peripheral tissues (skin, muscle, bone, viscera). The peripheral terminals of these sensory neurons are adapted so as to be activated only by intense or potentially damaging peripheral noxious stimuli. These receptors are functionally distinct from the low-threshold sensory fibers, which are normally activated only in response to nondamaging low-intensity innocuous stimuli. Nociceptor transduction mechanisms involve activation of any of the following:

1. Temperature-sensitive receptor ion-channel sensors [such as vanilloid (capsaicin) receptor subtype 1 (VR1) and vanilloid-receptor–like protein 1 (VRL1)]
2. Channels (yet to be identified) sensitive to intense mechanical deformation or stretch of the membrane
3. Chemosensitive receptors [such as VR1, dorsal root acid-sensing ionic channel (DRASIC) and ATP-gated ion channel type 3 (P2X3)] activated by protons, purines, amines, peptides or growth factors, and cytokines released from damaged tissue or inflammatory cells

2. Peripheral sensitization

The sensitivity of the peripheral terminal is not fixed, and its activation either by repeated peripheral stimulation or by changes in the chemical milieu of the terminal increases the excitability of the terminal and decreases the threshold for initiation of an action potential in the primary sensory neuron. This phenomenon is referred to as **peripheral sensitization**. Peripheral sensitization reflects changes in the channel kinetics caused both by transduction in ion channels themselves (autosensitization, resulting from prior activation) and by an increase in excitability of the terminal membrane (heterosensitization, initiated by sensitizing stimuli such as inflammatory mediators that do not activate the usual pain transducers).

Autosensitization of vanilloid receptors (VR1, VRL1), for instance, may represent both (a) conformational changes of the receptor secondary to the external heat stimuli and (b) the entry of calcium through the transducer itself, leading to activation of protein kinase C, which phosphorylates VR1. Heterosensitization is driven by sensitizing agents such as prostaglandin E_2, histamine, bradykinin, serotonin, and neurotrophic factors that can activate intracellular kinases. Intracellular kinases have the ability to phosphorylate and change the activity state of voltage-gated sodium channels such as SNS (the sensory-neuron–specific sodium channel PN3/Na$_v$1.8).

3. Central sensitization

In addition to changes in the sensitivity of the nociceptor peripheral terminal, post-injury pain hypersensitivity is also an expression of modulation of nociceptive synaptic transmission in the dorsal horn of the spinal cord. This is called **central sensitization**. Input from nociceptors to the spinal cord evokes an immediate sensation of pain that lasts for the duration of the noxious stimulus and also induces an activity-dependent functional plasticity in the dorsal horn that outlasts the stimulus. The increased excitability is triggered by peripheral nociceptor input, releasing excitatory amino acids and neurotransmitters that act on spinal cord postsynaptic receptors to produce inward currents, as well as activating signal transduction cascades in the neuron.

These processes result in activation of both serine/threonine kinases and tyrosine kinases, which, by phosphorylating membrane proteins, particularly the receptors for N-methyl-D-aspartate glutamate (NMDA) and alpha-amino-3-hydroxy-5-methyl-4-isoxazole propionic acid (AMPA)/kainate, increase membrane excitability by changing ion channel properties. This boost in excitability recruits existing subthreshold inputs to the dorsal horn neurons, thereby amplifying responses to noxious and non-noxious stimuli. The changes may be restricted to the activated synapse or spread to the adjacent synapse, and they are responsible for pain produced by low-threshold afferent inputs and the spread of pain hypersensitivity to regions beyond the tissue injury (secondary hyperalgesia).

Central sensitization is a major contributor to inflammatory and neuropathic pain, producing a largely NMDA-dependent, brush- or pinprick-evoked secondary hyperalgesia and a tactile allodynia. In inflammation, this activity-dependent central plasticity is driven by input from sensitized afferents innervating the inflamed tissue. After nerve injury, central sensitization can be driven by the **ectopic activity** in the injured fibers resulting from changes in the expression, distribution, or activity of ion channels. These central functional changes are contributed to by **changes or switches in the phenotype of sensory neurons**. Up to 30 molecules, mainly neuromodulators [such as galanin, vasoactive intestinal peptide (VIP), cholecystokinin (CCK), neuropeptide Y (NPY), brain-derived neurotrophic factor (BDNF), and nitric oxide synthase (NOS)] that alter synaptic drive and modify the response to basal stimulation, are regulated after nerve injury. In addition to the change in gene expression of the level of neuromodulators, novel expression also occurs, so that subpopulations of dorsal root ganglion (DRG) cells that do not normally express a neuromodulator, such as substance P or BDNF, begin to do so.

For example, substance P, which is normally expressed only in nociceptors, begins to be expressed in low-threshold sensory neurons after both inflammation and nerve injury. This means that although central sensitization is normally evoked only by nociceptor input, input from A fibers can also produce this phenomenon after nerve injury or inflammation. One example of this is the development of a progressive tactile pain hypersensitivity with the repeated touch of inflamed skin.

4. Disinhibition

In addition to the activity-dependent increase in membrane excitability triggered by peripheral input, a decrease in phasic and tonic inhibition can also produce changes in dorsal horn excitability. This **disinhibition** may result from a down-regulation of inhibitory transmitters or their receptors, and from a disruption of descending inhibitory pathways. Furthermore, nerve injury, by virtue of injury discharge and ectopic activity, may lead to cell death in the superficial lamina of the dorsal horn, where inhibitory interneurons are concentrated.

5. Structural reorganization

After nerve injury, another anatomic change occurs: the **structural reorganization of central connections**. This involves the sprouting or growth of the central terminals of low-threshold mechanoreceptors from their normal termination site in the deep dorsal horn into lamina II (See Chapter 1, figure 2), the site of termination of nociceptor C-fiber terminals. The sprouted low threshold A fibers make synaptic contact in lamina II with neurons that normally receive nociceptor input, and this new pattern of synaptic input provides an anatomic substrate for tactile pain hypersensitivity.

6. Overview

A complex system of mechanistic changes occurs then, following the activation of the somatosensory pathways by both peripheral inflammatory and nerve lesions. An increase in the gain of the nociceptive system, in the periphery and in the central nervous system, is caused by activity-dependent plasticity, and it manifests as a widely distributed but transient pain hypersensitivity. With time, the changes evolve so that a number of different mechanisms that induce pain hypersensitivity are recruited. Three different

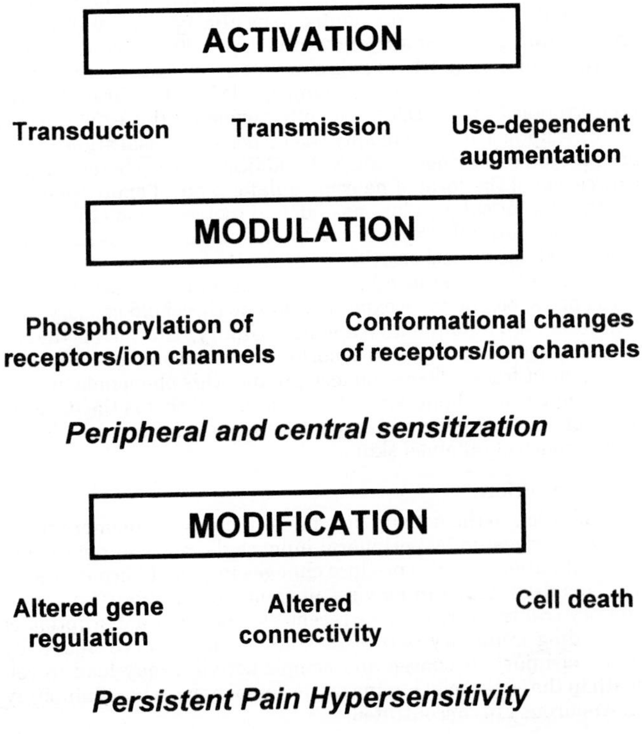

ACTIVATION

Transduction   **Transmission**   **Use-dependent augmentation**

MODULATION

Phosphorylation of receptors/ion channels   **Conformational changes of receptors/ion channels**

Peripheral and central sensitization

MODIFICATION

Altered gene regulation   **Altered connectivity**   **Cell death**

Persistent Pain Hypersensitivity

Figure 1.   The three forms of neural plasticity that can produce pain hypersensitivity are summarized, highlighting the molecular and cellular changes implicated in pain mechanisms. (Modified from Woolf CJ, Salter MW. Neuronal plasticity: increasing the gain in pain. *Science* 2000;288:1765–1769, with permission.)

forms (activation, modulation, and modification) of neural plasticity that produce pain hypersensitivity are summarized in Figure 1. Activation is directly linked to the noxious stimuli and it involves transduction and transmission of the signal. Modulation involves the peripheral and central sensitization processes. Modification of the system includes gene regulation, altered connectivity, and cell death. Persistent pain states may be associated with mechanisms that involve changes that are irreversible, such as cell death.

II. TOWARD A NEW CONCEPTUAL APPROACH FOR THE UNDERSTANDING OF PAIN

The current clinical evaluation of pain uses an etiologic or disease-based approach. This approach, however, should be modified to incorporate a mechanism-based diagnosis of pain. Identifying the causative disease is essential, particularly when disease-modifying treatment is required, but in the vast majority of patients with persistent pain, the disease or pathology cannot be treated, and the injury is not reversible. In these cases, it is helpful to consider pain as the disease, and to attempt to identify mechanisms responsible for the pain rather than to categorize the patient primarily on the basis of underlying disease.

Given that mechanisms that produce pain in normal and pathologic conditions are being identified with increasing frequency in the laboratory, it is appropriate to begin to assess how such mechanisms fit into the overall schema of pain production. The notion of **basal pain sensitivity**, a term that represents the current status of an individual's pain sensitivity, is fundamental. Basal pain sensitivity represents the pain experienced either spontaneously (i.e., in the absence of any identifiable stimulus) or evoked directly by, and within a short period of, a defined stimulus. In normal situations, there is no spontaneous or background pain, and pain is elicited only by intense or noxious stimuli. The amplitude of the pain, beyond a clear threshold level, is determined by the intensity of the stimulus, and the localization and timing of the sensation reflects the site and duration of the stimulus. This constitutes a state of pain **normosensitivity**. Normosensitivity is distinct from:

1. Pain **hypersensitivity**, in which pain may arise spontaneously, apparently in the absence of any peripheral stimulus
2. **Hyperalgesia**, in which the response to noxious stimuli is exaggerated
3. **Hyperpathia**, in which the pain may persist, radiate, or become excessively amplified
4. **Allodynia**, in which normally innocuous stimuli may produce pain

Normosensitivity is also distinct from those situations in which pain sensitivity is reduced, pain **hyposensitivity**, where suprathreshold noxious stimuli fail to elicit any pain response.

The aim of a mechanism-based approach is to first evaluate basal pain sensitivity by eliciting key aspects of the nature of the patient's symptoms. Figure 2 shows how basal pain sensitivity can be qualitatively assessed by selectively eliciting the nature of symptoms. This can be accomplished using a relatively brief, semi-directed interview (together with simple sensory testing to evoke symptoms) designed specifically to establish whether the patient's

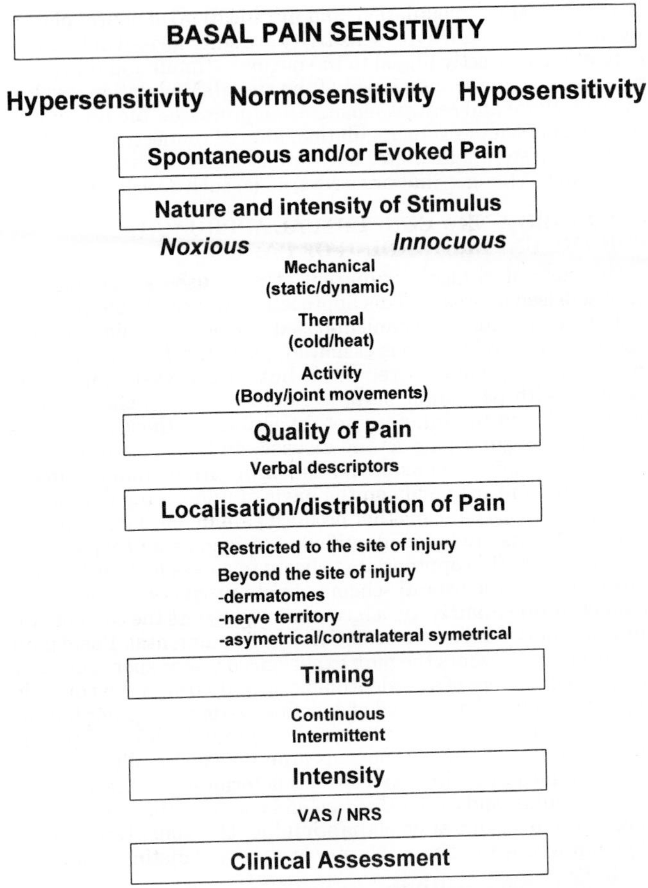

BASAL PAIN SENSITIVITY

Hypersensitivity   Normosensitivity   Hyposensitivity

Spontaneous and/or Evoked Pain

Nature and intensity of Stimulus

Noxious   *Innocuous*

Mechanical
(static/dynamic)

Thermal
(cold/heat)

Activity
(Body/joint movements)

Quality of Pain

Verbal descriptors

Localisation/distribution of Pain

Restricted to the site of injury

Beyond the site of injury
-dermatomes
-nerve territory
-asymetrical/contralateral symetrical

Timing

Continuous
Intermittent

Intensity

VAS / NRS

Clinical Assessment

Figure 2.   Canvas for an interview-based qualitative assessment of pain. (Modified from Woolf CJ, Decosterd I. Implications for recent advances in the understanding of pain pathophysiology for the assessment of pain in patients. *Pain* 1999;6:S141–S147, with permission.)

basal pain sensitivity is normal, above normal, or below normal, and the extent to which the pain is spontaneous or evoked. The goal of the assessment is to characterize the clusters of symptoms, their onset and evolution, and to identify when possible the mechanisms responsible for the symptoms. Careful questioning, rather than the usual global assessments, will produce a new sort of clinical pain record based on the nature of the reported pain, to supplement the standard history (Chapter 4) and physical examination. Of course, this new approach needs to be validated, but its simplicity is likely to be its strength, increasing its usefulness beyond tertiary referral centers. The approach may be adopted in the future to aid treatment selection, especially when treatment efficacy is closely correlated with pain mechanisms (see Section IV).

III. IMPLICATIONS FOR THERAPEUTIC APPROACHES

The conventional assessment of pain syndromes includes the causative disease, the anatomic referral pattern of the pain, and a quantitative evaluation [such as the visual analog scale (VAS)]. This approach groups patients into categories based on their disease syndromes, such as neuropathic pain, headache, osteoarthritic pain, or cancer pain. Contemporary preclinical basic science has successfully elucidated the molecular mechanisms of action of current analgesics (opiates, nonsteroidal anti-inflammatory drugs, and sodium channel blockers) and their effects on pain mechanisms. Yet there is an extremely poor correlation between the efficacy of analgesics and pain syndromes. The increasingly popular measure of the number needed to treat (NNT) is an efficacy index representing the number of patients who need to be treated with a certain drug to obtain one patient with a defined degree of pain relief. The NNT, which has been studied in different pain categories, is a good example of the lack of specificity and predictive value of the current pain classifications. The NNT measure of efficacy does not reveal any consistent differences across different pain conditions for distinct drug classes observed. The goal of a mechanism-based assessment of pain is to provide a classification in which the categorization of patients into mechanism-based subpopulations will aid the rational treatment of pain. Dividing pain into components that reflect some of the major pain mechanisms may help identify how and why certain treatments work, thus revealing useful correlations between pain mechanisms and treatments.

IV. IMPLICATIONS FOR EVALUATION OF EFFICACY OF NEW THERAPIES

A major problem in clinical studies of pain is that the high intra- and interpatient variability in pain scoring using global outcome measures makes it very difficult to evaluate the efficacy of novel analgesics. The usual explanations for this variability are the complexity of pain mechanisms, changes in the primary disease, and psychological factors. Another approach is therefore called for, one that provides new clinical outcome measures that enable an evaluation of whether new analgesics have an action on particular pain mechanisms.

If a new therapy is given to patients selected only on the basis of a particular disease (e.g., diabetic neuropathy), and the clinical outcome measure is a simple global pain measure (e.g., a VAS score of pain at rest), it is simply not possible to assess whether the treatment acts on a particular mechanism (e.g., central sensitization) and reduces a particular symptom (e.g., tactile or cold allodynia). Because the degree of central sensitization may differ considerably in this cohort of patients, any treatment that acts only on central sensitization will produce highly varied responses across the population. Once drugs are available that act specifically on novel pharmacologic targets such as the receptors and ion channels of DRG-specific VR1, P2X3, DRASIC, and SNS/SNS2 (SNS2 is sensory neuron-specific voltage-gated sodium channel NaN/Na$_v$1.9), patients will need to be selected on the basis of a reasonable assessment that their pain involves one of these targets. For example, since VR1 is involved in encoding heat pain, a VR1 antagonist would not be expected to have any effect on a patient with tactile allodynia. Selection of patients on the basis of categories, instead of on the basis of mechanisms, is likely to result in a cohort of patients whose pain mechanisms are quite different. Only a limited number of these patients can be expected to respond to a mechanism-specific drug treatment. Patients who do not respond to the treatment produce a false-negative result by diluting the benefit in a subgroup with the targeted mechanism.

V. CONCLUSION

In the last decade, neurobiology research has enormously increased our knowledge of the fundamental mechanisms responsible for producing chronic pain. On the other hand, changes in clinical pain management have been slow. The challenge now is to bridge the large gap between basic research and clinical practice by utilizing new inputs from basic science in the classification, assessment, diagnosis, and treatment of pain.

SELECTED READING

McCleskey EW, Gold MS. Ion channels of nociception. *Annu Rev Physiol* 1999;61:835–856.

Mogil JS, Yu L, Basbaum AI. Pain genes? Natural variation and transgenic mutants. *Annu Rev Neurosci* 2000;23:777–811.

Sindrup SH, Jensen TS. Efficacy of pharmacological treatments of neuropathic pain: an update and effect related to mechanism of drug action. *Pain* 1999;83:389–400.

Woolf CJ, Bennett GJ, Doherty M, et al. Towards a mechanism-based classification of pain? *Pain* 1998;77:227–229.

Woolf CJ, Decosterd I. Implications for recent advances in the understanding of pain pathophysiology for the assessment of pain in patients. *Pain* 1999;6:S141–S147.

Woolf CJ, Mannion RJ. Neuropathic pain: Aetiology, symptoms, mechanisms, and management. *Lancet* 1999;353:1959–1964.

Woolf CJ, Max MB. Mechanism-based pain diagnosis: Issues for analgesic drug development. *Anesthesiology* 2001 (in press).

Woolf CJ, Salter MW. Neuronal plasticity: increasing the gain in pain. *Science* 2000;288:1765–1769.

Yaksh TL. Spinal systems and pain processing: Development of novel analgesic drugs with mechanistically defined models. *Trends Pharmacol Sci* 1999;20:329–337.

3

The Placebo Effect

Brian W. Dubois and Paul J. Christo

Impatient at being kept awake by pain, I availed myself of the stoical means of concentration upon some indifferent object of thought, such as for instance the name of "Cicero" with its multifarious associations; in this way I found it possible to divert my attention, so that the pain was soon dulled.
—*Immanuel Kant, 1724–1804*

The word *placebo* was originally used to describe something that was pleasing, for example, a medical treatment that was used more to please the patient than to treat the medical condition. In present day medical terminology, a placebo is **a drug or therapy that simulates medical treatment but has no specific action on the condition being treated**. A placebo often provides a real therapeutic benefit even though it does not have a specific therapeutic action. It is well known that receiving medical treatment, in and of itself, often produces a "nonspecific" therapeutic benefit. It is unclear, however, how such a benefit arises and whether it occurs because patients expect relief from medical treatment or because their anxiety is reduced. Placebos have been administered deliberately (for example, in an attempt to satisfy patients who wish to pursue medical therapy), and they have been administered unintentionally, as in the use of therapies whose efficacy was later refuted. In one form or another, placebos have been used since the dawn of medical therapy.

Henry K. Beecher, the first chairman of anesthesia at the Massachusetts General Hospital, made some classic observations about pain plasticity, which have led to the present-day concept that pain and pain perception can be altered by a variety of central nervous system (CNS) factors. He first observed that after battle, soldiers experienced less pain and requested less morphine than did civilians hospitalized after surgery. He surmised that this effect was caused by lower levels of anxiety in the soldiers, who were relieved to be off the battlefield, in sharp contrast to the civilian patients whose concerns about surgery and hospitalization filled them with heightened anxiety. He had observed that a patient's state of mind could alter pain perception, and he studied other possible ways that a subject could conjure up feelings that would suppress pain.

In 1955, he published a classic study, "The Powerful Placebo," in which he analyzed the findings of 15 drug trials involving placebos in a thousand patients with various ailments. In the study, he noted a consistent therapeutic response to placebos for a variety of medical conditions. He surmised that patients' expectations of benefit were sufficient to achieve therapeutic benefit. As a result, Beecher advocated the use of placebos, blinding, and controls in medical studies. He had not only altered the standard for medical studies, he had also introduced psychosomatic medicine into modern medicine.

Since the publication of Beecher's classic study, placebos have been commonly used in studies in an attempt to separate out the "nonspecific" therapeutic benefits of medical treatment from true treatment efficacy. Many clinical and preclinical studies are conducted against a placebo-group baseline. The following are typical study designs involving placebos:

1. **The double-blinded, placebo-controlled study**, comparing a drug (or therapy) with a placebo when neither the patient nor the investigator knows what the patient is receiving.
2. **The single-blinded study**, comparing a drug (or therapy) with a placebo when the patient is blinded to what he is receiving but the investigator knows.
3. **The open-label study**, when both the patient and the investigator know what the patient is receiving.
4. **The crossover study**, when the patient sequentially receives both the placebo and the drug (or therapy), usually in a blinded fashion.

I. PLACEBOS AND THE NATURAL COURSE OF ILLNESS

Many diseases are characterized by periods of acute exacerbation followed by periods of remission or resolution. Common complaints such as backaches, headaches, muscle strains, earaches, and coughs usually improve spontaneously. The natural course of untreated illness must be appreciated to understand the true benefit of treatments.

The placebo effect, or the nonspecific therapeutic benefit derived from a placebo treatment, must be distinguished from the recovery or remission that occur during the natural course of disease. Most placebo-controlled studies do not include an untreated group, and consequently they cannot measure the magnitude of the true placebo effect in the study. By directly comparing the placebo-treated group with the untreated group, the placebo effect can be quantified for a given study.

Since most placebo-controlled studies do not include an untreated group, the reported placebo effect probably overestimates the true placebo effect. In fact, a published search by Ernst and Resch of clinical trials containing both an untreated group and a placebo group from the Medline literature (from 1986 to 1994) yielded only 12 reports, of which six dealt with pain relief. In the pain trials, the authors noted that placebo treatments were more effective in alleviating pain than no treatment. The untreated group, however, did improve, and this improvement, the authors note, must be appreciated to quantify the true placebo effect.

II. ACTIVE AGENTS

Active drugs or therapies have an efficacy greater than that shown by a placebo. The difference in efficacy between an active drug and a placebo defines the **specific therapeutic benefit** of the active drug. The greater the difference between the active drug and the placebo, the greater the specific therapeutic benefit of the active drug. The overall therapeutic effect of an active drug is therefore composed of two components: (a) the specific therapeutic benefit and (b) the nonspecific (placebo) effects of treatment. As Beecher put it, "The power attributed to morphine is presumably its drug effect plus a placebo effect." Any factor of treatment that potentially increases the nonspecific (placebo) component of therapy increases the overall perceived therapeutic effect of the active drug.

III. PLACEBO CHARACTERISTICS

1. The Placebo response rate

Beecher and others have examined the benefit of placebos in treating minor ailments such as headaches, nausea, anxiety, angina, backaches, and coughs. Beecher found that the number of patients given a placebo who had a response, defined as "a 50% or more relief of pain," varied widely, ranging from 15% to 53%. (The myth that the placebo response rate is approximately 30% originates from the gross averaging of these numbers.) Other investigators have also observed a wide range of placebo response rates, and some report response rates that are much higher than the 15% to 53%. High reported placebo response rates might overestimate the true placebo response if the remitting nature of the ailment is not appreciated.

The placebo response is very much influenced by patient perception and expectations. In fact, patients often feel better simply because medical treatment has been initiated. An impressive medical setting instills patient confidence and expectation of good medical treatment. The placebo response can be further augmented by a good physician–patient interaction. Physician expectations, and patients' perceptions of them, have also been shown to influence the placebo effect. For example, Gracely and colleagues, in a controlled double-blinded study of postoperative dental pain, showed that patients were influenced by subconscious signals received from their physicians. In the study, a first group of patients received a placebo, an opioid antagonist, or an opioid (an expected pain reliever), while a second group of patients received just the placebo or the opioid antagonist. Patients receiving the placebo in the second group had more pain than those receiving the placebo in the first group. It was argued that the clinicians' knowledge of the range of treatment alternatives (no opioid in the second group) was unconsciously communicated and perceived by the patients.

The placebo response has not been linked to any particular personality trait or personality type. As yet, there is no reliable way to predict who will respond to a placebo. Beecher, in his early studies, for example, could not find any response-rate difference that was based on sex or intelligence. In a recent study in a depressed patient population, Wilcox and colleagues looked at age, sex, marital status, education, duration of illness, and severity of illness to predict placebo response rates. No significant prediction of placebo response could be made on the basis of sex, age, education, or duration of illness. They did, however, find a slightly increased placebo response rate when the depression was less severe and when the patient was married.

2. Placebos and procedures

The placebo response is also seen with nondrug therapies, including medical devices and invasive procedures. For example, Hashish and colleagues have shown that ultrasound therapy reduces pain and swelling after dental surgery, but that it is no more effective than mock ultrasound therapy. A powerful placebo response to ligation of the internal mammary arteries for the treatment of angina became apparent after the treatment was widely popularized. The procedure was thought to improve coronary blood flow, and it was associated with a dramatic improvement in anginal symptoms and exercise tolerance in multiple non-placebo-controlled trials. Subsequent double-blinded studies using sham skin incisions with no ligation showed a similarly dramatic (70%) response in anginal symptoms and exercise tolerance. The ligation procedure has since been abandoned.

3. Placebo sag in chronic pain

Placebo sag is a decrease in the placebo response rate seen in patients who have experienced a number of treatment failures. Positive treatment experiences tend to augment the placebo response, whereas negative treatment experiences tend to cause an "extinction of the placebo response." Placebo sag has been described in patients with chronic pain, who frequently feel that previous pain therapies have failed them. Treatment of their pain becomes even more difficult, because not only are they less likely to respond to placebo but also they are less likely to respond to active medications (all of which have a placebo or nonspecific therapeutic treatment component to them).

4. The active placebo

During double-blinded placebo-controlled studies, patients (and evaluators) can sometimes differentiate placebos from active drugs on the basis of side effects. This is particularly true with psychiatric and pain treatments, when drugs have significant neurologic and cognitive effects. To enhance blindability in placebo-controlled trials, some investigators have proposed using active placebos. **An active placebo is a drug that simulates medical treatment (through side effects) but has no specific action on the condition being treated.** For example, certain antidepressants have significant anticholinergic properties. An active placebo for an antidepressant trial could be a substance with anticholinergic properties that does not have specific antidepressant properties.

5. The nocebo

Another observation made by Beecher was that "toxic" side effects may result from placebo drug administration, including "nausea, drowsiness, headache, fatigue, and dry mouth." These "noxious" side effects have subsequently been termed **nocebo effects**. Other investigators have noted these effects and have even described allergic-type reactions after placebo administration. Such side effects are augmented by heightened patient expectations of possible negative effects. Moreover, when patients expect little therapeutic benefit from therapy, they are at an increased risk of side effects. For example, it is reported that young healthy volunteers who feel they have little to gain from a treatment tend to experience more side effects.

IV. PLACEBO MECHANISMS

Many investigators feel that the placebo effect is caused by a reduction in patient anxiety and its consequent reduction in pain perception. Beecher, in fact, observed that placebos "are most effective when stress, anxiety, or pain is the greatest," and he noted the importance of a patient's "perception" and "reaction" to pain.

1. Cognitive theory

The cognitive theory states that the expectations of patients play an important role in the placebo response. Clinically, it seems clear that patients who expect a good response from treatment look for signs of a good response and try to dismiss any negative effects. Investigators have shown that patients' expectations of a drug's effects will alter their perception of those effects. For example, when patients were blindly given a psychostimulant, investigators showed that the stimulatory effects could be either exaggerated or diminished depending on whether the patient was told that the drug was a stimulant or a sedative.

2. Conditioning theory

The conditioning theory states that learning through association is important in the placebo response. Further, this theory proposes that the placebo response is a conditioned response that can be elicited by stimuli that, through prior conditioning, produce a reduction in symptoms. Evidence of this exists in both animals and humans. Ivan Pavlov, who described classical conditioning, demonstrated a conditioned placebo response in dogs. He reported that dogs, which previously received morphine when placed in an experimental chamber, displayed morphine-like effects when again placed in the experimental chamber. Since then, a number of investigators have published studies demonstrating conditioned responses to placebos in animals.

In humans, a learned placebo response to the analgesic effects of propoxyphene for the treatment of pain was demonstrated by Laska and Sunshine. In their study, patients were given the analgesic at different strengths. The patients who received the higher strength received greater analgesia. All patients were then given a placebo. The patients who had received the higher-strength analgesic thought the placebo was much more effective than the patients who had received the lower-strength analgesic. Here, the previous analgesic experience predicted the efficacy of the placebo.

3. Endogenous opioids

Endogenous opioids may be responsible for placebo analgesia, because naloxone, an opioid antagonist, has been shown to reverse placebo analgesia. Levine and colleagues, for example, examined the effects of naloxone on placebo analgesia in postoperative dental pain. They termed patients whose pain responded to placebo "placebo responders," and those patients whose pain worsened after placebo administration, "placebo nonresponders." When naloxone was given after placebo to patients in both groups, the placebo responders had a much greater increase in pain than the placebo nonresponders. This suggested that placebo-induced analgesia in the placebo-responder group was mediated by the release of endogenous opioids.

Ter Riet and colleagues recently reviewed the literature and found studies supporting naloxone reversibility of placebo-induced analgesia in both postoperative and experimentally induced pain. Another study that supports the role of endogenous opioids in the placebo response was conducted by Lipman and colleagues. These investigators measured endogenous opioid "peak B" fraction endorphin levels in cerebrospinal fluid after placebo administration in chronic pain patients. After placebo administration, they found that peak-B endorphin levels were significantly higher in placebo responders than in placebo nonresponders.

V. CONCLUSION

Because the placebo effect is a real therapeutic benefit, it is clear that the use of placebos to differentiate "real" pain and illness from "imagined" pain or illness is incorrect and inappropriate. The benefit of the placebo response, as well as a patient's trust, can easily be lost if placebos are used inappropriately. Even during the conduct of a trial, patients should be informed that they might receive a placebo. Although the placebo effect may be a confounding factor when determining new drug efficacy, it is of considerable benefit to the practicing clinician, and this should not be sacrificed. The effect is not simply a response to a dummy drug or procedure but is a response that can be triggered by many factors, such as the smell of a doctor's office, the sight of a needle, or the soothing words of a caregiver. By working to build good patient relationships, the placebo effect can be maximized. Maximizing the nonspecific (placebo) component of treatment increases the perceived therapeutic effect of both active and inactive treatments.

SELECTED READING

1. Beecher HK. The powerful placebo. *JAMA* 1955;159:1602–1606.
2. Ernst E, Resch KL. Concept of true and perceived placebo effects. *Br Med J* 1995;311:551–553.
3. Gracely RH, Duloner R, Wolskee PT, et al. Placebo and naloxone can alter post-surgical pain by separate mechanisms. *Nature* 1983;306:264–265.
4. Hashish I, Hai HK, Harvey W, et al. Reduction of postoperative pain and swelling by ultrasound treatment: A placebo effect. *Pain* 1988;33:303–311.
5. Heeg MF, Deutsch KF, Deutsch E. The placebo effect. *Eur J Nucl Med* 1997;24:1433–1440.
6. Laska E, Sunshine A. Anticipation of analgesia: A placebo effect. *Headache* 1973;13:1–11.

7. Levine JD, Gordon NC, Fields HL. The mechanism of placebo analgesia. *Lancet* 1978;2:654–657.
8. Lipmann JJ, Miller BE, Mays KS, et al. Peak B endorphin concentration in cerebrospinal fluid: Reduced in chronic pain patients and increased during the placebo effect. *Psychopharmacology* 1990;102:112–116.
9. Margo CE. The placebo effect. *Surv Ophthalmol* 1999;44:31–43.
10. Pavlov I. Conditioned reflexes. London: Oxford Press, 1927.
11. ter Riet G, de Craen AJM, deBoer A, Kessels AGH. Is placebo analgesia mediated by endogenous opioids? A systematic review. *Pain* 1998;76:273–275.
12. Turner JA, Deyo RA, Loeser JD, et al. The importance of placebo effects in pain treatment and research. *JAMA* 1994;271:1609–1614.
13. Wilcox CS, Cohn JB, Linden RD, et a. Predictors of placebo response: A retrospective study. *Psychopharmacol Bull* 1992;28:157–162.

II

Diagnosis of Pain

Diagnosis of Pain

The History and Clinical Examination

Jan Slezak and Asteghik Hacobian

To each his suff'rings: all are men,
Condemn'd alike to groan,
The tender for another's pain,
Th' unfeeling for his own.
—*Thomas Gray, 1716–1771*

The key to accurate diagnosis is a comprehensive history and detailed physical examination. Combined with a review of the patient's previous records and diagnostic studies, these lead to a diagnosis and appropriate treatment. In pain medicine, a majority of patients have seen multiple providers, have had various diagnostic tests and unsuccessful treatments, and are finally referred to the pain clinic as a last resort. With advances in research and better education of primary care providers, this trend is beginning to change, and more patients are being referred to pain management specialists earlier, with better outcomes as a result.

I. PATIENT INTERVIEW

1. Pain history

Development and timing

The pain history should reveal the location of the pain, the time of its onset, its intensity, its character, associated symptoms, and factors aggravating and relieving the pain.

It is important to know when and how the pain started. The pain onset should be described and recorded (e.g., sudden, gradual, rapid). If the pain started gradually, patients find identifying an exact time of onset difficult. In the case of a clear inciting event, the date and circumstances of onset of pain may point to the event. The condition of the patient at the onset of pain should be noted if possible. In cases of motor vehicle accidents or work-related injuries, the state of the patient before and at the time of the impact should be clearly understood and documented.

The time of the onset of the pain can be very important. If that interval is short, as in acute pain, the treatment should focus on the underlying cause. In chronic pain, the underlying cause has usually resolved and the treatment should focus on chronic pain management.

Intensity

Various methods are used to measure the intensity of pain, fully described in Chapter 6. Because the complaint of pain is purely subjective, it can be compared only to the sufferer's own pain over a period of time; it cannot be compared to another person's report of pain. Of the numerous scales for reporting the so-called level of pain, the most common is the visual analog scale (VAS) of pain intensity, in which patients are instructed to place a marker on a 100-mm continuous line between "no pain" and "worst imaginable pain." The mark is measured using a standard ruler and recorded as a numeric value between 0 and 100.

An alternative method of reporting the intensity of pain is the numeric rating scale. The patient directly assigns a number between 0 (no pain) and 10 (the worst pain imaginable). Another commonly used method is a verbal categorical scale, with intensity ranging from no pain through mild, moderate, and severe to the worst possible pain.

Character

The patient's description of the character of pain is quite helpful in distinguishing between different types of pain. For example, burning or "electric shocks" often describe neuropathic pain, whereas cramping usually represents nociceptive visceral pain (spasm, stenosis, or obstruction). Pain described as throbbing or pounding suggests vascular involvement.

Evolution

The pattern of pain-spread from the onset should also be noted. Some types of pain change location or spread further out from the original area of insult or injury. The direction of the spread also provides important clues to the diagnosis and ultimately to the treatment of the condition. For example, a complex regional pain syndrome can start in a limited area, such as a distal extremity, and then spread proximally, in some instances even to the contralateral side.

Associated symptoms

The examiner should ask about the presence of associated symptoms, including numbness, weakness, bowel and or bladder dysfunction, edema, cold sensation, or loss of use of an extremity because of pain.

Aggravating and relieving factors

Aggravating factors should be elicited, because they sometimes explain the pathophysiologic mechanisms of pain. Various stimuli can exacerbate pain. Exacerbating mechanical factors, such as different positions or activities (sitting, standing, walking, bending, and lifting) may help differentiate one cause of pain from another. Biochemical changes (e.g., glucose and electrolyte levels, hormonal imbalance), psychological factors (e.g., depression, stress, and other emotional problems), and environmental triggers (e.g., dietary influences, weather changes including barometric pressure changes) may surface as important diagnostic clues.

Relieving factors are also important. Certain positions will alleviate pain better than others (e.g., in most cases of neurogenic claudication, sitting is a relieving factor, whereas standing or walking worsens the pain). Pharmacologic therapies and "nerve blocks" affording relief to the patient help the clinician determine the diagnosis and select the appropriate treatment.

Previous treatment

All previously attempted treatment modalities should be listed at the interview. Knowing the history of the degree of pain relief, the duration of treatment, the dosages of prior medications, and adverse reactions helps to avoid repeating procedures or using pharmacologic management that has not helped in the past. The list should include all treatment modalities including physical therapy, occupational therapy, chiropractic manipulation, acupuncture, psychological help, and visits to other pain clinics.

2. Medical history

Review of systems

A complete review of all systems is an integral part of a comprehensive evaluation for chronic and acute pain. Some systems could be directly or indirectly related to the patient's presenting symptoms and some are important in the management or treatment of the painful condition. Examples are the patient with a history of bleeding problems who may not be a suitable candidate for certain injection therapies, and someone with impaired renal or hepatic function who may need adjustments in medication dosage.

Past medical history

All medical problems that the patient has had in the past should be reviewed, including conditions that were resolved. Previous trauma and any psychological or behavioral issues in the past or present should be recorded.

Past surgical history

A list of all operations and complications should be made, preferably in chronological order. As some painful chronic conditions are sequelae of surgical procedures, this information is important for diagnosis and management.

3. Drug history

Current medications

The practitioner must prescribe and intervene based on the knowledge of which medications the patient is taking, because complications, interactions, and side effects need to be taken into account. A list should be made of all medications currently being used by the patient, including pain medications. It should also include nonprescription and alternative medications (e.g., acetaminophen, aspirin, ibuprofen, and vitamins).

Allergies

Allergies, both to medications and to nonmedications (latex, food, environmental), should be noted. The nature of a specific allergic reaction to each medication or agent should be clearly documented.

4. Social history

General social history

Understanding the patient's social structure, support systems, and motivation is essential in analyzing psychosocial factors. Whether a patient is married, has children, and has a job makes a difference. Level of education, job satisfaction, and general attitude towards life are extremely important. Smoking, alcohol consumption, and history of drug or alcohol abuse are important in evaluating and designing treatment strategies. Lifestyle questions about how much time is taken for vacation or is spent in front of television, favorite recreations and hobbies, adequate exercise, and regular sleep, give the practitioner a more comprehensive overview of the patient.

Family history

A complete family history, including health status of the patient's parents, siblings, and offspring, offers important clues for understanding a patient's biologic and genetic profile. The existence of any unusual diseases in the family should be noted. A history of chronic pain and disability in family members (including the spouse) should be ascertained. Even clues that have no direct genetic or biologic basis may help by revealing coping mechanisms and codependent behavior.

Occupational history

The patient's highest level of education completed and degrees obtained should be identified. The specifics of the present job and as well as of previous employment should be noted. The amount of time spent on each job, reasons for leaving, any previous history of litigation, job satisfaction, whether the patient works full time or part time are important in establishing the occupational framework. Whether the patient has undergone disability evaluations, functional capacity assessment, or vocational rehabilitation is also relevant.

II. PATIENT EXAMINATION

The clinical examination is a fundamental and valuable diagnostic tool. Over the past few decades, advances in medicine and technology and a better understanding of the pathophysiology of pain have dramatically improved the evaluation process. The lack of a specific diagnosis in a majority of patients presenting to the pain clinic underscores the need for detail-oriented examinations.

The consequences of improper coding and inadequate documentation to support charges billed to Medicare for evaluation and management services include various sanctions. Complying with regulations by appropriate documentation not only will result in higher reimbursement but also will provide protection against fraud and abuse. The number of levels of evaluation and management services that can be coded depends on the complexity of the examination, which in turn reflects the nature of the presenting problem and the clinical judgment of the provider. Types of examinations include either general multisystem (10 organ systems: musculoskeletal, nervous, cardiovascular, respiratory, ear/nose/mouth/throat, eyes, genitourinary, hematologic/lymphatic/

immune, psychiatric, and integumentary) or single-organ-system examinations. In pain medicine, the most commonly examined systems are the musculoskeletal and nervous systems.

If interventional pain management is part of a diagnostic or therapeutic plan, the evaluation should reveal whether the patient has risk factors for the procedure being considered. Coagulopathy, untreated infection, or preexisting neurologic dysfunction should be documented prior to placement of a needle or catheter or implantation of a device. Extra caution is needed when administering medications such as (a) local anesthetics to a patient with seizure disorder, (b) neuraxial anesthetics to a patient who may tolerate vasodilatation poorly, or (c) glucocorticoids to a diabetic patient. Preanesthetic evaluation should assess ability to tolerate sedation or the anesthesia itself if indicated for a procedure.

The following sections outline a physical examination that incorporates the musculoskeletal and neurologic assessment relevant to pain practice. The examination starts with the evaluation of single systems and commonly proceeds from head to toe.

1. General examination

(i) Constitutional Factors

Height, weight, and vital signs (blood pressure, heart rate, respiratory rate, body temperature) should be measured and recorded. Appearance, development, deformities, nutrition, and grooming are noted. Scan the room for presence of assistive devices brought by the patient. Patients who smoke or drink heavily may carry an odor. Observing the patient who is unaware of being watched may reveal discrepancies that were not seen during the evaluation.

(ii) Pain behavior

Note facial expression, color, and grimacing. Speech patterns suggest emotional factors as well as intoxication with alcohol or prescription or nonprescription drugs. Some patients attempt to convince the practitioner how much pain they are suffering by augmenting their verbal presentation with grunting, moaning, twitching, grabbing the painful area, exaggerating the antalgic gait or posture, or tightening muscle groups. This, unfortunately, makes the objective examination more difficult.

(iii) Skin

Evaluate for color, temperature, rash, and soft-tissue edema. Trophic changes of skin, nails, and hair are frequently seen in advanced stages of complex regional pain syndrome.

2. Systems examination

(i) Cardiovascular System

A systolic murmur with propagation suggests aortic stenosis, and the patient may not tolerate the hypovolemia and tachycardia that accompany rapid vasodilatation (e.g., after administration of neuraxial local anesthetics or sympathetic or celiac plexus blockade). The patient with irregular rhythm may have atrial fibrillation and be anticoagulated. Feel the pulsation of arteries (diabetes, complex regional pain syndrome, thoracic outlet syndrome), venous filling, presence of varicosities, and capillary return.

(ii) **Lungs**

Examination of lungs may reveal abnormal breath sounds such as crackles, which may be a sign of congestive heart failure and low cardiac reserve. Rhonchi and wheezes are signs of chronic obstructive pulmonary disease. Caution in performing blocks around the chest cavity is advised, as there is an increased risk of causing pneumothorax.

(iii) **Musculoskeletal system**

The musculoskeletal system examination includes inspection of gait and posture. Deformities and deviation from symmetry are observed. After taking the history, the examiner usually has an idea from which body part the symptoms originate. If this is not the case, a brief survey of structures in the relevant region might be necessary. Positive tests then warrant further and more rigorous evaluation of the affected segment.

Palpation of soft tissues, bony structures, and stationary or moving joints may reveal temperature differences, presence of edema, fluid collections, gaps, crepitus, clicks, or tenderness. Functional comparison of the left and right sides, checking for normal curvature of the spine, and provocation of usual symptoms with maneuvers can help identify the mechanisms and location of the pathologic process.

Examination of range of motion may demonstrate hyper- or hypomobility of the joint. Testing active movement will determine range, muscle strength and willingness of the patient to cooperate. Passive movements, on the other hand, when performed properly, test for pain, range, and end-feel. Most difficulties arise when examining patients in constant pain, as they tend to respond to most maneuvers positively, therefore making the specificity of tests low.

For the patient with back pain, the suggested sequence of examinations is testing of range of motion of cervical, thoracic, and lumbosacral spine; sacroiliac and hip joints; and the straight leg raising test (see Chapter 27).

Specific tests:

Straight leg raising test

The straight leg raising (or Lasegue's Sign) test determines the mobility of the dura and dural sleeves from L4 to S2. The sensitivity of this test to diagnose lumbar disc herniation ranges between .6 and .97, with a specificity of .1 to .6. Tension on the sciatic nerve begins with 15 to 30 degrees of elevation in the supine position. This puts traction on the nerve roots from L4 to S2 and on the dura. The end of the range is normally restricted by hamstring muscle tension at 60 to 120 degrees. More than 60 degrees of elevation causes movement in the sacroiliac joint and therefore may be painful in sacroiliac joint disorders.

Basic sacroiliac tests

Sacroiliac tests are performed to determine when pain occurs in the buttock.

1. Push the ilia outward and downward in the supine position with the examiner's arms crossed. If gluteal pain results, the

test is repeated with patient's forearm placed under the lumbar spine to stabilize the lumbar joints.

2. Forcibly compress the ilia to the midline with the patient lying on the painless side. This stretches posterior sacroiliac ligaments.
3. Exert forward pressure on the center of the sacrum with the patient prone.
4. Patrick's or "FABER'S" test—Flex, abduct, and externally rotate femur while holding down contralateral anterior superior iliac spine. Stretches anterior sacroiliac ligament and reveals pain caused by ligamentous strain.
5. Force lateral rotation of the hip joint with knee held in 90 degrees of flexion and the patient in the supine position.

Spinal flexibility

Spinal flexion, extension, and rotation and lateral bending may be limited or painful, leading to a diagnosis of zygapophyseal joint, discogenic, muscular, or ligamentous pain.

Adson's test

Adson's test has been advocated for diagnosis of thoracic outlet syndrome. The examiner evaluates the change of radial artery pulsation in a standing patient with arms resting at the side. Ipsilateral head rotation during inspiration may cause vascular compression by the anterior scalene muscle. During the **modified Adson's test**, the patient's head is rotated to the contralateral side. Pulse change suggests compression by the middle scalene muscle. Both tests are regarded by some as unreliable, as the findings may be found positive in about 50% of the normal population.

Tinel test

The Tinel test involves percussion of the carpal tunnel. When it is positive, it gives rise to distal paresthesias. It can be performed at other locations (e.g., the cubital or tarsal tunnel), where it might be suggestive of nerve entrapment. **Phalen's test** is positive for carpal tunnel syndrome when a passive flexion in the wrist for 1 minute, followed by sudden extension, results in sensation of paresthesias.

(iv) **Neurologic examination**

Table 1 summarizes the localization of cervical and lumbar radicular nerves.

Evaluation of the **motor system** starts with observation of muscle bulk and tone and the presence of spasm. Muscle strength is tested in upper and lower extremities. Weakness might be caused by the patient's unwillingness to cooperate or trying to prevent pain provocation, or by poor effort, reflex neural inhibition in the painful limb, or an organic lesion. Further information is obtained by examination of **deep tendon reflexes**, clonus, and pathologic reflexes such as the Babinski. Evaluation of **coordination** and fine motor skills may reveal associated dysfunctions.

The integrity of **cranial nerve function** is tested by examination of visual fields, pupil and eye movement, facial sensation, facial symmetry and strength, hearing (using tuning fork, whisper

Table 1. Cervical and lumbar radicular localization

			Spinal nerve			
	C5	C6	C7	L4	L5	S1
Disc level	C4/5	C5/6	C6/7	L3/4 (L4/5)	L4/5 (L5/1)	L5/1
Sensory changes	Lateral upper arm	Lateral forearm and 1st, 2nd and ½ of 3rd digits	3rd digit	Medial leg and medial foot	Dorsal foot	Lateral foot
Deep tendon reflex	Biceps	Brachioradialis	Triceps	Patellar	None	Achilles
Muscles tested	Deltoid, biceps	Wrist extensors	Triceps, wrist and finger extensors	Foot inversion	Dorsiflexion of toes and foot	Plantar flexion and eversion

voice, or finger-rub), spontaneous and reflex palate movement, and tongue protrusion.

Sensation is tested to light touch (A-β fibers), pinprick (A-Δ fibers), hot and cold stimuli (A-Δ and C fibers). Tactile sensation can be evaluated quantitatively with von Frey filaments. The sharp end of a broken sterile wooden Q-tip is a convenient and safe tool for testing sensation to pinprick. The following are often observed in neuropathic pain conditions:

Hyperesthesia–increased sensitivity to stimulation, excluding the special senses

Dysesthesia–an unpleasant abnormal sensation, either spontaneous or evoked

Allodynia–pain caused by a stimulus that normally does not provoke pain

Hyperalgesia–an increased response to a stimulus that is normally painful

Hyperpathia–a painful syndrome characterized by an abnormally painful reaction to stimulus (especially a repetitive one), as well as increased threshold

Summation–a repetitive pinprick stimulus applied at intervals of more than 3 seconds, with a gradually increasing sensation of pain with each stimulus

(v) Mental status examination

The mental status examination is a part of the neuropsychiatric assessment. Examine level of consciousness, orientation, speech, mood, affect, attitude, and thought content. **The Mini-Mental Status Exam** (MMSE) of Folstein is a useful guide for documenting level of mental function. There are five areas of mental status tested: orientation, registration, attention and calculation, recall, and language. Each correct answer is given one point. A maximum score on the Folstein is 30. A score of less than 23 is abnormal and suggests cognitive impairment.

III. INCONSISTENCIES IN THE HISTORY AND PHYSICAL EXAMINATION

Inconsistencies in the history and physical examination, vague description of symptoms, and evidence of intense suffering, together with inappropriate pain behavior, may suggest symptom exaggeration, malingering for compensation, and other gains or psychogenic pain. The frequently cited **Waddell** nonorganic signs may raise suspicion in patients with lower back pain. It may be warranted to proceed with the SF-36 or another instrument designed to identify underlying problems or issues. The Waddell nonorganic signs are grouped into five categories:

a. Tenderness
   - Widespread superficial sensitivity to light touch over lumbar spine
   - Bone tenderness over a large lumbar area
b. Simulation
   - Axial loading, during which light pressure is applied to the skull in the upright position
   - Simulated rotation of lumbar spine with the shoulders and pelvis remaining in the same plane

c. Distraction
   - Greater than 40 degrees difference in sitting versus supine straight leg raising
d. Regional disturbance
   - Motor: generalized giving way or cogwheeling resistance in manual muscle testing of lower extremities
   - Sensory: nondermatomal loss of sensation to pinprick in lower extremities
e. Overreaction
   - Disproportionate pain response to testing (pain behavior with assisted movement using cane or walker, rigid or slow movement, rubbing or grasping the affected area for more than 3 seconds, grimacing, sighing with shoulders rising and falling)

IV. CONCLUSION

The history and physical examinations are the foundations for pain evaluation and treatment and essential elements of good pain management. They need to be tailored to the individual patient, the complexity of the pain problem, and the medical condition of the patient. The standard history and physical examinations outlined here can be applied to most patients presenting in the pain clinic.

SELECTED READING

1. Benzon H, ed. *Essentials of pain medicine and regional anesthesia.* Philadelphia: Churchill-Livingstone, 1999.
2. Kanner R, ed. *Pain management secrets.* Philadelphia: Hanley & Belfus, 1997.
3. Ombregt L, ed. *A system of orthopaedic medicine.* London: WB Saunders, 1997.
4. Raj P, ed. *Pain medicine: A comprehensive review.* St. Louis: Mosby Year Book, 1996.
5. Tollison D, ed. *Handbook of pain management.* Baltimore: Williams & Wilkins, 1994.

5

Diagnostic Imaging and Pain Management

Onassis A. Caneris

I have a little shadow that goes in and out with me,
And what can be the use of him is more than I can see.
He is very, very like me from the heels up to the head;
And I see him jump before me when I jump into my bed.
—*Robert Louis Stevenson, 1850–1894*

I. Imaging techniques and studies
  1. Plain film radiology
  2. Fluoroscopy
  3. Computed tomography
  4. Magnetic resonance imaging
  5. Myelography
  6. Bone scans and nuclear medicine
  7. Discography
  8. Positron-emission tomography
II. Headache
  1. Primary headache
  2. Secondary headache
III. Craniofacial pain syndromes
  1. Trigeminal neuralgia
  2. Glossopharyngeal neuralgia
IV. Central pain syndromes
  1. Thalamic pain syndromes
  2. Spinal cord injury
V. Vertebral axis pain
  1. Plain x-ray evaluation in low back pain
  2. MRI and low back pain
  3. Pain after lumbar surgery
  4. Arachnoiditis
  5. Metastatic disease of the spine
  6. Infectious processes of the vertebral spine
VI. Conclusion

In recent years, there have been tremendous advances in understanding the pathophysiology and mechanisms of pain; concomitantly, there have been enormous advances in diagnostic imaging. Diagnostic imaging is an essential tool for the pain practitioner, who uses it to understand, diagnose, and treat pain. Although plain x-rays remain the mainstay of diagnostic imaging, advanced modalities including computed tomography (CT), magnetic resonance imaging (MRI), and nuclear medicine studies have proved extremely valuable diagnostic tools for patients with pain. Over the past decade, the use of new technologies has resulted in a 50% increase in healthcare costs. It becomes increasingly important for the pain physician to have a clear understanding of imaging studies and to optimize the use of diagnostic imaging. Consultation with a radiologist or imaging specialist often aids in choosing the most cost-effective test for establishing a diagnosis and in understanding the underlying pathology.

I. IMAGING TECHNIQUES AND STUDIES

1. Plain film radiology

Plain x-rays (static x-rays) generate two-dimensional (2D) images that primarily display skeletal tissue, but in addition soft tissue anatomy is either seen or inferred. Contemporary x-ray technology generally produces high-quality images with minimal radiation exposure. X-rays are produced as electrons from a cathode are accelerated by electrical current toward an anode target. The x-ray beam is differentially absorbed as it passes through a portion of the patient and then goes on to expose film. Radiopaque contrast materials given orally, locally, intravenously, and intrathecally may be used to aid the study. Most contrast materials used with plain x-rays are iodine-based. Plain x-rays remain the first-line examination for many conditions.

2. Fluoroscopy

The principles of fluoroscopy are the same as those of plain x-rays. The primary difference is that the transmitted radiation is viewed on a fluorescent screen rather than on a static film, and the patient can be imaged in real time. The image is generally amplified by an image intensifier. Fluoroscopy can be used both in diagnostic studies and in assisting with therapeutic treatment.

3. Computed tomography

The prototype CT scanner was developed in the 1960s. First-generation scanners took days to collect data and then hours to reconstruct the images. In the early 1970s, CT scanning for imaging the brain became available. Today's fourth-generation scanners have significantly improved quality, and the imaging time is significantly shortened. In CT imaging, the x-ray tube produces a beam of energy that passes through a single section of the patient. This beam is then detected by a circular array of detectors on the opposite side. Both the detector and the x-ray source rotate around an axis of the patient and produce exposures at small intervals of rotation. Subsequently, computer reconstruction results in a display of the targeted area. The resolution can be as small as 0.5 mm. Intravenous contrast can be used to enhance the imaging of vascular structures as well as normal tissues.

CT scanning offers the advantage of three-dimensional (3D) images, but they are generally in standard cross-sectional or axial planes. Quantitative CT scanning is particularly useful in measuring bone density for the assessment of osteoporosis. 3D CT also allows postreconstruction images to be rotated at various angles. CT displays soft tissues fairly well and is used for soft tissue imaging if MRI (which provides superior soft tissue contrast) is not available, or if the patient cannot tolerate MRI because of claustrophobia or because it is a more lengthy process.

4. Magnetic resonance imaging

As early as the 1940s and 1950s, nuclear magnetic resonance (NMR) was used to image chemical compounds by exposing them to strong magnetic fields. By the mid 1980s, clinical NMR had become common, and the name was changed to magnetic resonance imaging because of public anxiety engendered by the word *nuclear*.

A significant difference between MRI scanning and CT and x-rays is that MRI uses no ionizing radiation. In MRI, signals are obtained by subjecting the tissues to strong magnetic fields, which influence hydrogen ions in the tissues to align in a certain direction. Tiny radiofrequency signals are emitted as the hydrogen ions "relax" when the magnetic field is removed. The image represents the intensities of the electromagnetic signals emitted from the hydrogen nuclei in the patient. A tissue such as fat, which is rich in hydrogen ions, gives a bright signal, whereas bone gives a void, or essentially no signal. Abnormal tissue generally has more free water and displays different MR characteristics.

The MR signal is a complex function of the concentration of deflected normal hydrogen ions, buildup and relaxation times of the magnetic field (T1 and T2 respectively), flow or motion within the sample, and the MR sequence protocol. Three types of MR sequences are used: spin echo, gradient echo, and inversion recovery. MRI is easily able to provide multiplanar images. Its advantage over CT is its superior contrast of soft tissues, especially neural tissue. The addition of gadolinium as a contrast material aids in defining tumors and inflammatory processes.

5. Myelography

Injection of radiocontrast material into the intrathecal space, followed by imaging using conventional x-ray techniques or CT, provides diagnostic information about potential structural abnormalities affecting the spinal nerves. When noninvasive imaging with either MRI or CT does not provide adequate information, myelography, which was once the gold standard for assessing the spine, remains an option for diagnosing structural spine disease. It is also useful for imaging patients who have had spinal instrumentation, which tends to produce extensive artifact on CT.

Postmyelogram CT imaging is sometimes useful for detecting subtle spinal nerve impingement caused by far-posterior lateral intervertebral disc herniation that has been missed by MRI. Its disadvantages are that it is invasive and, unlike MRI, it utilizes ionizing radiation.

6. Bone scans and nuclear medicine

The field of nuclear medicine followed the discovery of radioactivity in 1896. There are three types of radioactive emissions: positive particles (alpha particles); negative particles (beta particles); and high-penetration gamma radiation. The scintillation events are detected by a scintillation camera and mapped in 2D space. Nuclear medicine uses the tracer principle, which essentially tags certain physiologic substances in the body and measures its distribution and flow or its presence in a target system. A radiopharmaceutical agent is injected into the patient and the radioactive decay is detected by a detection device, for example, a gamma counter.

Bone scans are commonly used to evaluate complaints of skeletal pain. Radiopharmaceuticals labeled with technetium-99m localize areas of increased bone turnover and blood flow that represent increased rates of osteoblastic activity. Bone scans are more sensitive than x-rays in detecting skeletal pathology. One third of patients with pain and known malignant disease with normal x-rays have metastatic lesions on bone scans. The specificity of bone scans is not high, which can sometimes be a problem.

7. Discography

Discography involves injecting the nucleus pulposus of an intervertebral disc with contrast material under fluoroscopic guidance. This can provide objective structural and anatomic information regarding the intervertebral disc. In addition, it can provide subjective information as to whether a particular disc is the source of a patient's axial lumbar pain.

8. Positron-emission tomography

In positron-emission tomography (PET), positron emissions are detected with a circular array of detectors. The number of decays is displayed to produce an image of specific metabolic processes. PET is an excellent tool for quantification of various metabolic and physiologic changes and processes, making it a functional imaging device. The collection of literature about PET scanning and functional neuroimaging of pain processes is increasing.

II. HEADACHE

Headache is a frequent presentation in both the primary care physician's office and the pain clinic. The pain specialist must become familiar with the indications for imaging in the assessment of patients with headache. The vast majority of patients who complain of headache and have normal neurologic examinations have a normal CT imaging study.

In a large prospective study of 195 headache patients with normal neurologic examinations, only a minority (9%) had abnormal CT scans (seven had tumor, five had hydrocephalus, three had arteriovenous malformations, two had hemorrhages, and one had cerebral infarction). In a retrospective study of 505 patients with headache without regard to neurologic examination, 35 patients (7%) had abnormal imaging studies. In a study of 350 patients who complained of headache and were prospectively studied with contrast scans, seven patients (2%) had positive scans. Positive pathology included metastasis, sinusitis with epidural abscess, meningiomas, and subdural hemorrhage. In all patients with positive scans, abnormal neurologic exams were present.

An overview of the available data suggests that of 100,000 patients who complain of headache as a sole symptom and have a normal neurologic examination, less than one has a tumor or other significant pathology on cranial imaging studies. It becomes evident that a careful history and neurologic examination are crucial for deciding whether a patient is at risk and whether to order a diagnostic test. Imaging studies ordered without good clinical indication are usually unhelpful and certainly expensive.

1. Primary headache

In patients who present with a history characteristic of primary headache without additional neurologic symptoms and with normal neurologic examinations, it is exceedingly rare to find imaging abnormalities. In a study of 435 patients with symptoms characteristic of classic migraine, contrast-enhanced CT scans were reviewed; one patient was found to have a choroid plexus tumor and no other abnormalities were found. The patient continued to have classic migraines after neurosurgical removal of this tumor, and it was most likely an incidental finding. In a study of 90 patients with "chronic headaches" lasting more than 1 week, CT scanning of all patients found no significant abnormalities. Patients were followed clinically and developed no significant problems.

2. Secondary headache

Several other clinical scenarios warrant discussion. In patients without history of headaches, presenting with the "worst headache of my life," acute subarachnoid hemorrhage needs to be considered. In such cases, emergent noncontrast CT scanning is the imaging evaluation of choice. Noncontrast CT scanning is extremely sensitive for identifying the presence of acute blood. Additionally, in patients who complain of new headache and fever, lumbar puncture may be indicated. A noncontrast CT scan to exclude a space- occupying lesion, which would be a contraindication for lumbar puncture, is indicated before proceeding.

Noncontrast CT scanning is also indicated in acute trauma, because it best identifies acute hemorrhage and lesions of the bone. Contrast CT scanning is indicated when there is clinical suspicion of vascular lesions, neoplastic lesions, or inflammatory conditions. Plain x-rays are not helpful in evaluating headache. In the nonacute setting, MRI scanning has a high degree of sensitivity for intracranial pathology. Diagnostic criteria and imaging for secondary headache are discussed in Chapter 28.

Neoplasia

Of patients with newly diagnosed brain tumors, 40% present with a chief complaint of headache. Obstructing the flow of cerebrospinal fluid (CSF), thus increasing intracranial pressure, can produce headaches. Not infrequently, larger parenchymal tumors may initially not produce headache. In patients presenting with headache and focal or lateralizing neurologic symptoms, MRI with contrast material would be the imaging study of choice.

Carotid artery dissection

Symptoms of carotid artery dissection include new-onset unilateral headache with associated anterior cervical pain. Fluctuating hemispheric neurologic deficits as well as Horner's syndrome may also be present. Carotid dissections are most common in association with trauma; fibromuscular dysplasia may also predispose to carotid dissection. The most common location for dissection is several centimeters above the carotid bifurcation.

Arterial angiography is usually most effective in making the diagnosis, but MRI and magnetic resonance angiography (MRA) may also be helpful, particularly in subsequent follow-up examinations. MRI scanning demonstrates high signal intensity, which usually represents a clot or low arterial flow.

Cerebrovenous and sinus occlusive disease

The most common presenting symptom with either venous or sinus occlusive disease is headache; more than 75% of these patients generally complain of headache. Occlusive disease frequently results in increased intracranial pressure. Cerebral ischemia may also result. Cavernous sinus thrombosis produces severe retro-orbital or periorbital pain with proptosis and ophthalmoparesis. Traditional contrast angiography is in most circumstances the imaging study of choice, but traditional angiography is being replaced by MRA and MRI.

Hydrocephalus

Both CT and MRI are appropriate in the evaluation of hydro-cephalus. Aqueductal stenosis is seen on imaging studies represented by dilatation of the lateral ventricles and the third ventricle, with a normal appearance of the fourth ventricle; MRI is the imaging study of choice.

In pseudotumor cerebri, imaging studies tend to be normal. Diagnosis is made by examination of the CSF with careful manometry and identification of increased intracranial pressure.

Low Pressure Headache

Postural headaches can be seen as a result of diminished intracranial pressure. These headaches are most commonly seen after lumbar puncture, but they can also be seen after trauma or can occur "spontaneously." CT and MRI tend to be normal. Isotope cysternography may demonstrate the site of dural leakage of CSF.

Chiari Malformation

Patients with Chiari malformations very frequently present with headache as a primary symptom. Additional neurologic complaints are often associated. MRI is the modality of choice for imaging Chiari malformations. Three types are identified. In type 1, the cerebellar tonsils are displaced caudally into the cervical spinal canal. In type 2, there is additional caudal displacement of the lower cerebellum as well as the brainstem; anatomic abnormalities are seen in the fourth ventricle, and there is associated meningomyelocele. In type 3, either encephalocele or spina bifida is also present.

III. CRANIOFACIAL PAIN SYNDROMES

1. Trigeminal neuralgia

Severe unilateral paroxysmal lancinating pain in the distribution of the trigeminal nerve is characteristic of trigeminal neuralgia. Trigeminal neuralgia is idiopathic. Imaging studies are generally negative. In patients with trigeminal neuropathy and trigeminal neuropathic pain in which atypical features exist, it is important to evaluate for other diagnostic possibilities. MRI is the imaging modality of choice. Occasionally, vascular malformations, aneurysms, and tumors cause trigeminal neuropathy. Multiple sclerosis is sometimes associated with neuropathic facial pain, in which case lesions of increased T2-weighted signal intensity on MRI may be seen in the trigeminal brainstem dorsal root entry zones.

2. Glossopharyngeal neuralgia

The characteristic pain of glossopharyngeal neuralgia is similar to that of trigeminal neuralgia, but it is located unilaterally in the posterior tongue throughout the tonsillar area and sometimes at the auricular area. It also is most frequently idiopathic. In isolated glossopharyngeal neuralgia, imaging studies are rarely positive. In patients with evidence of associated pathology, particularly at the brainstem, MRI with contrast medium is the imaging study of choice.

IV. CENTRAL PAIN SYNDROMES

Central neuropathic pain can result after there has been injury to the primary somatosensory nervous system. Constant burning neuropathic pain is typically seen. Infarction, trauma, and radiation are frequent causes.

1. Thalamic pain syndromes

Injury to the thalamus, specifically the ventral posterolateral nucleus of the thalamus, results in constant burning pain in the contralateral hemi-corpus, including the face, arm, trunk, and leg, although variations in the distribution of pain do exist. This most frequently results from thalamic infarction but can also be the result of hemorrhage, trauma, or space-occupying lesions, including tumor, infection, and abscess. Imaging reveals signal abnormalities in the thalamus contralateral to the pain. A "pseudo-thalamic pain syndrome" can result after injury to the thalamocortical white matter tract. Clinical presentation is the same, but MRI reveals abnormalities in the thalamocortical radiations. In exceptional cases, the MR image is normal but pathology be delineated using functional imaging studies.

2. Spinal cord injury

Injury to the spinal cord at any level can result in a central pain syndrome. Damage to the spinothalamic tract frequently results in central neuropathic pain. Significant central neuropathic pain accompanies spinal cord injury in 25% of patients. Underlying pathology may be trauma, space-occupying lesions including neoplasms, demyelinating process including multiple sclerosis, and syringomyelia. MRI is the imaging modality of choice. In multiple sclerosis, lesions of increased T2-weighted signal intensity are seen in the white matter tracts of the spinal cord. In syringomyelia, MRI reveals a central cavity that shows high signal intensity on T2-weighted images and diminished signal on T1-weighted images.

V. VERTEBRAL AXIS PAIN

Low back pain is an extremely common presentation to both the primary care physician and the pain clinic. Underlying pathologic processes affecting the lumbar spine include disc degeneration, degrees of intervertebral disc herniation, osteoarthrosis of the facet joints, fracture of a vertebra, dislocation of a vertebra, spondylolisthesis, and osteoporosis. Degenerative changes causing low back pain may be difficult to distinguish from other common causes, including pain of muscular origin and pain of additional soft tissue origin. Less common alternative causes include intradural and extradural neoplasms, infections, and congenital abnormalities of the spine. The history and physical examination are the basis of the evaluation, but imaging studies may be needed to make a definitive diagnosis.

The primary rationale for radiographic imaging of low back pain is to exclude or define serious pathology. The majority of low back pain originates from soft tissues, and imaging studies are often not helpful. In older patients, imaging studies frequently reveal abnormalities that may or may not be responsible for the patient's pain syndrome. Plain x-rays can be helpful in diagnosing spondylolysis (pars interarticularis defects, usually at L5 or sometimes L4), ankylosing spondylitis, fractures, and occasionally degenerative disc disease. When neurologic signs or symptoms are present, including those of sciatica, MRI is the imaging modality of choice. MRI without contrast material can detect herniation of lumbar discs with compression of nerve roots causing radicular symptoms.

In patients with a previous history of lumbar surgery, it is imperative to also obtain a contrast-enhanced study, which helps differentiate recurrence of disc herniation from epidural scar tissue; the latter is detected by T1-weighted signal enhancement after administration of contrast. In patients with a clinical complaint of lumbar claudication and suspected spinal stenosis, both CT and MRI are appropriate. CT offers the advantage of superior imaging of bony hypertrophic changes of the lumbar spine.

1. Plain x-ray evaluation of low back pain

Plain x-ray provides an adequate assessment of the configuration and alignment of the lumbar vertebral spine with a high degree of accuracy. There have been a number of natural history and comparative studies evaluating the usefulness of plain x-rays in evaluating low back pain. In a large retrospective study reviewing 1,000 lumbar spine radiographs from patients who complained of low back pain, more than one half of the radiographs were normal. In another study of 780 patients, only 2.4% had unique diagnostic findings on plain radiographs.

Most episodes of low back pain resolve within 7 weeks of onset. It is generally felt that the risks and cost of taking radiographs for all patients at a first presentation of low back pain do not justify the possible small associated benefit. General recommendations for radiographs in patients with low back pain are as follows:

- For patients with a first episode of low back pain, present for less than 7 weeks, who have not been treated or who are improving with treatment, no radiographs of the lumbar spine are indicated unless an atypical clinical finding or special psychological or social circumstances exist. Atypical history includes age over 65, history suggesting a high risk for osteoporosis, symptoms of persistent sensory deficit, pain worsening despite treatment, intense pain at rest, fever, chills, unexplained weight loss, and recurrent back pain with no radiographs within the past 2 years. Atypical physical findings include significant motor deficit and unexplained deformity.
- For patients with recurrent low back pain, radiographs are not indicated if a previous radiographic study had been done within 2 years.
- Patients with a history of a brief, self-limited previous episode of low back pain do not require radiographs within the first 7 weeks of a current episode if they are improving.

In general, anteroposterior and lateral views are the only views that should be done initially. In patients with chronic pain or additional history and physical findings that suggest stenosis or instability, flexion and extension films may be indicated.

2. MRI and low back pain

MRI has a very high sensitivity for detecting pathology of the lumbar spine. A poor correlation exists between the severity of pain symptoms and the extent of morphologic changes seen on MRI studies: a significant percentage of normal individuals without lumbar pain have degenerative changes on MRI (as many as 50% to 60%) and even disc herniation (as many as 20%). Careful attention must be paid to correlating clinical symptoms with radiographic findings; otherwise, imaging findings may be used inappropriately to justify unneeded intervention or treatment.

Age-related morphologic changes occur in the lumbar spine throughout life. There is a decrease in water and glycosaminoglycans in the intervertebral disc, and there is also an increase in collagen. On MRI, this is seen as loss of signal intensity on T2-weighted images, a reduction in the height of vertebral bodies, a reduction in the height of the intervertebral discs, and a reduction in the caliber of the spinal canal. The onset of degenerative processes of the lumbosacral spine seem to be consistently marked by tears of the annulus fibrosis, as well as by MRI and histologic changes of the vertebral bone marrow adjacent to the intervertebral spaces. Facet degeneration rarely occurs in the absence of disc degeneration, and it seems likely that facet osteoarthropathy results from the added stress of increased loading after disc space narrowing has occurred. Multiple studies have found an association between degenerated disc and facet osteoarthritis using imaging criteria.

In patients with radicular symptoms, the clinical evaluation can usually predict the spinal nerve involved. The actual spinal pathology, however, cannot be predicted with clinical evaluation alone, and MRI examination can be of great assistance. A spinal nerve can be compressed by a disc at either the traversing segment by central disc herniation or at the exiting segment by a lateral disc herniation. In these circumstances, imaging is beneficial for defining the site of pathology. Symptomatic patients may have neuroimaging abnormalities at more than one spinal level.

3. Pain after lumbar surgery

In patients who have had previous back surgery and now complain of recurrent radicular pain, the differential diagnosis includes the following:

- Incorrect original diagnosis or concomitant disease
- Spinal nerve or dorsal root ganglion pathology, including axonal injury or persistent neurapraxic injury
- Retained or recurrent intervertebral disc fragment
- Epidural fibrosis
- Central sensitization
- Complex regional pain syndrome

Postoperative fibrosis is a natural consequence of surgical procedures. Numerous reports suggest that fibrosis and adhesions cause compression or tethering of the spinal nerves and their roots, which in turn causes recurrent radicular pain and physical impairment. The literature repeatedly suggests that fibrosis is the major cause of recurrent symptoms when no alternative bony or disc pathology can be found. It has also been suggested that fibrosis may be causal in as much as 25% of all patients with failed back surgery syndrome.

Recurrent radicular pain is defined as pain in a patient who had a successful outcome from the primary surgery at 1 month postoperatively but has had recurrence of radicular pain within 6 months postoperatively. A significant association between the size of the peridural scar and incidence of pain has been demonstrated in this group of patients.

In patients who have had lumbar surgery and present with recurrent radicular pain, it is essential to obtain an MRI scan without and with contrast. This assists in differentiating between a recurrent or retained disc fragment and epidural scarring.

The criteria used to identify epidural fibrosis by MRI include the following:

- Epidural scar is isointense to hypointense relative to the intervertebral disc on T1-weighted images on an MRI scan.
- Peridural scar tends to form in a curvilinear pattern surrounding the dural tube, with homogenous intensity.
- Traction of the dural tube toward the side of the soft tissue is more characteristic of scar.
- Scar tissue is seen to consistently enhance immediately after the injection of contrast material, regardless of its location.

The criteria used to identify recurrent herniated disc by MRI include the following:

- Recurrent herniated disc material is isointense to the intervertebral disc on T1-weighted images. There tends to be a more variable appearance on T2-weighted images.
- Recurrent herniations tend to have a polypoid configuration with a smooth outer margin.
- Recurrent disc material does not enhance within the first 10 to 20 minutes after administration of contrast material.

4. Arachnoiditis

Arachnoiditis, which is distinct from epidural scar formation, involves inflammatory and scar tissue within the dura surrounding the spinal nerves. The MRI characteristics of arachnoiditis show three different possible patterns. The first is centrally clumped spinal nerve roots in the thecal sac seen on T1-weighted images; the second is peripheral adhesions of roots to the thecal sac; the third is an increased soft tissue signal within the thecal sac below the conus. Arachnoiditis typically presents as polyradicular lower extremity pain.

5. Metastatic disease of the spine

Severe back pain is a common presentation of metastatic disease of the lumbar spine. The most common tumors that metastasize to bone and thus the lumbar spine are lung, prostate, and breast. Multiple myeloma and breast cancer typically are osteolytic, whereas prostate tends to cause osteosclerotic changes. Bone scans are very sensitive for detecting metastatic involvement of the lumbar spine. The correlation between the severity of bone scan and the intensity of pain is generally poor.

When spinal cord compression resulting from epidural metastatic disease is suspected, MRI is the imaging modality of choice and contrast enhancement is recommended. Back pain is a common presentation of spinal cord compression. When significant reduction of vertebral body height is seen, concomitant epidural involvement is common. Disruption of the pedicle on imaging suggests metastatic disease and, when seen on a plain radiograph, warrants thorough investigation.

6. Infectious processes of the vertebral spine

Plain x-rays can be utilized to assess osteomyelitis. Characteristic changes include loss of end-plate definition, associated soft tissue swelling, destruction of vertebral bodies, and loss of intervertebral disc height. MRI detects involvement of the disc space. Occasionally, MRI is negative and radionucleotide imaging studies can be helpful in establishing the diagnosis. The characteristics of osteomyelitis as seen on MRI include decreased signal intensity, a loss of delineation and demarcation of the vertebral end plate on T1-weighted images; and increased signal intensity in the intervertebral disc on T2-weighted images.

VI. CONCLUSION

Imaging studies are indispensable tools for the pain physician, who must use them not only as appropriate diagnostic tools but also in a cost-effective manner. Consultation with the department of radiology may be helpful when a diagnosis is uncertain.

SELECTED READING

1. Atlas SW, ed. *Magnetic resonance imaging of the brain and spine.* New York: Raven Press, 1996.
2. Modic MT, Masaryk TJ, Ross JS, eds. *Magnetic resonance imaging of the spine.* Chicago: Year Book Medical, 1989.
3. Osborn AG. *Diagnostic neuroradiology.* St Louis: Mosby. 1994.

6

Assessment of Pain

Alyssa A. LeBel

When you can measure what you are speaking about, and express it in numbers, you know something about it; but when you cannot express it in numbers, your knowledge is of a meager and unsatisfactory kind: it may be the beginning of knowledge, but you have scarcely, in your thoughts, advanced to the stage of science.
—*William Thompson Lord Kelvin, 1824–1907*

Pain is a complex multidimensional symptom determined not only by tissue injury and nociception but also by previous pain experience, personal beliefs, effect, motivation, environment, and, at times, pending litigation. **There is no objective measurement of pain**. Self-report is the most valid measure of the individual experience of pain. The pain history is key to the assessment of pain and includes the patient's description of pain intensity, quality, location, timing, and duration, as well as ameliorating and exacerbating conditions.

Frequently, pain cannot be seen, defined, or felt by the examiner, and the physician must assess the pain from a combination of factors. The most important of these is the patient's report of pain, but other factors such as personality and culture, psychological status, the potential of secondary gain, and the possibility of drug-seeking behavior also deserve consideration. Reports of pain may not correlate with the degree of disability or findings on physical examination. It is important to remember, however, that to our patients and their families, distress, suffering, and pain behaviors are often not distinguished from the pain itself.

Acute pain diagnosis and measurement require frequent and consistent assessment as part of daily clinical care to ensure rapid titration of therapy and preemptive interventions. Chronic pain is often more diagnostically challenging than acute pain, but it is no less compelling. Application of a structured history and comprehensive physical examination will define treatable problems and identify complicating factors. Somatic, visceral, or neuropathic pain, or a combination of these problems, suggests specific diagnoses and interventions. An understanding of pain pathophysiology guides rational and appropriate treatment.

I. PAIN HISTORY

The general medical history may contribute significantly, and it is always included as part of the pain assessment (see Chapter 4). The specific pain history includes three main issues—intensity, location, and pathophysiology. The following questions help define them:

- What is the time course of the pain?
- Where is the pain?
- What is the intensity of the pain?
- What factors relieve or exacerbate the pain?
- What are the possible generators of the pain?

1. Pain assessment tools

Pain cannot be objectively measured, and its intensity is very difficult and often frustrating to try to pinpoint. Several tests and scales are available. Some of the more commonly used are discussed here.

Unidimensional self-report scales

In practice, self-report scales serve as very simple, useful, and valid methods for assessing and monitoring patients' pain.

VERBAL DESCRIPTOR SCALES. The patient is asked to describe his or her pain by choosing from a list of adjectives that reflect gradations of pain intensity. The five-word scale consists of *mild, discomforting, distressing, horrible,* and *excruciating*. Disadvantages of this scale include the limited selection of descriptors and the fact that patients tend to select moderate descriptors rather than the extremes.

VERBAL NUMERIC RATING SCALES. These are the simplest and most frequently used scales. On a numeric scale (most commonly 0 to 10, with 0 being "no pain" and 10 being "the worst pain imaginable"), the patient picks a number to describe the pain. Advantages of numeric scales are their simplicity, reproducibility, easy comprehensibility, and sensitivity to small changes in pain. Children as young as 5 years who are able to count and have some concept of numbers (e.g., "8 is larger than 4") may use this scale.

VISUAL ANALOG SCALES. These are similar to the verbal numeric rating scales, except that the patient marks on a measured line, one end of which is labeled "no pain" and the other end, "worst pain imaginable," where the pain falls. Visual scales are more valid for research purposes, but they are less used clinically because they are more time consuming to conduct than verbal scales.

"FACES" PAIN RATING SCALE. Evaluating pain in children can be very difficult because of the child's inability to describe pain or understand pain assessment forms. This scale depicts six sketches of facial features, each with a numeric value, 0 to 5, ranging from a happy, smiling face to a sad, teary face (Fig. 1). To extrapolate this scale to the visual analog scale, multiply the chosen value by two. This scale may also be beneficial for mentally impaired patients. Children as young as 3 years may reliably use this scale.

Multidimensional instruments

Multidimensional instruments provide more complex information about the patient's pain and are especially useful for assess-

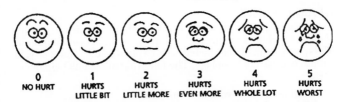

0	1	2	3	4	5
NO HURT	HURTS LITTLE BIT	HURTS LITTLE MORE	HURTS EVEN MORE	HURTS WHOLE LOT	HURTS WORST

Figure 1.   Wong-Baker's "faces" pain rating scale. Explain to the person that each face is for someone who feels happy because he has no pain (hurt) or sad because he has some or a lot of pain. Face 0 is very happy because he doesn't hurt at all. Face 1 hurts just a little bit. Face 2 hurts a little more. Face 3 hurts even more. Face 4 hurts a whole lot. Face 5 hurts as much as you can imagine, although you don't have to be crying to feel this bad.

ment of chronic pain. As they are time consuming, they are most frequently used in outpatient and research settings.

McGill Pain Questionnaire (MPQ)

The MPQ is the most frequently used multidimensional test. Descriptive words from three major dimensions of pain (sensory, affective, and evaluative) are further subdivided into 20 subclasses, each containing words that represent varying degrees of pain. Three scores are obtained, one for each dimension, as well as a total score. Studies have shown the MPQ to be a reliable instrument in clinical research.

Brief Pain Inventory (BPI)

In the BPI, patients are asked to rate the severity of their pain at its "worst," "least," and "average" within the past 24 hours, as well as at the time the rating is made. It also asks patients to represent the location of their pain on a schematic diagram of the body. The BPI correlates with scores of activity, sleep, and social interactions. It is cross-cultural and a useful method for clinical studies (Fig. 2).

Massachusetts General Hospital (MGH) Pain Center pain assessment form

The MGH form (Fig. 3) combines many of the preceding assessment instruments and is given to all patients on initial consultations at the MGH Pain Center. It elicits information about pain intensity, its location (via a body diagram), quality of pain, therapies tried, and past and present medications. It takes 10 to 15 minutes to complete and is an extremely valuable instrument. Its disadvantages are that it is time consuming to complete and it is not applicable if there are language constraints.

Pain Diaries

A diary of a patient's pain is useful in evaluating the relationship between pain and daily activity. Pain can be described using the numeric rating scale, during activities such as walking, standing, sitting, and routine chores. Blocks of time are usually hourly. Medication use, alcohol use, emotional responses, and family responses may also be helpful information to record. Pain diaries may reflect a patient's pain more accurately than a retrospective description that may significantly over- or underestimate pain.

2. Pain location

Knowing the location and distribution of pain is extremely important for understanding the pathophysiology of the pain complaint. Body diagrams, found in some of the assessment instruments, can prove very useful. Not only can the clinician view the patient's perception of the topographic area of pain but the patient may demonstrate psychological distress by an inability to localize the pain or by magnifying it and projecting it to other areas of the body.

Is the pain localized or referred? Localized pain is pain that is confined to its site of origin without radiation or migration. Referred pain usually arises from visceral or deep structures and radiates to other areas of the body. A classic example of referred pain is shoulder pain from phrenic nerve irritation (causes include liver metastases from pancreatic cancer) (Table 1).

Is pain superficial/peripheral or visceral? Superficial pain, arising from tissues rich in nociceptors, such as skin, teeth, and mucous membranes, is easily localized and limited to the affected part of the body. Visceral pain arises from internal organs, which contain relatively few nociceptors. Visceral afferent information may converge with superficial afferent input at the spinal level, referring the perception of visceral pain to a distant dermatome. Visceral pain is diffuse and often poorly localized. In addition, it often has an associated autonomic component, such as diaphoresis, capillary vasodilation, hypertension, or tachycardia.

3. Pain etiology

By taking a complete history and answering the preceding two questions, the clinician can begin to formulate the causes of the pain. The rest of the history, as well as the physical examination, can be tailored to systematically explore aspects of pain, such as symptoms and physical signs, common to the particular type of pain in question.

It is possible to describe different types of pain, and they tend to present differently (e.g., nociceptive pain is associated with tissue injury caused by trauma, surgery, inflammation or tumor; neuropathic pain is invariably associated with sensory change; radicular pain is often associated with radiculopathy). The history and physical examination help to identify these differences. Because the different types of pain tend to respond to different treatments, the identification of pain type during pain assessment is important. The types can be categorized as follows:

- **Nociceptive pain** arises from activation of nociceptors. Nociceptors are found in all tissues except the central nervous system (CNS); the pain is clinically proportional to the degree of activation of afferent pain fibers and can be acute or chronic (e.g., somatic pain, cancer pain, postoperative pain).
- **Neuropathic pain** is caused by nerve injury or disease, or by involvement of nerves in other disease processes such as tumor or inflammation. Neuropathic pain may occur in the periphery or in the CNS.

(*text continues on page 65*)

STUDY ID# _____   HOSPITAL# _____

DO NOT WRITE ABOVE THIS LINE
Brief Pain Inventory (Short Form)

Date: ___ /___ /___   Time: _____

Name: _____   _____   _____
         Last   First   Middle Initial

1) Throughout our lives, most of us have had pain from time to time (such as minor headaches, sprains, and toothaches). Have you had pain other than these everyday kinds of pain today?

                1. Yes   2. No

2) On the diagram, shade in the areas where you feel pain. Put an X on the area that hurts the most.

    Right   Left   Left   Right

3) Please rate your pain by circling the one number that best describes your pain at its **worst** in the last 24 hours.

0	1	2	3	4	5	6	7	8	9	10
No Pain									Pain as bad as you can imagine	

4) Please rate your pain by circling the one number that best describes your pain at its **least** in the last 24 hours.

0	1	2	3	4	5	6	7	8	9	10
No Pain									Pain as bad as you can imagine	

5) Please rate your pain by circling the one number that best describes your pain on the **average.**

0	1	2	3	4	5	6	7	8	9	10
No Pain									Pain as bad as you can imagine	

6) Please rate your pain by circling the one number that tells how much pain you have **right now.**

0	1	2	3	4	5	6	7	8	9	10
No Pain									Pain as bad as you can imagine	

7) What treatments or medications are you receiving for your pain?

8) In the last 24 hours, how much relief have pain treatments or medications provided? Please circle the one percentage that most shows how much relief you have received.

0%	10%	20%	30%	40%	50%	60%	70%	80%	90%	100%
No Relief										Complete Relief

9) Circle the one number that describes how, during the past 24 hours, pain has interfered with your:

A. General activity

0	1	2	3	4	5	6	7	8	9	10
Does not interfere									Completely Interferes	

B. Mood

0	1	2	3	4	5	6	7	8	9	10
Does not interfere									Completely Interferes	

C. Walking ability

0	1	2	3	4	5	6	7	8	9	10
Does not interfere									Completely Interferes	

D. Normal work (includes both work outside the home and housework)

0	1	2	3	4	5	6	7	8	9	10
Does not interfere									Completely Interferes	

E. Relations with other people

0	1	2	3	4	5	6	7	8	9	10
Does not interfere									Completely Interferes	

F. Sleep

0	1	2	3	4	5	6	7	8	9	10
Does not interfere									Completely Interferes	

G. Enjoyment of life

0	1	2	3	4	5	6	7	8	9	10
Does not interfere									Completely Interferes	

Pain Research Group • Department of Neurology • University of Wisconsin-Madison

Figure 2.   Brief pain inventory (see text). Reprinted with permission from the University of Wisconsin–Madison, Department of Neurology, Pain Research Group.

M.G.H. PAIN CENTER
PAIN ASSESSMENT FORM

Information About the Pain

1. What is the problem you would like us to help you with?

2. Please mark the event or events that led to your present pain: (If you experience more than one kind of pain, please write in separate sets of answers for each type of pain you have.)

_____ Accident   _____ Cancer

_____ Other injury _____ _____ No obvious cause

_____ Following an operation _____ Other disease _____

_____ Other _____

3. For how long have you had this pain?

4. How often does the pain occur?
_____ Continuously (nonstop)

_____ Several times a day

_____ Once or twice a day

_____ Several times a week

_____ Less than 3 or 4 times per month

5. How has the *intensity* of the pain changed throughout the time you have had it?

_____ Increased _____ Decreased _____ Stayed the same

6. The following five words represent pain of increasing intensity:

1	2	3
Mild	Discomforting	Distressing

4	5
Horrible	Excruciating

To answer each question below, write the *number* of the most appropriate word in the space beside the question.

a. Which word describes your pain at its worst? _____
b. Which word describes your pain at its least? _____
c. Which word describes your pain right now? _____
d. Which word describes how your pain is most of the time? _____

7. Location of the Pain
(please shadow in the affected areas).

8. Quality of the Pain

Below is list of words that are often used to describe pain. After each descriptive word, indicate with a checkmark whether this word describes a particular quality of your pain and, if it does, the intensity of that quality.

	None (not at all)	Mild	Moderate	Severe
Throbbing	0)	1)	2)	3)
Shooting	0)	1)	2)	3)
Stabbing	0)	1)	2)	3)
Sharp	0)	1)	2)	3)
Cramping	0)	1)	2)	3)
Gnawing	0)	1)	2)	3)
Hot-Burning	0)	1)	2)	3)
Aching	0)	1)	2)	3)
Heavy	0)	1)	2)	3)
Tender	0)	1)	2)	3)
Splitting	0)	1)	2)	3)
Tiring/Exhausting	0)	1)	2)	3)
Sickening	0)	1)	2)	3)
Fearful	0)	1)	2)	3)
Punishing/Cruel	0)	1)	2)	3)

9. Which of the following have an effect on your pain? Please indicate whether it makes the pain better, worse, or has *no effect*.

_____ Heat   _____ Cold   _____ Noise
_____ Sitting   _____ Standing   _____ Lying down
_____ Walking   _____ Fatigue   _____ Particular position
_____ Coughing _____ Anxiety/emotions   or movement
_____ Vibration _____ Massage/rubbing   explain: _____
_____ Climate   _____ Alcoholic beverages _____ Caffeinated drinks
                                            (coffee, tea, colas)

10. How does the pain affect your activity in these different areas:
Work-school–
Household chores–
Social interactions–
Leisure–
Sexual activity–

11. What is your current employment status?

12. Do you have pending a settlement about disability, workers' compensation, or a legal matter?

_____ yes _____ no

If yes, briefly explain: _____

13. What treatments have you tried for your pain?
_____ Surgery   _____ TENS unit
_____ Nerve block   _____ Exercise program
_____ Brace   _____ Trigger point injection
_____ Physical therapy   _____ Acupuncture
_____ Relaxation training _____ Chiropractic therapy
_____ Biofeedback   _____ Psychotherapy/counseling
Other _____   _____ Hypnosis
                           _____ Massage

14. What specialists have you seen for your pain (e.g., orthopedic surgeon, neurologist, neurosurgeon, psychiatrist)?

15. Pain Medications and Other Treatments

A. What are the medications you are currently taking for pain?

	Drug	Dose	Frequency
1.			
2.			
3.			
4.			

B. What other medications have you taken in the past for pain?

	Drug	Effect on Pain
1.		
2.		
3.		
4.		

C. Are you allergic to any medications (including local anesthetics)?

     Drug   *Type of Reaction*

D. What other medications are you currently taking?

16. Name, address, and phone number of your primary care physician:

17. Name, address, and phone number of the physician who referred you to us:

Figure 3. The Massachusetts General Hospital (MGH) Pain Center's pain assessment form.

- **Sympathetically mediated pain** is accompanied (at some point) by evidence of edema, changes in skin blood flow, abnormal sudomotor activity in the regional of pain, allodynia, hyperalgesia, or hyperpathia.
- **Deafferentation pain** is chronic and results from loss of afferent input to the CNS. The pain may arise in the periphery (e.g., peripheral nerve avulsion) or in the CNS (e.g., spinal cord lesions, multiple sclerosis).
- **Neuralgia pain** is lancinating and associated with nerve damage or irritation along the distribution of a single nerve (e.g., trigeminal) or nerves.
- **Radicular pain** is evoked by stimulation of nociceptive afferent fibers in spinal nerves, their roots, or ganglia, or by other neuropathic mechanisms. The symptom is caused by ectopic impulse generation. It is distinct from radiculopathy, but the two often arise together.
- **Central pain** arises from a lesion in the CNS, usually involving the spinothalamic cortical pathways (i.e., thalamic infarct). The pain is usually constant, with a burning, electrical quality, and it is exacerbated by activity or changes in the weather. Hyperesthesia and hyperpathia and/or allodynia are invariably present, and the pain is highly resistant to treatment.
- **Psychogenic pain** is inconsistent with the likely anatomic distribution of the presumed generator, or it exists with no apparent organic pathology despite extensive evaluation.
- **Referred pain** often originates from a visceral organ (see Table 1). It may be felt in body regions remote from the site of pathology. The mechanism may be the spinal convergence of visceral and somatic afferent fibers on spinothalamic neurons. Common manifestations are cutaneous and deep hyperalgesia, autonomic hyperactivity, tenderness, and muscular contractions.

Table 1. Examples of referred pain

Origin of pain	Region of pain referral
Head (dura mater or vessels)	
Anterior cranial fossa	Ipsilateral forehead
Middle cranial fossa	Ipsilateral supraorbital region, temples
Posterior cranial fossa	Ipsilateral ear, postauricular region, occiput
Pharynx	Ipsilateral ear
Chest	
Esophagus	Substernal region
Heart	Left arm, epigastric
Abdomen	
Visceral pain	Segmental muscle spasms
Cholecystitis	Upper abdominal muscles
Appendicitis	Lower abdominal muscles
Renal colic	L2–L3 segments
Subphrenic region	Shoulder pain
Liver	Right phrenic region
Kidney	Lower thorax and back
Ureter	
Upper (renal pelvis)	Groin, testis, or ovary
Terminal	Scrotum/labia
Pelvis	
Prostate	Lower back
Uterus	Lower back
Ovary	Anterior thigh
Lower extremity	
Peroneal entrapment at fibula	Dorsum of foot
Other	
Unilateral cordotomy	Pain applied to analgesic side produces pain in symmetrical contralateral body part

Adapted from Brass LM, Stys K. *Handbook of neurological lists.* New York: Churchill-Livingstone, 1991, with permission.

II. PHYSICAL EXAMINATION

A complete examination is required, including a general physical examination followed by a specific pain evaluation, and neurologic, musculoskeletal, and mental status assessments. It is important not to limit the examination to the painful location and surrounding tissues and structures.

1. General physical examination

This physical examination consists of the usual head-to-toe examination as described in Chapter 4. It is important to note the following points:

a. Appearance—obese, emaciated, histrionic, flat effect
b. Posture—splinting, scoliosis, kyphosis
c. Gait—antalgic, hemiparetic, using assistive devices
d. Expression—grimacing, tense, diaphoretic, anxious
e. Vital signs—sympathetic overactivity (tachycardia, hypertension), temperature asymmetries

It is also important to watch how a patient dresses and moves. Favoring an extremity or protecting a part of the body may not be appreciated unless the relevant movements are elicited. Some elements of the comprehensive examination may be missed if a clinician is fearful of invading the patient's privacy.

2. Specific pain evaluation

After the general examination, the clinician evaluates the painful areas of the body. The history often directs the search for physical findings. Inspection of the skin may reveal changes in color, flushing, edema, hair loss, presence or absence of sweat, atrophy, or muscle spasm. Inspection of nails may show dystrophic changes. Nerve root injury may be manifest as goose flesh (cutis anserina) in the affected dermatome. Palpation allows mapping of the painful area and detection of any change in pain intensity within the area, as well as during the examination, and helps to define pain type and trigger points. Patient responses, both verbal and nonverbal, should be noted, as well as the appropriateness of the responses and their correlation with affect. Factors that reproduce, worsen, or decrease the pain are sought.

While conducting the physical examination, it is important to identify any changes in sensory and pain processing that may have occurred. These changes may be manifest as anesthesia, hypoesthesia, hyperesthesia, analgesia, hypoalgesia, allodynia, hyperalgesia, or hyperpathia.

3. Neurologic examination

Subtle physical findings are often found only during the neurologic examination. It is essential to conduct a comprehensive neurologic examination when first assessing a patient with pain, to identify associated, and possibly treatable, neurologic disease. The examination can be performed in 5 to 10 minutes. Later in the course of treatment, the neurologic examination can be more focused and briefer.

Mental function is assessed by evaluating the patient's orientation to person, place, and time, short- and long-term memory, choice of words used to describe symptoms and answer questions, and educational background.

The **cranial nerves** should be examined, especially in patients complaining of head, neck, and shoulder pain symptoms. Table 2 lists the function of each cranial nerve.

A simple assessment of **spinal nerve function** should also be performed. Spinal nerve sensation is determined by the use of cotton or tissue paper for light touch, and pinprick for sharp pain and proprioception. Potentially painful peripheral neuropathies are listed in Table 3. Spinal nerve motor function is determined by deep tendon reflexes, the presence or absence of the Babinski reflex, and tests of muscle strength. Table 4 lists sensory and motor manifestations of common root syndromes.

Table 2. Neurologic examination of cranial nerves

Cranial nerves	Function
I—Olfactory nerve	Smell
II—Optic	Vision
III—Oculomotor	
Parasympathetic	Sphincter muscle of iris, ciliary muscle
Motor	Superior, inferior, and medial rectus muscles; inferior oblique and levator palpebrae superioris muscle
IV—Trochlear	Superior oblique
V—Trigeminal	
Motor	Muscles of mastication
Sensory	Face, mucosa of nose, mouth, dura, and cornea
VI—Abducens	Lateral rectus muscle
VII—Facial	
Motor	Muscles of expression
Parasympathetic	Lacrimal gland, salivary glands and mucous membranes of mouth
Sensory	Sensation to parts of external ear, auditory canal, and tympanic membrane
	Taste to anterior two thirds of tongue
VIII—Vestibulocochlear	Equilibrium and hearing
IX—Glossopharyngeal	
Parasympathetic	Parotid gland
Motor	Stylopharyngeal muscle
Sensory	Sensation to posterior one third of tongue, pharynx, middle ear, and dura
X—Vagus	
Parasympathetic	Viscera of thorax and abdomen
Motor	Muscles of pharynx and larynx
Sensory somatic	Dura and auditory canal
Sensory visceral	Viscera of thorax and abdomen
XI—Accessory	
Motor	Muscles of larynx, sternocleidomastoid and trapezius
XII—Hypoglossal	Intrinsic muscles of tongue, genioglossus, hypoglossus, and styloglossus

Table 3.   Painful sensory neuropathies

Endocrinologic
  Diabetes mellitus
  Hypothyroidism
Metabolic
  Uremia
  Thiamine deficiency
  Acute intermittent porphyria
Toxic
  Vincristine
  Acrylamide
  Heavy metals
  Organic solvents
Infectious/inflammatory
  HIV-related painful neuropathies
  Herpes zoster—acute and chronic postherpetic neuralgia
  Guillain-Barré syndrome
  Chronic inflammatory polyneuropathy
Immunologic
  Polyarteritis nodosa
  Cryoglobulinemia
  Systemic lupus erythematosus
Physical
  Brachial plexopathies
  Compressive
Neoplastic
  Multiple myeloma
  Cancer (including nonmetastatic effects and carcinomatosis)
Genetic
  Fabry's Disease
  Tangier disease
  Familial dysautonomias (Riley-Day syndrome, inherited sensory
    neuropathy III)
  Amyloidosis

Coordination is assessed by testing balance, rapid hand movement, finger-to-nose motion, toe-to-heel motion, gait, and Romberg's test. Cerebellar dysfunction can often be detected during these maneuvers. Table 5 lists pain disturbances, caused by various disease processes, that can affect gait.

Pain of psychogenic origin usually results in a neurologic examination whose findings are not typical of organic pathology. Abnormal pain distributions, such as glove or stocking patterns and exact hemianesthesia, are common in patients with psychogenic pain.

4. Musculoskeletal system examination

Abnormalities of the musculoskeletal system are often evident on inspection of the patient's posture and muscular symmetry. Muscle atrophy usually indicates disuse. Flaccidity indicates extreme weakness, usually from paralysis, and abnormal movements indicate neurologic damage or impaired proprioception. Limited

Table 4.   Pain-induced disturbances of gait

Diagnosis	Symptoms
Intermittent claudication,	Pain on walking a specific distance, arterial insufficiency
	Pain sooner with increasing intensity of work
	Pain disappears after rest
	Pain localized to calf
Cauda equina (neurogenic claudication, spinal stenosis)	Pain on walking after varying distances
	Patient usually elderly
	Usually bilateral
	Radicular in character
	Pain localized to saddle area, upper thigh, and calf
	Pain in back on sneezing
	Pain does not usually disappear on cessation of walking
	Pain improved when leaning forward
Hip disease	Pain worse on first few steps
Inguinal region	Pain increased on prolonged standing
	Usually after appendectomy, hernia repair
Meralgia paresthetica	Pain in the lateral aspect of the thigh
Long bones	Localized pain
	Evidence of tumor/osteoporosis, Paget's disease, pathologic fracture
	After surgical procedure—anterior compartment syndrome
Feet	
Foot deformities	Pain after walking or standing
Calcaneal spur	
Achilles tendinitis	
Tarsal tunnel syndrome	Pain in the plantar aspect of foot (prevents walking)

Adapted from Mumenthaler M. *Neurologic Differential Diagnosis.* New York: Thieme-Stratton, 1925:118–119, with permission.

range of motion of a major joint can indicate pain, disc disease, or arthritis. Palpation of muscles helps in evaluating range of motion and in determining whether trigger points are present. Coordination and strength are also tested.

5. Assessment of psychological factors

Complete assessment of pain includes analysis of the psychological aspects of pain and the effects of pain on behavior and emotional stability. Such assessment is challenging, because many patients are unaware of or reluctant to present psychological

Table 5. Common painful root syndromes

Root	Sensory loss	Motor changes	
		Weakness	Decreased deep tendon reflexes
Upper extremity			
C5	Lateral aspect of upper arm	Deltoid and biceps	None/biceps
C6	Thumb and index finger	Biceps and brachioradialis	Brachioradialis and biceps
C7	Middle finger	Triceps and pronator teres	Triceps
Lower extremity			
L4	Medial calf	Quadriceps	Knee
L5	Medial half of foot and lateral calf	Peroneal, anterior and posterior tibial and toe extension	Internal hamstring
S1	Lower posterior calf and lateral foot	Plantar flexion	Ankle

issues. It is also more socially acceptable to seek medical than psychiatric care.

Initially, the use of a descriptive pain questionnaire, such as the MPQ, may provide some evidence of a patient's affective responses to pain. For example, whereas words such as *aching* and *tingling* refer to sensory aspects of pain, words such as *agonizing* and *dreadful* suggest negative feelings and do not aid in characterizing the pain sensation. For a fuller description of psychological evaluation in pain management, see Chapter 15.

A patient's personality greatly influences his or her response to pain and choice of coping strategies. Some patients may benefit from the use of strategies of control, such as distraction and relaxation. Patients who have an underlying anxiety disorder may be more likely to seek high doses of analgesics. Therefore, inquiry regarding a patient's history of coping with stress is often useful.

As part of the pain history, the clinician should include questions about some of the common symptoms in patients with chronic pain: depressed mood, sleep disturbance, preoccupation with somatic symptoms, reduced activity, reduced libido, and fatigue. Standardized questionnaires, such as the Minnesota Multiphasic Personality Inventory (MMPI), may expand the assessment. On this inventory, patients with chronic pain characteristically score very high on the depression, hysteria, and hypochondriasis scales. However, the MMPI may reflect functional limitation secondary to pain as well as psychological abnormality associated with chronic pain, limiting its interpretation for some patients suspected of having psychogenic pain.

A number of psychological processes and syndromes predispose patients to chronic pain. Predisposing disorders include major depression, somatization disorder, conversion disorder, hypochondriasis, and psychogenic pain disorder. The diagnosis of somatization disorder is quite specific, although many patients with chronic pain may **somatize** (i.e., focus on somatic complaints). This diagnosis requires a history of physical symptoms of several years' duration, beginning before the age of 30 years and including complaints of at least 14 specific symptoms for women and 12 for men. These symptoms are not adequately explained by physical disorder, injury, or toxic reaction.

Psychogenic pain may occur in susceptible individuals. In some patients, pain may ameliorate more unpleasant feelings, such as depression, guilt, or anxiety, and distract the patient from environmental stress factors. Features from the patient's history that suggest a psychogenic component to chronic pain include the following:

- Multiple locations of pain at different times
- Pain problems dating since adolescence
- Pain without obvious somatic cause (especially in the facial or perineal area)
- Multiple, elective surgical procedures
- Substance abuse (by patient and/or significant other)
- Social or work failure

Psychogenic pain is clearly distinct from malingering. Malingerers have an obvious, identifiable environmental goal in producing symptoms, such as evading law enforcement, avoiding work, or obtaining financial compensation. Patients with psychogenic pain make illness and hospitalization their primary goals. Being a patient is their primary way of life. Such patients are unable to stop symptom production when it is no longer obviously beneficial.

The physical examination in patients with psychological factors exacerbating pain may be perplexing. Some findings may not correspond to known anatomic or physiologic information. Examples of such findings include the following:

- Manual testing inconsistent with patient observation during sitting, turning, and dressing
- Grasping with three fingers
- Antagonist muscle contraction on attempted movement
- Decreased tremor during mental arithmetic exercises
- A positive Romberg's sign with one eye closed
- Vibration absent on one side of midline (skull, sternum)
- Inconsistency of timed vibration when affected side is tested first
- Patterned miscount of touches
- Difficulty touching the good limb with the bad
- A slight difference in sensation on one side of the body

Useful neurologic signs are deep tendon reflexes, motor tone and bulk, and the plantar response. Observation is critical. Pain drawings at multiple time intervals are also useful in evaluating a patient with chronic pain of unclear etiology.

III. DIAGNOSTIC STUDIES

The diagnosis and understanding of a patient's pain complaint can usually be obtained after a thorough history and physical examination. Diagnostic and physiologic studies are used to support a clinician's suspicion, as well as to assist in the diagnosis. Some of the more common studies used for pain assessment include the following.

Conventional radiography is used to diagnose bony abnormalities, such as pathologic fractures seen in bony metastases, spine pathology (including spondylolisthesis, stenosis, and osteophyte formation), and bone tumors. Some soft-tissue tumors and bowel abnormalities can also be seen. Radiographs of the painful area have usually been obtained by the referring physician.

A **CT scan** is most often used to define bony abnormalities, and **MRI** best shows soft-tissue pathology. Spinal stenosis, disc herniation or bulge, nerve root compression, and tumors in all tissues can be diagnosed, as well as some causes of central pain, such as CNS infarcts or plaques of demyelination.

Diagnostic blocks may differentiate somatic from visceral pain and confirm the anatomic location of peripheral nerve pain. They may help localize painful pathology or contribute to the diagnosis of complex regional pain syndrome (CRPS). They are also necessary precedents to neurolytic blocks for malignant pain or radiofrequency lesions. Diagnostic blocks are described in detail in Chapter 12.

Drug challenges are used to predict drug treatment utility and to help in the assessment of pain etiology. For example, brief intravenous infusions of opioids, lidocaine, and phentolamine are used to predict opioid sensitivity in nonmalignant chronic pain, to predict sensitivity to sodium channel blockade in neuropathic pain, and to assess the potential reversibility of the sympathetic component of pain in CRPS. The value of this type of testing in predicting treatment efficacy is debatable. In most reports, chronic treatment has been limited to responders, which precludes validation of the infusion as a predictive test.

Various **neurophysiologic tests** are used to help in the diagnosis of pain syndromes and related neurologic disease (see Chapter 7). The neurophysiologic tests most commonly used in pain clinics are categorized as quantitative sensory testing (QST), and these tests specifically evaluate patients' responses to carefully quantified physical stimuli.

Thermography is a noninvasive way of displaying the body's thermal patterns. A normal thermal pattern is relatively symmetric. Tissue pathology is associated with chemical and metabolic changes that may cause abnormal thermal patterns by altering vascularity, such as in CRPS. The differences in patterns of color are not specific for underlying central or peripheral pathology.

Myelography is the injection of radiopaque dye into the subarachnoid space to radiographically visualize spinal cord/column abnormalities, such as disc herniation, nerve root impingement, arachnoiditis, and spinal stenosis. Major disadvantages of this procedure are postdural-puncture headache and meningeal irritation.

Bone scanning is the use of a radioactive compound to detect bone lesions, including neoplastic, infectious, arthritic, and traumatic lesions; Paget's disease; and the osteodystrophy of reflex sympathetic dystrophy. The radioactive compound accumulates in areas of increased bone growth or turnover. The test is very sensitive for subtle bone abnormalities that may not appear on conventional radiographs.

Small punch **skin biopsy** (immunolabeled to show the cutaneous sensory nerve endings) is a new tool with which to directly visualize the cutaneous endings of pain neurons. Although currently available at only a few centers, this technique is replacing sural nerve biopsy for the diagnosis of sensory neuropathies. The technique appears to be helpful for diagnosing focal painful nerve injuries. Research has shown that various painful neuropathic conditions are associated with loss of nociceptive innervation in painful skin. Skin biopsies are only minimally invasive, can be repeated, and can be performed in areas other than those innervated by the sural nerve.

Functional brain imaging, such as by positron emission tomography or functional MRI, is an investigative tool at present with provocative findings regarding the cortical and subcortical processing of pain information. Functional MRI shows pain to be a remarkably distributed system at the cortical level.

IV. CONCLUSION

The assessment of pain can be challenging and intensive, but it is an essential component of pain management, and it allows the pain physician to devise optimal treatment for some of medicine's most complex patients. The patient must be treated as a complete person and not just as a painful location. Believing the patient and establishing rapport are of the utmost importance. A systematic approach, grounded in a knowledge of anatomy and physiology, will assist the clinician in determining the pathophysiology of the patient's pain complaint. Then, therapy can be formulated, promptly initiated, and easily reassessed.

SELECTED READING

1. Beecher HK. *Measurement of subjective responses.* New York: Oxford University Press, 1959.
2. Boivie J, Hansson P, Lindblom U. Touch, temperature and pain in health and disease: Mechanisms and assessments. Progress in pain research and management, volume 3. Seattle: IASP Press, 1994.
3. Carlsson AM. Assessment of chronic pain. I: Aspects of the reliability and validity of the visual analogue scale. *Pain* 1983;16:87–101.
4. Gracely RH. Evaluation of multidimensional pain scales. *Pain* 1992;48:297–300.
5. Katz J. Psychophysical correlates of phantom limb experience. *J Neurol Neurosurg Psychiatry* 1992;55:811–821.
6. Lowe NK, Walder SM, McCallum RC. Confirming the theoretical structure of the McGill pain questionnaire in acute clinical pain. *Pain* 1991;46:53–60.
7. McGrath PA. *Pain in children: Nature, assessment and treatment.* New York: Guilford Press, 1990.
8. Melzack R. The McGill pain questionnaire: Major properties and scoring methods. *Pain* 1975;1:277–299.
9. Melzack R, Katz J. Pain measurement in persons in pain. In: Wall PD, Melzack R, eds. *Textbook of pain*, 4th ed. New York: Churchill-Livingstone, 1999.
10. Price DD, Bush FM, Long S, et al. A comparison of pain measurement characteristics of mechanical visual analogue and simple numerical rating scales. *Pain* 1994;56:217–226.

Neurophysiologic Testing in Pain Management

Annabel D. Edwards

As to pain, I am almost ready to say the physician who has not felt it is imperfectly educated.
—R. Weir Mitchell

Specialized neurophysiologic testing techniques have been used at the Massachusetts General Hospital (MGH) Pain Center for more than 5 years. This chapter will review neurophysiologic testing and its utility in pain practice and research.

I. NEUROPHYSIOLOGIC TESTING IN PAIN PRACTICE

Pain signals are communicated through the peripheral and central nervous systems and interpreted supraspinally. Parts of the nervous system that are not normally involved in pain transmission, such as the sensory, sympathetic, and parasympathetic systems, can become involved in pain processes in certain disease states and after injury or sensitization. Thus, activities in the various afferent systems overlap, connect, or change functionally both anatomically and at the cellular and molecular levels, creating a particularly complex challenge for the diagnosis and treatment of pain problems. Neurophysiologic testing is useful because it does the following:

- Helps to detect underlying pathology
- Helps to define mechanisms
- Helps to anatomically localize pain instigators
- Helps to focus treatments on mechanisms
- Helps to predict if patients will respond to particular treatments by clarifying mechanisms
- Used sequentially, helps to monitor disease progress and response to treatment

- May have medicolegal applications
- Advances pain research by providing quantitative and reproducible measures of pain and its various mechanisms

In clinical practice, neurophysiologic testing is useful when a diagnosis is elusive, or when a pain problem has been refractory to treatment. Testing may uncover the mechanism of the pain and direct treatment appropriately. Neurophysiologic testing is time consuming and not widely available, and it is not appropriate for all pain patients. To get maximal benefit from this testing in the clinical setting, patients and tests should be selected on the basis of a reasonable likelihood that the testing will help direct treatment. Figure 1 summarizes the utility of various tests in different parts of the nervous system.

II. USEFUL TESTS

Quantitative sensory testing (QST) is a useful clinical and research tool that has been adopted in many pain centers. Other neurophysiologic tests have less applicability to pain practice but are used occasionally to aid diagnosis. In most centers, the latter are carried out exclusively in the neurology clinic.

1. Quantitative sensory testing

Quantitative sensory testing is a noninvasive form of somatosensory testing, and the tests are relatively simple to perform. QST provides information on the activity of the entire afferent pain pathway from the periphery (receptor) to the brain (supratentorium). It tests high-threshold pain and temperature-sensing mechanisms by measuring subjective responses to quantified sensory and painful stimuli applied to the skin. Measured stimuli (most commonly thermal) are used to invoke pain responses and identify alterations in threshold such as those that occur in abnormal pain states such as allodynia and hyperalgesia (see Chapter 1).

Tests that fit into the QST category measure responses to thermal, mechanical (light touch and pinprick), vibratory, and electrical stimuli. These tests are geared mainly to explore the function of the primary nociceptive afferents (Aδ and C fibers) as well as Aβ fibers. Because these fibers respond to specific types of stimuli, tests are chosen to match them (see Fig. 1). Common findings and their association with various pain processes are listed in Table 1.

QST utilizes subjective responses to accurately calibrated sensory stimuli. Thus, although the stimuli are quantitative, the responses are susceptible to factors that depend on the patient and can result in confusion and inaccuracy, such as the following:

- Unwillingness or inability to pay attention and to respond accurately
- Distractions and discomfort during testing
- Inability to understand directions and use equipment
- Medical problems (known and unknown)
- Use of medications

Other potential confounding factors include faulty equipment, failure to adhere to standard protocols, and the lack of normative data for particular testing sites. Tremendous variation exists between centers in the methods and interpretations used. An important challenge for pain clinicians and researchers is to reach a

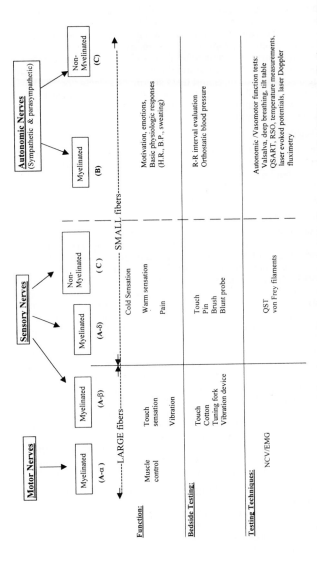

Figure 1. Peripheral nervous system. NCV, nerve conduction velocity; EMG, electromyography; QST, quantitative sensory testing; QSART, quantitative sudomotor axon reflex testing; RSO, resting sweat output.

Table 1. Pain processes and their association with test findings

Pain processes	Test findings
Painful neuropathies (including CRPS II)	Thermal hypesthesia, hyperesthesia, hypalgesia, or hyperalgesia
Peripheral sensitization	Heat hyperalgesia and inflammation
CRPS I	Cold or heat hyperalgesia without hypesthesia or hyperesthesia
Central sensitization	Tactile allodynia, mechanical hyperalgesia
Postherpetic neuralgia	Thermal hypoesthesia and hyperalgesia (anesthesia dolorosa)
Sympathetically mediated (CRPS I and II)	Changes in sudomotor reflexes (QSART) sweat output (RSO), and vasomotor function

CRPS, complex regional pain syndrome; QSART, quantitative sudomotor axon reflex testing; RSO, resting sweat output.

consensus on testing methodology so that results are broadly applicable across patient populations.

QST devices and techniques have developed rapidly over the last few years. Several companies specialize in making accurate devices. The most common devices create quantified stimuli including temperature (hot and cold), vibration, electrical stimuli, and punctate pressure. These stimuli are more reproducible and measurable than are the standard screening stimuli because they are delivered by well-calibrated systems.

2. Nerve conduction velocity and electromyography

Although electromyography (EMG) is not a test of sensory or pain function, it is commonly used in conjunction with sensory nerve conduction velocity (NCV) studies to provide information about the function of the peripheral nervous system and to aid in the diagnosis of disease processes underlying pain. These tests are invasive (involving the placement of electrodes into nervous tissue and muscle), do not measure central nervous system (CNS) activity, and are sensitive only to large fiber activity (i.e., sensory and motor, not pain).

However, the tests are useful for localizing the specific anatomic site of a lesion that might be causing pain. In fact, three of the most common conditions identifiable by EMG and NCV (peripheral neuropathy, radiculopathy, and carpal tunnel syndrome) frequently present with pain. The tests involve stimulating the periphery electrically, and measuring the amplitude and latency of the responses in various proximal locations (up to the level of the dorsal root ganglion and anterior horn cells). EMG and NCV help to localize the lesion and determine whether it is axonal or demyelinating; whether it is motor, sensory, or mixed; whether it is focal, multifocal, or diffuse; and the age, severity, and prognosis of the lesion.

Referral of pain patients for NCV and EMG testing is appropriate when the diagnosis of neurologic dysfunction associated with pain is unclear or unconfirmed.

3. Quantitative sudomotor axon reflex testing and resting sweat output

An increasingly used somatosensory modality is quantitative sudomotor axon reflex testing (QSART). QSART is sensitive and reproducible in demonstrating small fiber neuropathies, which it does by testing a specific neuronal pathway and the sweat response it produces. This activity is subserved by the autonomic nervous system, which plays an important role in pain modulation and perception, especially in small fiber neuropathies and in complex regional pain syndrome (CRPS), in which pain processes derive a significant contribution from sympathetic activity (neuronal or humeral).

Recent evidence suggests that sweat test activity correlates well with symptoms in CRPS. Patients with painful diabetic neuropathy also display increased sweat activity related to sympathetic over activity. The resting sweat output (RSO) test is similar to the QSART, but it measures only resting activity, which is an indication of spontaneous sympathetic activity.

4. Other tests

Vasomotor function tests

Vasomotor function tests are another way of demonstrating autonomic lability. They include bilateral temperature measurement, the Valsalva maneuver, deep breathing, the tilt test (measuring heart rate and blood pressure), and blood flow variations. The tests take a great deal of time, patience, and experience to conduct reliably, and they are less applicable in pain practice than in general neurologic and medical practice. However, they are occasionally indicated in patients with pain, especially when a diagnosis is needed before provocative tests can be arranged or when provocative tests are not available.

Single-unit nerve studies

Single-unit nerve studies, performed in academic centers, define abnormalities of specific fiber types (e.g., C-fiber activity that cannot be defined using conventional nerve conduction studies).

Laser doppler fluximetry

Laser Doppler fluximetry is a technique that evaluates superficial capillary flow in the face and extremities, thereby revealing asymmetries in sympathetically mediated vascular tone in areas of autonomic dysfunction.

Laser-evoked potentials

This new test is not widely available. It is noninvasive and measures the function of pain pathways in neuropathic pain. The skin is heated by a laser probe that activates Aδ and C fibers. Electrical activity is measured at the skull and Aδ and C-fiber activities are identified by their respective latencies (late and ultra-late).

III. QST EQUIPMENT

1. Thermal stimuli

Because pain and temperature sensitivities are closely related (both being transmitted to higher centers by small, high-threshold fibers—C fibers—with contributions from Aδ fibers) via the lateral spinothalamic tracts, thermal sensory tests are an excellent measure of neural pathology producing pain. To test thermal stimuli in the clinical setting, a device is used that can create temperature changes at a set rate and within specific limits to avoid heat or cold burns. (For research purposes, the device allows more extreme temperature settings.)

A thermode, which is placed flat against the skin, creates an area of temperature change. The size of the thermode must be selected for the individual since variations in size alter the results. Site selection is critical, and the literature contains many recommendations for sites based on areas of pain. For example, to test S1, the thermode is placed on the dorsum of the foot just proximal to the fourth and fifth toes and spaced equally between them.

Protocols have been developed for various forms of patient testing. These include specifics about how the equipment is programmed, as well as what questions are asked of the patients during testing. For example, the usual starting temperature of the thermode is 32°C. The temperature is changed at the rate of 1° per second. The patient is asked to push a button when a temperature change is first detected and again when the sensation becomes painful. These details are crucial to maintaining a common language among practitioners and researchers.

The thresholds measured are called warm sensation (WS), cold sensation (CS), heat pain (HP), and cold pain (CP). Normal thresholds are not exact, although in most cases, the normal for WS (i.e., the amount of temperature change it takes to detect an increased temperature from baseline) and CS (i.e., the amount of temperature change it takes to detect a decreased temperature from baseline) is within 1° or 2°C from the start. Heat pain usually occurs near 45°C. Cold pain seems to vary the most but usually does not occur until around 10°C or lower. The QST device can also be used to create non-noxious warm and cool stimuli to identify heat and cold allodynia.

2. Vibration stimuli

The vibration test assesses larger Aβ fiber function. The vibration device must make solid, even, and balanced contact with the skin. The pressure applied to the skin must be reliably controlled, as excess pressure can change the function of the nerves. These devices typically have a vibratory range of about 0 to 130 microns and an ability to deliver stimuli at a rate of from 0.1 to 4 microns per second. Site selection is critical, and sites are recommended in the literature. For example, vibration testing for S1 would be done on the plantar surface of the foot, between the fourth and fifth toes on the metatarsal head.

3. Mechanical stimuli

The most commonly used device for quantifying mechanical stimuli is a set of von Frey filaments. These are monofilaments of different thicknesses, which, when placed on the skin and made to bend, create a reproducible and reliable calibrated force. They are arranged in order of increasing mechanical force, starting at around 1.65 to 6.65. These numbers represent the common logarithms of the forces (expressed in 0.1 g) required to bow the filaments. A lowered or raised pain threshold can be detected, as can areas of primary and secondary hyperalgesia.

These filaments are commonly used in research and occasionally in clinical practice. Although full testing can be extremely time consuming, a few standardized filaments can be selected to represent a relevant range for routine clinical purposes (e.g., to test for loss of sensation in peripheral neuropathy).

Another mechanical test involves the use of a pin that is rhythmically applied to the skin with just enough force to cause a slight prick sensation. It is touched to the skin about every 2 seconds (but no more than 3 seconds). In normal skin, the repetitive C-fiber stimulation does not escalate the pain, whereas in patients with hyperalgesia, the repetitive stimulation results in increasingly more discomfort within about eight repetitions.

Tactile allodynia can be identified using a light touch stimulus, for example the examiner's fingers, a cotton-tipped applicator, or a camel's hair paintbrush. The patient's responses to such stimuli are compared from side to side as well as with other body areas.

4. Electrical stimuli

The use of electrical stimuli is a research tool only. In this modality, electrodes placed on the skin deliver stimuli at three different frequencies: 2000 Hz, 250 Hz, and 5 Hz. This is not considered a "normal" stimulus (i.e., it is not what the sensory nerve was meant to respond to), and it does not activate the nociceptor, but it is thought to activate a specific fiber type at each frequency: large myelinated Aβ fibers at 2000 Hz, Aδ fibers at 250 Hz, and small unmyelinated C fibers at 5 Hz.

IV. USES OF QST IN THE MGH PAIN CENTER

1. Clinical applications

The primary uses of QST in the clinical practice of the MGH Pain Center include clarification and confirmation of mechanisms, pain diagnoses, and documentation of responses to treatment. It is also helpful in certain difficult and refractory cases to document changes in treatment efficacy so that adjustments can be made on the basis of formal testing rather than on the basis of subjective assessment by the physician. The tests used most often for clinical assessments at the MGH Pain Center are the following:

- Thermal thresholds to warmth and coolness
- Pain thresholds to heat and cold
- Vibration-detection thresholds
- Sensation to pinprick
- Thresholds to mechanical sensation and pain by von Frey filaments

2. Research applications

Tests used for research at MGH include those used clinically and the following:

- Perception and pain thresholds to controlled electrical current
- Blood flow changes as measured by laser Doppler

Because QST devices are so accurate, the stimuli are consistently repeatable, and normative data rapidly are being amassed, these testing techniques have a solid role in research. Mapping of the brain areas involved in the perception of different types of pain (using evoked potentials, functional magnetic resonance imaging, magnetoencephalography, and positron-emission tomography) is just one way in which these tests can be applied. Responses to new techniques such as spinal cord stimulation can also be monitored using QST. The pain field is an exciting area for research, and QST provides a useful tool for quantifying pain stimuli and identifying pain mechanisms.

V. CONCLUSION

This chapter describes some of the neurophysiologic tests used in pain management. Some of these tests (chiefly those used to aid in the diagnosis of disease) need to be conducted by experienced personnel and are usually available only in a hospital setting, not in pain clinics. The most useful tests in the pain clinic are those incorporated in QST.

Because QST is essentially noninvasive and causes little discomfort, it is widely applicable. Although the tests are time consuming, which restricts their clinical use, they are a valid means of assessing treatment efficacy at a time when it is becoming mandatory to monitor treatment effects They are also a useful research tool.

SELECTED READING

1. Eisenach JC, Hood DD, Curry R. Relative potency of epidural to intrathecal clonidine differs between acute thermal pain and capsaicin-induced allodynia. *Pain* 2000;84:57–64.
2. Haanpaa M, Laippala P, Nurmikko T. Pain and somatosensory dysfunction in acute herpes zoster. *Clin J Pain* 1999;15:78–84.
3. Hilz MJ, Stemper B, Axelrod FB, et al. Quantitative thermal perception testing in adults. *J Clin Neurophysiol* 1999;16:462–471.
4. Peripheral Neuropathy Association. Quantitative sensory testing: A consensus report from the Peripheral Neuropathy Association. *Neurology* 1993;43:1050–1052.
5. Quantitative sensory testing in the evaluation of chronic neuropathic pain conditions. *MEDOC Advanced Medical Systems*, vol. 1. 1998.
6. Thimineur M, Sood P, Kravitz E, et al. Central nervous system abnormalities in complex regional pain syndrome (CRPS): Clinical and quantitative evidence of medullary dysfunction. *Clin J Pain* 1998;14: 256–267.
7. Tobin K, Giuliani MJ, Lacomis D. Comparison of different modalities for detection of small fiber neuropathy. *Clin Neurophysiol* 1999;110:1909–1912.
8. Yarnitsky D. Quantitative sensory testing. *Muscle Nerve* 1997;20: 198–204.

Therapeutic Options: Pharmacologic Approaches

Nonsteroidal Anti-inflammatory Drugs

Jane Ballantyne

Take an aspirin and call me in the morning.
—*Twentieth-century physician*

The nonsteroidal anti-inflammatory drugs (NSAIDs), including aspirin, are the most widely used analgesics in the United States and worldwide. Traditionally considered to be weak analgesics, they have achieved popularity as treatment for headaches, menstrual cramps, arthritis, and a wide range of minor aches and pains. Recently, NSAIDs have also become popular for use in the surgical population, especially since the advent of injectable preparations. Because of their predominantly peripheral site of action, they are used in combination with opioids and other centrally acting analgesics, and they are used in combination therapies for severe pain, both acute and chronic. In pain clinics, NSAIDs are often underutilized because of their inadequacy as a sole therapy for severe pain; their potential for providing useful adjunctive analgesia is easily forgotten. This chapter reviews the use of NSAIDs for acute and chronic pain: indications, efficacy, side effects, and contraindications.

I. PHARMACOLOGY

The NSAIDs are a heterogeneous group of compounds consisting of one or more aromatic rings connected to an acidic functional group (Fig. 1). The chemical families of commonly used NSAIDs are outlined in Table 1. The NSAIDs are weak organic acids (pKa 3 to 5.5), act mainly in the periphery, bind extensively to plasma albumin (95% to 99% bound), do not readily cross the blood–brain

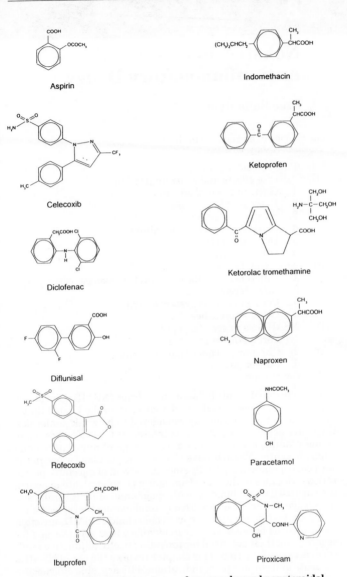

Figure 1.   Chemical structures of commonly used nonsteroidal anti-inflammatory drugs.

**Table 1. Classification of commonly
used antipyretic analgesics**

I. Carboxylic acid and enolic acid groups (pK$_a$ 3–5.5)
  A. Carboxylic acid containing
  salicylates
  *aspirin, diflunisal, salicylic acid, salsalate, sodium salicylate,
    choline magnesium trisalicylate*
  2-propionic acid derivatives
  *naproxen, ibuprofen, ketoprofen, flurbiprofen, fenoprofen,
    carprofen, nabumetone^a*
  indoleacetic acid derivatives
  indomethacin, suldinac
  phenylacetic acid derivatives
  diclofenac, alclofenac, fenclofenac
  pyrroleacetic acid derivatives
  ketorolac, tolmetin
  N-phenylanthranilic acid derivatives
  mefenamic acid
  B. Enolic acid containing
  enolic acid pyrazolone derivatives
  phenylbutazone, aminopyrine, antipyrine, piroxicam
II. Benzenesulfonic acid derivatives
  celecoxib, rofecoxib
III. Phenol group (pK$_a$ 9–10)
  para-amino-phenol derivatives
  paracetamol / acetaminophen, phenacetin

---

^{a}A nonacidic prodrug metabolized to a structural analogue of naproxen, and
thought to be associated with less GI toxicity than the acidic NSAIDs.

barrier, are extensively metabolized by the liver, and have low
renal clearance (<10%).

Acetaminophen is not strictly an anti-inflammatory drug, but it
is included because it shares many of the properties of the NSAIDs.
In contrast to the true NSAIDs, it is nonacidic and a phenol derivative, and it readily crosses the blood–brain barrier. Its action re-
sides mainly in the central nervous system, where prostaglandin
inhibition produces analgesia and antipyresis. Its peripheral and
anti-inflammatory effects are weak.

NSAIDs are powerful inhibitors of prostaglandin synthesis
through their effect on cyclooxygenase (COX) (Fig. 2). Prostaglandins have many effects, and the therapeutic and toxic effects of
NSAIDs can be accounted for by their ability to inhibit prostaglandin and thromboxane synthesis (Table 2). Prostaglandins themselves are not thought to be important pain mediators, but they do
cause hyperalgesia by sensitizing peripheral nociceptors to the
effects of various mediators of pain and inflammation, such as somatostatin, bradykinin, and histamine. Thus, NSAIDs are used
primarily to treat hyperalgesia or secondary pain, particularly pain
resulting from inflammation.

In the last decade, two isoforms of COX have been recognized.
An inducible isoenzyme (COX-2), in addition to the constitutive

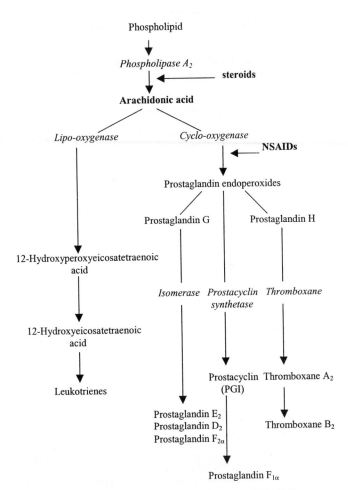

Figure 2.   A schematic diagram showing the metabolism of phospholipids and arachidonic acid. NSAIDs inhibit cyclooxygenase and thereby suppress the synthesis of prostaglandin E, prostacyclin, and thromboxane, altering the balance between these eicosanoids and the leukotrienes.

enzyme (COX-1), has been identified. COX-1 is expressed in most tissues under physiologic conditions, whereas COX-2 is induced by mediators of inflammation under pathologic conditions (Fig. 3). Investigators have studied the relative inhibitory effects of NSAIDs on COX-1 and COX-2 activities. It appears that the risk of certain side effects correlates with the ability of NSAIDs to inhibit COX-1, whereas the anti-inflammatory effects are a result of their ability to inhibit COX-2. Clinical trials and clinical experience to date

Table 2.   Prostaglandin and thromboxane actions

fever vascular smooth muscle relaxation (predominant) (PGI_1, PGE) and contraction (PGF_1, TXA)

increase capillary permeability (LTB)

contract uterine smooth muscle (PGE, PGF_2)

bronchial smooth muscle relaxation (PGE) and contraction (PGF_2, TXA, LTC, LTD)

increase GI contraction and motility (PGE_1, PGI)

protect GI tract by inhibiting gastric acid secretion and enhancing gastric mucus secretion (PGE_1, PGI)

regulate renal blood flow and sodium/potassium exchange (PGE_1, PGI)

markedly potentiate the effects of other mediators of inflammation and pain (serotonin, bradykinin, histamine) (PGE_1, PGI)

sensitize nociceptors (PGE_1, PGI)

inhibit platelet aggregation (PGI)

enhance platelet aggregation (TXA)

constrict vascular smooth muscle (TXA)

Key to abbreviations: PGI = prostacyclin; PGE and PGF = prostaglandin E and F; TXA = thromboxane A; LTB, LTC and LTD = leukotriene B,C and D

have confirmed the efficacy and favorable side-effect profile of these drugs, particularly with regard to their effect on the gastric mucosa.

II. ADVERSE EFFECTS AND CONTRAINDICATIONS

Unfortunately, the NSAIDs are not free of bothersome, and sometimes even dangerous, adverse effects (Table 3). Many patients cannot tolerate these drugs because of their gastrointestinal (GI) effects. Several hundred deaths per year are the result of GI

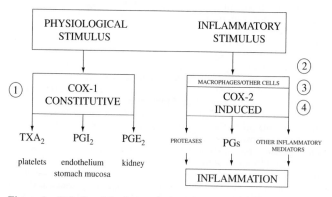

Figure 3.   Relationships between the pathways leading to the generation of prostaglandins, thromboxanes, and other eicosanoids by COX-1 or COX-2.

Table 3. Principal adverse effects of long-term NSAID therapy

dyspepsia, peptic ulcer disease

diarrhea, gastrointestinal hemorrhage

renal dysfunction and failure—acute papillary necrosis, chronic interstitial nephritis, decreased renal blood flow, decreased glomerular filtration rate, salt and water retention

inhibition of platelet aggregation; increased bleeding time

altered liver function tests, jaundice

drug interactions

impaired cartilage repair in osteoarthritis

---

bleeding induced by chronic NSAID use, the elderly being particularly susceptible. After the introduction of the injectable nonsteroidal *ketorolac*, the drug became very popular for postoperative pain. There followed a rash of reported problems with the drug, the most serious of these being catastrophic GI bleeding. It is unclear, as yet, whether these problems were the result of the inappropriately high dose initially recommended by the manufacturers (now reduced by 50%) or the sudden widespread use of a potent NSAID in the vulnerable postoperative patient population.

Yet these events do suggest caution in the use of NSAIDs in postoperative patients, particularly after major surgery. As GI complications are the most troublesome adverse effects, the introduction of a new class of NSAIDs, the selective COX-2 inhibitors, which have been shown to be associated with significantly fewer GI complications, is an exciting advance.

1. Gastrointestinal effects

Prostaglandins inhibit acid secretion by blocking the activation of parietal cells by histamine. At the same time, they are cytoprotective in that they stimulate mucus production from the upper GI tract. By inhibiting prostaglandins, NSAIDs cause gastroduodenal mucosal lesions and ulcers. Gastritis, resulting in abdominal pain, nausea, and vomiting and sometimes diarrhea, is an extremely common side effect of NSAIDs that occurs particularly in persons with a propensity to peptic ulceration; it occasionally results in catastrophic GI bleeding and death. It is accepted practice to withhold NSAIDs from patients with known peptic ulcer disease.

The risk of GI toxicity can be scored using the ARAMIS (American Rheumatism Association Medical Information System) scoring system (Table 4). This system provides a guide for assessing patients' suitability for NSAID treatment, or their suitability for concomitant prophylactic treatment. Prostaglandin analogs such as *misoprostol*, parietal cell inhibitors (acid inhibitors) such as *omeprazole*, and histamine antagonists such as *ranitidine* and *cimetidine* can provide useful prophylaxis against NSAID-induced GI symptoms. The selective COX-2 inhibitors, being associated with less GI toxicity than standard NSAIDs, are a good choice for patients with a history of GI symptoms or sensitivity to NSAIDs. However, they are expensive ($4.80 per day for *celecoxib*, $2.20 per

Table 4.   The ARAMIS model for estimating the risk of gastric ulceration while taking nonselective NSAIDs

Step 1	Start at a score of 0
Step 2	Add 0.3 for every 5 years of patient age over 50
Step 3	Add 1.2 if the patient is receiving a corticosteroid
Step 4	Add 1.4 if the patient has reported a previous NSAID-related GI side effect
Step 5	Add 0.5 if the patient has substantial disability

Note: A score greater than 1.5 is considered a high risk and a contraindication for the use of nonselective NSAIDs at MGH.

The ARAMIS rating system is an evidenced based scale which assesses risk in patient populations. It has been validated prospectively. The scale is for chronic use over a 12 month period.

day for *rofecoxib*, versus $0.24 per day for generic *ibuprofen*), and many payers require that physicians prescribe the much cheaper combination of a standard NSAID with prophylaxis, which is thought to be equally effective in terms of efficacy and freedom from GI toxicity.

2. Decreased hemostasis

The decreased hemostasis associated with NSAIDs is largely the result of platelet dysfunction. Cyclooxygenase inhibition also inhibits the endogenous procoagulant thromboxane. Platelets are especially susceptible to cyclooxygenase inhibition because they have little or no capacity for protein biosynthesis and thus cannot regenerate the enzyme. The literature confirms that bleeding time is consistently prolonged in patients receiving long-term NSAID treatment, but the consensus is that such prolongation is not excessive, and that values remain below the upper limits of normal. However, NSAIDs are usually withheld from patients with a coagulopathy and from patients on anticoagulant therapy. Before surgery, NSAIDs are usually stopped for at least 24 hours, or 10 to 14 days in the case of aspirin, whose platelet effects are not as rapidly reversed as those of other NSAIDs because of irreversible covalent binding to COX. It is still unclear whether the selective COX-2 inhibitors damage platelet function to the same extent, but early studies suggest that they do not.

3. Surgical bleeding

The degree of risk of perioperative bleeding in patients treated with NSAIDs is not very clear. Some studies show increased blood loss in patients treated with NSAIDs, whereas others fail to show this effect. Increased bleeding in NSAID-treated patients undergoing major abdominal surgery, hysterectomy, and tonsillectomy has been reported. Several reports of perioperative bleeding associated with the use of ketorolac have recently appeared. Most commonly, this is GI bleeding, but there are also reports of hematoma formation and hemarthrosis after knee surgery. As mentioned earlier, it is as yet unclear whether the high reported incidence of GI hemorrhage associated with ketorolac is a function of the excessively high doses used before the manufacturers recommended a lower dose or whether this problem will still occur after decreasing the dose.

4. Renal dysfunction and failure

Prostaglandins in the kidney contribute to the maintenance of renal blood flow and glomerular filtration, to the modulation of renin release and tubular ion transport, and to the excretion of water. In normal, sodium-repleted, well-hydrated individuals, the role of prostaglandins in the kidney is less important than it is in patients with abnormal renal function, hypovolemia, or abnormal serum electrolytes, in whom local synthesis of vasodilating prostaglandins is important in maintaining renal homeostasis. In these patients, NSAID administration may decrease the glomerular filtration rate and result in the release of renin from the juxtaglomerular cells, leading to further reduction in renal blood flow and a disturbance of renal function. The most common clinical picture is of a small and rapidly reversible fall in the glomerular filtration rate, which occasionally progresses to acute renal failure. Sodium and water retention, hyperkalemia, hypertension, papillary necrosis, and the nephrotic syndrome are other possible consequences of the renal disturbance.

Although NSAID-induced renal dysfunction is extremely rare in healthy patients, it is a significant risk for patients with renal compromise, this risk increasing with prolonged and excessive NSAID use. The elderly, and patients with chronic renal dysfunction, congestive heart failure, ascites, or hypovolemia, and patients treated with nephrotoxic drugs such as the aminoglycosides and vancomycin, are at particular risk. Early clinical studies suggest that the selective COX-2 inhibitors have renal effects similar to those of nonselective NSAIDs. Thus, this new class of drugs does not appear to spare the kidneys.

Recent opinion, in contrast to the traditional view, suggests that renal effects can occur after only a few days (not weeks) of NSAID treatment. Does this mean that patients undergoing major surgery, who are liable to become hypovolemic during the perioperative period, have an increased risk of renal toxicity from NSAIDs, even with short-term use? Our experience to date with ketorolac is that it appears to be safe to the kidneys in healthy patients, without preoperative renal risk factors, undergoing minimally invasive surgery not associated with significant fluid shifts or major blood loss. It is a sensible precaution, however, to reserve NSAIDs for the postoperative period in patients undergoing major surgery, thus avoiding preoperative or intraoperative administration in those who face the possibility of blood loss, hypotension, and hypovolemia.

5. Drug interactions

NSAIDs are highly bound to albumin in plasma, and adverse drug interactions could potentially occur because of this high degree of binding. However, NSAIDs do not seem to alter the effects of the oral hypoglycemic drugs or warfarin. Warfarin doses may need to be altered because of the platelet effects of NSAIDs, and concomitant use may be contraindicated. Reduced doses of NSAIDs are recommended in severely hypoalbuminemic patients. NSAIDs may also reduce the diuretic and natriuretic effects of furosemide, as well as the antihypertensive effects of the thiazide diuretics, β-adrenergic antagonists, and angiotensin-converting enzyme inhibitors, probably because of inhibition of renal or vascular prostaglandin synthesis.

6. Other adverse effects

Other adverse effects are less common. The incidence of immune-related hypersensitivity is low, the most serious effect being dose-dependent, potentially fatal **hepatic necrosis**. **Asthma** can occur in susceptive individuals, not due to hypersensitivity but rather to blockade of the cyclooxygenase pathway leading to exaggerated leukotriene effects. Some patients display intolerance to NSAIDs in the form of **vasomotor rhinitis**, **angioneurotic edema**, generalized **urticaria**, **asthma**, **laryngeal edema**, **hypotension**, and even **shock**. Despite the resemblance to anaphylaxis, these reactions do not appear to be immunologically based.

Prolonged or excessive use of *acetaminophen* (>10g/day) can cause potentially fatal centrilobular hepatic necrosis. For this reason, acetaminophen (alone or in combination preparations such as *Percocet*), should not be used for prolonged, chronic pain therapy. NSAIDs are known to **impede cartilage repair**, which has become a problem for some patients who have osteoarthritis and take NSAIDs for long periods of time (i.e., years).

NSAIDs **adversely affect osteogenesis** in animals. Although impaired bone remodeling and delayed fracture healing have not been firmly established in humans, many surgeons prefer to avoid the use of NSAIDs in patients who have undergone bone fusion, particularly in the spine. NSAIDs have been associated with **decreased healing of GI anastomoses**, but this association is rare and not confirmed in humans.

By way of summary, contraindications are listed in Table 5.

III. NEW NSAIDs

Over the last few decades, NSAIDs have proved themselves to be highly effective, popular, and useful analgesics, but they are plagued by their side effects. It is not surprising, therefore, that pharmaceutical companies are committing huge resources to the search for NSAID formulations with more favorable side-effect profiles. Several approaches are taken.

Table 5.   Contraindications to NSAID use

---

history of peptic ulcer disease or intolerance to NSAIDs

bleeding, bleeding diatheses or anticoagulant therapy

renal failure, renal dysfunction or risk factors for renal dysfunction
(*i.e. hypovolemia, sodium depletion, congestive heart failure, hepatic cirrhosis, concurrent use of nephrotoxic drugs including aminoglycocides*)

old age, particularly in the presence of any of the above[a]

prophylactic use in major surgery (*i.e. pre- or intra-operative use, particularly if there is a potential for bleeding*)

---

[a] the elderly (>60 years) appear to be especially vulnerable to the effects of prostaglandin inhibition by NSAIDs.

1. Differential inhibition of cyclooxygenase isoenzymes

The most advanced development is that of cyclooxygenase isoenzyme-specific inhibitors. The first of this group of drugs (*celecoxib*) became available in the United States in 1999, and *rofecoxib* is now also available. These two drugs and *meloxicam* have been used in Europe for several years.

In large clinical trials, COX-2 inhibitors have been shown to be at least as effective as existing NSAIDs, with a significantly improved side-effect profile. The improved safety is largely the result of a marked decrease in the incidence and severity of GI complications. COX-2 seems to play an important role in human renal function, and as a group, the selective COX-2 inhibitors do not appear to spare the kidneys when compared with standard NSAIDs. However, there are some differences that may favor the selective COX-2 inhibitors, and studies to date have not fully elucidated the renal effects of these newer NSAIDs. Platelet function does seem to be preserved.

Another notable benefit of these drugs is that they appear to have no effect on cartilaginous repair. They have also been shown to inhibit colorectal tumor cell growth, and early trials indicate that they may prove to be a useful treatment for delaying premature labor.

2. New stereoisomers

Pure enantiomers of 2-propionic acid derivatives have recently been isolated, allowing study of their individual properties. It is already clear that the R- and S-enantiomers act differently, both in the periphery and in the central nervous system, and that it may be possible to develop clinically useful analgesics, free from significant peripheral prostaglandin inhibition and thus free from GI and renal toxicity.

3. Central nervous system activity

Although acid NSAIDs do not readily cross the blood–brain barrier, and a large proportion of the NSAID effect is in the periphery, a central contribution to NSAID effects appears established. Several mechanisms for this effect have been proposed, including prostaglandin inhibition in neural tissue, inhibition of nitric oxide systems via inhibition of N-methyl-D-aspartate (NMDA) and substance P systems, interaction with G proteins, modulation of neurotransmitter release, and amelioration of glutamate receptor–directed gene expression. This is an exciting area that could lead to the development of NSAIDs with a more useful central nervous system effect, for administration either neuraxially or systemically.

4. Other approaches

Other strategies under study include coupling NSAIDs to nitric oxide–releasing compounds, preassociation of NSAIDs with zwitterionic phospholipids to prevent NSAID–mucosal interactions, and concomitant administration of trefoil peptides to stimulate mucosal defense pathways. The clinical feasibility of these strategies remains to be determined.

IV. NSAID USE IN SPECIFIC POPULATIONS

Physicians commonly prescribe NSAIDs for acute and chronic pain, particularly for pain resulting from surgery and trauma and pain caused by joint disease. Commonly used NSAIDs and their dosages are presented in Appendix VIII. They are also available over the counter and are widely used as household analgesics. Thus, not only are physicians responsible for appropriate prescribing of NSAIDs, they also need to advise patients about the safe and appropriate use of over-the-counter preparations. These factors are will be discussed further.

1. Perioperative patients

(i) *Domestic use—cautions*

NSAIDs are the most ubiquitous of drugs. Most are available without prescription. They are widely used for minor aches and pains, for headaches, for menstrual cramps, and for the chronic arthritides. Patients should be advised to stop taking NSAIDs before surgery, chiefly because of their platelet effects and their propensity to increase surgical bleeding. Aspirin, whose platelet effects are not reversible, should be stopped for 10 to 14 days before elective surgery. Other NSAIDs have rapidly reversible platelet effects, and 24 hours cessation is probably sufficient, although a 2- to 3-day cessation is usually advised. Acetaminophen, which has only mild peripheral effects and does not affect platelets, can be substituted. Spinal and epidural instrumentation and catheter placement appear to be safe even if aspirin and other NSAIDs are not discontinued.

(ii) *Postoperative and acute pain*

NSAIDs are extremely useful, and often underutilized, for acute and postoperative pain. Broadly, there are two indications in this population: (a) as a sole analgesic for mild pain, and (b) as an adjunct to other analgesics in severe pain.

a) *Mild Pain*

The efficacy of NSAIDs for mild acute pain is well established by countless randomized controlled trials. However, until recently, their widespread applicability for postoperative pain was limited because of the lack of availability of parenteral formulations and the limitations this placed on the use of NSAIDs in patients who cannot take oral medications. Prompted by the availability of rectal and parenteral preparations, the value of NSAID treatment in postoperative patients has now been realized, and both enteral and parenteral preparations are being used preoperatively, intraoperatively, and postoperatively, providing useful postoperative analgesia.

The use of NSAIDs allows for complete avoidance, or minimal use, of opioids during and after minor surgery, thus avoiding the opioid-induced side effects (nausea and somnolence) that commonly delay recovery and discharge. NSAID side effects are rare in the relatively healthy day surgery population, and with short-term use. NSAIDs (unless contraindicated) are arguably the treatment of choice for pain after minor surgery, and late in the postoperative course after major surgery.

Acetaminophen is a popular choice, particularly in infants, as it avoids GI irritation. Combinations of opioid and acetaminophen are also widely prescribed for mild to moderate acute and postoperative pain.

b) *Adjunct use and opioid sparing*

For more severe acute pain, NSAIDs alone may be ineffective, but in conjunction with other modes of pain treatment they have an important role. Opioids will probably always hold a place in the management of acute somatic pain because they are highly effective, and they are the only analgesics that have no ceiling effect. However, their side effects, particularly respiratory depression, severely limit their use. There are many ways to reduce opioid requirement, including the use of local nerve blocks, the use of epidural and intrathecal anesthesia and analgesia, and the use of nonopioid analgesics, including NSAIDs. A multimodal approach, using a combination of appropriate pain treatments, appears to be the best way to achieve synergy between different modes of treatment and to reduce the side effects of each.

Multiple controlled trials confirm the opioid-sparing effects of NSAID usage in postoperative pain. Whether this reduction in opioid consumption can be translated into a significant difference in the incidence of opioid-associated side effects or in improved overall outcome is less clear. Certainly there are groups of patients in whom opioid treatment and opioid side effects are particularly undesirable, including the very young, those with pre-existing ventilatory compromise, and those with a strong history of opioid-induced side effects. These patients are not widely studied in trials, yet they are the patients for whom NSAIDs may be particularly advantageous.

The adjunctive use of NSAIDs is also useful in patients receiving epidural treatment for postoperative pain. Trials of NSAIDs for this indication have yet to appear in the literature in great numbers, but in practice, the addition of an NSAID to epidural opioid therapy often makes the difference between adequate and inadequate pain control.

c) *Adverse effects*

The adverse effects of NSAIDs in surgical patients are summarized in Table 6.

d) *Timing of administration*

There is no consensus regarding timing of NSAID doses in patients undergoing surgery, even though speed of onset influences the usefulness of the drugs. In studies that specifically examine the issue of timing of doses and effects, the benefit of NSAIDs was not seen until 4 hours or more after the parenteral administration of an NSAID (ketorolac or other), and effectiveness continued to improve even after administration. Is it advisable, then, to start NSAID treatment preoperatively?

Pretreatment demonstrated superior efficacy when it was assessed in dental patients. However, in a large meta-analysis of the general surgical population, no measurable difference was found between the same dose given preoperatively and given postoperatively. Moreover, as discussed, NSAID pretreatment may be ill ad-

Table 6. Adverse effects of NSAIDs in surgical patients

gastrointestinal hemorrhage
  (occasionally catastrophic)

renal dysfunction or failure

decreased hemostasis and hematoma formation

asthma in susceptible individuals
  *(due to blockade of the cyclo-oxygenase pathway, leading to
  exaggerated effects of the metabolites of the lipo-oxygenase pathway (i.e. leukotrienes)*

anaphylaxis
  *(risk of immune-related anaphylactoid reactions is small,
  although some individuals suffer anaphylaxis-like symptoms
  that are unrelated to an immune process)*

decreased healing of gastrointestinal anastomoses

delayed fracture healing
  (not established in humans, but demonstrated in animals)

vised before major surgery because of the risks of hypovolemia, hypotension, bleeding, and renal compromise. The question of when to treat is a complex one that needs to be addressed by research into the clinical benefit versus cost benefit of pretreatment with NSAIDs. Currently, it is probably better to offer preoperative oral NSAIDs to patients undergoing minor surgery, and to reserve injectable NSAIDs for the end of surgery or for postoperative use.

e) *Ketorolac*

Ketorolac was introduced in the United States in 1990, and it was the first NSAID to have approval from the U.S. Food and Drug Administration for parenteral use in postoperative patients. Ketorolac differs from other NSAIDs in two respects: not only is it injectable, it is also highly efficacious, with efficacy close to that of morphine. For these reasons, it has been widely adopted for use in acute and postoperative pain.

Unfortunately, ketorolac also has side effects, and there are many reported cases of problems associated with its use, possibly caused by inappropriately high doses or by failure to recognize contraindications. The most common and serious side effects have been GI bleeding, other bleeding problems, and reversible renal dysfunction.

Ketorolac has been found to be as effective as morphine and other opioids for surgery ranging from simple outpatient procedures to major operations. At the same time, investigators have demonstrated the efficacy of other NSAIDs, traditionally considered weak analgesics, to be equal to that of ketorolac for mild pain. Were it not that ketorolac is markedly more expensive than other NSAIDs ($6.50 versus a few cents per dose) and suitable only for short-term use, the efficacy of ketorolac might dictate that it be the NSAID of choice for postoperative pain in most situations. However, cost and side effects limit it's usefulness. Whenever oral dosing is possible, other NSAIDs, not ketorolac, should be considered the first-line NSAID treatment for mild to moderate pain. For more severe pain, other NSAIDs may be inadequate and unhelpful, and then ketorolac contributes significantly to the attenuation of pain.

2. Chronic noncancer pain patients

By far the most common indication for NSAIDs, and the biggest market for drug companies, is **joint pain**. Other indications for NSAID use in patients with chronic noncancer pain are **myalgias**, **headache**, and **mild to moderate pain of any etiology**.

(i) *Joint pain*

The NSAIDs are the first-line pharmacologic treatment for inflammatory joint diseases, including osteoarthritis, rheumatoid arthritis, ankylosing spondylitis, and scleroderma. They are used to treat both pain and inflammation in these diseases. So effective are they at improving the quality of life for these patients that the significant risk of GI toxicity is accepted, despite the occurrence of several deaths per year from catastrophic GI bleeding in this population. As discussed, the race is on to develop effective antiinflammatory analgesics that are free from GI toxicity. The new selective COX-2 inhibitors hold the greatest hope for these patients at present, and they are rapidly gaining popularity. The treatment of large-joint pain is largely the province of rheumatologists and primary physicians, and these patients rarely present to pain clinics unless they have intractable back or neck pain.

(ii) *Other indications*

NSAIDs are useful therapy for **myalgias**, including **fibromyalgia**, and for other muscle pains that may occur in conjunction with joint pain, particularly back pain. In noncancer patients, perhaps the most common indication for NSAIDs in pain clinics is **headache**. Acetaminophen and NSAIDs are useful first-line treatments for both migraine and tension headaches. If nausea is a prominent feature of a patient's headaches, an antiemetic can be added, or the gastric route can be avoided by using a rectal or parenteral preparation. Intramuscular ketorolac is useful in some patients. Even if therapy with an NSAID alone is not sufficient for headaches, its combination with other treatments such as vasoconstrictors (caffeine, ergotamine, sumatriptan) is often useful. In addition, NSAIDs can be tried as a first line treatment for any **mild to moderate pain**.

The choice of NSAID for any indication is largely a matter of trial and error. The older, cheaper NSAIDs (aspirin, *indomethacin*, and *phenylbutazone*) are often poorly tolerated because of their GI effects. They also need frequent doses. Aspirin is the oldest and cheapest of the NSAIDs, and it maintains its place as a useful analgesic despite its side-effect profile. Several formulations (e.g., buffered and enteric coated) are available that are less toxic to the GI tract. Ibuprofen, the most popular of the newer NSAIDs, is less toxic than the older drugs but still needs 4- to 6-hour dosing to maintain therapeutic levels. *Naproxen* and *diflunisal* are widely used for chronic pain because they are long acting and need only twice-daily dosing. *Nabumetone* (a nonacidic prodrug metabolized to a structural analog of naproxen) is minimally toxic to the GI tract and has been the treatment of choice when GI side effects are a problem. The COX-2 inhibitors (celecoxib and rofecoxib) are also minimally toxic to the GI tract. The COX-2 inhibitors may become the NSAIDs of choice if they hold to their promise of being effective and having a superior side-effect profile. Despite these logical considerations, it is often necessary to try out different NSAIDs before finding the best drug for an individual patient.

3. Cancer patients

In cancer pain patients, acetaminophen and NSAIDs are used as a first-line therapy for mild to moderate pain, in combination with opioids for more severe pain, and especially for bone and inflammatory pain in advanced cancer.

(i) *The World Health Organization guidelines*

In 1986, the World Health Organization (WHO) released a set of guidelines called Cancer Pain Relief. The central component is the "three-step analgesic ladder" (see Chapter 32, figure 1), which became the guiding principal for cancer pain treatment in many parts of the world. The three-step analgesic ladder recommends initial treatment with nonopioid analgesics, alone or with adjuvants (e.g., anticonvulsants, antidepressants); advancing to mild opioids, alone or in combination with nonopioid analgesics and adjuvants; and finally to potent opioids, alone or in combination. Although new drugs and techniques have in some measure altered the way we might wish to treat cancer pain, the basic principles in the WHO guideline are still sound for cancer pain treatment.

Since the advent of more potent NSAIDs, the question arises whether the second step in the ladder (the use of opioid with or without nonopioid analgesic, with or without adjuvant) should be abandoned in favor of simply continuing the first step (the use of nonopioid analgesics with or without adjuvant) for mild to moderate pain. However, there is still a safety issue, and at present, opioid plus nonopioid combinations maintain their place for mild to moderate cancer pain, because these combinations exhibit synergy and have the ability to reduce the side effects of each drug. The advent of an even more potent and safer NSAID may well change the way we treat moderately severe, or even severe, cancer pain.

(ii) *The role of NSAIDs in advanced cancer*

In advanced cancer, NSAIDs are particularly useful for **bone pain** (caused by distention of the periosteum by metastases), for **soft tissue pain** (caused by compression or distention of tissues), and for **visceral pain** (caused by irritation of the pleura or peritoneum). Of particular concern in these patients is the platelet effect of NSAIDs and the risk of inducing bleeding. Many of these patients suffer general debilitation, with resultant effects on protein synthesis, including the synthesis of clotting factors. They commonly have thrombocytopenia or pancytopenia as a result of the underlying malignancy or prior therapy.

The nonacetylated salicylates (*salsalate, sodium salicylate, choline magnesium trisalicylate*) are often substituted for other NSAIDs in patients at risk, because they do not profoundly affect platelet aggregation and do not alter bleeding time. Whether the selective COX-2 inhibitors will prove to be safe in cancer patients with a bleeding risk is as yet unclear.

V. CONCLUSION

NSAIDs are useful analgesics with a predominantly peripheral action that can provide sole treatment for mild pain, or that can complement the central effects of opioids and neuraxial analgesics for more severe pain. Were it not for their side effects, which are occasionally catastrophic, NSAIDs would be more widely used. Several developments in NSAID pharmacology are leading toward the introduction of more efficacious and safer drugs that will undoubtedly influence pain treatment for both acute and chronic pain.

SELECTED READING

1. Kenny GNC. Potential renal, haematological and allergic adverse effects associated with nonsteroidal anti-inflammatory drugs. *Drugs* 1992;44(suppl 5):31–37.
2. Laneuville O, Breuer DK, Dewitt DL, et al. Differential inhibition of human prostaglandin endoperoxide H synthases-1 and -2 by nonsteroidal anti-inflammatory drugs. *J Pharmacol Exp Ther* 1994; 271:927–934.
3. Mather LE. Do the pharmacodynamics of the nonsteroidal anti-inflammatory drugs suggest a role in the management of postoperative pain? *Drugs* 1992;44(suppl 5):1–13.
4. McCormack K. The spinal actions of NSAIDs and the dissociation between anti-inflammatory and analgesic effects. *Drugs* 1994;47: 28–45.
5. Moote C. Efficacy of nonsteroidal anti-inflammatory drugs in the management of postoperative pain. *Drugs* 1992;44(suppl 5):14–30.
6. Souter AJ, Fredman B, White PF. Controversies in the perioperative use of nonsteroidal antiinflammatory drugs. *Anesth Analg* 1994; 79:1178–1190.
7. Vane JR, Botting RM. Mechanism of action of aspirin-like drugs. *Semin Arthritis Rheum* 1997;26(suppl 1):2–10.
8. Wolfe MM. Future trends in the development of safer nonsteroidal anti-inflammatory drugs. *Am J Med* 1998;105:44S–52S.

Opioids

Jeffrey Uppington

Among the remedies which it has pleased Almighty God to give to man to relieve his sufferings, none is so universal and so efficacious as opium.
—*Thomas Sydenham, 1624–1689*

Opioids are the core pharmacologic treatment for pain. They are the mainstay for the treatment of both acute and cancer pain, and although controversy still exists over their use in chronic non-malignant pain, they are increasingly used for this indication also. They are the only pain medications that have no ceiling effect, and are therefore the only systemic treatment for severe accelerating pain. Any person treating pain should understand the effects and proper usage of these important drugs.

I. TERMINOLOGY

Opiates are drugs derived from opium, which is obtained from the juice of the poppy *Papaver somniferum*. They include morphine, codeine, and various semisynthetic congeners derived from them and another component of opium, thebaine. The term *opioid* applies to substances with morphine-like activity, including agonists and antagonists as well as naturally occurring and synthetic opioid peptides. *Endorphin* is a generic term applying to the endogenous opioid peptides. There are three families of endogenous opioids—the endorphins, the enkephalins, and the dynorphins. The word *narcotic*, derived from the Greek word for stupor, originally referred to any drug that induced sleep, but it later became associated with the strong opiate analgesics. The term is no longer useful pharmacologically as it is being increasingly used in the legal and regulatory context to refer to a wide variety of abused substances.

II. ENDOGENOUS OPIOIDS

Each of the three families of opioid neuropeptides (endorphins, enkephalins, and dynorphins) is derived from a distinct precursor polypeptide and has a distinct anatomic distribution. Like peptide hormones, endogenous opioids have biologically inactive precursors that generate active agents only after enzymatic cleavage. The precursor for beta-endorphin, pro-opiomelanocortin, also contains peptide sequences for adrenocorticotropin (ACTH) and melanocyte-stimulating hormone (MSH), illustrating the close relationship between endogenous opioids and hormone systems.

III. CLASSIFICATION OF OPIOIDS

Opioids can be classified as naturally occurring, semisynthetic, and synthetic (Table 1). Morphine, codeine, papaverine, and thebaine are naturally occurring. The semisynthetic drugs are derived from morphine, codeine, and thebaine. The synthetic drugs structurally resemble morphine but do not occur in nature. They are produced by gradually reducing the number of rings from the five-ring structure of morphine, through the four-ring morphinans and

Table 1.   Classification of opioids

Naturally occurring
   Morphine
   Papaverine
   Codeine
   Thebaine

Semisynthetic
   Heroin
   Hydromorphone
   Hydrocodone
   Buprenorphine
   Oxycodone

Synthetic
   Morphinan series (levorphanol, butorphanol)
   Diphenylpropylamine series (methadone)
   Benzomorphinan series (pentazocine)
   Phenylpiperidine series (meperidine, fentanyl, sufentanil, alfentanil)

the three-ring benzomorphinans, to the two-ring phenylpiperidines (Fig. 1).

There are alternative classifications of opioids. The drugs may be grouped according to the specific receptors they act on (see later). Another useful distinction is whether they are agonists, antagonists, or some combination of the two (Table 2).

IV. OPIOID RECEPTORS

Opioids act via specific receptors on cell membranes. Specific opioid receptors have been proposed on the basis of a mixture of clinical and laboratory observations. The structure of opioid receptors is currently understood at cellular, molecular, and genetic levels, although the existence of some receptor types proposed on clinical grounds has not yet been confirmed in the laboratory. There are five proposed classes of opioid receptor: mu, delta, kappa, sigma, and epsilon.

1. Mu receptors

It seems likely that morphine and morphine-like drugs produce analgesia primarily through interaction with mu receptors. These receptors are present in large quantities in the periaqueductal gray matter (brain) and the substantia gelatinosa (spinal cord). Activation of mu receptors results in analgesia, euphoria, respiratory depression, nausea and vomiting, decreased gastrointestinal (GI) motility, tolerance, and dependence. Using selective antagonists, two distinct subgroups of the mu receptor have been identified: mu_1, found supraspinally, and mu_2, found in the spine. Both respiratory depression and constipation (reduced GI motility) are thought to be mediated through mu_2 receptors. The concept of a selective mu_1 agonist, which could theoretically produce analgesia without respiratory depression, is intriguing but unrealized. Beta-endorphin has a high affinity for mu receptors, as do the enkephalins. Dynorphin also binds to the mu receptor, but not as avidly as it does to the $kappa_1$ receptor.

2. Kappa receptors

Activation of these receptors also causes analgesia, but it causes less respiratory depression than activation of mu receptors. Kappa-

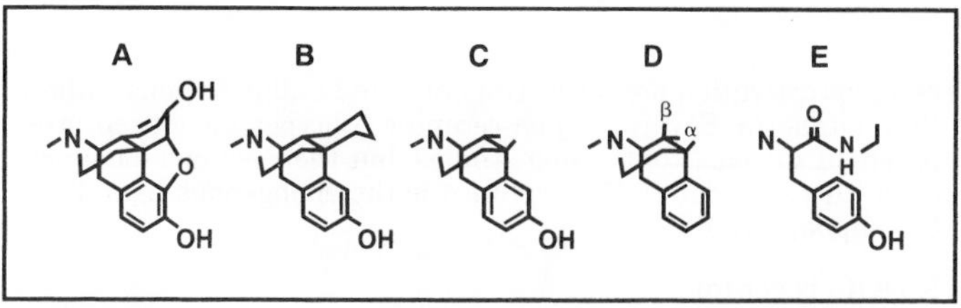

Figure 1.   Structure of morphine-like opioids. A: Morphine.
B: Morphinan. C: Benzomorphan. D: Phenylpiperidine.
E: Tyramine moiety of endogenous opioids. Note the progressive removal of ring structures from five-ring morphine to two-ring phenylpiperidine. (Reproduced with permission from Carr DB. Opioids. *Int Anesthesiol Clin* 1988;26:273.)

Table 2.   Alternative classification of opioids

Class	Definition	Example
Agonist	A drug that, when bound to the receptor, stimulates the receptor to the maximum level; by definition, the intrinsic activity of a full agonist is unity.	Morphine
Antagonist	A drug that, when bound to the receptor, fails completely to produce any stimulation of that receptor; by definition, the intrinsic activity of a pure antagonist is zero.	Naloxone
Partial agonist	A drug that, when bound to the receptor, stimulates the receptor to a level below the maximum level; by definition, the intrinsic activity of a partial agonist lies between zero and unity.	Buprenorphine (partial mu agonist)
Mixed agonist–antagonist	A drug that acts simultaneously on different subtypes, with the potential for agonist action on one or more subtypes and antagonist action on one or more subtypes.	Nalbuphine (partial mu agonist, kappa agonist, delta antagonist)

From Melzack, Wall 1994.

receptor activation produces dysphoria and hallucinations rather than euphoria. Several kappa-receptor subtypes have been proposed on the basis of binding studies, but their actions have not been fully elucidated. Dynorphin A is the endogenous ligand for the kappa$_1$ receptor.

3. Delta receptors

Using selective agonists and antagonists, studies have established delta-receptor analgesia both spinally and supraspinally, although the spinal system appears more robust. Delta$_1$- and delta$_2$-receptors have been proposed on the basis of differential sensitivity to several antagonists. The enkephalins are the endogenous ligands for the delta-receptors.

4. Sigma receptors

The sigma receptor may not be a true opioid receptor, as its actions are not antagonized by naloxone. There is some evidence that it may be the receptor for phencyclidine ("angel dust"). Although the psychotomimetic effects of drugs such as pentazocine were initially attributed to sigma receptors, the status of these sites is presently uncertain.

5. Epsilon receptor

This has been postulated as the specific receptor for beta-endorphin, although beta-endorphin is known to act at both mu and delta receptors.

6. Cloned receptors

The mu, delta, and kappa receptors have been cloned and their genes identified. They are the only opioid receptors that have been cloned, despite an intensive search for genes corresponding to opioid-receptor subtypes. The cloned opioid receptors have characteristics of typical G-protein-coupled receptors. There are seven hydrophobic regions that span the cell membrane, with three extracellular and three intracellular loops. There are an intracellular carboxy-terminal tail and an extracellular amino-terminal tail. The amino acid sequences of the different opioid receptors are approximately 65% identical to each other. The regions of highest similarity are the sequences predicted to lie in the seven transmembrane-spanning regions and intracellular loops. The extracellular regions that differ in amino acid sequence may contain the unique ligand-binding domains for each receptor (Fig. 2).

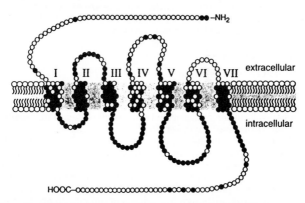

Figure 2. Amino acid sequence identity among the three cloned opioid receptors. Comparison of the amino acid sequences of the cloned mouse δ and κ receptors and the rat p receptor reveals that approximately 65% of the residues are either identical or similar. Amino acid residues that are identical or similar among the receptors are in *black*, and those that are not similar are in *open circles*. Note that the intracellular loops and transmembrane-spanning regions I, II, III, V, and VII are very similar in amino acid sequence. In contrast, the amino and carboxy termini are very different, as are extracellular loops two and three and transmembrane-spanning region IV. From Goodman and Gilman. The Pharmacological Basis of Therapeutics, 9th ed. 1996.

7. Receptor mechanisms

Opioid receptors are coupled to G proteins and are thus able to affect protein phosphorylation via second messenger systems, thereby altering ion channel conductance. Opioids act both pre- and postsynaptically. Presynaptically, they inhibit the release of neurotransmitters, including substance P and glutamate. Postsynaptically, they can inhibit neurons by opening potassium channels that hyperpolarize the cell. There is evidence that opioids produce both short- and long-term effects on neural function, and they may play a distinct role during early embryonic development.

Administration of opioids significantly reduces the facilitation of nociceptive processing (e.g., "windup"). Opioids (including endogenous opioids) can also affect opioid gene regulation, with possible short- and long-term effects and local as well as distal effects.

8. Alternative opioid mechanisms

Not all nociceptive mechanisms are mediated by opiate receptors. It is known that N-methyl-D-aspartate (NMDA)-sensitive glutamate receptors are involved in nociceptive transmission in the spinal dorsal horn. Norepinephrine, serotonin, and sodium channels are also involved, and it is possible that a central nitric oxide–cyclic guanosine monophosphate signaling pathway may help mediate nociception.

It appears that some opioid actions are not mediated by opioid receptors. This observation is potentially important for understanding pain and analgesic mechanisms. Thus, methadone, meperidine, and tramadol inhibit serotonin and norepinephrine reuptake. Methadone, meperidine, and other opioids are antagonists of the NMDA amino acid excitatory pathway. Meperidine blocks sodium channels and has local anesthetic properties.

V. OPIOID EFFECTS

1. Central nervous system

(i) *Analgesia, mood, and consciousness*

Opioids selectively relieve pain without affecting other sensory modalities. Pain can be described as a specific sensation (burning, shooting, throbbing), or in terms of suffering (excruciating, miserable). Opioids alter the sensation of pain as well as the affective response. Patients often say that their pain is still present but that they feel more comfortable. Occasionally, patients experience euphoria or dysphoria, more so when these drugs are used for recreational purposes. Useful analgesia occurs without loss of consciousness, although high doses of opioids do produce unconsciousness, and drowsiness is a common side effect.

(ii) *Respiratory depression*

Opioids of the morphine type depress respiration by acting directly on the respiratory centers in the brainstem. Equianalgesic doses of morphine-like opioids have the same degree of respiratory depression as morphine itself. The effect is chiefly via mu receptors (probably the mu_2 subpopulation). Partial agonists and agonist–antagonist opioids are less likely to cause severe respiratory depression, as are the selective kappa agonists.

Therapeutic doses of morphine depress all phases of respiration, respiratory rate, and minute volume. At the same time, the responsiveness to carbon dioxide (CO_2) is decreased and thus the CO_2 response curve is shifted upward and to the right. The degree of respiratory depression is dependent on opioid dose and other factors, and apnea is a true risk. Pain and stimulation counteract respiratory depression, whereas sedative drugs such as the benzodiazepines potentiate the respiratory depression. Natural sleep also reduces CO_2 responsiveness and is additive to the opioid effect. Unexpected respiratory depression may occur in relation to variations in serum concentration, concomitant drug use, and varying degrees of pain and stimulation. Naloxone effectively reverses the respiratory depression.

(iii) *Nausea and vomiting*

Nausea and vomiting from opioids is the result of the direct stimulation of the chemoreceptor trigger zone (CRTZ). The CRTZ is situated in the area postrema in the floor of the fourth medulla. There is also an associated increase in vestibular sensitivity, so that opioid-induced nausea tends to be exacerbated by movement. Treatment includes opioid dosage reduction, antidopaminergics [e.g., droperidol, prochlorperazine edisylate (Compazine), metoclopramide], anticholinergics (e.g., scopolamine), or serotonin antagonists (e.g., ondansetron).

(iv) *Cough*

Opioids depress the cough center in the medulla. There is no obligatory relationship between cough suppression and respiratory depression, and effective antitussive agents are available that do not depress respiration in clinical doses, such as dextromethorphan. The antitussive receptors are less sensitive to naloxone than receptors involved in analgesia.

(v) *Miosis*

Mu and kappa agonists constrict the pupil by an excitation of the Edinger-Westphal nucleus (parasympathetic) of the oculomotor nerve. Tolerance to the miotic effects occurs with long-term opioid use, but addicts with high circulating blood concentrations exhibit small pupils. The pupillary effects of opioids are altered by concomitant use of other drugs including general anesthetics. Morphine reduces intraocular pressure.

(vi) *Convulsions*

In animals, high doses of morphine and related opioids cause convulsions. The drugs stimulate hippocampal pyramidal cells, probably by inhibiting release of gamma-aminobutyric acid (GABA) at the synaptic level. Selective delta-agonists may do the same. In humans, convulsions are rarely seen because seizure-producing doses are extremely high and not administered. However, meperidine is particularly prone to produce seizure activity through its metabolite normeperidine, accumulation of which is most likely to occur in patients with renal dysfunction and in the elderly. Meperidine-induced seizures are relatively common, and for that reason the use of meperidine is discouraged, particularly in susceptible patients, for chronic pain. Naloxone can be used to treat seizures, but it is more effective at treating convulsions caused by morphine and related drugs than by meperidine.

(vii) *Hypothalamic effects*

Opioids can cause decreases in body temperature. The chief mechanism is alteration of the equilibrium point of the hypothalamic heat-regulating mechanism, although opioid-induced vasodilation may worsen the effect. Although shivering is not observed consistently after opioid anesthesia, it does occur frequently after inhalation anesthesia. Small doses of opioid (particularly meperidine) can attenuate or abolish the shivering through a mechanism that is poorly understood.

2. Neuroendocrine effects

Opioids have a number of neuroendocrine effects. High-dose opioid therapy reduces stress hormone release (glucocorticoids and catecholamines). It is not at all clear to what extent and under what conditions this is a desirable effect. Evidence is emerging that high-dose opioids may also suppress immune responses, which clearly is not a desirable effect. Opioids suppress hypothalamic releasing factors, thus suppressing the release of luteinizing hormone (LH), follicle-stimulating hormone (FSH), adrenocorticotropin (ACTH), and beta-endorphin. Cortisol and testosterone levels are thereby reduced. In women, the menstrual cycle may be disrupted, and testosterone levels may be reduced in men. Some opioids also reduce growth hormone production. During chronic opioid administration, tolerance to these effects develops. Thus heroin addicts maintained on methadone normalize their disrupted menstrual cycles (women), and plasma concentrations of LH and testosterone (men) return to normal.

3. Gastrointestinal system

Stomach

Gastric motility is decreased, prolonging gastric emptying and increasing the risk of esophageal reflux. The passage of gastric contents through the duodenum is usually delayed. Mu agonists usually decrease gastric acid secretion, but stimulation can occur. Indirect effects, such as increased secretion of pancreatic somatostatin, predominate.

Small intestine

Biliary, pancreatic, and intestinal secretions are diminished, and the digestion of food is delayed. The duodenum is affected more than the ilium. Water is absorbed more completely and the viscosity of bowel contents increase.

Large intestine

Peristaltic propulsive waves are decreased or abolished in the colon. Bowel tone increases. Water is absorbed, which desiccates the feces and slows their passage. In postoperative patients, prolonged ileus is a problem. In patients taking chronic opioids, constipation is common and these patients should take stimulant laxatives.

Biliary tract

The sphincter of Oddi constricts, and bile duct pressure may increase. Despite this, little clinical effect is seen. Naloxone reverses the effects, as does glucagon. Atropine and nitroglycerine only partially reverse the effects. Morphine and morphine-like drugs are thought to have a worse effect than meperidine and its derivatives, but the validity of this finding is in doubt.

4. Cardiovascular system

Opioids exhibit a number of actions on the cardiovascular system. Histamine release and peripheral vasodilation accompany morphine use and that of some other opioids. High doses of any opioid will reduce sympathetic output and thus allow a greater preponderance of parasympathetic effects. The pulse rate may be slowed by stimulation of the vagal center, especially with high doses. There is little direct effect on the myocardium, but the peripheral effects may reduce myocardial oxygen consumption, left ventricular end diastolic pressure, and cardiac work. High doses, low blood volume, and combination with other drugs such as phenothiazines accentuate the hypotensive effects.

5. Tolerance, dependence, and addiction

These phenomena are discussed in detail in Chapters 30 and 35, but as it is important to understand these phenomena when prescribing opioids, a brief overview is included here. Whereas tolerance and dependence are likely (almost inevitable) consequences of chronic opioid use, addiction is a behavioral problem that arises only in certain individuals. Tolerance is the need for increasing doses to achieve the same analgesic effect, and it is a form of tachyphylaxis. Tolerance to side effects also occurs. Changing from one opioid to another is often effective in reducing tolerance because of incomplete cross-tolerance between opioids (see Chapter 32).

Dependence, or physical dependence, arises when continuous exposure to a drug is necessary to avoid withdrawal symptoms. Slow weaning of opiate drugs usually prevents a withdrawal syndrome from appearing.

Addiction implies socially destructive drug-seeking behavior, and it arises in certain individuals who are predisposed to it. Addiction rarely occurs in patients treated with opioids for acute or cancer pain, but the risk of addiction should always be considered when prescribing opioids for chronic nonmalignant pain (see Chapter 30).

In the treatment of acute and cancer pain, it is often necessary to reassure patients that the risk of their developing addiction is extremely low, and that tolerance and dependence are not addiction.

6. Other effects

(i) *Chest wall rigidity*

Rapid infusion of a large bolus injection of potent opioids can induce increased muscle tone, mainly of the chest wall and abdomen. The opioids most associated with this phenomenon are fentanyl, sufentanil, and alfentanil. The mechanism of the muscle rigidity is not clear, but it is resolved with muscle relaxants or opioid antagonists.

(ii) *Ureter and bladder*

The ureteral tone and amplitude of contraction may increase with therapeutic doses of opioids. The urinary voiding reflex is inhibited, and external sphincter tone and bladder volume increase. Urinary retention may result. Tolerance to these effects usually occurs over time.

(iii) *Skin*

Therapeutic doses of morphine can produce dilation of the cutaneous blood vessels. Histamine release is the likely cause. Histamine release also probably accounts for the local urticaria sometimes seen after injection. Pruritus may occur, particularly after neuraxial administration of opioids. Naloxone does not abolish the histamine effects, but it does reverse itching. Antihistamines are also effective for opioid-induced itching, even if the presumed mechanism of effect is central (as in neuraxial administration).

VI. PRECAUTIONS

Hepatic and renal diseases

In hepatic and renal disease processes, because of decreased metabolism and elimination of opioids, some concerns arise:

- Active metabolites of morphine and codeine, especially morphine-6-glucuronide, may accumulate.
- Meperidine administration can lead to accumulation of normeperidine, causing CNS excitation with tremors or seizures.
- Repeated doses of propoxyphene may cause naloxone insensitive cardiac toxicity secondary to its metabolite norpropoxyphene.

Respiratory disease

Caution is advisable when using opioids whenever respiratory reserve is diminished (e.g., emphysema, kyphoscoliosis, severe obesity). Opioids that release histamine may precipitate bronchospasm, especially in asthmatics. Depression of the cough reflex may be deleterious in patients with copious secretions (e.g., those with pneumonia, bronchiectasis, prior thoracotomy).

Head injury

An increase in PCO_2 from respiratory depression can lead to elevated intracerebral pressure. Meiosis, vomiting, and mental clouding, which are important clinical signs in the evaluation of head injury, may be obscured.

Allergic reactions

True allergies to opioid medications are rare but do occur. More commonly, patients mistakenly believe they are allergic because they have suffered a side effect. Wheals at the injection site are from histamine release.

Drug interactions

Opioid effects may be potentiated by concomitant drug use, and these effects are not unusual. In particular, the sedative and respiratory depressant effects of opioids may be exaggerated by concomitant administration of drugs with sedative properties (e.g., antihistamines, anxiolytics, antiemetics). On the other hand, opioid sedative and respiratory depressant effects may be offset by stimulants (e.g., amphetamines, analeptics). The only specific dangerous interaction is that between meperidine and the monoamine oxidase inhibitors (MAOIs). This results in a potentially fatal excitatory reaction with delirium, hyperpyrexia, and convulsions, and it is caused by central serotonergic overactivity secondary to blockage of neuronal uptake of serotonin by meperidine.

VII. ROUTES OF ADMINISTRATION

Opioids may be administered by a number of routes, although the oral route is the route of choice in most situations. Some relatively new routes have been described.

Oral

There is usually a significant first-pass effect, so that the oral dose of opioids needs to be higher than the parenteral dose (commonly 3 : 1). For example, the bioavailability of oral morphine is only about 25%. The duration of oral opioids is prolonged by their slow absorption through the GI tract. Sustained-release forms are available that further prolong the action. The oral route is simple because of its accessibility, and it is relatively safe because of the slow absorption of the drug. Opioids are also relatively easy to titrate using this route.

Parenteral

The clinical parenteral routes of administration are the intravenous, intramuscular, and subcutaneous routes. Patient-controlled analgesia (PCA) may be used for all these routes, although the intravenous route is most common. PCA via the subcutaneous route is chosen for home care.

Transdermal

Passive diffusion of certain drugs through the skin is possible. A drug is delivered via patches that contain a drug reservoir and a controlling membrane. Fentanyl has been used in this way for several years, and patches are available that deliver doses from 25 to 100 μg/hr. After the initial placement of the patch, it may take 12 hours for the maximal blood level to be reached, after which analgesia persists for up to 72 hours (although less in some patients). Patches are changed every 2 to 3 days. The liver is bypassed, blood levels are fairly constant, and the system is convenient and comfortable. The great disadvantage of the transdermal route is that rapid titration is impossible (either up or down). However, for patients with stable pain, especially patients who cannot take oral medications, the patches are useful. This is also a useful way to give fentanyl, which is a highly specific mu receptor agonist thought to be particularly effective for neuropathic pain.

Neuraxial

The epidural, intrathecal, and intraventricular routes of administration allow smaller doses, prolonged duration of action, and minimal systemic side effects. The aim of this form of administration is to produce a specific spinal effect called selective spinal analgesia. Delayed respiratory depression may occur with larger doses, particularly with morphine, which is extremely non-lipophilic and therefore subject to rostral flow in the watery cerebro spinal fluid where this drug tends to accumulate. This occurs when the drug reaches the respiratory center in the brainstem. The more lipophilic opioids tend to diffuse across lipid bilayers more readily, and they generally do not travel rostrally (see Chapter 21). Neuraxial opioids are used commonly to treat postoperative pain and less commonly to treat cancer pain.

Rectal

Morphine may be given rectally and suppositories are available. Plasma morphine concentration after oral and rectal routes suggests that the oral-to-rectal potency ratio for morphine is 1:1. Thus, oral and rectal doses are the same. Slow-release morphine tablets have been given rectally when patients are no longer able to swallow tablets.

Transmucosal

The more lipophilic opioids are readily absorbed through buccal, nasal, or gingival mucosa. First-pass effects in the liver are avoided and rapid onset of action is possible. Buprenorphine, butorphanol, fentanyl (fentanyl lollipop), and sufentanil have all been given via this route.

VIII. PRINCIPLES OF OPIOID THERAPY

1. "Mild" versus "strong"

There is really no such thing as a mild opioid, since all opioids can be titrated to achieve equianalgesic effects and there is no ceiling effect to any opioid. However, certain opioids have traditionally been considered mild either because dosing is limited by side effects (e.g., codeine's constipating effect), or more often because they have been offered by the pharmaceutical companies in combined preparations in which the secondary drug (e.g., acetaminophen or aspirin) limits dosing (e.g., Percocet, Percodan, Vicodin, Tylenol #3). These combination therapies are useful for short-term management of mild to moderate pain such as acute pain after surgery or trauma, but they are less useful in long-term pain management because of their dose limitations.

In fact, physicians are moving away from the World Health Organization (WHO) concept of using these drugs as second-level therapy in the treatment of cancer pain (see Chapter 32) because of the inability to titrate them. Most authorities now encourage the earlier adoption of small doses of "strong" opioids (i.e., any single opioid) in preference to combination therapies for the treatment of chronic and cancer pain. Clearly, adjuncts can be given at the same time, but giving these as a separate preparation allows the opioid to be titrated to need.

2. The titration principle

For many reasons, not the least of which is to avoid side effects, particularly respiratory depression, the best principle for giving opioids is to start low (standard starting doses of opioids for acute pain are presented in tables in Chapter 21, and for chronic pain in Appendix VI) and titrate up (or down) in increments until optimal (i.e., maximal analgesia with acceptable side effects). The size of the starting dose and the size and timing of incremental increases clearly depend on the patient's opioid sensitivity, which will depend in turn on the patient's medical condition and whether tolerance has developed.

The only exception to this principle is when PCA or intravenous infusions are used to treat acute severe pain. In these cases, it is safer to give a monitored bolus to achieve comfort, then maintain comfort using standard or near-standard PCA or infusion doses. This is safer than rapidly increasing PCA or infusion doses in an effort to achieve pain relief in patients who not only are opioid naive but also have probably been given multiple centrally acting depressant drugs in the course of treatment. Once these patients become comfortable and can sleep, overdose may occur if a high-dose infusion or frequent large bolus dosing is allowed to continue.

3. Choice of opioid

Combination mild opioids such as Percocet, Vicodin, and Tylenol #3 are acceptable choices for mild to moderate short-term pain, especially considering physicians' familiarity with their use. Demerol is often avoided, especially for long-term use, because of the possibility of normeperidine toxicity and because its euphoric effects result in its being often favored by addicts. Likewise, propoxyphene (Darvon, Darvocet) is avoided because of the possibility of norpropoxyphene toxicity (see the section "Precautions") and because its analgesic effect at standard doses is weak. Long-term morphine use should be avoided in patients with renal dysfunction, including the elderly (>80 years) because of the likelihood of morphine-6-glucuronide accumulation.

Partial agonists (e.g., buprenorphine) and mixed agonist/antagonists (e.g., pentazocine, nalorphine) are sometimes chosen because of their low potential for abuse and respiratory depression. However, pure agonists are preferred, particularly in chronic pain patients, because of their superior efficacy and because they are more easily titrated. Also, difficulties arise in switching opioids when mixed agonists/antagonists are used and the effects of one drug (e.g., an analgesia) are reversed by another.

Otherwise, any opioid is suitable, and preference is often dictated by physician familiarity and by patient choice. It is worth asking patients if they have received opioids in the past and have a preference, because efficacy and side effects are often patient dependent and idiosyncratic.

4. Short-acting versus long-acting

Several choices of long-acting opioids are now available (MS Contin, OxyContin, Duragesic, methadone) making the use of long-acting opioids highly feasible. In the treatment of chronic pain, it is preferable to base therapy on a long-acting preparations and to use short-acting drugs for "breakthrough" pain (i.e., pain that breaks through the analgesia achieved by a long-acting medication and does so because of factors such as activity, anxiety, or time of day). In fact, in the treatment of chronic nonmalignant pain (CNMP), it is often preferable to avoid short-acting medication altogether. Long-acting opioid therapy is associated with less euphoria and dysphoria (and therefore has less addictive potential), which is another reason for preferring it in chronic pain states. As a general principle in chronic pain management, long-acting therapy is maximized and short-acting pain is minimized. In CNMP, short-acting opioids are avoided so the patients can learn to use other means to control their breakthrough pain. Long-acting preparations may also be useful in the treatment of resolving acute pain, when analgesic needs are predictable and the patient would prefer twice-daily to more frequent dosing.

5. Prescribing opioids

In the hospital setting, prescribing opioids is relatively easy and regulatory restrictions apply particularly to the pharmacy and to those actually administering the drugs (nurses and anesthesiologists). Hospital personnel are generally comfortable with using opioids within regulatory guidelines and restrictions. Prescribing opioids for home use is much more difficult. Each state has its own regulations and the prescribing physician must be familiar with these. The federal U.S. Drug Enforcement Administration guidelines for the prescription of controlled substances are presented in Appendix VI. The U.S. Food and Drug Administration drug schedules are presented in Appendix VII. The Massachusetts General Hospital (MGH) guidelines for prescribing opioids for CNMP are presented in Appendix V.

6. Controlling side effects

Respiratory depression is rightly the most feared of the opioid side effects. Hypoxia, apnea, and even death can occur with opioid use. However, this is much more likely to occur when opioids are used for acute rather than chronic pain. Obeying the principles of acute pain management (Section V) and the opioid titration principle (discussed earlier) will avoid respiratory depression in most cases. Nausea and vomiting are also far less likely to be troublesome when opioids are used for chronic rather than acute pain.

When side effects do occur, they can be treated either by reducing opioid dose, by switching opioid, or by giving an antiemetic. Constipation is a common complication of chronic opioid treatment, so preventive treatment should always be offered in conjunction with chronic opioid therapy. This should be with stimulant laxatives (e.g., Senokot, Lactulose), not with bulk-forming laxatives, which do not solve the problem of slow transit time and may actually worsen the situation. Other side effects are uncommon and should be treated by dose reduction or symptomatically if necessary.

7. Treating overdose

Overdose may result from clinical overdose, accidental overdose in addicts, or a suicide attempt. Death is nearly always attributable to respiratory failure, but if this is being treated with ventilation, very high doses of opioid are safely tolerated. Blood pressure may fall progressively, the patient is flaccid and cannot be roused. Noncardiogenic pulmonary edema is possible and frank convulsions may occur with very large doses. The pupils are pinpoint, unless hypoxia intervenes, and then they may dilate.

Treatment is supportive, with ventilation and careful fluid management. Naloxone may be given to reverse the respiratory depression, but large doses given quickly can precipitate withdrawal or rebound increases in sympathetic nervous system activity. The safest approach is to dilute the standard 0.4 mg naloxone with 10 mL of fluid and titrate carefully to effect. It should be remembered that naloxone has a short duration (a shorter half-life than most agonists) and re-narcotization can occur. Repeat doses of naloxone or an infusion may be needed.

IX. SPECIFIC OPIOIDS

The structures of some commonly used opioid agonists, partial agonists, and antagonists are shown in Figure 3. Opioid conversion doses are shown in Appendix VIII.

Morphine

Morphine remains the standard with which all other opioids are compared. It is widely used, and it is recommended as a standard by the WHO because of its wide availability and low cost. One third of morphine is bound to plasma protein and the unbound fraction is ionized at physiologic pH; thus the drug is very hydrophilic. Therefore, although it is distributed widely in the body, it has limited ability to penetrate tissues. It is for this reason that morphine given epidurally or intraspinally can spread rostrally in cerebrospinal fluid and cause delayed respiratory depression.

Morphine is metabolized by the liver. The major metabolites are morphine-3-glucuronide and morphine-6-glucuronide. Whereas morphine-3-glucuronide is inactive, morphine-6-glucuronide is more potent than morphine itself and has a longer half-life. The glucuronides are excreted by the kidneys and patients with renal dysfunction can accumulate morphine-6-glucuronide and develop prolonged opioid effects, including respiratory depression. On the other hand, patients in liver failure tolerate morphine up to the point of hepatic pre-coma because glucuronidation is rarely impaired. Intravenous (IV) injection of morphine results in rapid peak plasma levels, but peak effector site (brain and spinal cord receptors) concentrations occur 15 to 30 minutes later, so there is a relatively slow onset of peak central nervous system (CNS) effects. Plasma half-life after an IV bolus is 2 to 3 hours. The initial dose given intramuscularly (IM) or subcutaneously (SC) is highly variable, although 10 mg for a 70-kg healthy patient is reasonable. The high first-pass effect means that the oral dose is approximately three times that of the parenteral dose or more. Preservative-free morphine (Duramorph) given in small doses epidurally (1 to 4 mg) or intrathecally (0.1 to 0.4 mg) can produce profound analgesia of long duration (up to 12 to 24 hours). These are conservative doses given at MGH for patients who are in unmonitored beds. Higher doses (up to 10 mg epidurally or 1 mg intrathecally) can be given to monitored patients in intensive care or step-down units.

Preparations

- Morphine sulfate injections, 1, 5, 8, 10, 15, and 30 mg/mL; oral tablets, 8, 10, 15, and 30 mg; rectal suppositories, 5, 10, 20, and 30 mg.
- Morphine sulfate controlled release (MS Contin) tablets, 15, 30, 60, and 100 mg; Oramorph SR tablets, 30, 60, and 100 mg.

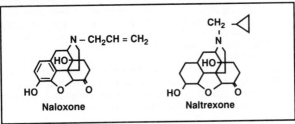

Figure 3.   Structures of opioid agonists, partial antagonists, and antagonists.

- Morphine sulfate immediate release (MDIR, Roxanol, Rescudose, MS/L) oral solution, 2 and 4 mg/mL; oral concentrate, 20 mg/mL; tablets and capsules, 15 and 30 mg.
- Morphine sulfate preservative-free solution (Duramorph and Astramorph) for intravenous, epidural, or intrathecal use, 0.5 and 1.0 mg/mL.
- Morphine sulfate preservative free (Infumorph) for continuous microinfusions for implantable epidural or intrathecal pumps, 10 and 25 mg/mL.

Formulations containing morphine for the treatment of diarrhea include paregoric and laudanum.

Codeine

Codeine is less potent than morphine but it has a high oral-to-parenteral potency ratio. Codeine is largely metabolized by the liver, and the byproducts are excreted by the kidney. About 10% of codeine is demethylated to morphine. Its analgesic action is probably related to this conversion. It has a significant antitussive action, probably involving receptors that bind codeine itself. The plasma half-life is 2 to 4 hours. Codeine is available in combination with acetaminophen or aspirin.

Preparations
- Codeine phosphate injections, 15, 30, and 60 mg/mL; tablets, 15, 30, and 60 mg; oral solution, 3 mg/mL.
- Codeine sulfate tablets, 15, 30, and 60 mg.

Hydrocodone

Hydrocodone is a semisynthetic codeine derivative with analgesic and antitussive properties, used most commonly in combination with acetaminophen in Vicodin.

Preparation
- Hydrocodone bitartrate (Vicodin) tablet, 7.5 mg with acetaminophen 750 mg.

Heroin

Heroin, or diacetylmorphine, is an atypical pro-drug. It has no direct action itself on the opioid receptor, but is rapidly metabolized to 6-monoacetylmorphine and subsequently to morphine. It is not available for clinical use in the United States, but is available in Canada and the United Kingdom. Although many have touted heroin as having advantages over morphine, all present evidence suggests that this is not so. It does come in a preservative-free powder and it has a high solubility, so high concentrations can be made, but other potent soluble drugs such as hydromorphone can be substituted.

Hydromorphone

This semisynthetic derivative of morphine is 10 times more potent than its parent compound. After parenteral injection, levels rise rapidly but there is a slower onset of CNS effects. Plasma half-life is 2 to 3 hours after an IV dose. IM injection delays peak plasma levels and CNS effects. Oral dosing takes 45 minutes or so for peak effects. Typical doses are 2 to 6 mg orally and 1.5 mg parenterally every 3 to 4 hours.

Preparations

- Hydromorphone hydrochloride (Dilaudid) injections, 1, 2, and 4 mg/mL; tablets, 1, 2, 3, 4, and 8 mg; suppository, 3 mg; cough syrup, 1 mg in 5 mL; oral liquid, 1 mg/mL.
- Hydromorphone hydrochloride (Dilaudid HP) highly concentrated for opioid-tolerant patients, 10 mg/mL.

Oxycodone

Oxycodone is a synthetic thebaine derivative with a profile and potency similar to that of morphine. It has typically been used in combination with nonopioids (Percocet, Percodan), but more recently it has been formulated as a long-acting preparation (OxyContin), which has popularized its use in cancer and other pain states. Immediate-release oxycodone has also become more popular, partly because it makes sense to prescribe it for breakthrough pain in patients taking OxyContin and partly because it is now perceived as a strong, titratable opioid rather than as a weak, nontitratable opioid (in combination therapies). OxyContin and oxycodone are a useful substitute for MS Contin and immediate-release morphine, particularly in the elderly who are sensitive to morphine-induced sedation and mental status change and to morphine-6-glucuronide accumulation.

Preparations

- Oxycodone hydrochloride immediate release (OxyIR) capsule, 5 mg; (OxyFAST) concentrated oral liquid, 20 mg/mL.
- Oxycodone hydrochloride controlled release (Oxycontin) tablets, 10, 20, 40, and 80 mg.
- Oxycodone hydrochloride (Percocet) tablet, 5mg with 325 mg acetaminophen; (Tylox) capsule 5 mg with 500 mg acetaminophen.
- Oxycodone hydrochloride (Roxicet) oral solution, 5 mg with 325 acetaminophen per 5 mL.
- Oxycodone hydrochloride (Percodan) tablet, 5 mg with 325 mg aspirin.
- Oxycodone hydrochloride (Roxicodone) tablet, 5 mg; oral solution, 5 mg in 5 mL; (Intensol) concentrated oral solution, 20 mg/mL.

Meperidine

Meperidine is 70% protein bound, which is more highly protein bound than morphine. Parenteral and oral doses are similar. The analgesic effects of meperidine are detectable approximately 15 minutes after an oral dose, reach their peak effect in 1 to 2 hours, and then gradually subside over several hours. Onset after parenteral administration of the same dose is within 10 minutes, and the peak is in 1 hour. Clinical duration of effective analgesia is between 2 to 4 hours. The usual initial dose is between 50 and 100 mg. The drug has vagolytic activities, and it is the only opioid that may produce tachycardia. Meperidine is eventually metabolized to normeperidine.

This metabolite has a half-life of 15 to 20 hours and is eliminated by both the kidney and the liver. Decreased renal or hepatic function can cause normeperidine to accumulate. The half-life is extended in the elderly. Thus in some individuals, there can be metabolite buildup. Normeperidine is toxic and large doses can cause tremors, muscle twitches, dilated pupils, hyperactive reflexes, and convulsions. If meperidine is combined with monoamine oxidase inhibitors (MAOIs), a number of reactions may be seen, including severe respiratory depression or excitation, delusions, hyperpyrexia, and convulsions. Meperidine has weak local anesthetic activities. This drug is generally avoided except for short-term use because of the risk of normeperidine toxicity and because of its high abuse potential.

Preparations

- Meperidine hydrochloride (Demerol) injection, 25, 50, 75, and 100 mg/mL; tablets, 50 and 100 mg; syrup, 50 mg in 5 mL; (Mepergan) injection, 25 mg/mL with 25 mg promethazine.

Cogeners of meperidine are diphenoxylate hydrochloride (Lomotil) and loperamide hydrochloride (Imodium), which are used to treat diarrhea.

Levorphanol

This drug is a morpinium, and it is the only example in this series that is commercially available. It has a long duration of action and pharmacologic effects that resemble morphine, except it may be associated with less nausea and vomiting. The average dose is 2 mg (SC or orally) and this would be expected to last 6 to 8 hours. The oral-to-parenteral potency ratio is comparable to that of oxycodone and codeine. Levorphanol may be crushed so that it can be administered via nasogastric tube. It is occasionally useful in cancer patients who feel nauseated by morphine and who benefit from the longer-lasting effect, although it has largely been superseded by oxycodone and OxyContin.

Preparations

- Levorphanol tartrate (Levo-Dromoran) injection, 2 mg/mL; tablet, 2 mg.

Methadone

Methadone is the only opioid with prolonged activity not achieved by controlled release formulation. It is a synthetic opioid with properties similar to those of morphine. Sedation and respiratory depression can outlast the analgesic action. In addition to its mu agonist effect, it is an NMDA inhibitor and an inhibitor of serotonin and norepinephrine reuptake. This is thought to confer real benefit in terms of reducing tolerance, a property that can be useful in opioid rotations (see Chapter 32). Abstinence symptoms are said to be less than morphine, and because of this and its long duration of action, it is used for detoxification or maintenance treatment for opioid addicts. For pain relief, oral doses may vary from 2.5 to 15 mg, parenteral doses from 2.5 to 10 mg and, for addict maintenance, 40 to 100 mg daily. After an oral dose, analgesia occurs in 30 to 60 minutes. After a parenteral dose, analgesia occurs in 10 to

20 minutes, with peak effects in 1 to 2 hours. The drug is eliminated slowly, which makes it liable to accumulate. Rapid titration (up and down) is not possible, so that this drug is best reserved for patients with stable pain. Although methadone is cheap, many physicians are uncomfortable prescribing it for outpatients because of its lack of titratability.

Preparations
- Methadone hydrochloride (Dolophine) injection, 10 tablets, 5 and 10 mg (40-mg specialized dose for opioid addiction); oral solutions, 1, 2, and 10 mg/mL.

Fentanyl

This is a phenylpiperidine that is 50 to 80 times as potent as morphine. It can be used as an analgesic (2 to 10 µg/kg) or anesthetic (20 to 100 µg/kg). Onset after parenteral administration is very rapid. Maximal analgesia and respiratory depression may not peak until 20 to 30 minutes after IM injection or several minutes after IV usage. Fentanyl may also be given intrathecally, epidurally, via mucous membranes, or through the skin. Transdermal fentanyl is extremely useful as a treatment for chronic pain, especially cancer pain, when the oral route cannot be used. Several fentanyl derivatives (sufentanil, alfentanil, and remifentanil) are used in anesthetic practice but not in pain practice.

Preparations
- Fentanyl citrate (Sublimaze) injection, 50 µg/mL.
- Fentanyl transdermal system (Duragesic) patches, 25, 50, 75, and 100 µg/hr.

Buprenorphine

Buprenorphine is a highly lipophilic, semisynthetic opioid with partial activity at the mu receptor and very little activity at the kappa and sigma receptors. It has a high affinity but low intrinsic activity at the mu receptor. It has qualitatively similar effects to morphine in terms of analgesia, CNS, and cardiovascular system effects. However, since it is a partial agonist, it has a pharmacologic ceiling. Buprenorphine 0.4 mg is the equivalent of 10 mg of morphine IM, but buprenorphine has a longer duration of action. The dose for analgesia is 0.3 mg IM or IV every 6 hours. After IM administration, initial effects are seen at 15 minutes with a peak at 1 hour. IV administration results in shorter onset and peak times. Sublingual doses of 0.4 mg produce effective pain relief.

Preparation
- Buprenorphine hydrochloride (Buprenex) injection, 0.3 mg/mL.

Nalbuphine

Nalbuphine is an agonist–antagonist; the chief agonist effects are at the kappa site. Nalbuphine has a ceiling effect on analgesia and respiratory depression, and doses above about 30 mg have no further effect. Dysphoria due to sigma activation may occur. Sedative effects are similar to those of morphine. Sweating and headache may occur. The usual dose in the adult is 10 mg every 3 to 6 hours parenterally, when the onset of effect is 5 to 10 minutes and the duration of action is 3 to 6 hours.

Preparations

- Nalbuphine hydrochloride (Nubain) injections, 10 and 20 mg/mL.

Tramadol

Tramadol is a synthetic, centrally acting analgesic with an unusual mode of action. It has weak opioid activity at mu, delta, and kappa receptors, with a 20-fold preference for the mu receptor. It also has nonopioid analgesic activity via norepinephrine and serotonin reuptake inhibition. In the United States, tramadol is available only as an oral preparation. It has a low potential for addiction and respiratory depression. Its main use is in mild to moderate pain, but it can be used to treat severe pain (usually together with other nonopioid analgesics) in patients who cannot tolerate standard opioids. It is usually given as 25 to 100 mg every 4 to 6 hours orally, but the maximum daily dose should not exceed 400 mg. Dosing is limited by side effects, especially dizziness and vertigo.

Preparations

- Tramadol hydrochloride (Ultram) scored tablet, 50 mg.

Naloxone

Naloxone is an opioid antagonist with greatest affinity for the mu receptor but acting at all opioid receptors. Small doses given intravenously or intramuscularly either prevent or promptly reverse the effects of mu-receptor agonists. In addition to reversing analgesia, patients with respiratory depression show an increase in respiratory rate within 1 to 2 minutes. Sedative effects are also reversed and blood pressure, if low, returns to normal. The duration of action is 1 to 4 hours and the plasma half-life is about 1 hour. Abrupt reversal of narcotic depression with large doses of naloxone may result in nausea and vomiting, tachycardia, sweating, hypertension, tremulousness, seizures, and cardiac arrest. These effects are at least partially attributable to a sudden surge of sympathetic activity as is seen in opioid withdrawal states. Other side effects that have been reported include hypotension, ventricular tachycardia and fibrillation, and pulmonary edema.

To avoid these serious and potentially dangerous side effects, it is advisable to reverse the effects of opioids slowly with repeated small doses of naloxone, titrating the dose to effect. This can easily be accomplished by diluting one 0.4-mg ampule in 10 ml (0.04 mg/mL) and injecting 1 to 2 ml (0.04 to 0.08 mg) every 1 to 2 minutes. In this way, it is sometimes possible to reverse respiratory depression while retaining analgesia.

Naloxone is readily absorbed from the GI tract, but the drug is almost completely metabolized by the liver before it reaches the circulation. Parenteral administration is thus needed for systemic effects. The drug may be used orally to treat constipation, utilizing its localized effect on opioid receptors in the gut. Generally, doses range from 0.8 to 4.0 mg (2 to 10 ampoules) every 4 hours, four times, or until a bowel movement has occurred.

Preparations

- Naloxone hydrochloride (Narcan) injections, 0.02, 0.4, and 1.0 mg/mL.

CONCLUSION

Opioids are the most effective analgesics known, which is not surprising, as we now know that endogenous opioids are responsible for natural analgesic states and that opiate drugs produce analgesia by binding to endogenous opioid receptors. Unfortunately, there are several barriers to their use, not the least of which is the risk of respiratory depression—a potentially lethal side effect of opioids. Another important barrier is the social stigma attached to opioids because of their use as recreational drugs. Careful education of healthcare providers, patients, and patients' relatives is often needed to allow them to understand the therapeutic value of opioids and the difference between this use and recreational use.

The opioids are not benign drugs and should be used with knowledge of their complex actions and adverse effects. At the same time, they are essential tools in pain management and in medicine in general, so that an understanding of opioid effects is important.

SELECTED READING

Borsook D. Opioids and neurological effects. *Curr Opin Anaesthesiol* 1994;7:352–357.

Carr D, Lipkowski A. Mechanisms of opioid analgesic actions. In: Rogers MC, Tinker JM, Corrino BG, Longneckes DE, eds. *Principles and practice of anesthesiology*. St. Louis: Mosby–Year Book, 1993.

Cowan A. Mechanisms of opioid activity. *Curr Opin Anaesthesiol* 1992;5:529–534.

Fields HL. *Pain*. New York: McGraw-Hill, 1987:251–279.

Lambert DG. Opioid receptors. *Curr Opin Anaesthesiol* 1995;8: 317–322.

Malan TP Jr. Opioid pharmacology in anesthesia pain management. *ASA refresher lectures*. 2000:422.

Physicians Desk Reference. Oradell, NJ: Medical Economics [annual].

Reisine T, Pasternak G. Opioid analgesics and antagonists. In: Hardman JG, Limbird LE, et al., eds. *Goodman and Gilman's the pharmacological basis of therapeutics*, 9th ed. New York: McGraw-Hill, 1996.

Twycross RG. Opioids. In: Wall PD, Melzack R, eds. *Textbook of pain*, 3rd ed. New York: Churchill-Livingstone, 1994.

Wall PD, Melzack R, eds. *Textbook of Pain*, 3rd ed. New York: Churchill-Livingstone, 1994.

Adjuvant Treatments

Robert S. Cluff

My heart aches, and a drowsy numbness pains
My senses, as though of hemlock I had drunk,
Or emptied some dull opiate to the drains
One minute past, and Lethe-ward had sunk.
—*"Ode to a Nightingale," John Keats, 1795–1821*

The opioids and the anti-inflammatory agents are the primary analgesics used in pain management. These drugs have the unique property of providing immediate (i.e., within minutes to hours) pain relief. The opioids are the only drugs indicated for the treatment of moderate to severe pain. The anti-inflammatory drugs are useful for the treatment of osteoarthritis and rheumatoid arthritis, as well as various mild to moderate acute and chronic pain conditions, and as adjuncts in the case of severe pain. The remaining categories of analgesic drugs, called adjuvant analgesics, have primary indications [U.S. Food and Drug Administration (FDA) approved] for non-pain diagnoses, their analgesic effects being secondary. These non-pain diagnoses include epilepsy, depression, and cardiac arrhythmia. Characteristically, the adjuvant drugs do not provide immediate pain relief; rather, their effects are noticeable only after days or weeks of therapy.

The many categories of drugs in the adjuvant class include the cyclic antidepressants, the selective serotonin reuptake inhibitors, the monoamine reuptake inhibitors, the sodium channel blockers, the GABAergics, the benzodiazepines, and the alpha adrenergics. This chapter will focus on the use of anticonvulsants, local anesthetics, corticosteroids, and antispasmodics in the treatment of chronic (including cancer) pain. The psychotropic medications are described in Chapter 11, and analgesics for headache are described in Chapter 28. A brief review of all the adjuvant analgesics is presented in Appendix VIII.

I. GENERAL CONSIDERATIONS

The decision to begin a particular analgesic medication for any patient involves many issues. Each decision is based partly on previous experience (e.g., previous success with mexiletine for peripheral neuropathy). The potential benefit of a drug must be weighed against its side effects. The patient should be made aware of evidence of the drug's efficacy and should have realistic expectations for improvement. A check of the patient's medical background is needed to identify any areas of susceptibility, and the patient's current medications are reviewed for drug interactions.

Often, the side effects of an adjunctive agent are noticed within days of initiating treatment. However, the analgesic effect is often not apparent for 1 to 2 weeks. The possible utility, as well as the adverse side effects, should be considered, and appropriate patient selection is of key importance. For example, although the sedative effect of a tricyclic antidepressant can be utilized to improve sleep while treating pain, tricyclic use would be relatively contraindicated in an 80-year-old patient with Parkinson's disease because of increased risk of falls, decreased cognitive capacity, and constipation.

Knowledge of a drug's mechanism of action can direct treatment strategies if the cause of the pain is known (e.g., a sodium channel blocker in neuropathic pain). Over the past several years, the treatment algorithm for chronic pain has seen a shift toward a mechanism-based approach. This concept is underscored in the following statement:

As we approach the new millennium, it is clear that we are on the brink of a major change in clinical pain management. We are poised to move from a treatment paradigm that has been almost entirely empirical to one that will be derived from an understanding of the actual mechanisms involved in the pathogenesis of pain. . . . The implications of this are immense and will necessitate major changes . . . to a mechanism-based classification. . . . The aim in the future will be to identify in individual patients what mechanisms are responsible for their pain and to target treatment specifically at those mechanisms. (Clifford Woolf, 1999)

This approach will make it possible to match a medication (with a known mechanism of action) to a pain syndrome in which this physiologic mechanism has been disrupted. The use of a sodium channel blocker in peripheral neuropathic pain is an example (upregulation of sodium channels with spontaneous activation). In addition, this approach will allow pairing of medications with different mechanisms of action to provide synergistic effects. Last, it will allow agents with the same mechanism of action to be used interchangeably, so that a drug that is effective but not tolerated because of side effects can be avoided.

II. AN EVIDENCE-BASED APPROACH

Objective data from randomized controlled trials (RCTs) provide us with an evidence-based approach that is more scientific than relying on anecdotal reports. RCTs assess the efficacy of an agent versus a placebo or an established therapy. The best studies are those that include each of the following:

1. A homogeneous population
2. An established diagnosis with objective criteria (e.g., dermatomal scarring and sensory loss in postherpetic neuralgia)
3. An appropriate duration of treatment
4. Use of placebo

The use of homogeneous study populations enables mechanism-based targeting of specific therapies. The number of subjects needed to show a statistical difference between the two study groups must be derived and used in the recruitment process. Table 1 presents a summary of adjuvant analgesics and the pain conditions for which they are effective, as demonstrated in RCTs.

Despite the attractiveness of the mechanistic approach to both pain treatment and pain research, the literature is at present devoid of RCTs with outcome measures that distinguish between various pain qualities.

Postherpetic neuralgia, a devastating chronic pain entity, is ideally suited for mechanistic pain trials. This painful disease has a known cause, a preponderance of cases occurring in otherwise healthy people over the age of 60, and consistent symptomatology. Patients usually complain of one of three types of pain: (a) a constant deep aching or burning pain, (b) an intermittent spontaneous pain with a lancinating or jabbing quality, and (c) a dysesthetic pain provoked by light tactile stimulation (allodynia). The reduction of a distinct pain quality in response to a particular drug should allow more targeted treatment of specific pain types.

In a recent article, Max challenges the feasibility of this concept. He lists difficulties in this approach in both the clinical and the research arenas. Even so, he states that the concept deserves further attention, and he suggests a "coordinated approach by academic and industry pain scientists, FDA regulators of analgesics, and industry" to facilitate the research that is needed to make this concept a reality.

Table 1.   Adjuvant analgesic indications[a]

Adjuvant	Indicated diagnoses
Amitriptyline	Diabetic neuropathy, postherpetic neuralgia, postoperative breast pain, fibromyalgia, central pain, tension headache
Nortriptyline	Central pain
Desipramine	Peripheral neuropathy
Clomipramine	Central pain
Mexiletine	Peripheral neuropathy
Carbamazepine	Trigeminal neuralgia
Gabapentin	Diabetic neuropathy, postherpetic neuralgia, migraine headache
Valproic acid	Trigeminal neuralgia
Lamotrigine	Trigeminal neuralgia, peripheral neuropathy
Tizanidine	Trigeminal neuralgia
Lidocaine ointment	Postherpetic neuralgia
Lidocaine patch	Postherpetic neuralgia
Capsaicin	Postherpetic neuralgia
Prednisolone	Rheumatoid arthritis

[a] In randomized controlled trials.

III. ANTICONVULSANTS

Anticonvulsants are a heterogeneous group of drugs used in the treatment of seizures, some of which have proven analgesic effect in pain patients. Anticonvulsants appear to benefit patients suffering from neuropathic pain—that is, pain related to direct injury of the peripheral or central nervous system. Six anticonvulsants are useful in neuropathic pain states—gabapentin, carbamazepine, valproic acid, clonazepam, phenytoin, and lamotrigine.

Gabapentin has quickly become widely used in the treatment of multiple pain syndromes, partly because of its lack of drug–drug interactions and mild side-effect profile. In 1998, data were presented from three multicenter placebo-controlled trials that demonstrated the efficacy of this drug in migraine headache, peripheral neuropathy, and postherpetic neuralgia. These findings demonstrate the utility of this agent in both neuropathic and non-neuropathic pain.

Although the mechanisms of action of the six anticonvulsants differ, the mechanisms underlying their anticonvulsant effect most likely contribute to their analgesic effect (e.g., the pathophysiology of epilepsy and neuropathic pain may be similar). Anticonvulsants have great side-effect potential, and their individual side-effect profiles are quite different, as described later (see also Appendix VIII).

1. Indications

The following are indications for anticonvulsants in patients with chronic pain:

- Neuralgia—trigeminal, glossopharyngeal, and postherpetic
- Neuralgia secondary to peripheral nervous system and central nervous system infiltration by cancer
- Central pain states (e.g., thalamic pain syndrome and post-stroke pain)
- Postsympathectomy pain
- Post-traumatic neuralgia
- Porphyria, Fabry's disease, and others
- Painful diabetic neuropathy
- Paroxysmal pain in multiple sclerosis
- Migraine headaches
- Phantom limb pain and postamputation stump pain
- Peripheral neuropathy secondary to a variety of disease states [e.g., alcoholism, amyloidosis, diabetes mellitus, human immunodeficiency virus (HIV) and acquired immunodeficiency syndrome (AIDS), malabsorption]

2. Clinical guidelines

(i) *Dosing regimens*

Anticonvulsants are most effective in the management of paroxysmal lancinating dysesthesias associated with neuropathic pain syndromes; they are less useful for continuous neuropathic pain. Although carbamazepine is considered the drug of choice for the treatment of trigeminal neuralgia, its significant potential for side effects may limit its use to this indication and to the management of painful conditions refractory to other therapies.

In addition to a complete history and physical examination, a complete blood count and liver function baseline tests are recommended before starting an anticonvulsant.

A 4- to 6-week trial is the minimum required to adequately assess the analgesic efficacy of a new anticonvulsant. The patient is given dosage instructions along with a titration schedule. In general when beginning a new anticonvulsant analgesic, the phrase "Start low and go slow" is adhered to. This allows the body to adjust to the new drug and decreases the likelihood of significant side effects. Doses are generally increased until therapeutic effects or limiting adverse effects are observed, or until plasma concentrations approach toxic levels.

A review of previous analgesic drug trials is valuable, with special attention paid to pain relief and side effects. Serum levels do not appear to correlate well with pain response, but the potential for many side effects and toxicity mandates periodic evaluation of the serum level. Both physician and patient must understand that this process may take months to years (i.e., several medication trials).

(ii) *Choice of drug*

Because of its favorable side effect profile, gabapentin is often used as a first-line agent for various forms of neuropathic pain. Lamotrigine is a sodium channel blocker that may provide effective relief of chronic pain, but because of the risk of serious rash (including Stevens-Johnson syndrome), this agent is used only if other agents fail. A trial of carbamazepine or phenytoin is usually initiated prior to trials of valproic acid or clonazepam, because of superior controlled-trial and anecdotal support for the former two agents.

(iii) *Initial dose and maintenance*

As a general principle, a standard initial dose is chosen. The choice of a stable dose is determined by subsequent titration on the basis of serum levels, analgesic efficacy, and side effects. In some patients, attempts at tapering and discontinuation are successful, but often therapy is maintained at the therapeutic dose initially chosen. These medications should not be discontinued abruptly but should be tapered over a period of time to avoid withdrawal symptoms.

3. Drug characteristics

(i) *Phenytoin*

MECHANISM OF ACTION.   Phenytoin is believed to have a stabilizing effect on neuronal membranes and can alter sodium, calcium, and potassium flux.

PHARMACOLOGY.   Phenytoin has variable absorptions when administered orally. Its peak serum level is reached between 3 and 12 hours after the dose, but generally in 4 to 8 hours. It is highly protein bound and has approximately a 10% free fraction. This percentage varies with the serum protein level: low serum protein levels that are otherwise therapeutic might result in an elevated free fraction and toxicity. Metabolism is hepatic, with a serum half-life of approximately 24 hours.

RECOMMENDED DOSAGE. In an average adult patient, start with 100 mg three times a day (tid), check the blood level in 3 weeks, and follow the clinical response. A blood level over 20 µg/mL is considered to be toxic. Phenytoin should be taken after meals to avoid gastrointestinal (GI) irritation.

ADVERSE EFFECTS.   Cerebellar–vestibular dysfunction, allergic reactions (skin rash), GI irritation, hepatotoxicity, and fetal hydantoin syndrome can occur with phenytoin. Folic acid deficiency can also occur, resulting in peripheral neuropathy and megaloblastic anemia. Other side effects include gingival hyperplasia (requiring meticulous oral hygiene) and hyperglycemia or glycosuria. These two side effects are related to fibrocyte stimulation and to phenytoin-induced inhibition of insulin secretion, respectively.

(ii) *Carbamazepine*

MECHANISM OF ACTION.   Carbamazepine is chemically and pharmacologically related to the tricyclic antidepressants. It inhibits norepinephrine uptake, and it prevents repeated discharges in neurons. Carbamazepine most likely blocks sodium channels, as do phenytoin and lamotrigine. This observation is consistent with its ability to relieve lancinating pain in states of neuralgia.

PHARMACOLOGY.   Carbamazepine is absorbed slowly and unpredictably after oral intake. Peak concentrations are seen in 2 to 8 hours. It is moderately protein bound and has active metabolites. Metabolism is hepatic, and excretion is urinary. It has a serum half-life of 10 to 20 hours, averaging 14 hours.

RECOMMENDED DOSAGE.   Start at 200 mg/day and increase by 200 mg every 1 to 3 days to a maximum of 1,500 mg/day. If side effects are encountered, the dose should be decreased to the previous level for several days, and then gradually increased. Therapeutic doses usually range from 800 to 1,200 mg/day. Carbamazepine is a gastric irritant and therefore should be taken with food.

ADVERSE EFFECTS.   Sedation, nausea, diplopia, and vertigo are the side effects that occur most frequently with this drug. Hematologic abnormalities such as aplastic anemia, agranulocytosis, pancytopenia, and thrombocytopenia can occur. Other side effects include jaundice (hepatocellular and cholestatic), oliguria, hypertension, and acute left ventricular heart failure.

Complete blood counts (CBCs) and liver function studies should be obtained. In general, CBCs are obtained at baseline, followed by every 2 weeks for a month, monthly for 3 months, twice over the following year, and then yearly. A patient who, in the course of treatment, exhibits low or decreased white blood cell or platelet counts should be monitored closely. Discontinuation of the drug should be considered if any evidence of significant bone marrow depression develops. Liver function studies should always be obtained for patients with a history of liver dysfunction. Carbamazepine should be discontinued immediately in cases of aggravated liver dysfunction or acute liver disease.

(iii) *Valproic acid*

MECHANISM OF ACTION.   Valproic acid is believed to increase the inhibitory activity of gamma-aminobutyric acid (GABA) through interference with GABA transaminase.

PHARMACOLOGY.   Valproic acid has a rapid oral absorption, with peak concentrations in 1 to 4 hours. It is highly protein bound; it undergoes hepatic metabolism and is excreted renally. Its half-life is 10 to 12 hours in serum.

RECOMMENDED DOSAGE. Start at 15 mg/kg per day in divided doses. Increase weekly by 5 to 10 mg/kg per day until it becomes clinically therapeutic or the maximum dose of 60 mg/kg is reached. Baseline and periodic liver function tests are recommended because of previous reports of fatal hepatic failure. Reversible liver enzyme dysfunction occurs more commonly.

ADVERSE EFFECTS. GI symptoms such as nausea, vomiting, anorexia, and diarrhea can occur, but they improve with time. Sedation, tremors, and ataxia are occasionally seen, as are platelet aggregation effects. Hepatotoxicity can also occur.

(iv) *Clonazepam*

MECHANISM OF ACTION. Clonazepam is a benzodiazepine with anticonvulsant activity. It appears to act through enhancement of GABA inhibitory activity, which results in decreased firing of neurons.

PHARMACOLOGY. Clonazepam has good oral absorption, with a peak serum concentration in 1 to 4 hours. It is moderately protein bound; it undergoes hepatic metabolism to inactive metabolites and it is excreted renally. It has a serum half-life of approximately 24 hours.

RECOMMENDED DOSAGE. Start with 0.5 mg tid and increase by 0.5 mg every 3 to 4 days until an adequate response is achieved or a maximal dosage of 6 mg/day is attained. The usual therapeutic pain dosage range is 1 to 4 mg/day. Because of its sedative effect, clonazepam should be taken at bedtime.

ADVERSE EFFECTS. Lethargy and sedation, two common side effects, usually subside over time. Ataxia and dizziness are sometimes noted early in the course of drug therapy, but they improve with continued use.

Psychologic disinhibitory changes occur and are manifested as mood disturbances and delirium. A withdrawal syndrome, including seizures, can occur with abrupt discontinuation of therapy.

(v) *Gabapentin*

MECHANISM OF ACTION. The mechanism of analgesic effect for this drug is not known. Although this drug's structure resembles that of the neurotransmitter GABA, it does not interact with GABA receptors, inhibit GABA degradation, or convert into GABA. It is believed that gabapentin increases the total brain concentration of GABA, but the mechanism of this effect is unknown. In addition, this drug binds to a calcium channel subunit that may play a role in analgesia.

PHARMACOLOGY. Gabapentin is not appreciably metabolized in humans. Its bioavailability is inversely proportional to dose, especially at low doses (e.g., 100 to 400 mg). At the recommended dosage schedule (300 to 600 mg, tid) the differences in bioavailability are not significant (average, about 60%). Food has no effect on the rate or extent of absorption. Gabapentin circulates largely unbound (<3% bound to plasma proteins). It is eliminated from the systemic circulation by renal excretion as unchanged drug. Elimination half-life is 5 to 7 hours, and this is unaltered by dose or following multiple doses. Plasma clearance is directly proportional to creatinine clearance.

RECOMMENDED DOSAGE.   Start with a 300-mg capsule at bedtime for 1 to 2 days. If the bedtime dose is tolerated, begin three-times-daily dosing. The dosage should be increased by 300-mg increments until either pain relief or intolerable side effects are experienced. If maximal three-times-daily dosing (900 mg tid) does not provide relief, four-times-daily dosing is a reasonable next step. Starting at 100 mg tid is appropriate in patients with a history of therapy failure as a result of intolerable side effects. Absorption of individual doses is dependent on GI enzymes and decreases abruptly at doses greater than 900 mg (excess gabapentin is eliminated in the stool). Dosage adjustments are required in patients with renal impairment (Table 2). Change in dose is not required in patients with hepatic insufficiency. When discontinuing the drug, it should be tapered gradually over at least 7 days.

ADVERSE EFFECTS.   Somnolence, dizziness, ataxia, fatigue, inability to concentrate, GI disturbances, and nystagmus are the most commonly observed adverse events with gabapentin treatment. Pedal edema is listed in one study as occurring in only 1.7% of subjects, although practitioners report that it is often responsible for drug termination.

(vi) *Lamotrigine*

MECHANISM OF ACTION.   Lamotrigine (Lamictal) is an antiepileptic drug that is structurally unrelated to other drugs in current use. Lamotrigine acts by stabilizing the slow inactivated conformation of type IIa neuronal sodium channels, resulting in inhibition of repetitive firing of action potentials under conditions of sustained neuronal depolarization. No impairment of neuronal function occurs under normal firing conditions. By this mechanism, lamotrigine is believed to suppress the excessive release of excitatory amino acids (principally glutamate a neurotransmitter implicated in central sensitization and wind-up). By inhibiting the pathologic release of glutamate, lamotrigine has the potential to be antinociceptive and to prevent the mechanisms responsible for the establishment of chronic pain.

PHARMACOLOGY.   Lamotrigine is rapidly and completely absorbed after oral administration with negligible first-pass metabolism (absolute bioavailabilty, about 98%). The bioavailability is

Table 2.   Neurontin dosage based on renal function

Renal function, creatinine clearance (mL/min)	Total daily dose (mg/day)	Dose regimen (mg)
>60	1,200	400 TID
30–60	600	300 BID
15–30	300	300 QD
<15	150	300 QOD
Hemodialysis	—	200–300[a]

[a] Loading dose of 300–400 mg in patients who have never received Neurontin, then 200–300 mg Neurontin following each 4 hours of hemodialysis
Adapted from the Physicians Desk Reference, 2000, with permission.

not affected by food. Peak plasma concentrations occur from 1.4 to 4.8 hours after drug administration. Data from *in vitro* studies indicate that lamotrigine is not highly protein bound, and therefore clinically significant interactions with other drugs through competition for protein binding sites are unlikely. Lamotrigine is metabolized by the liver through glucuronic acid conjugation.

RECOMMENDED DOSAGE. Because of an increased risk of rash (see the section "Adverse Effects"), dose escalation with lamotrigine is very gradual and should not exceed (at least initially) 50 mg in 2 weeks. It is advisable to start at 25 mg bid for 2 weeks and increase by 25-mg increments every 2 weeks until reaching 100 mg bid at week 6. After 2 weeks at 100 mg bid, it is reasonable to increase the dose by 25 mg bid weekly until the target dose of 200 mg bid is achieved. The recommended maximum dosage is between 400 and 500 mg/day divided into bid dosing.

ADVERSE EFFECTS. Dizziness, ataxia, somnolence, headache, diplopia, blurred vision, and nausea and vomiting are the most commonly observed side effects of lamotrigine. Although the incidence of rash is uncommon, it can be life threatening. The appearance of any systemic skin changes warrants evaluation by a physician, and lamotrigine should be immediately discontinued unless otherwise stated by that physician. Serious rash requiring hospitalization and discontinuation of lamotrigine, including Stevens-Johnson syndrome and toxic epidermal necrolysis, has occurred in association with lamotrigine therapy. Rare deaths have been reported, but these have been too few to permit a precise estimate of the rate.

IV. LOCAL ANESTHETICS

The use of local anesthetics as blocking agents—subcutaneous, along the nerve roots, or at the spinal cord—is well known. However, the use of systemic local anesthetics as adjuvant analgesics is not as common. Intravenous lidocaine has been found to be useful in the treatment of some neuropathic pain conditions, including continuous and lancinating dysesthesias. Other conditions include neuropathic pain due to herpes zoster, phantom limb pain, diabetic neuropathy, and various other pain complaints resulting from neuropathies.

The mechanism of pain relief appears to be the stabilization of nerve membranes. This occurs as a result of the blockade of sodium channels, which prevents the influx of sodium. The rapid influx of sodium is responsible for the initiation and propagation of depolarization in nerve fibers, which may in turn be perceived as pain.

A trial of intravenous lidocaine is often used to assess (in a timely manner) the efficacy of sodium channel blockade in a particular chronic pain disease. Prior to the trial, a baseline electrocardiogram (ECG) and liver function tests should be obtained. Galer et al. demonstrated the value of the lidocaine infusion to achieve successful relief of pain with subsequent use of mexiletine, an oral sodium channel blocker.

The lidocaine infusion procedure involves administering 1 to 2 mg/kg of lidocaine intravenously over 10 to 15 minutes while the patient is adequately monitored. The dose is usually 100 mg for adult patients. Verbal analog scores are obtained before, during, and after the test. Patients commonly experience tinnitus, perioral numbness, a metallic taste in the mouth, and dizziness during the trial. A 50% or greater reduction in pain warrants a trial of mexiletine.

Mexiletine (Mexitil) has a favorable side-effect profile and is the most commonly used oral sodium channel blockers. Mexiletine is started at 150 mg at bedtime for about a week. If tolerated, it is increased to 150 mg tid. If pain relief is inadequate, the dose can be slowly escalated (every 5 to 7 days) to the maximum of 1,200 mg/day. This results in remarkable pain relief in some patients. Possible adverse effects include arrhythmias, syncope, hypotension, ataxia, tremors, nervousness, upper GI distress, dizziness, hepatotoxicity, skin rash, visual changes, and fever and chills.

V. CORTICOSTEROIDS

Corticosteroids are useful as adjuvant analgesics, either alone or in combination with opioids. The exact mechanism of action is not clear. A peripheral effect is apparently the result of a reduction of inflammation, and a central effect may occur through altered neurotransmitter levels. In addition, corticosteroids are believed to reduce neuronal excitability by affecting cell membranes directly.

Steroids are used primarily in the management of pain resulting from rheumatic disease and cancer. They may reduce pain resulting from metastatic bone tumors, spinal cord compression, plexopathies, lymphedema, hepatomegaly, and some types of primary tumors. High doses of steroids can be tried for 1 week. If there is not a positive response, therapy should be terminated. If there is a useful therapeutic response, therapy should be continued but tapered to the lowest dosage that maintains the response. Prednisone (100 mg every day), methylprednisolone (100 mg every day), or prednisolone (7.5 mg every day) can be tried for 1 week and then tapered.

Steroid tapers (e.g., Medrol Dosepacks) are often useful in nonmalignant pain of acute onset (e.g., back pain) or for an exacerbation of a chronic pain state. The standard taper of oral methylprednisolone is from 24 to 0 mg over a period of 7 days.

The numerous adverse effects of steroids are well known and range from osteoporosis and infections to gastric ulcerations, perforations, and Cushing's disease. These are not first-line medications, and explicit risk–benefit analysis should precede their administration. As a general principle, steroids should not be used in combination with the nonsteroidal anti-inflammatory drugs.

VI. ANTISPASMODICS

The two antispasmodic agents routinely used to treat chronic pain are lioresal (Baclofen) and cyclobenzaprine (Flexeril). Tizanidine (Zanaflex) is a relatively new agent with a mechanism of action similar to that of clonidine, an adjuvant analgesic often used in the treatment of sympathetically maintained pain.

(i) *Baclofen*

Baclofen is an antispasmodic drug that is often used in the treatment of spasticity associated with multiple sclerosis and spinal cord lesions. However, it is believed to possess some analgesic properties, which may augment opioid-induced analgesia. This apparently occurs through its GABA-B agonist actions. Baclofen appears to be useful in the treatment of painful spasticity, trigeminal neuralgia, and other forms of neuropathic pain, particularly lancinating pain. It should be avoided in patients with seizure disorders and impaired renal function.

Baclofen is usually started at 5 mg tid orally. Each dose can be increased by 5 mg every 3 days, to a maximum of 80 mg/day. Baclofen is also administered intrathecally, and pump systems are sometimes implanted for continuous infusion therapy in selected patients. Common side effects include drowsiness, fatigue, vertigo, orthostatic hypotension, headaches, hypotonia, psychiatric disturbances, insomnia, slurred speech, ataxia, rash, urinary frequency, and GI distress. These can be avoided through slow titration and avoidance of abrupt discontinuation.

(ii) *Flexeril*

Flexeril relieves muscle spasm of local origin without interfering with muscle function. It is ineffective in muscle spasm resulting from central nervous system disease. Flexeril is indicated as an adjunct to rest and physical therapy for relief of muscle spasm associated with acute, painful musculoskeletal conditions. Relief of muscle spasm results in relief of pain, tenderness, movement limitation, and activity restriction. Flexeril is closely related to the tricyclic antidepressants and its side-effect profile closely resembles that of the tricyclics. Common side effects are drowsiness, dry mouth, and dizziness. Tachycardia, hypertension, syncope, and GI upset have also been reported. Flexeril should not be used in conjunction with a monoamine oxidase inhibitor. Other contraindications are similar to those of the tricyclics and include cardiac arrhythmias, hyperthyroidism, and urinary obstructions. The usual dosage is 10 mg tid, with a range of 20 to 40 mg/day in divided doses. Flexeril use should not exceed 2 to 3 weeks.

(iii) *Zanaflex*

Zanaflex is an alpha-2-agonist that decreases sympathetic transmission at the level of the dorsal horn. Its antispasmodic action is attributed to reduced facilitation of the spinal motor neurons. Following oral administration, Zanaflex is completely absorbed. Its half-life is approximately 2.5 hours and its duration of action is short (3 to 5 hours). It is indicated for sympathetically maintained pain, as well as for pain described as lancinating, electrical, or burning. Adverse effects most commonly seen with use of Zanaflex include dry mouth, sedation, asthenia (weakness, fatigue, and/or tiredness), and dizziness. Dosage is started at 1 to 2 mg at bedtime, followed by 1 mg tid. The usual daily dose for chronic pain is 4 to 12 mg. Maximum dose should not exceed 36 mg/day.

VII. CLONIDINE

Clonidine stimulates alpha adrenoreceptors in the brainstem, thereby decreasing sympathetic outflow from the central nervous system with a resultant decrease in peripheral resistance, heart rate, and blood pressure. Its unique mechanism of action explains why it is the only transdermal or oral agent that employs the mechanistic treatment approach for sympathetically maintained pain.

The transdermal patch (Catapres-TTS) is the preferred mode of administration, as it produces more consistent blood levels. Dosing with the patch starts with the TTS-1 and can increase to a maximum of two TTS-3 patches applied every 7 days. The patch should be applied to a hairless area of intact skin of the upper arm or chest. Subsequent patches should be applied to a different site and the prior one removed to prevent skin irritation. The most common adverse events include dry mouth, drowsiness, fatigue, headache, lethargy, and sedation. Dizziness is not uncommon, especially in those with low baseline blood pressures.

VIII. TOPICAL AGENTS

Disorders responsive to topical therapy include complex regional pain syndromes and peripheral polyneuropathy. Transdermal analgesic therapy is often used in patients who cannot tolerate oral administration irrespective of the pain condition (e.g., the Duragesic patch). Postherpetic neuralgia (PHN) is an ideal chronic pain syndrome to treat with topical agents for several reasons. Most PHN patients have clearly demarcated areas of affected skin, and they obtain relief of pain from modest amounts of a topical preparation and suffer few accompanying side effects.

Three categories of topical agents have received the most attention: capsaicin preparations, local anesthetics, and nonsteroidal anti-inflammatory drug preparations. All three have been demonstrated in controlled trials to be effective analgesics in PHN patients. Anecdotally, many drugs are being mixed into creams and ointments by compounding pharmacies for the treatment of superficial pain (e.g., ketoprofen, 100 mg/mL, plus bupivacaine, 50 mg/mL, plus ketamine 50 mg/mL). An endless number of mixtures could potentially be used. Combining agents that have different mechanisms of action may increase the likelihood of significant benefit. Use of these agents requires caution, however, as applying the mixture too often or to a large surface area may result in toxicity.

IX. CONCLUSION

The adjuvant analgesics include a great number of drugs with various mechanisms of action. As the name implies, they were originally used as "add on" therapy, in combination with an opioid or an anti-inflammatory agent. Presently, they are often the first choice for analgesic therapy. Although little progress has been made in matching drug mechanism of action to pain pathophysiology, there has been some success anecdotally. For instance, although neuropathic pain appears to be resistant to pharmacologic treatment in general, certain drugs (e.g., sodium channel blockers) do seem to be effective. RCTs provide us with the best evidence available to determine treatment strategy. Treatment approaches need to be based on scientific evidence, yet each patient is unique; therefore, treatment needs to be adjusted to the individual. This is just one of the challenges faced when treating patients with chronic pain.

SELECTED READING

1. Benedetti C, Butler SH. Systemic analgesics. In: Bonica JJ, ed. *The management of pain*, vol. 2. Philadelphia: Lea & Febinger, 1990: 1640–1675.

2. Galer BS, Harle J, Rowbotham MC. Response to intravenous lido-caine infusion predicts subsequent responses to oral mexiletine: A prospective study. *J Pain Symptom Manage* 1996;12:161–167.

3. Max MB. Is mechanism-based pain treatment attainable? Clinical trial issues. *J Pain* 2000;1(suppl 1):2–9.

4. McQuay H, Carroll D, Jadad AR, et al. Anticonvulsant drugs for management of pain: A systematic review. *Br Med J* 1995;311: 1047–1052.

5. Munglani R, Hill RG; Other drugs including sympathetic blockers. In: Wall PD, Melzack R, eds. *Textbook of pain*, 4th ed. New York: Churchill-Livingstone, 2000:1233–1250.

6. Woolf CJ, Decosterd I. Implications of recent advances in the un-derstanding of pain pathophysiology for the assessment of pain in patients. *Pain* 1999;82:1–7.

Psychopharmacology for the Pain Specialist

Daniel M. Rockers and Scott M. Fishman

It was a most repugnant undertaking to have to treat a group of complaints which, as all authors are agreed, are typified by instability, irregularity, fantasy, unpredictability—complaints which are governed by no law or rule, and whose diverse manifestations are connected to no serious theoretical formulation.

—From "Traite Clinique et Therapeutique de l'Hysterie," Paul Briquet

Knowledge of psychopharmacology is important for a pain practitioner because of the significant overlap of psychiatric diagnoses with chronic pain conditions, and because the common psychopharmacologic medication groups are used as analgesics. Many of these agents have multiple mechanisms of action, which accounts for their dual effects. In this chapter, psychotropic medications and their role in pain treatment are reviewed. Because of the high comorbidity of depression and pain, antidepressants—the largest category—are covered first. Next, medications that directly affect cognitive functioning—antipsychotics or neuroleptics—are reviewed. Mood stabilizers, used to treat bipolar disorder and derivative conditions, are next. Anxiolytics and psychostimulants conclude the section.

I. ANTIDEPRESSANTS

In the majority of cases, patients with chronic pain are prescribed an antidepressant or have already been taking one. Antidepressants often serve a dual role: treating a mood disorder as well as independently addressing pain symptoms.

The earliest forms of the currently used antidepressants were tricyclic antidepressants (TCAs) and monoamine oxidase inhibitors (MAOIs), each with inhibitory actions on norepinephrine (NE) and serotonin (5-HT) reuptake. These were the drugs of choice for treating depression until the 1980s, when the selective serotonin reuptake inhibitors (SSRIs) were found to possess substantial antidepressant efficacy. The SSRIs revolutionized the treatment of depression by offering efficacy with greatly reduced side-effect profiles.

Over the past decade, numerous atypical antidepressants have been developed, including norepinephrine and dopamine reuptake inhibitors (NDRIs), serotonin-norepinephrine reuptake inhibitors (SNRIs), and serotonin-2 antagonist/reuptake inhibitors (SARIs). These newer agents are currently undergoing clinical trials to assess their relative efficacy when compared with that of standard TCAs and SSRIs. When first reported to be analgesic, TCAs were thought to work via relieving the depression component of pain. It is now well known that relieving depression by any method is likely to decrease pain. Not all antidepressants, however, have independent analgesic properties.

1. Cyclic antidepressants

Indications

TCAs are approved by the U.S. Food and Drug Administration (FDA) for the treatment of major depressive disorders, and for the treatment of secondary depression in other disorders. In treating chronic pain, they are considered to have independent analgesic effects. A reasonable goal for using TCAs as analgesics is decreasing pain intensity from unbearable to bearable. Some mild side effects may be unavoidable in exchange for analgesia.

Mechanisms

All tricyclics inhibit both serotonergic and noradrenergic reuptake; and these effects are seen early, whereas clinical benefits often begin 2 to 3 weeks after initiation of treatment.

Misconceptions

Misconceptions about TCAs as analgesics are common. For instance, there is not a clear therapeutic window of dosages above and below which analgesia is diminished. Another misconception is that analgesia requires only low doses of TCA. Evidence suggests that analgesia is maximized with increased doses as well as with time. The time course of TCA analgesia varies between 1 and 120 days, suggesting that initial early analgesia is maximized over time. Duration of TCA analgesia also persists over time with maintenance of therapy. Thus, when clinicians choose to use TCAs as analgesics, they are encouraged to be patient with effects that may increase over weeks and to push the dosage upward, as long as side effects are tolerated, to increase efficacy.

Adverse reactions

The main side effects of cyclic antidepressant drugs include anticholinergic reactions (constipation and dry mouth) and cardiovascular effects. Other effects include orthostasis, sedation, extrapyramidal syndromes (tics, tremor, dyskinesia), weight gain, and sexual dysfunction. Prior to initiating treatment, routine laboratory screening may include a complete blood count, electrolytes (disturbances such as hypokalemia can precipitate cardiac arrhythmias), blood urea nitrogen, creatinine, and liver function tests. Some possible side effects of TCAs include jaundice, leukopenia, and rashes.

Other screening may include an electrocardiogram: although tricyclics are antiarrhythmic at therapeutic dosages, at supratherapeutic dosages they can be cardiotoxic. They can increase myocardial irritability, induce hypotension and tachycardia, decrease contractility, and increase conduction delays. Relative contraindications include second-degree heart block, structural heart disease, right bundle branch, and left bundle branch block. As patients with any of these disorders may develop bradyarrhythmia when prescribed tricyclics, they should be started on low doses that increase gradually, and they should be monitored by a cardiologist. Recent myocardial infarction is an absolute contraindication, as is closed-angle glaucoma.

TCAs interact with multiple neurotransmitter systems and as a result present with a wider side-effect profile than SSRIs. Combining TCAs with opioids can lead to decreased intestinal motility, already a problem for many patients taking opioids. Additive anticholinergic and opioid effects on the bowels can lead to treatment-resistant constipation or ileus.

Withdrawal may manifest as anxiety, fever, sweating, myalgia, headache, nausea, vomiting, dizziness, dyskinesia, or akathisia. Overdose with TCAs can be lethal. Toxicity results from anticholinergic effects and central nervous system (CNS) effects (including seizures and coma). The most hazardous side effect is cardiac toxicity, especially QRS complex widening. TCA overdose is a leading cause of drug-related overdose sequelae and death. Since three to five times the therapeutic dose of a TCA is potentially lethal, this low therapeutic index (ratio of toxic to therapeutic dose) should make prescribers vigilant. This is probably a large part of the reason SSRIs are often chosen over TCAs as first-line antidepressants.

Dosages and monitoring

As a general principle, dosing should start at the low end of the dose range and be titrated upward in 10- to 25-mg increments per week until a therapeutic level is reached (Table 1). As this minimizes side effects, patients are less likely to reject the therapy. Titration may need to be more rapid when TCAs are used for depression. Although somewhat controversial, it is generally agreed that plasma levels may be clinically valuable when using imipramine, desipramine, or nortriptyline to treat depression. Controversy on this issue stems from unclear correlation of plasma levels with clinical effects. Plasma levels of nortriptyline may be especially useful, because a therapeutic level may exist at a dose (e.g., 150 mg) above which the drug is actually less effective.

The effects of all antidepressants are often delayed. They may be seen anywhere from 2 to 6 weeks after beginning a trial at therapeutic dosages. If the drug is found to be effective, the patient should continue the medication for 6 to 12 months to prevent relapse. The dosage should not be decreased during the maintenance phase of treatment. If a patient has had multiple recurrences of illness, an indefinite length of treatment may be indicated.

Table 1. Tricyclic antidepressants

Medication	Proprietary Name	Dosage Range (mg/day)	Anticholinergic Activity	Central Action	Hypotension	Sedation
Tertiary amines						
Imipramine[a]	Tofranil	10–300	Moderate	N/S	Moderate	Moderate
Amitriptyline[a]	Elavil	10–300	Strong	S(N)	Strong	Strong
Clomipramine[a]	Anafranil	25–300	Moderate	S(N)	Strong	Mild
Doxepin	Sinequan	10–300	Moderate	S	Strong	Mild
Secondary amines						
Desipramine[a]	Norpramin	10–300	Minimal	N	Mild	Minimal
Nortriptyline[a]	Pamelor	10–200	Mild	N/S	Moderate	Mild
Protriptyline	Vivactil	10–60	Moderate	N	Minimal	Mild
Amoxapine	Asendin	50–400	Minimal	N	Mild	Minimal

[a] Commonly used for neuropathic pain

S, serotonergic; N, norepinephrinergic; (N), weakly norepinephrinergic in quantitative sensory testing.

2. Monoamine oxidase inhibitors

Indications

MAOIs (Table 2) are approved for use in major depression, double depression (dysthymia superimposed on major depression), psychotic depression, social phobia, and simple phobias, and they are often also used to treat anxiety, panic disorder, and obsessive-compulsive disorder. They are not considered first-line agents in the treatment of major depression because of their high incidence of side effects, dietary restrictions, and lethality in overdose. "Atypical" subtypes of depression involving mood reactivity, increased appetite, hypersomnia, leaden paralysis, and rejection sensitivity may respond better to MAOIs than to other agents.

Mechanisms

MAOIs work by binding to the enzyme monoamine oxidase, thus inhibiting the breakdown of monoamines at the synaptic junction. This results in increased concentration and availability of the neurotransmitters epinephrine, norepinephrine, and dopamine at various storage sites in the central and sympathetic nervous system.

MAOIs require up to 2 weeks to achieve maximal MAO inhibition, and clinical effects may not be seen for 2 to 4 weeks, although an energizing effect may occur within a few days following initiation of treatment. Table 2 offers some dosage guidelines for MAOIs. Unlike standard TCAs and SSRIs, MAOIs have a short half-life and require twice-daily dosing; this factor can be significant.

Adverse reactions

Patients taking MAOIs should avoid foods high in tyramine content, such as cheeses, yeast supplements, and aged alcohols, as they may precipitate a hypertensive crisis. Symptoms include occipital headache, neck stiffness or soreness, dilated pupils, tachycardia or bradycardia, and constricting chest pain. MAOIs should be used with caution in patients with cerebrovascular disease, cardiovascular disease, or hypertension.

Side effects include constipation, anorexia, nausea, vomiting, dry mouth, urinary retention, drowsiness, headache, dizziness, and weakness. As with SSRIs and TCAs, sexual dysfunction may occur, manifested as impotence, anorgasmia, decreased libido, ejaculation difficulties, and, rarely, priapism.

TCAs and SSRIs should be used very cautiously with MAOIs: fatalities have been reported in patients taking fluoxetine with MAOIs. Concomitant use of MAOIs and SSRIs or meperidine runs a risk for development of serotonin syndrome. Symptoms of sero-

Table 2.   Monoamine oxidase inhibitors

Medication	Proprietary Name	Dosage Range (mg/day)
Isocarboxacid	Marplan	30–50
Phenelzine	Nardil	45–90
Tranylcypromine	Parnate	20–60

tonin syndrome include CNS irritability, myoclonus, diaphoresis, and elevated temperature. Severe cases may result in death. Patients should discontinue MAOIs for at least 2 weeks before beginning an SSRI.

Dosages and monitoring

It appears that optimal antidepressant efficacy occurs when MAOIs are given at doses that reduce MAO activity by at least 80% (see Table 2). Liver function tests should be monitored periodically, as MAOIs are associated with hepatotoxicity. With long-term use, MAOIs may impair their own metabolism. Unfortunately, MAOI serum levels are not useful for guiding therapy.

3. Selective serotonin reuptake inhibitors

Indications

Since the introduction of fluoxetine (Prozac) in 1987, several other SSRIs have been introduced and have revolutionized first-line therapy for depression (Table 3). Although SSRIs were initially introduced for use in major depressive disorder, the FDA has approved the use of these agents for other indications, including panic disorder, bulimia nervosa, and obsessive-compulsive disorder. In addition, SSRIs are often used by clinicians for a variety of other conditions, including premenstrual syndrome, chronic fatigue syndrome, intermittent explosive disorder, and chronic pain management.

Mechanisms

SSRIs act via specific mechanisms in the CNS and may have fewer side effects than other antidepressants as a result. The immediate effect of the SSRIs on the CNS is blockade of the presynaptic serotonin reuptake pump. Although there are reports of SSRI-induced analgesia, to date these are largely anecdotal. The only controlled trial [by Max (1992)] did not find these agents to possess independent analgesia.

Adverse reactions

SSRIs have fewer side effects than many other antidepressants because they have minimal effects on neurotransmitters other than serotonin, although they may cause some undesirable symptoms. Possible CNS effects include headaches, stimulation or sedation, fine tremor, tinnitus, and rare extrapyramidal symptoms including dystonia, akathisia, dyskinesia, and possibly tar-

Table 3. Selective serotonin reuptake inhibitors

Medication	Proprietary Name	Dosage Range (mg/day)
Fluoxetine	Prozac	10–80
Fluvoxamine	Luvox	50–300
Paroxetine	Paxil	10–50
Sertraline	Zoloft	50–200
Venlafaxine	Effexor	75–225

dive dyskinesia. Cardiovascular effects are rare, but there are reports of tachycardia, bradycardia, palpitations, and vasoconstriction. Gastrointestinal effects include nausea, vomiting, anorexia, bloating, and diarrhea. The limited sedation associated with these agents makes them ideal additions for patients who are on sedating analgesics and experiencing pain. Other serotonergic drugs should be avoided or used with caution because of the possibility that serotonergic syndrome may develop. Approximately 10% to 15 % of patients taking an SSRI experience sexual side effects of decreased libido, impotence, ejaculatory disturbances, and anorgasmia.

Dosages and monitoring

No initial laboratory workup is required. Dosage titration is usually based on clinical response and side effects. Beneficial effects are usually not seen prior to 2 to 3 weeks. Dosages must be tapered slowly to avoid withdrawal symptoms.

4. Atypical antidepressants

Other classes of antidepressants have been developed to target specific neurotransmitter interactions at the synaptic level. They maximize therapeutic benefits while minimizing side effects. Included are norepinephrine and NDRIs such as bupropion (Wellbutrin), SNRIs such as venlafaxine (Effexor), and SARIs represented by trazodone (Desyrel).

Bupropion, an NDRI, is metabolized to hydroxybupropion, a powerful inhibitor of both noradrenergic and dopaminergic pumps. This agent differs from most other antidepressants in that it has psychostimulant properties. There have been no controlled clinical trials of its efficacy in the treatment of chronic pain; however, its stimulating properties offer advantages in treating depression in patients on sedating drugs such as opioids.

Treatment should be initiated at 75 to 100 mg once per day, starting in the morning to avoid potential insomnia. It can then be given twice daily and the dose can be gradually increased, although never above 450 mg/day or 150 mg in a single dose. A new sustained-release form is available, saving the practitioner from concern about dosage splitting. Seizures occur in approximately 0.4% of patients at dosages less than 450 mg/day, and in 4% of patients when dosages range from 450 to 600 mg/day. Therefore, dosages above 450 mg/day should be avoided. Bupropion should also be avoided in patients with seizure disorder or those taking medications that may cause seizures. The most common adverse effects are headache, insomnia, upper respiratory complaints, nausea, restlessness, agitation, and irritability. In overdose, dosages as high as 4,200 mg have been taken without death.

Venlafaxine is an SNRI with some anecdotal evidence of efficacy in the treatment of chronic pain. Potential analgesia is suggested by its profile of dual inhibition of serotonin and norepinephrine reuptake, which is similar to that of proven analgesic antidepressants such as imipramine, amitriptyline, and desipramine. Venlafaxine differs from these agents in its lack of anticholinergic, antiadrenergic, and antihistaminergic side effects, a difference that has unknown bearing on analgesia.

Although venlafaxine is available in extended-release form, it is traditionally given in two or three divided daily doses beginning at 75 mg/day and increased to as high as 375 mg/day. No laboratory studies are indicated and serum levels of venlafaxine are clinically useful. Side effects include nausea, headache, somnolence, dry mouth, dizziness, nervousness, constipation, anxiety, anorexia, blurred vision, and sexual dysfunction. No reports of fatal overdose have been reported. Venlafaxine should not be used in conjunction with MAOIs, and it may affect the hepatic metabolism of other medications.

Trazodone and **nefazodone** are SARIs by virtue of blocking serotonin-2 receptors as well as serotonin reuptake. These agents are used for depression and insomnia. Their usefulness in the treatment of chronic pain is undetermined, but given the incidence of insomnia in pain patients, they are likely to have at least a potential adjuvant role. Trazodone is less effective for the treatment of depression than nefazodone, although trazodone may be more sedating.

Dosages should begin as low as 50 mg/day but can be increased to as high as 600 mg/day in twice-daily divided doses. No laboratory studies are indicated before beginning SARIs, and plasma levels are not clinically useful. Side effects include sedation, orthostatic hypotension, dizziness, headache, nausea, dry mouth, and gastrointestinal (GI) upset. There are no anticholinergic effects of SARIs. Rare cases of cardiac arrhythmias have been reported. An infrequent but serious side effect is priapism (1/1,000 to 1/10,000), and patients should be warned of this prior to starting treatment. There have been no reported cases of death following overdose with SARIs taken alone.

SARIs should not be used in conjunction with MAOIs. Also, use with astemizole or terfenadine may decrease hepatic P450 metabolism of these compounds, resulting in cardiac arrhythmias. Finally, SARIs may increase serum levels of triazolam (Halcion) and alprazolam (Xanax).

II. ANTIPSYCHOTICS

Indications

Antipsychotics are used to treat various psychoses and schizophrenia, as well as psychotic symptoms such as paranoid disorders, schizophreniform disorder, brief psychoses, and psychoses associated with mood disorders. They have been used to treat pain as well as personality disturbances, although the potentially permanent side effect of tardive dyskinesia makes chronic usage inadvisable.

Antipsychotics are also known as neuroleptics because of the often-irreversible side effects they produce. Because neuroleptic agents poses some degree of independent analgesia, they can have a role in chronic pain when used for very short periods of time. Their potential efficacy may be further realized with the advent of new antipsychotic agents that may have greatly reduced side effect profiles. Should the risk of tardive dyskinesia be eliminated, chronic usage of these agents would be markedly safer and thus the analgesia they offer may be more attractive as an adjunct in the treatment of chronic pain.

1. Typical neuroleptics

Mechanisms

Typical neuroleptics (Table 4) function as antipsychotics as a result of their dopaminergic antagonism, particularly at postsynaptic D2 receptors, probably in pathways from the midbrain to the limbic system and the temporal and frontal lobes. Typical neuroleptics also may affect cholinergic, alpha-1-adrenergic, and histaminic systems. These actions are responsible for many of the significant side effects of typical neuroleptics.

Adverse reactions

Antipsychotics carry a risk of extrapyramidal symptoms including acute dystonia, akathisia, pseudoparkinsonism, and tardive dyskinesia; those with the least anticholinergic effects have the greatest risk. Neuroleptics also have effects on numerous hormonal systems. Prolactin may be elevated by neuroleptics, with possible effects that include amenorrhea, galactorrhea, and false-positive pregnancy tests in women and gynecomastia and galactorrhea in men. Neuroleptics may cause hypothalamic dysfunction (leading to the syndrome of inappropriate antidiuretic hormone and to temperature regulation difficulties) or disrupt serum glucose levels. Neuroleptic malignant syndrome is a particularly serious, albeit rare, event.

Table 4. Typical neuroleptics

Medication	Proprietary Name
Phenothiazine	
Aliphatic	
Chlorpromazine	Thorazine
Piperidine	
Mesoridazine	Senentil
Thioridazine	Mellaril
Piperazine	
Fluphenazine	Prolixin
Perphenazine	Trilafon
Trifluoperazine	Stelazine
Thioxanthenes	
Thiothixene	Navane
Butyrophenone	
Haloperidol	Haldol
Diphenylbutylpiperidines	
Pimozide	Orap
Dibenzoxazepine	
Loxapine	Daxolin, Loxitane
Dihydroindolone	
Molindone	Moban
Dibenzodiazepine	Clozaril
Clozapine	

Anticholinergic activity may cause dry membranes, blurred vision, constipation, urinary retention, and confusion or delirium. Histaminic effects include sedation, cognitive impairment, and weight gain. A combination of dopaminergic, anticholinergic, and alpha-1-adrenergic effects may cause sexual dysfunction. In addition, neuroleptics may lower the seizure threshold, seen most in lower-potency agents such as chlorpromazine (Thorazine) and least in high-potency agents such as haloperidol. Cardiovascular effects include hypotension, tachycardia, dizziness, fainting, nonspecific electrocardiographic changes, and rarely arrhythmias, including *torsades de pointes*, and sudden cardiac death.

2. ATYPICAL NEUROLEPTICS

Dosages and monitoring

No routine laboratory tests are necessary for the prescribing of antipsychotic agents. The physician should be aware of the emergence of extrapyramidal side effects and should warn patients about potential tardive dyskinesia.

Mechanisms

The atypical neuroleptics include agents such as risperidone (Risperdal), clozapine (Clozaril), and olanzapine (Zyprexa) (Table 5). These agents have D2 antagonism but to a lesser degree than typical neuroleptics. Additionally, they appear to block serotonin-2 receptors and, to variable degrees, the D4 receptor. Atypical neuroleptics may be more efficacious than typical neuroleptics, particularly with negative psychotic symptoms. However, no controlled studies of the use of atypical neuroleptics in the treatment of chronic pain have been conducted. One advantage of atypical neuroleptics over typical neuroleptics is the lower incidence of extrapyramidal side effects.

Adverse effects

Clozapine is considered a second-line treatment because of the possibility of fatal agranulocytosis in about 1% of patients. Olanzapine is similar in structure and mechanism to clozapine. Olanzapine has a low drug interaction potential and reduced incidence of extrapyramidal side effects. No incidents of leukopenia have been reported for olanzapine. Risperidone also has reduced incidence of extrapyramidal side effects and, like olanzapine, is not associated with agranulocytosis. Olanzapine appears to be more sedating than risperidone; risperidone can cause insomnia.

Table 5. Atypical neuroleptics

Medication	Proprietary Name
Risperidone	Risperdol
Clozapine	Clozaril
Olanzapine	Zyprexa

III. MOOD STABILIZERS

Indications

Mood stabilizers are used to treat bipolar disorder, which involves alternating periods and degrees of mania and depression. Lithium is the classic agent for treating bipolar disorder, but recently many other agents such as anticonvulsants (valproic acid, carbamazepine, gabapentin, and clonazepam) have gained popularity. The overlap of this group of drugs with those used to treat neuropathic pain is striking, and the meaning of this has not yet been clarified.

Whereas bipolar disorder is not overly common in the patient with chronic pain, it does occur and can be worsened by drugs that are commonly in the arsenal for pain. Analgesic agents that may provoke mania include antidepressants as well as steroids. However, several agents that are specifically effective against neuropathic pain also are helpful in treating bipolar disorder (i.e., carbamazepine and gabapentin) and are thus clear choices for treatment of comorbid bipolar disorder and chronic pain.

Lithium

Lithium has been used extensively for treatment of migraine and cluster headaches. However, there is no evidence of efficacy in the treatment of any other type of chronic pain. Lithium remains the most commonly used agent for treating bipolar disorder. A narrow therapeutic index and its frequent side effects limit its use.

Anticonvulsants

At present, it appears that all commonly used neuropathic analgesics are anticonvulsants, in that these agents are either directly used as antiseizure agents or otherwise as antiarrhythmics or local anesthetics. Anticonvulsant drugs, including carbamazepine (Tegretol), valproate (Depakote), phenytoin (Dilantin), gabapentin (Neurontin), and clonazepam (Klonopin) are widely used for treating chronic pain, neuropathic pain in particular. This same group of drugs is being used more and more widely in treating psychiatric disorders.

Mechanisms

The mechanisms of action of this diverse group are certainly varied, but all are thought to act as membrane stabilizers. Phenytoin and carbamazepine slow the rate of recovery of voltage-activated sodium ion channels from inactivity. Valproic acid is believed to increase gamma-aminobutyric acid (GABA) concentrations in the brain, clonazepam stimulates GABAergic pathways, and the action of gabapentin is unknown (although it functions as a GABA analog, it does not act as GABA receptors). The mechanism of lithium's therapeutic effects is unknown, but it is postulated to be either endocrine, neurotransmissive, circadian, or cellular. Lithium is not a sedative, depressant, or euphoriant. Possible side effects include blood dyscrasias (although less common than with carbamazepine) and hepatitis.

IV. ANXIOLYTICS

Anxiety disorders may occur in a large percentage of patients with chronic pain. These disorders include panic disorder, generalized anxiety disorder, obsessive-compulsive disorder, and post-traumatic stress disorder. These often present with somatic symptoms including chest pain, GI upset, and neurologic symptoms (headache, dizziness, syncope, and paresthesias). Treatment of chronic pain that is comorbid with an anxiety disorder should include anxiolysis as part of the analgesic strategy.

1. Benzodiazepines

Benzodiazepines are the most popular medication for anxiety and in fact are the most widely prescribed medication of any type. Clonazepam is considered both a psychotropic agent (anxiolytic) and a neurologic agent (anticonvulsant). This suggests its possible usefulness in the pain clinic pharmacologic armamentarium.

Indications

Benzodiazepines are approved for use with anxiety disorders, alcohol withdrawal seizures, and insomnia. They have also been used to treat akathisia, agitation (including mania), depression, catatonia, and muscle spasm.

Mechanisms

Benzodiazepines depress the CNS at the levels of the limbic system, brainstem reticular activating formation, and cortex by binding to and facilitating the action of GABA. Although they are not primary analgesics, benzodiazepines often have a role in the analgesic regimen.

Adverse reactions

The most common side effect of benzodiazepines is sedation and respiratory depression. Rapid withdrawal from benzodiazepines can result in rebound insomnia, anxiety, delirium, or other withdrawal symptoms. Severe withdrawal reactions include seizures, psychosis, and death. Discontinue dosages by gradually tapering.

Dosages and monitoring

As with any medication in which tolerance develops, dosage ranges tend to be open-ended. In overdose, benzodiazepines are rarely fatal if taken alone, although they may cause respiratory depression. If taken with alcohol or barbiturates, however, benzodiazepines can be fatal, with symptoms including hypotension, depressed respiration, and coma. The choice of a specific benzodiazepine is often based on onset of action and half-life (Table 6). In general, short-acting agents are used to treat insomnia and acute anxiety, whereas long-acting agents are used to treat chronic conditions.

2. Buspirone (buSpar)

Although not known to be efficacious for the treatment of pain, buspirone can be an effective anxiolytic. Buspirone acts as a 5-HT-1A agonist. Buspirone may potentiate the antidepressant and antiobsessional effects of SSRIs. It is also being studied for use in post-traumatic stress disorder.

No laboratory studies are required before initiating treatment with buspirone. Patients may take 5 to 30 mg/day in divided doses, starting at 5 mg three times a day and increasing to as high as

Table 6. Benzodiazepines: onset and half life

Medication	Proprietary Name	Onset	Half-life (hrs)
Alprazolam	Xanax	Intermediate	6–20
Chlordiazepoxide	Librium	Intermediate	30–100
Clonazepam	Klonopin	Intermediate	18–50
Clorazepate	Tranxene	Rapid	30–100
Diazepam	Valium	Rapid	30–100
Estazolam	Prosom	Intermediate	10–24
Flurazepam	Dalmane	Rapid-intermediate	50–160
Lorazepam	Ativan	Intermediate	10–20
Midazolam	Versed	Intermediate	2–3
Oxazepam	Serax	Intermediate-slow	8–12
Quazepam	Doral	Rapid-intermediate	50–160
Temazepam	Restoril	Intermediate	8–20
Triazolam	Halcion	Intermediate	1.5–5

10 mg three times a day. Anxiolytic effects require 1 to 4 weeks to appear. Buspirone has relatively few side effects; less than 10% of patients experience headache, dizziness, lightheadedness, fatigue, paresthesias, and GI upset. Buspirone has a low potential for abuse or addiction and it does not impair psychomotor or cognitive functions. There have been no reports of withdrawal symptoms or death from overdose. However, buspirone should be used with caution in patients taking MAOIs, as this combination may result in elevated blood pressure. Also, buspirone inhibits the metabolism of benzodiazepines and haloperidol.

V. PSYCHOSTIMULANTS

Indications

Although approved indications for psychostimulants include attention deficit disorder, Parkinson's disease, and narcolepsy, they are also used for treatment-resistant depression, to augment antidepressants, and in the treatment of sedation or fatigue in terminal illness. They are the only immediate-acting "antidepressants." Although they have been used as so-called diet pills, they can improve appetite in cancer treatment. Additionally, psychostimulants are used to counter iatrogenic sedation, most commonly caused by opioid analgesics. Common psychostimulants include dextroamphetamine, methylphenidate, and magnesium pemoline.

Mechanisms

At normal dosages, amphetamines stimulate the release of norepinephrine. As the dosage increases, they cause the release of dopamine, which accounts for the behavioral changes and the reinforcing properties. At excessive dosages, amphetamines cause the release of serotonin, which may be associated with the amphetamine psychosis. Methylphenidate blocks the reuptake of dopamine. Magnesium pemoline exhibits effects similar to those of amphetamines and methylphenidate. The stimulant effects appear to be mediated through dopaminergic mechanisms, but weak sympathomimetic effects are also involved. Tachyphylaxis associated with psychostimulants results from their being indirect agonists. Thus, by stimulating the release of endogenous neurotransmitters, they deplete the stores of these mediators.

Adverse reactions

Risk factors include hypertension and tachyarrhythmias, and tension. Liver disease is a contraindication (pemoline is not used as a first-line treatment because of reports of late-onset hepatotoxicity), as are functional psychosis, anxiety, and anorexia. A 20% to 50% incidence of tics occurs in patients with Tourette's syndrome. Other adverse effects commonly seen include anorexia, irritation, sadness, and clingy behavior.

Dosages and monitoring

Psychostimulants should be used cautiously in patients with existing drug or alcohol abuse problems. Start at a low dosage and then increase gradually over several days (Table 7). Because of its short half-life, methylphenidate must be dosed twice daily (it is also available in extended release form). Patients should not stop taking the drug abruptly.

VI. CONCLUSION

Treating pain often requires the use of medications that impact both nociceptive and non-nociceptive processes. Without adequate familiarity with psychopharmacologic agents, the pain specialist risks having a limited analgesic repertoire and may overlook potentially beneficial possibilities as well as potential adverse complications of polypharmacy. The ongoing revolution in development

Table 7.   Psychostimulants: dosage and cautions

Generic Name	Proprietary Name	Dosage	Cautions
Dextroamphe-tamine	Dexedrine, Dextrostat	5–60 mg/day	Abuse potential
Methyl-phenidate	Ritalin	10–30 mg/day	Same abuse potential as amphetamines Tourette's is a contraindication.
Magnesium pemoline	Cylert	37.5–112.5 mg/day; dose depends on age	Long half-life (9–14 hrs) means once-a-day dosing is possible. Not used as first-line because of association with hepatotoxicity

of psychoactive drugs will surely impact pain management, and drugs will very likely gain increased prominence in the arsenal against pain.

SELECTED READING

1. Bezchlibnyk-Butler KZ, Jeffries JJ, Martin BA, eds. *Clinical handbook of psychotropic drugs*, 4th ed. Seattle: Hogrefe Huber, 1994.
2. Bloom FE, Kupfer DJ, eds. *Psychopharmacology: The fourth generation of progress*. New York: Raven Press, 1995.
3. Ciraulo DA, Shader RI, Greenblatt DJ, Creelman W, eds. *Drug interactions in psychiatry*, 2nd ed. Baltimore: Williams & Wilkins, 1995.
4. Guze B, Richeimer S, Szuba M, eds. *The psychiatric drug handbook*. St. Louis: Mosby–Year Book, 1995.
5. Hyman SE, Arana GW, Rosenbaum JF, eds. *Handbook of psychiatric drug therapy*, 3rd ed. Boston: Little, Brown, 1995.
6. Kaplan HI, Sadock BJ, eds. *Comprehensive textbook of psychiatry*, 6th ed. Philadelphia: Williams & Wilkins, 1995.
7. Magni G. The use of antidepressants in the treatment of chronic pain: A review of the current evidence. *Drugs* 1991;42:730–748.
8. Sindrup SH, Brosen K, Gram LF. Antidepressants in pain treatment: Antidepressant or analgesic effect? *Clin Neuropharmacol* 1992;15(suppl 1):636A–637A.
9. Stahl SM. *Essential psychopharmacology: Neuroscientific basis and clinical applications*. Boston: Cambridge University Press, 1996.
10. Zitman FG, Linssen AC, Edelbroek PM, Van Kempen GM. Clinical effectiveness of antidepressants and antipsychotics in chronic benign pain. *Clin Neuropharmacol* 1992;15(suppl 1):377A–378A.
11. Max MB, Lynch SA, Muir J, Shouf SE, Smoller B, Dubner R. Effects of desipramine, amitriptyline, and fluoxetine on pain in diabetic neuropathy. *N Engl J Med* 1992;326:1250–1256.

Therapeutic Options: Nonpharmacologic Approaches

Diagnostic and Therapeutic Procedures in Pain Management

Salahadin Abdi and YiLi Zhou

This chapter outlines the major diagnostic and therapeutic procedures performed at the Massachusetts General Hospital (MGH) Pain Center. We have found these procedures to be valuable and to have a good safety record. Many of these techniques were developed by Donald Todd, who founded the Pain Unit in 1948. They have been refined over the years and are now effective, reliable, and reasonably free of unwanted effects, and we continue to use them and teach them to our fellows and residents.

The specific nerve blocks described involve the use of C-arm fluoroscopy, which reflects standard practice at MGH.

I. GENERAL PRINCIPLES

1. Diagnostic versus therapeutic procedures

Before starting a procedure, the clinician determines whether to perform a diagnostic or a therapeutic procedure and prepares the patients accordingly. Diagnostic blocks are utilized for the following reasons:

- To evaluate and compare the roles of the sympathetic and somatosensory nerves in maintaining pain (differential nerve blocks)
- To identify the particular nerve(s) that carry pain, or to alter neuromuscular function (selective nerve blocks)

For example, we may want to know the answers to the following questions. Is there a significant sympathetic component to a painful limb syndrome? Which of several bulging vertebral discs is actually causing pain by its impingement on a nerve root? Are degenerating facet joints causing a low back pain syndrome? Or, which intercostal nerve(s) are causing pain in a patient with chest wall metastases?

Diagnostic nerve blocks help to identify the source of pain and to structure a treatment plan. The treatment plan could involve medical treatment (e.g., emphasis on neuropathic pain medications), further nerve blocks (e.g., a series of sympathetic blocks with physical therapy), permanent neurolysis (e.g., radiofrequency lesioning of nerves in the facet joint, alcohol ablation of intercostal nerves or celiac plexus), or referral to a surgeon for surgical decompression of a disc.

In performing a diagnostic block for sympathetic pain, the clinician must choose a site at which the anesthetic is unlikely to affect somatic nerves, as this would interfere with interpretation (e.g., stellate and lumbar sympathetic ganglion, versus intrapleural and epidural). In the case of somatic pain, very small, concentrated amounts of anesthetic are used at each site so that the blocks are localized to specific nerves. This degree of accuracy requires C-arm fluoroscopic guidance.

Before a diagnostic block is performed, the clinician must be sure that the patient has sustained and reproducible pain and must document what activities or stimuli evoke the pain. These factors can then be reassessed after the block and compared to the pre-block state. Finally, the clinician must confirm (by objective testing) that the block was actually accomplished.

The use of placebo agents (e.g., saline instead of local anesthetic) for diagnostic procedures is unethical and strongly discouraged. This practice is likely to be helpful only in identifying placebo responders, not in identifying those with "real" versus psychogenic pain. Furthermore, the practice may damage the patient–physician relationship, and it may reduce the placebo effect of future treatments (see Chapter 3).

2. Pre-block management

Patients are requested to consume only light meals on the day of a procedure, and to take only clear liquids for 4 hours prior to the procedure. Baseline vital signs (including pain scale) are obtained at arrival in the clinic. If indicated, an 18- or 20-gauge intravenous (IV) catheter with Hep-Lock is placed. An IV is routinely placed in patients undergoing procedures that are associated with a risk of sympathectomy and hypotension (e.g., stellate ganglion block, lumbar sympathetic nerve block, cervical epidural steroid injection). The medical condition of the patient could also dictate that an IV should be placed (e.g., extreme anxiety, history of vasovagal syncope, significant cardiovascular disease). In general, premedication is avoided so that the baseline pain is not altered and so that patient cooperation is maintained.

The patient is positioned appropriately, and monitors are placed as needed. Decisions about the level of monitoring needed are made on an individual basis using criteria similar to those for IV placement. The usual monitors are noninvasive blood pressure, electrocardiogram (EKG), and pulse oximetry. Baseline verbal analog scores (VAS) and range of motion estimates are obtained before starting the procedure.

3. Choice of injectant

Local anesthetic

For most diagnostic nerve or plexus blocks, a mixture of equal parts of 1% lidocaine and 0.5% bupivacaine is used (giving a final concentration of 0.5% lidocaine and 0.25% bupivacaine). This adequately blocks sympathetic and somatic nerves, and a sufficient volume can be used without toxicity. Lidocaine provides rapid onset of effect, whereas bupivacaine provides a useful prolongation of the effect so that patients can make observations that may have diagnostic value. It is not necessary to use epinephrine-containing solutions in the pain clinic setting. In fact, in emotionally labile patients [e.g., those with complex regional pain syndrome I (CRPS-I)], epinephrine may cause a panic attack and is best avoided.

Steroids

The steroids currently used are depot preparations of methylprednisolone (Depo-Medrol) and triamcinolone (Aristocort, which may be irritating, and Kenalog, which is less irritating but allergenic). The doses generally range between 40 and 80 mg for epidural injection and between 20 and 40 mg for selective nerve root injection. We typically use 80 mg of triamcinolone for epidural injection and 20 mg for selective nerve root injection.

Neurolytic agents

Alcohol (50% to 95%) and phenol (6% to 10%) are the two agents commonly used for neurolysis. Alcohol has been extensively used as a neurolytic agent because it is effective and easy to inject. It is used as the neurolytic agent of choice for injecting into the trigeminal ganglion, celiac plexus, and lumbar sympathetic chain. Occasionally, neuritis with intense burning pain is seen after alcohol neurolysis. We inject local anesthetics prior to the neurolytic to localize the target nerve or plexus and to minimize the incidence of neuritis. The analgesic effect of phenol is almost equal to that of alcohol, but it does not produce neuritis, which is its advantage. It is extremely viscous and difficult to inject (needing a larger-bore needle and slow injection). Neither agent is isobaric in cerebrospinal fluid (CSF) (alcohol is hypobaric, phenol hyperbaric); therefore, patients need to be positioned appropriately according to the baricity of the agent chosen. Neurolytic blocks have a delayed effect (beginning within 1 week) that generally lasts for up to 1 year.

4. Defining landmarks

The needle insertion point is usually designated by measurement or by palpation, using x-ray (C-arm fluoroscopy) guidance. It is also helpful to use a "tunnel-view" technique to help define the correct needle angle, and to identify any bony obstructions to the passage of the needle (e.g., ribs) as it is guided toward the target for injection. First, rest the point of a metal clamp (e.g., a Kelly clamp) over the target site as seen on the radiograph, then over the skin insertion site. The position of the C-arm is then angled so that the tip of the clamp rests at the skin insertion point as well as at the target point. The chosen point is marked on the skin by firmly pressing the hub of a 15-gauge needle onto the skin for 30 to 60 seconds (the old fashioned way), or by using a special skin marker. The needle is then inserted through the skin mark in a direction parallel to the x-ray beam, toward the target point. Using this tunnel-view technique, the needle should reach the target without hitting the bone or other important structures. There are now commercially available laser-guided C-arms that help define the correct needle trajectory and obviate the use of markings.

5. Post-block management

Once the procedure is over, patients recover in the recovery room. When they meet standard recovery room discharge criteria, they are discharged home with an escort.

II. SPECIFIC BLOCKS

1. Epidural steroid injections

The intended effect of steroids is to reduce the inflammation, swelling, and scarring that arise as a consequence of disc extrusion and nerve pressure (or inflammation and scarring that occur elsewhere in the body, such as in tendonitis). Pathology studies have shown that steroids reduce the bulk of a scar by diminishing its hyaline portion while leaving the fibrous skeleton intact.

Indications
- Acute herniated or bulging disc
- Herniated nucleus pulposus, with nerve root irritation or compression
- Spinal stenosis
- Spondylolisthesis
- Scoliosis
- Chronic degenerative disc disease

Potential complications
- Dural puncture, with possible total spinal block
- Postdural puncture headache
- Epidural hematoma
- Epidural abscess; cutaneous infections; meningitis
- Intrathecal steroid injection, with potential complications such as anterior spinal artery syndrome, arachnoiditis, meningitis, urinary retention, and conus medullaris syndrome, as well as a lack of effect
- Spinal cord injury and paralysis

Block treatment protocol
We usually offer three epidural injections at 4-week intervals, as needed to ascertain a response. A steroid-free period of 6 months avoids possible ligamentous atrophy from steroid injections. The three-injection cycle of steroids may then be repeated if needed.

Patient position
The patient is prone, with feet over the end of the table and a bunched-up pillow under the abdomen (between iliac crests and costal margin) to reverse lumbar lordosis and for comfort. For the cervical approach, the pillow is placed under the chest (see later).

Supply a small support under the head if it is requested. The arms are relaxed over the sides of the table.

a) Lumbar translaminar approach

Technique

1. Locate the appropriate interspinous process space with the C-arm, using the tip of a Kelly clamp as marker. Mark spot on skin with the hub of a 15-gauge needle.
2. Prepare skin with Betadine and drape widely.
3. Begin intra- and subcutaneous 1% lidocaine infiltration slowly, and in small amount. Deep interspinous infiltration to full length of a 1½-inch, 22-gauge needle.
4. Insert 3½-inch, 22-gauge spinal needle in the plane of the C-arm (usually a little cephalad) down to the ligament.
5. Attach a well-lubricated 10-mL syringe to the needle, with 4 mL of air or saline in it. Holding the syringe (not the needle) with one hand, and pressing firmly with finger or thumb of the other hand on plunger, maintain positive pressure constantly while rapidly oscillating the plunger. Advance the needle slowly and steadily until a sudden loss of resistance is achieved (allow only a minimum of air to escape).
6. If depth of the needle (before the loss of resistance) seems inappropriate, withdraw needle 3 mm and repeat.
7. Inject 1 to 2 mL of dye (Omnipaque-240); confirm with fluoroscopy that the dye is spread inside the epidural space.
8. Inject 2 mL of 40 mg/mL triamcinolone with 0.5 mL to 2 mL of 0.5% bupivacaine, diluted with saline if desired.
9. Replace stylet in needle (to avoid tracking steroid through skin) and withdraw the needle.
10. With gauze pressure on needle hole, slide skin back and forth to stop bleeding, and close tract.
11. Apply adhesive bandage to be removed on reaching home.
12. Slowly sit the patient up; do not leave unattended until safely in wheelchair, as legs may be weak and buckle.

b) Lumbar paramedian approach

Technique

1. Skin wheal is made about 1 cm lateral and 1 cm caudad from the spinous process.
2. Remember, there is no interspinous ligament to provide resistance to air or saline. Resistance is encountered only when the ligamentum flavum is reached.
3. Proceed as in midline approach.

c) Lumbar transforaminal approach

This approach is useful if symptoms are mainly radicular, and if previous midline injections have not helped. Dose is usually reduced to 40 mg triamcinolone. Dilution is not needed.

d) Caudal epidural injection

This approach is useful if the patient has had multiple laminectomies that have resulted in severe scarring and an alteration of the normal anatomy. A total volume of 20 to 30 mL is needed to fill the caudal canal and reach the L5-S1 junction. The standard sacral hiatus approach is used. Using a lateral view on fluoroscopy will ensure needle placement in the sacral canal (Fig. 1).

e) Posterior S1 foramen approach

This approach is useful if epidural space is not otherwise accessible, and especially when symptoms are confined to the S1 or S2 level. About 5 to 15 mL (total volume) is needed to reach the L5-S1 junction, a common site of disease.

f) Cervical epidural injection

Cervical epidural is used for the treatment of neck and shoulder pain associated with cervical radiculopathy.

Technique

1. Place the patient in a prone position with a pillow under the chest to straighten the neck and open the cervical interspinous space.
2. Cervical interspinous space is identified with fluoroscopy.
3. A 1½-inch, 25-gauge spinal needle is inserted cephalad, parallel to the cervical spinous process at the midline.
4. Loss-of-resistance technique is used as described for lumbar epidural steroid injection.

A

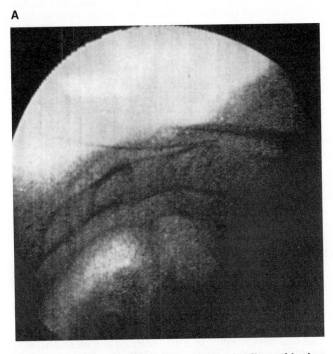

Figure 1.   Caudal epidural injection. A: Lateral radiographic view. B: Diagrammatic representation.

B

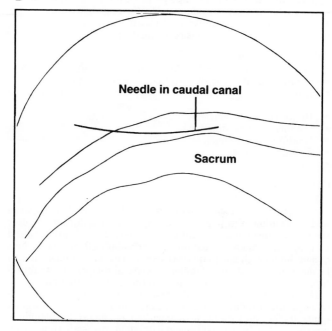

Figure 1.   *Continued.*

5. After negative aspiration, 0.5 to 1.0 mL of dye is injected to confirm correct needle position with anteroposterior (AP) and lateral views on fluoroscopy.
6. Inject 0.5 to 1.0 mL of solution including 20 to 40 mg of triamcinolone into epidural space without local anesthetics.
7. Use extreme caution to avoid injection into subarachnoid space and injury to cervical spine.

2. Central nerve blocks

(i) *Epidural blocks (catheters)*

We do not routinely employ cervical epidural catheters at MGH; therefore, this section focuses on lumbar and thoracic epidural catheter techniques. Epidurally administered local anesthetics block both somatic and sympathetic nerves. However, a predominantly sympathetic block, continuous or intermittent, can be achieved using dilute local anesthetic solutions (e.g., 0.1% to 0.25% bupivacaine). Somatic blockade is achieved by increasing the local anesthetic concentration (e.g., to 0.25% to 0.5% bupivacaine). For prolonged use, tunneled epidural catheters are placed.

Indications

• Pain syndromes resulting from peripheral vascular insufficiency, including ischemic vasospastic pain

- Sympathetically maintained pain, unilateral or bilateral
- Acute herpes zoster and postherpetic neuralgia
- Acute thoracic or lumbar strain with radiculopathy
- Regional pain syndromes resulting from malignancy

Potential complications
- Dural puncture and possible postdural puncture headache
- Subarachnoid injection with high spinal anesthesia
- Intravascular injection (e.g., into epidural veins), with possible seizures
- Broken epidural catheter
- Potential neural damage
- Epidural hematoma
- Epidural abscess
- Arachnoiditis

Catheter treatment management

Pain relief is achieved using a continuous infusion of 0.1% bupivacaine, up to 10 mL/hour, sometimes with the addition of opioids and/or clonidine. Vital signs are closely monitored during and after the initial bolus injection or infusion. If the catheter is to be utilized for continuous block, the patient is either admitted for several days or sent home with adequate instructions. Hospital admission may be desirable for intensive, in-house physical therapy. Diet and activity recommendations are based on the clinical situation.

If the catheter is to be used for cancer pain relief, 0.1% bupivacaine solution should be tried initially, but if pain relief is inadequate, 0.25% bupivacaine, with or without opioids and/or clonidine, may be needed. Infusions of opioid without local anesthetic are used in cancer patients in whom local anesthetics produce undesirable effects. Vital signs are monitored as described earlier. Activity and diet are as tolerated. If prolonged infusions are required, the catheter is tunneled subcutaneously at the time of placement.

a) Lumbar epidural catheters

Midline Approach

Technique
1. Patient lies in the lateral position, with maximal flexion of the back and with knees to the abdomen.
2. Obese patients should sit bent forward, with knees to the abdomen, or legs resting on a stool. This helps identify the midline and may widen the posterior interspinous space.
3. The spinal cord terminates at L1 or L2 in the adult; therefore, the spinous process, intervertebral space, and midline are carefully palpated below this level. An appropriate interspace is located.
4. The overlying skin is prepared with antiseptic solution (such as alcohol or Betadine), and a sterile, fenestrated drape is placed over the site.
5. A skin wheal is made with a ½-inch 25-gauge needle, using 1% lidocaine, and deeper infiltration is performed with a 1½-inch 22-gauge needle.
6. A 17- or 18-gauge Tuohy needle is directed perpendicularly or slightly cephalad in the interspinous space, bevel pointing cephalad, and advanced to the ligamentum flavum.

7. The stylet is removed, and a syringe containing 3 to 4 mL of air or saline is attached to the Tuohy needle. The needle is advanced, with rapid oscillation of the plunger of the syringe, until there is a loss of resistance. Loss of resistance may also be detected with continuous pressure on the plunger, advancing until pressure is lost. We do not recommend the hanging-drop method, as we have noted a higher incidence of dural punctures.

8. Medication or saline can be injected into the Tuohy needle to distend the epidural space. The catheter is advanced through the needle, no more than 5 cm into the epidural space.

9. The Tuohy needle is removed while the catheter is maintained in position. The distance between the catheter mark and the skin is measured to ensure that the catheter has not been moved during the needle removal.

10. The catheter is then secured to the skin with a transparent dressing and tested for intravascular or intrathecal placement with 3 mL of 2% lidocaine with epinephrine. Aspiration is also performed for blood or cerebrospinal fluid.

11. To decrease displacement of catheter tip, it is wise to bring the excess catheter around the flank to the epigastrium, rather than up the back and over the shoulder, as in operative cases. This is because flexing of the spine tends to pull the catheter back from the epidural space.

12. The catheter is then ready for use, either with bolus or continuous infusions.

Paramedian approach

Technique

1. A skin wheal is made 1 cm lateral and 2 cm caudad to the interspinous space chosen.

2. A 17- or 18-gauge Tuohy needle is aimed from the lateral skin wheal to the top of the target interspace (i.e., the needle is aimed medially and slightly cephalad).

3. The needle is advanced to the ligamentum flavum, and an air- or saline-filled syringe is attached.

4. After obtaining a loss of resistance, the catheter is threaded and the Tuohy needle is removed; after negative aspiration, the catheter is tested and secured, as earlier.

Tunneling

Technique

1. Place epidural catheter as described before.

2. Anesthetize a subcutaneous track, horizontally across one side of the back.

3. Tunnel a long, 14-gauge, 5½-inch IV catheter through the track, starting at the distal point and emerging in the same skin nick as the epidural catheter (Note: Do not puncture epidural catheter with IV needle.)

4. Remove needle from IV catheter and thread epidural catheter through IV catheter.

5. Remove IV catheter and secure epidural catheter at lateral skin exit wound, with transparent dressing.

6. The epidural catheter is tested (as before) and used for intermittent boluses or continuous infusion.

b) Thoracic epidural catheters

This procedure is performed as for lumbar epidural catheters. The choice of catheter location may vary, but the technique varies only in that additional care is required in approaching the epidural space, as the distances are less than those for the lumbar approach. Further, the needle must be aimed in a more cephalad direction to traverse the sloping thoracic interspinous space. Management and complications are similar to those of the lumbar epidural catheters.

(ii) *Selective nerve root blocks*

For the purpose of identifying a specific nerve root as a possible source of pain, only a small amount of local anesthetic (1 mL) is needed. This ensures that only the target nerve root is blocked and reduces the possibility of epidural spread of the local anesthetic. The forcible injection of local anesthetic (particularly of large volumes) directly into a nerve may disrupt it. The needle itself can also produce nerve damage if it pierces the nerve repeatedly. Nerve damage produced in this way can ultimately cause neuropathic pain. Selective blockade of thoracic nerve roots is not described or used at MGH because of the high risk of pneumothorax associated with these blocks. Intercostal nerve blocks are used instead (see II, 5).

Indications

- To determine the nerve root(s) involved in a pain syndrome. The surgeon can then proceed with more confidence in removing a disc, or in decompressing the root that carries the pain.
- To inject local anesthetics and/or steroid at the site of a scarred or compressed root, when pain has not been relieved by other approaches (e.g., epidural injection). This is particularly useful in lumbar and cervical radicular pain syndromes.

a) Cervical paravertebral nerve blocks

The cervical nerves leave the spine above their respective vertebrae, and the C1 root has no cutaneous sensory function. The C2 root emerges laterally, between the C1 and the C2 vertebrae, passes over the articular process of C1, and emerges between the posterior arches of C1 and C2. It is distributed mainly to the greater occipital nerve.

C2 nerve root block

The C2 root is best blocked as it passes over the posterior surface of the superior articular process of C2. Generally, it is simpler to block the occipital nerve, if that fulfills the need. With C-arm fluoroscopy guidance, and the patient in prone position, the needle is directed vertically down to the articular process, where a paresthesia may be obtained.

C3 through C6 nerve root blocks

Technique

1. Patient is positioned supine, flat (no pillow), head in neutral position or rotated away from side to be blocked. Anatomy is more symmetrical in neutral position, but it is more difficult to

palpate the site and to guide the needle. With the head rotated (it may be necessary to elevate shoulder on padding), it is easier to view the intervertebral foramen and to guide the needle into the foramen, but the anatomy of the neck becomes spiral (Fig. 2).

2. Using C-arm fluoroscopy, a skin mark is made over the posterior border of the intervertebral foramen image and slightly cephalad to it. Approaching the cervical nerve in its foramen from a posterior position avoids encountering the cervical plexus, since this lies lateral and anterior to the transverse processes.

3. A 2½-inch, 22-gauge spinal needle is advanced so as to encounter the superior surface of the groove in the transverse process that supports the nerve. The needle is then deviated toward the intervertebral opening until a paresthesia is obtained (Fig. 3).

4. The C-arm is then rotated to the AP position to observe the medial progress of needle. The needle point should not go beyond the cephalad-directed lip on the lateral border of the body of the vertebra, which marks lateral extent of epidural space. The needle point should also be at least halfway into the mass of the transverse process image to avoid spread of anesthetic to other roots (Fig. 4).

5. A single nerve root can be anesthetized with 1 to 2 mL of a mixture of equal parts of 1% lidocaine and 0.5% bupivacaine with 1:400,000 epinephrine. Inject 0.25 to 0.5 mL at a time.

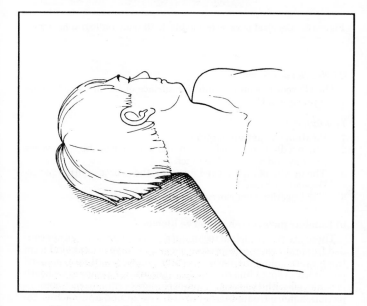

Figure 2.   Cervical paravertebral block. Patient position.

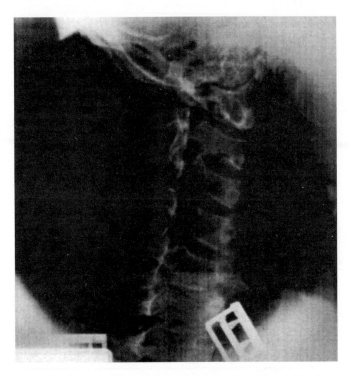

Figure 3.   Cervical paravertebral block. Oblique radiographic view.

C7 Nerve root block

The C7 root lies on the anterior surface of the flattened transverse process of C7.

Technique
1. Position the patient supine.
2. The needle is inserted lateral and superior to the transverse process and advanced to touch it.
3. The needle is then moved about on the process until a paresthesia is achieved.
4. The injection is performed as described before.

b) Lumbar paravertebral nerve blocks

There are two principal techniques: direct the needle either caudad from the transverse process above the nerve or cephalad from the process below the nerve. Greater accuracy and an increased possibility of spreading solution along or into the perineural sheath is achieved with the second approach; however, subarachnoid injection is more frequently a hazard. The second approach is described here.

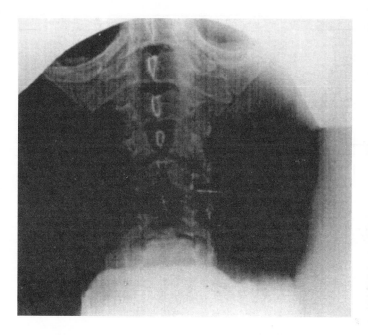

Figure 4. Cervical paravertebral block. Anteroposterior radiographic view.

When using this technique in the lumbar region (as opposed to the thoracic region), it is so easy to enter and inject the epidural or intrathecal spaces that the diagnostic value of a single nerve root block is questionable. However, the technique is chosen for its greater success rate and accuracy, as it is easy to obtain a paresthesia when the needle encounters a nerve as it emerges just caudad to the pedicle of the vertebra.

L1 through L4 nerve root blocks

Technique

1. Patient is positioned prone, with pillow under belly, using C-arm (Fig. 5).
2. Visualize the caudad border of the desired vertebral pedicle and mark this target skin projection.
3. Needle is inserted 5 cm lateral to midline (4 to 7 cm, depending on body mass), so as to encounter caudad border of transverse process above the target nerve.
4. The needle is then advanced from the transverse process, caudad and medially toward the pedicle of the vertebra, which projects as an oval shadow on an AP view of the spine. Lateral C-arm view will show the depth of the needle in relation to intervertebral foramen (Fig. 6).

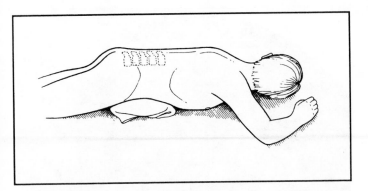

Figure 5.   Lumbar paravertebral block. Patient position (used also for lumbar sympathetic and lumbar epidural injections).

5.   Inject 0.2 mL of contrast dye to confirm the correct needle placement.
6.   Once optimal needle placement is confirmed, inject 1 to 2 mL of solution, in 0.25-mL increments. For therapeutic purposes, 40 mg of triamcinolone (Aristocort or Kenalog) is adequate.

L5 nerve root block

Because of the close proximity of the L5 transverse process to the sacrum, it is often difficult to maneuver the needle in this narrow space from an insertion point 5 cm lateral to the midline. Hence, a more lateral insertion point is usually more successful, so that the needle passes either caudad or anteriorly, to a posteriorly inclined transverse process.

Technique
1.   Patient is positioned prone, with a pillow under lower belly.
2.   The skin entry site is well anesthetized.
3.   A 3½-inch, 22-gauge spinal needle is inserted 8 cm lateral to the midline, just above the iliac crest under C-arm fluoroscopy guidance.
4.   It is advanced medially and somewhat caudad, to strike the L5 transverse process.
5.   The needle is then redirected slightly caudad and anteriorly, to encounter the posterior surface of the lateral body of L5, just caudad to the pedicle and about 2 cm deeper.
6.   The point is maneuvered as for other lumbar nerves, to achieve an optimal proximity to the nerve root. Dye (0.3 mL) is injected.
7.   The position and dye distribution are checked using a lateral C-arm view; 1 to 2 mL of local anesthetic, in 0.25-mL increments, is injected.

a) Sacral paravertebral nerve block

For diagnostic sacral nerve root blocks, it is necessary to inject at a site where each root is anatomically separated from adjacent

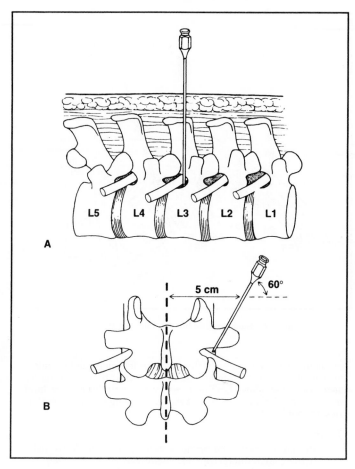

**Figure 6.   Lumbar paravertebral block. A: Lateral view.
B: Anteroposterior view.**

roots. This site is the anterior sacral foramen, where the anterior primary division emerges from the sacral epidural space to join the lumbosacral plexus in the posterior pelvis (Fig. 7). If, on the other hand, the aim is to concentrate steroid near the affected sacral root (but not exclusively to one root), sacral epidural injections can be made as soon as the needle is through the posterior foramen. At S1, the epidural space is about 2 cm deep; at S2, 1½ cm deep; at S3, 1 cm; and at S4, ¼ cm deep.

S1 nerve root block

Scan the sacral area briefly with the C-arm at different angles (remember, the sacrum takes off posteriorly from the lumbar spine

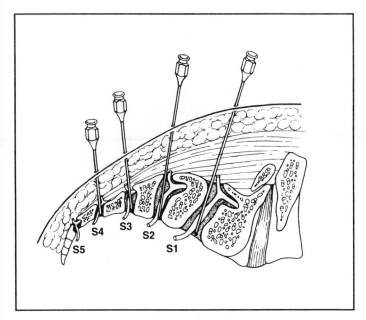

Figure 7.   Sacral nerve blocks. Parasagittal section.

at about 45 degrees) to see if the posterior foramen can be made to overlie the anterior foramen. Usually, only the anterior foramen is seen. Bowel shadows (gas or feces) may partially obscure landmarks, but attempts to clean out the bowel using enemas or cathartics are not helpful.

Technique

1. Patient is positioned prone with a pillow under lower belly, using C-arm fluoroscopy for visualization.
2. Using a 3½-inch, 22-gauge spinal needle, insert needle at the level of the L5 vertebra (C-arm in straight AP direction), just lateral to image of anterior S1 foramen.
3. The needle is advanced at 45 degrees caudally, to strike the posterior surface of the sacrum.
4. The needle is then moved about until it falls through the posterior foramen.
5. The posterior foramen is usually found somewhat cephalad and lateral to the superomedial border of the elliptical image of the anterior foramen.
6. For epidural injections, the needle point is advanced 1 cm through the posterior foramen.
7. To block the S1 root, the needle is advanced another 1 cm, until a paresthesia is achieved, at the anterior foramen (Fig. 8).
8. If no paresthesia is achieved after two or three thrusts of the needle, it must be withdrawn and inserted through a new

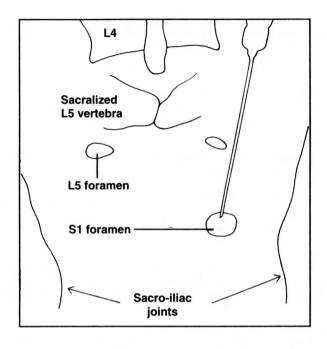

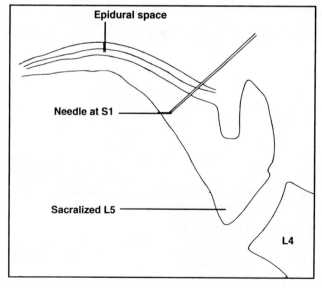

Figure 8.   First sacral (S1) nerve block. A: Anteroposterior diagrammatic representation. B: Lateral diagrammatic representation.

skin wheal, 1 cm either medial or lateral to the initial wheal. One of these three positions usually achieves a paresthesia.
9.   Inject 1 to 2 mL of contrast dye to confirm correct position of the needle.
10. Inject 1 to 2 mL of solution, 0.25 mL at a time.

S2 through S4 nerve root blocks

Remember that the sacrum is curved, and needles will appear in a radial array, starting from the S1 root.

Technique
1.   Patient is positioned prone, with a pillow under lower belly, using C-arm for visualization.
2.   Skin wheals are made slightly lateral to image of anterior foramen, and vertical to it.
3.   As described earlier, anterior foramina and paresthesias will be found about 1.5 cm, 1.0 cm, and 0.5 cm through the posterior foramina of S2, S3, and S4, respectively.

S5 nerve root block

In most individuals, there is no S5 posterior or anterior foramen. This is not an accurate block, nor is accuracy often required. The S5 root can be anesthetized (without paresthesias) by passing a needle just inferior and lateral to the tip of the sacrum (Fig. 9).

3. Sympathetic nerve blocks

These techniques attempt to isolate the sympathetic from the somatic nerves. The following techniques are specifically for use with C-arm fluoroscopy. Nonfluoroscopic techniques have been widely reported, but C-arm fluoroscopy increases the success rate of upper extremity sympathetic blocks from between 27% and 70% to about 90%.

Block treatment protocol

In treating CRPS with sympathetic blocks, our practice is to give one block per week, for 3 weeks. If, in conjunction with physical therapy, the blocks allow the disease to improve, they are continued. If the duration of relief from the blocks is too short and symptoms fails to improve, a 1-week continuous block with in-hospital care is performed. If improvement is sustained after the week's hospital stay but symptoms recur, a second or even third attempt at hospitalized continuous catheter treatment is tried. If this fails, a surgical sympathectomy may be recommended. If a 4- to 6-week sympathetic ablation is desired, then aqueous phenol may be used. Spinal cord stimulation is a recent alternative treatment.

Confirmation of sympathetic blockade

Confirmation is an essential element of both diagnostic and therapeutic blocks. Since there are no sensory measures of block efficacy, other means are needed.

SKIN TEMPERATURE.   This is simple to measure with a thermocouple, best placed on the pads of the fingers or on the toe tips, to record maximum temperature swings. This measurement applies, of course, only to blocks involving the upper or lower extremities.

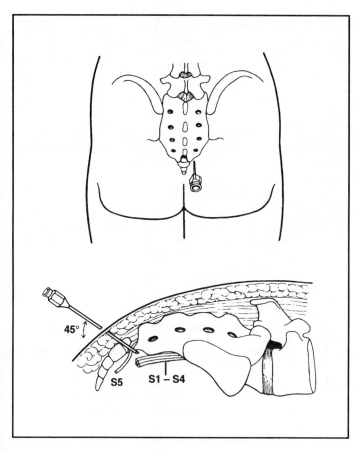

Figure 9.   Fifth sacral (S5) nerve block.

No clear-cut means of assessing the completeness of sympathetic block of the trunk has been devised.

Temperature tests are best performed in a cool room (68° to 70°F) with patient fasting for more than 2 hours, with arms and legs exposed to air. This allows the baseline skin temperature to stabilize at close to room temperature. Contralateral temperatures should be simultaneously measured for comparison. A complete sympathetic block should cause a rise in temperature from 72°F (22°C) to 93°F (34°C) in a patient with normal peripheral circulation. With vascular insufficiency (unusual in reflex sympathetic dystrophy), skin temperature does not fall as low as 72° or rise as high as 93°. Other signs of sympathetic block should appear, such as flushing and dry skin.

PSYCHOGALVANIC RESPONSE (PGR) OR GALVANIC SKIN RESPONSE. A more clear-cut endpoint is provided by this response. It is easily performed using a standard EKG as a galvanometer. Any two opposing leads (e.g., RA–LA as lead I, which is simple) are placed on palm and dorsum of hand, or on sole and dorsum of foot, depending on extremity involved. Other leads are attached at random for stability of recording (preferably not in EKG configuration to avoid EKG tracing). To "discharge" the sympathetic nerves, the stimulus of a single deep breath, sudden unexpected noise, or painful stimulus is used. If the sympathetic pathway is intact, a biphasic response occurs seconds later, returning to baseline in about 5 seconds (Fig. 10). If the sympathetic nerves are completely blocked, there is no response (flat line). The response may not be present in very old people or diabetics with peripheral neuropathy. The electrophysiologic mechanism is not understood.

Evaluation of block efficacy:

In sympathetically maintained pain, there should be immediate, complete pain relief, lasting hours to weeks. Partial relief is thought to indicate a sympathetic element to the pain. However, in some patients with a clinical diagnosis of CRPS-I, there is no relief. The results of sympathetic blocks indicate whether blocking procedures would be useful in therapy.

(i) *Stellate ganglion block*

Indications

- Diagnosis and therapy of sympathetically maintained pain (SMP)
- Peripheral vasospastic disease (e.g., Raynaud's phenomenon)
- Acute herpes zoster
- Acute post-traumatic or postoperative vascular insufficiency of face, neck, or upper extremities

Potential complications

- Transient nerve paralysis of the recurrent laryngeal nerve (hoarseness) or phrenic nerve (shortness of breath)

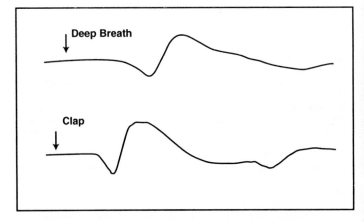

Figure 10.   Psychogalvanic reflex galvanometer (EKG) tracing.

- Pneumothorax
- Hematoma
- Subarachnoid or epidural anesthesia by injection into the dural sleeve of the cervical root
- Seizures, as a result of intravascular injection of local anesthetic, including vertebral artery
- Brachial plexus blockade

Prolongation of block

Using a stellate ganglion catheter, the stellate ganglion block can be prolonged. Occasionally, this is an advantage for patients who have failed to respond to repeat blocks and physical therapy because it facilitates aggressive in-patient physical therapy. Intrapleural catheter treatment can also provide prolonged sympathetic blockade to the upper extremity. However, these treatments require in-patient admission, and they are rarely offered today because of restrictions placed on the treatments by insurers.

Technique

1. Position the patient supine with the neck extended and a pillow under the shoulders. Neck extension makes the cervical spine more superficial and easier to reach; and it draws the esophagus behind the trachea so it is less easily pierced by a left-sided approach.
2. Palpate the space between carotid pulsation and the lateral trachea, as low as possible in the neck.
3. Make a skin wheal over the medial edge of carotid pulsation at this level, usually at C6 or C7 over the transverse process, by C-arm fluoroscopy.
4. Direct a 2½-inch, 22-gauge spinal needle caudally and medially toward the junction of the lateral portion of the bodies of C7 and T1. Figure 10 shows the level of the stellate ganglion.
5. When bone is encountered, check the position (it should feel like the hard, flat top of a table), withdraw the needle 1 mm, and inject 5 to 10 mL 0.25% bupivacaine or 0.5% lidocaine, or a mixture of the two.
6. The 10-mL solution will conveniently spread (as dye would show) from C1 to T4.
7. Because there is no anatomic guide to the depth of the appropriate fascial plane (Figs. 11 and 12), a certain percentage of blocks (about 10%) will be missed.
8. Because of the medial placement (3 to 5 mm medial to stellate ganglion), complications of vertebral artery injection, brachial plexus block, and pneumothorax are not common. Recurrent laryngeal nerve block does occur, especially if the needle passes close to the trachea.
9. Horner's syndrome (ptosis, miosis, enophthalmos, often with anhidrosis and nasal congestion) is commonly produced, but this does not preclude the need for testing the upper extremity sympathetic nerve block. The appearance of Horner's syndrome does not ensure an adequate block of the upper extremity.
10. If only the cervical portion of the sympathetic nerves need to be blocked, then the procedure is more easily done at C6 or C5, but the C-arm should be employed for accuracy.

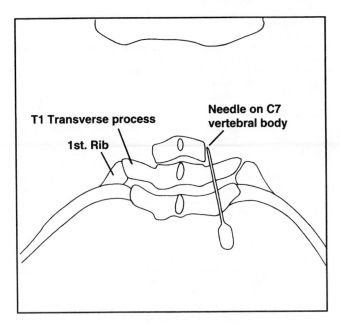

Figure 11.   Stellate ganglion block. Diagrammatic representation.

11.   Patients who underwent a stellate ganglion block are given
      sips of water to detect possible aspiration, prior to feeding. If
      hoarseness is present, oral intake should be avoided. Other
      potential complications should be sought prior to discharge.

(ii) *Lumbar sympathetic blocks*

   Because the principal spinal segmental sympathetic supply to
the lower extremities comes mainly from L1, L2, and L3, it seems
logical to place a needle at L2, relying on volume and diffusion of
local anesthetics to cover the whole outflow.

Indications
• Diagnosis and therapy of sympathetically maintained pain
  syndromes of the lower extremities
• Evaluation of potential benefit of neurolytic sympathectomy
• Acute peripheral vascular insufficiency
• Acute herpes zoster of the lower extremities
• Some peripheral neuropathic pain syndromes of the lower ex-
  tremities (sympathetically maintained pain syndromes)

Potential complications
• Intravascular injection
• Great vessel perforation and retroperitoneal hematoma
• Puncture of abdominal viscera
• Injection into ureters, kidneys, or peritoneal cavity

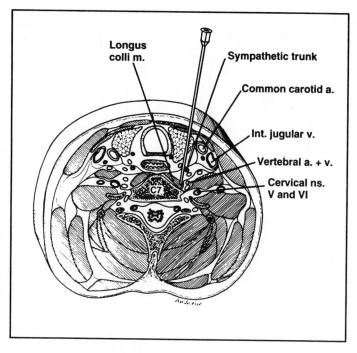

Figure 12. Cross-section of the neck at C7 level for stellate ganglion block.

- Inadvertent epidural, subarachnoid, or lumbar plexus injection
- Transient backache and stiffness

Technique

1. Accurate placement of the needle requires fluoroscopy.
2. Position the patient prone, with a pillow beneath the epigastrium.
3. Identify the lateral cephalad border of the body of the L2 vertebra (this point should be cephalad to the transverse process to avoid spinal nerves).
4. Mark skin projection.
5. Using fluoroscopy, make another mark 8 cm lateral to spinous process of L2, slightly cephalad to the first mark.
6. Check to see that the mark is over, or medial to, the twelfth rib. If not, move medially.
7. Infiltrate lidocaine through the second skin mark down to the body of the vertebra.
8. A 20-gauge, 12.5-cm (5-inch) needle is inserted down to the first target (the lateral-cephalad portion of the body of L2).
9. Withdraw, redirect laterally, with needle bevel facing medially, and advance so that the needle slides easily by the lateral surface of the vertebra (Fig. 13).

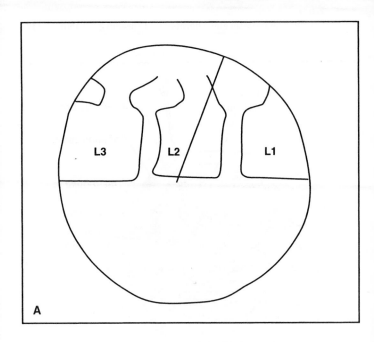

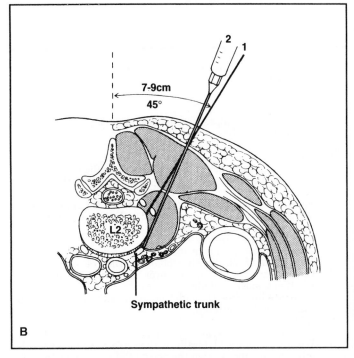

Figure 13. Lumbar sympathetic block. A: Diagrammatic representation. B: Cross-section at L2 level.

10. Rotate the C-arm to the lateral view, and advance the needle 1 to 2 mm anterior to the anterior margin of L2.
11. Inject a total volume of 20 to 30 mL 0.5% lidocaine and 0.25% bupivacaine.

Within minutes, flushing and warming of foot should occur and skin temperature should rise. Sometimes, if the patient is very apprehensive and hyperreactive, the skin temperature does not rise for 20 to 30 minutes, presumably because circulating epinephrine maintains vasoconstriction. Once patient relaxes in the recovery room, the foot usually warms up.

4. Visceral nerve blocks

(i) *Celiac plexus block*

Because the celiac plexus is a network surrounding the celiac artery and the adjacent anterior aorta, the objective is to deposit solution anterior to the aorta. A variety of approaches are possible:

- Bilateral, posterior, asymmetrical approach with C-arm fluoroscopy guidance, described later. The right-sided needle is passed between the inferior vena cava and the aorta toward its anterior surface, and the left-sided needle is passed tangential to the aorta (Fig. 14). (Note: Neurolytic substances should never be injected in the vicinity of the spine without C-arm and preliminary dye guidance.)

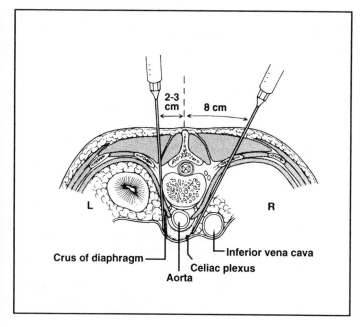

Figure 14. Celiac plexus block. Cross-section at L1 level.

- Posterior approach with transfixion of the aorta
- Anterior approach using a computed tomography scanner or ultrasound, placing needle on anterior aorta

Indications
- Treatment of pain for pancreatic cancer (and sometimes herpetic or gastric cancer)
- Pain of chronic relapsing pancreatitis (the combination of local anesthetic and steroid is sometimes helpful)
- Diagnosis and therapy of sympathetically mediated abdominal, retroperitoneal, or flank pain

Potential complications
- Intravascular injection
- Great vessel perforation and retroperitoneal hematoma
- Puncture of a viscus
- Injection into kidneys, pancreas, peritoneal cavity, or liver
- Epidural, subarachnoid, or lumbar plexus injection, possibly with neurolytic agents
- Acute abdominal and chest discomfort, lasting about 30 minutes
- Orthostatic hypotension, as a result of profound sympathetic neural blockade, lasting for 48 hours or more, following a neurolytic injection
- Thrombosis or pressure occlusion of the spinal branch of the aorta, with resultant paraplegia (extremely rare)

Post-block management
Regular monitoring of vital signs following a celiac plexus block for up to 4 hours with a local anesthetic block, and 24 hours or longer with a neurolytic block, may be necessary. Evaluation for the other potential complications is also necessary.

a) Diagnostic block
Technique
1. Patient in prone position, pillow under epigastrium.

Right side
1. Mark the skin, as in lumbar sympathetic block, but at the L1 level (instead of L2).
2. A 20-gauge, 15-cm stylet needle is passed to the upper lateral portion of the body of L1, deviated laterally and caudad about 2.5 cm anteriorly to the anterior surface of L1 vertebral body.
3. Proceed while aspirating carefully.

Left Side
1. A 20-gauge, 15-cm stylet needle is inserted to the back, 2 to 3 cm lateral to the spinous process of L1, aiming at the upper lateral margin of the L1 body, using C-arm fluoroscopy visualization.
2. The needle is carefully carried down to, and passed beyond, the lateral edge of the L1 vertebral body until a pulsating resistance is reached (the aorta) or the needle advances 2 cm anteriorly to L1.

3. After negative aspiration and a 2-mL test dose, 20 to 25 mL of 0.5% lidocaine or 0.25% bupivacaine (or a mixture of both) is injected on each side.

b) Neurolytic block

Technique

1. Prior to performing a neurolytic block, a diagnostic block should be done (a day before if the scheduling condition of the patient allows) to demonstrate pain relief. If this is only done just prior to the alcohol block, placebo effect and duration of relief cannot be evaluated.
2. Inject 10 mL of 1% lidocaine on either side.
3. This is followed by 5 mL of water-soluble dye (Omnipaque, diluted 50% with saline). Ideally a sausage-like pattern around the aorta is produced, but layering either anterior or posterior to the aorta is satisfactory. If the dye streaks diagonally toward the diaphragm, it is in the crus of the diaphragm, and alcohol injection would be ineffective. If the dye follows posteriorly toward the intervertebral foramen, the needle needs to be repositioned to avoid alcohol contacting somatic nerves.
4. After a 20-minute wait to allow dispersal of lidocaine and dye (disappearance can be confirmed using fluoroscopy), 25 mL of 50% alcohol (absolute alcohol diluted with saline) is injected on each side.
5. Usually, 10 mL of lidocaine protects against the irritative effect of the alcohol, but the patient may experience a brief aching in the epigastrium or back.

(ii) *Hypogastric plexus*

The superior hypogastric plexus lies anterior to the L5 vertebra, innervating the organs in the pelvis and pelvic floor, including the vagina, vulva, uterus, rectum, bladder, perineum, prostate.

Indications
- Pelvic cancer pain
- Nonmalignant pelvic pain

Complications
- Hematoma
- Infection
- Impotence
- Peripheral vascular occlusion

Technique

1. With patient in the prone position, the L4-5 interspace is identified using fluoroscopy.
2. A skin wheel is made with local anesthetic 5 to 7 cm from the midline at the L4-5 interspace.
3. Insert a 7-inch, 22-gauge, short-beveled needle through the skin wheel, aiming at the anterolateral aspect of the bottom of the L5 vertebral body.
4. Guide the needle with fluoroscopy to avoid hitting the iliac crest and the L5 transverse process.

5. The contralateral needle is inserted in the same way under fluoroscopic guidance.
6. Inject 2 to 4 mL of water-soluble contrast. In the AP view, the dye should be just anterior to the L5-S1 intervertebral space. In the lateral view, a smooth posterior contour, corresponding to the anterior psoas fascia, indicates proper needle position.
7. For a diagnostic block, 5 to 10 mL of 0.25% bupivacaine is injected bilaterally after negative aspiration.
8. For neurolytic block, 10 mL of 10% phenol is used unilaterally or bilaterally. A diagnostic block should be performed before the neurolytic block.

5. Peripheral nerve blocks

(i) *Trigeminal nerve blocks*

Trigeminal nerve blocks are commonly used for the treatment of trigeminal neuralgia. At MGH, this procedure is performed by neurosurgeons. Under monitored sedation, the patient is placed in a supine position with the neck extended. At a point 2.5 cm lateral to the corner of the mouth, the skin is prepared and draped in a standard sterile fashion. After anesthetizing the skin with 1% lidocaine, a 20-gauge, 13-cm Hinck needle is advanced through the anesthetized skin, in the direction of the fixed pupil in a cephalad trajectory into the foramen ovale. At this point, there is often a free flow of CSF when the stylet is removed. After radiographic confirmation of needle position, 0.1-mL aliquots of a preservative-free local anesthetic (1% lidocaine or 0.5% bupivacaine) or a neurolytic agent is injected. The patient is left in the supine position if alcohol is to be injected. If phenol is chosen for the injection, the patient is moved into a sitting position with the chin on the chest so that the solution gravitates around the maxillary and mandibular divisions of the nerve and thus spares the ophthalmic division. A similar approach can be utilized to place radiofrequency and cryotherapy probes.

(ii) *Occipital nerve block*

Occipital neuralgia results from stretching or entrapment of the occipital nerve. The nerve may become trapped in fascia overlying the posterior surface of C2 or in occipital ligamentous attachments.

Indication

Occipital neuralgia as in either tension headaches or following injury (e.g., auto accidents with whiplash, falls, or work injuries)

Technique

1. Position the patient sitting on a stool, elbows leaning on a table, and forehead in hands.
2. Palpate the posterior occipital protuberance and move 1.5 to 2 cm laterally and feel for occipital artery pulsation and groove (Fig. 15).
3. Inject 2 to 3 mL 0.5% bupivacaine with 10 to 20 mg triamcinolone, down to the bone and fan out. Occipital nerve analgesia should occur very rapidly.
4. Inject some of the solution more caudally, for occipital muscle attachment pain and spasm, which often responds to steroid injections.

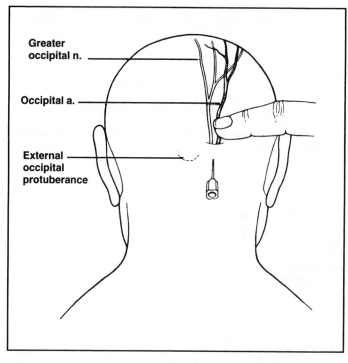

Figure 15. Occipital nerve block.

(iii) *Suprascapular nerve block*

Indications

- Shoulder pain secondary to rotator cuff lesions, osteoarthritis of the shoulder, or adhesive capsulitis ("frozen shoulder")
- Shoulder arthroscopy and other orthopedic manipulations of the shoulder

Potential complications

- Pneumothorax
- Infection
- Intravascular injection
- Seizure
- Muscle atrophy

Technique

1. Position the patient sitting.
2. A 22-gauge, $1\frac{1}{2}$-inch needle is inserted 1 to 2 cm superior to the midpoint of the spine of the scapula and advanced toward the suprascapular notch until a paresthesia is elicited.
3. Inject 5 to 10 mL of local anesthetics with or without steroids.

4.   Position the hand ipsilateral to the block onto the contralateral shoulder: this can move the scapula away from the posterior chest wall and reduce the risk of pneumothorax.

(iv) *Intercostal nerve blocks*

Indications
- Rib fractures—acute, traumatic, and pathologic
- Chest wall metastases, or tumor
- Post-thoracotomy pain or pain caused by percutaneous drainage tubes
- Diagnostic or therapeutic blocks for abdominal pain or abdominal wall pain

Potential complications
- Pneumothorax
- Intravascular injection
- Seizures
- Infection
- Bleeding

Technique
1.   Position the patient in a semilateral position, with sites to be injected made prominent by a pillow under the opposite chest wall.
2.   The injection site is the posterior axillary line, to 5 to 7 cm lateral to the vertebral spinous processes. [The posterior division cannot be reached without injecting by the paravertebral approach because of the hazard of pneumothorax (see II, 2)]
3.   Produce a skin wheal at the injection site. With a 25-gauge, $\frac{1}{2}$-inch (or longer, if necessary) needle, enter vertically to the skin, and "walk" the needle to just below the rib and forward 2 mm. Inject 3 mL 0.5% bupivacaine with epinephrine at each rib (Fig. 16). (Note: Anesthetic is absorbed rapidly into the systemic circulation because of the vascularity of the injection site.)
4.   Neurolytic intercostal block: first block the nerve proximally with 0.5% bupivacaine, then inject 2 to 3 mL 100% ethyl alcohol, lateral to the anesthetized site (alcohol injection is initially very painful).

(vi) *Lateral femoral cutaneous nerve block*

Lateral femoral cutaneous nerve pain is believed to be associated with obesity or pregnancy or the wearing of a tight belt. It is thought to be caused by entrapment of the lateral femoral cutaneous nerve as it passes through the inguinal ligament. Neurolytic blocks are not recommended; however, surgical dissection may be considered.

Indication

Meralgia paresthetica: burning pain, numbness and tingling in the anterolateral aspect of the thigh

Technique
1.   Position the patient supine.

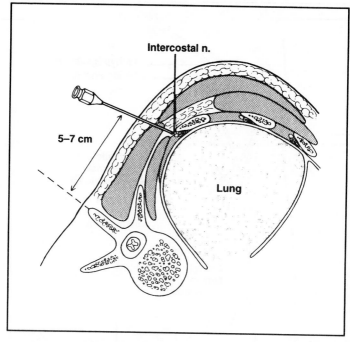

Figure 16.   Intercostal nerve block. Patient in semilateral position.

2.   Palpate the anterior superior iliac spine, and insert a 1½-inch, 25- or 22-gauge needle 2 cm medial and 2 cm caudal to it (Fig. 17).
3.   Proceed through the fascia (feel a "pop"), and inject 10 mL of 0.5% bupivacaine with 30 mg triamcinolone fanwise, from the medial surface of the iliac spine medially to beneath the insertion point.

Evaluation of block

Analgesia of the upper two thirds of the anterolateral thigh should be produced.

(vii) *Ilioinguinal nerve block*

Indications
•   Postherniorrhaphy pain, which is usually caused by trauma to the genitofemoral nerve in the floor of the inguinal canal
•   Diagnostic block, prior to surgical dissection or neurolytic block (Note: hazardous) (Fig. 17)
•   Testicular pain, with or without history of trauma or surgery

Technique
1.   Position the patient supine.
2.   Produce a skin wheal with local anesthetic, 2 cm medial to the anterior superior iliac spine.

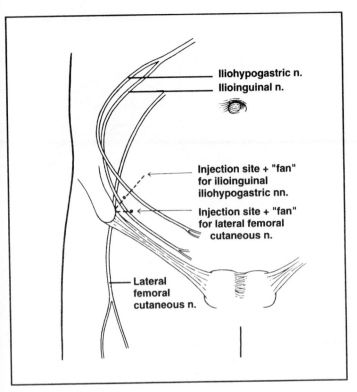

Figure 17.   Lateral femoral cutaneous, ilioinguinal, and iliohypogastric nerve blocks.

3.   Infiltrate all layers of muscle toward the umbilicus with a 1½-inch, 22-gauge needle and 10 to 20 mL of 0.5% bupivacaine, for a distance of 10 cm.

Evaluation of block
   Variable distribution of analgesia is noted in the medial thigh and groin, which should relieve the groin pain if the ilioinguinal nerve is involved.

(viii) *Genitofemoral nerve block*
Indication
   Groin or testicular pain unrelieved by ilioinguinal block. (Lumbar sympathetic block is another reasonable treatment for testicular pain.)

Technique
1.   Position patient in supine position.
2.   Inject 5 mL of 0.5% bupivacaine around the spermatic cord, at the base of the scrotum.

Evaluation of block

If pain relief occurs but returns, the next option is either to repeat the block as frequently as required or to do a cryoneurolysis or even a rhizotomy of L1 and L2.

III. FACET JOINT BLOCKS

Back pain may result from the effects of degenerative arthropathy (as a part of diffuse degenerative joint disease) (Fig. 18) and trauma such as whiplash injury on the zygapophysial joints. A facet joint block can be performed as a diagnostic aid for the orthopedic surgeon deciding whether to perform spinal fusion. Inject local anesthetic into a joint to determine if it is the source of back pain. It may be worthwhile to inject steroid into the joints, although this usually provides relief for only up to 2 weeks. A facet joint block can also be used as a predictive tool, prior to denervating the joint with alcohol, or prior to radiofrequency lesioning of the joint nerve (the

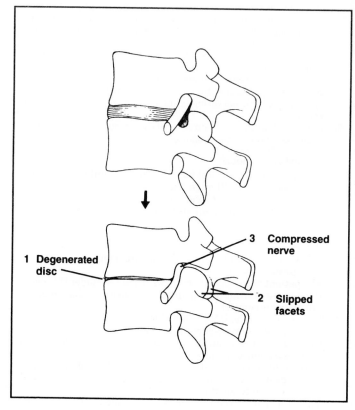

Figure 18. Consequences of disc degeneration.

nerve of Luschka, the medial branch of posterior primary ramus) at the same level and one above.

a) Lumbar facet block

Prior to beginning the block, the pain should be evaluated by putting the patient through a range of back motions. Extension characteristically produces facet pain.

Technique

1. Place the patient in a prone position with the C-arm fluoroscopy in oblique position.
2. Rotate the C-arm to get the best view into the joint: The "Scotty dog" x-ray image is characteristic—the vertically oriented joint image is behind the dogs ear.
3. Usually, an entry point 2 cm lateral to midline leads into the joint. However, entering directly over the joint image or even lateral to it may be required, depending on arthritic overgrowth of the joint.
4. A 22-gauge, $3\frac{1}{2}$-inch spinal needle is carried with minimal local anesthetic to the edge of the joint. The needle is then "walked" in 1-mm steps medial or laterally, cephalad or caudad, until it drops into the joint. A characteristic curve is seen at the distal end of the needle, showing that it is following the joint, usually medially.
5. An intact joint will accept up to 1 mL of fluid to anesthetize the joint (0.5% bupivacaine). If the joint capsule is disrupted, it will have a much greater capacity. Be careful not to inject more than 1 mL, preferably in 0.5-mL increments, or the fluid will spread to other innervating branches and cause a false-positive response.
6. Relief that outlasts the duration of the anesthetic (1 to 2 hours) suggests a nonspecific response.

b) Cervical facet block

The reasons to use cervical facet blocks are similar to those for lumbar facet blocks, although the former are especially useful when abnormally moving facet joints are identified by previous continuous fluoroscopy. Whiplash injuries tend to disrupt facet motion.

Technique

1. An IV catheter is placed, vital signs are monitored, and fluoroscopy is employed.
2. The patient is positioned prone, with a pillow under the chest, the neck somewhat flexed, and the forehead resting on an IV fluid bag for comfort.
3. With C-arm in the PA direction, enter at a point directly over the transverse process mass, usually 1.5 to 2.0 cm lateral to the midline, and about three vertebrae caudad to the desired level (see angle of joints).
4. With minimal local anesthetic, a 22-gauge, $3\frac{1}{2}$-inch spinal needle is advanced at about a 30-degree angle with the skin until bone is encountered at the desired level.
5. The joint space is then visualized by placing the C-arm in lateral position, and the needle is "walked" 1 mm at a time until

it drops into joint. The final position of the needle tip is halfway through the joint.

6. The lateral-medial position of the needle needs to be checked again with the C-arm in AP view. The needle point should be in the middle of the transverse process mass. (Slipping too far medially produces epidural or spinal anesthesia.)

7. Again, 1-mL 0.5% bupivacaine in 0.5-mL increments is sufficient to anesthetize the joint.

8. If the joint is the source of pain, motion of neck that was painful before the block should immediately disappear following the block.

c) Lumbar medial branch block

Each lumbar facet joint is innervated by a medial branch of the posterior primary rami of the lumbar nerve at the same level and another medial branch from one level above. For example, the L4-L5 facet joint is innervated by the medial branches of the posterior primary rami of the L4 and L3 nerve roots. The L5-S1 facet joint, however, is innervated by the medial branch of the L4 posterior primary rami and the dorsal ramus of the L5 nerve root. It has been found that medial branch radiofrequency lesioning provides longer pain relief than intrafacet joint steroid injection. Thus it is more common now to do medial branch blocks (twice), followed by radiofrequency lesioning if the patient's pain is significantly reduced by both medial branch blocks.

Technique

1. Place the patient in a prone position.

2. The position of the C-arm is adjusted in the PA view first, to square the endplate of the vertebral body at the level of the target nerve to be blocked. The C-arm is then rotated to an oblique view until the vertical line of the facet joint is at the middle of the endplate.

3. Lidocaine, 3 mL of 1%, is used to anesthetize the skin and the needle pathway, except for the area near the target point.

4. The target point of the block is just caudal to the most medial portion of the L2 through the L5 transverse processes for the L1 through the L4 medial branches, respectively (i.e., high at the "Scotty dog's eye"). For the dorsal ramus of L5, the target point of the needle is at the junction of the sacral ala and the superior articular process. The PA view is used for the block of the L5 dorsal ramus.

5. A 25-gauge, 90-mm spinal needle with a curve at the tip is used. The point of needle insertion on the skin is selected above and lateral to the target point, usually just above the tip of target transverse process. The needle is inserted in a caudal, ventral, and medial direction using a tunnel-view technique.

6. Insertion is terminated once the tip of the needle strikes the bone of the target point. In the AP view, the needle tip should be slightly medial to the lateral margin of the silhouette of the superior articular process.

7. Once the needle is in correct position, 0.1 to 0.3 mL of contrast medium is injected to test that venous uptake does not occur. If it does, the needle must be readjusted by 1 or 2 mm and the test repeated. If there is no venous uptake, 0.5 mL of 1% lidocaine is injected onto the target nerve.

d) Cervical medial branch block

The C2-3 facet joint, the highest cervical facet joint, is innervated mainly by the third occipital nerve, which runs in an AP direction across the lateral surface of the C2-3 facet joint. The medial branches of the C3 and C4 dorsal rami innervate the C3-4 facet joint. Each of these medial branches runs anteroposteriorly, hugging the midpoint of the articular pillar. The rest of the cervical facet joints have innervations the similar to those of the C3-4 facet joint from the medial branches at their respective levels.

Potential complications
- Infection
- Injury and injection into carotid artery and vertebral arteries
- Seizure
- Damage to brachial plexus
- Spinal cord injury
- Epidural or spinal injection

Technique
1. The patient lies in the lateral position.
2. PA and lateral fluoroscopic views are used to identify the cervical articular pillars and facet joints.
3. A 25-gauge, 1.5-inch spinal needle is used.
4. The target point for the block is slightly anterior to the midpoint of C2-3 facet joint in the lateral view and on the surface of the C2-3 facet joint in the PA view.
5. To block the deeper medial branches of C3 and the medial branches of C4 to C7, the end of the needle point is at the midpoint of the pyramid of the articular pillars in the lateral view and on the lateral surface of the articular pillar in the PA view. The target point for the C7 medial branch block is high on the apex of the superior articular process of C7.
6. Needle insertion should be carefully guided by fluoroscopy.
7. Once the needle reaches the target, and after negative aspiration, 0.5 mL of 1% lidocaine is injected.

IV. SACROILIAC JOINT BLOCK

Although the sacroiliac (SI) joint is not a facet joint, its block technique is very similar to that of facet joint injection. The temptation to inject this joint is great because tenderness over the SI joint is a very common finding in patients with low back pain. In fact, this was the reason back pain used to be treated by SI fusion, before Mixter and Barr demonstrated that the herniated disc was a cause of sciatica in the early 1930s. As the joint is well innervated, it is no wonder that this can be the source of acute or chronic low back pain.

Indications
- Since the clinical presentation is very variable (pain in the gluteal area with or without radiation to posterior thigh or knee, or even down to the ankle), SI joint injection is used for the diagnosis and therapy of low back or sacral pain.

Potential complications
- Infection

- Penetration of pelvic viscus if needle traverses the joint (a remote possibility)

Technique

1. As the joint region is easily palpable, its injection would seem simple. Actually, it is not, and C-arm guidance is needed.
2. The patient should be in prone position, with the C-arm rotated to the oblique position until the images of the anterior and posterior joints overlap.
3. The insertion point is usually at the caudal tip of the joint.
4. A 22-gauge, 3½-inch spinal needle is carried deeply into the joint. The needle tip shows the same deviation it does in the lumbar facet under C-arm visualization (Fig. 19).
5. To anesthetize this joint, 2 to 3 cc of 0.5% bupivacaine should be adequate. Steroid is an option.

V. TRIGGER POINT INJECTIONS

Trigger point injections are utilized to relieve pain associated with myofascial pain syndrome, which is characterized by spontaneous and evoked pain of affected muscles. It is commonly possible to palpate the band type of muscle spasms, also known as trigger points, that trigger pain. These points are usually very tender (also known as tender points). This syndrome can be either primary or secondary to underlying diseases such as facet arthropa-

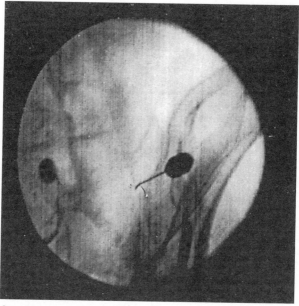

A

Figure 19. Sacroiliac joint injection. A: Oblique radiographic view. B: Diagrammatic representation.

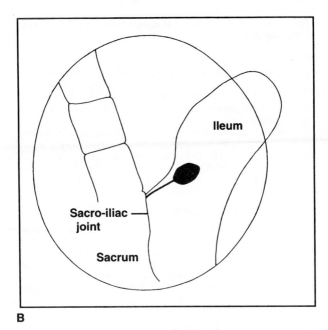

B

Figure 19.   *Continued.*

thy, sacroiliac arthropathy, and disc herniation. The reproduction of pain during injections into the muscle and the relief of pain post injection is the hallmark of this type of pain. Even though we routinely inject local anesthetics into the trigger points, some physicians use just dry needling, or steroids with or without the local anesthetics; others use normal saline.

Technique

Inject 1 to 2 mL of 0.25% bupivacaine, with or without 5 to 10 mg triamcinolone, into and around the trigger point, using a 25-gauge, 1½-inch needle, and aspirating before injecting. Repeat as needed, and wherever required.

VI. ADDITIONAL DIAGNOSTIC AND THERAPEUTIC TECHNIQUES

In addition to administering local anesthetics with or without steroids locally or regionally, anesthetic (lidocaine) can be administered locally, or adrenergic blockers systemically.

a) Intravenous lidocaine injection

Lidocaine is an amide local anesthetic and a sodium channel blocker that is given by controlled IV infusion to test the analgesic response and predict the possible efficacy of mexiletine (an oral sodium channel blocker). Although many positive responders demonstrate a good response to mexiletine, the true predictive value of this test is uncertain because it has not yet been shown that that negative responders do not respond to mexiletine.

Indications
- Neuropathic pain syndromes, particularly with continuous or lancinating dysesthesias, (e.g., diabetic neuropathy, phantom limb pain, stump pain, and neuralgia)

Pretest management
1. The patient is asked to eat lightly prior to the procedure, and to abstain for the 4 hours immediately preceding the procedure.
2. A baseline EKG and are obtained. Myocardial conduction abnormalities and abnormally elevated liver function test results are contraindications to oral mexiletine.

Potential complications
- Cardiac arrhythmias
- Syncope
- Hypotension
- Ataxia
- Tremors
- Dizziness
- Nervousness
- Rash
- Visual changes
- Seizures
- Anaphylaxis or an anaphylactic reaction

Technique
1. Blood pressure, EKG, and oxygen saturation are monitored continuously.
2. Patient is supine on a bed, and an 18- or 20-gauge IV catheter is placed in an upper extremity.
3. Pre-block VAS pain rating is obtained. Pain must exist at the time of the test for the efficacy of the infusion to be evaluated.
4. Lidocaine, 1 to 2 mg/kg (without epinephrine), is injected over 10 to 15 minutes (usually 100 mg for the average adult). If tinnitus, perioral numbness, metallic oral taste, or dizziness is experienced, injection speed should be reduced, and then restarted with resolution of the symptoms.

Evaluation of procedure
- VAS scores are obtained before, during, and after the infusion.
- A 50% or greater reduction in pain suggests that a trial of oral mexiletine is worthwhile.
- Specificity of response can be tested by injecting 10 mL of normal saline prior to the IV lidocaine and then obtaining VAS scores.

After the infusion, the patient is observed for 30 minutes in the sitting position and then allowed to ambulate. If the status is stable, the IV catheter is removed and the patient is discharged.

b) Intravenous phentolamine infusion

Phentolamine is an alpha-1-adrenergic blocking agent, which is given IV as a test for sympathetically mediated pain.

Indications
- Diagnosis, and occasionally therapy, of sympathetically maintained pain when sympathetic blocks are contraindicated (e.g., in anticoagulated patients, for infection of needle entry site)

Pre-block management
1. Patients are requested to eat lightly up to 4 hours prior to the procedure.
2. They are evaluated for cardiac disease or other conditions that may be affected by hypotension.

Potential complications
- Hypotension, mild to profound, possibly leading to hypoperfusion states
- Dizziness, lightheadedness
- Reflex tachycardia
- Syncope

Technique
This procedure is performed at our institution according to the protocol described by Raja and colleagues.

1. With the patient supine, EKG, blood pressure, and oxygen saturation monitors are placed.
2. An 18- or 20-gauge IV catheter is placed.
3. Baseline pain levels are recorded (VAS scores).
4. A bolus of 500 mL of lactated Ringer's solution is administered via a continuous infusion. This helps counteract hypotension and can act as a placebo test.
5. Stimulus-independent pain evaluations (VAS scores), and stimulus-evoked pain evaluations (e.g., VAS, mechanical test, cold test) are performed and recorded.
6. Propranolol, 2 mg IV, is administered to counteract reflex tachycardia.
7. Phentolamine, 35 to 70 mg IV in 250 mL normal saline, is infused over 20 minutes, without the patient's direct knowledge of initiation of the infusion.

Evaluation of procedure:
Pain testing and vital signs are evaluated for another half hour, prior to discharge. Relief of pain indicates that the pain was sympathetically maintained. If the pain is not relieved, either corroborative blocks or sympathetically independent pain may be considered, but the diagnosis is not definitively excluded.

Post-block management
Patients are observed for 30 minutes after the block, and somatosensory and pain evaluations are conducted. Patients are then allowed to sit and stand up, slowly, as tolerated. If they are stable, they are discharged; if not, they are observed for as long as necessary, prior to discharge with an escort.

c) Intravenous regional sympathetic blocks (Bier blocks)
Background
Bier blocks are done in an attempt to create a sympathetic block in an extremity (i.e., a peripheral block). Several medications can

be used, including guanethidine, bretylium, labetalol, prazosin, clonidine, and reserpine. Intravenous guanethidine and reserpine are not readily available in the United States. At MGH, we use the mixed alpha and beta antagonist labetalol.

Indications
* Therapeutic sympathetic blockade of an upper or lower extremity
* Diagnostic blockade when patients refuse needle blocks or are on anticoagulants, or when needle blocks are contraindicated or have been unsuccessful

Pre-block management
1. Patients are instructed to abstain from food for up to 4 hours prior to the procedure.
2. Baseline vital signs (EKG, blood pressure, oxygen saturation) are obtained.

Potential complications
* Hypotension, mild to profound, particularly when deflating the pneumatic cuff, or with a leaking cuff
* Dizziness
* Ischemia or neuropathy in the affected limb, usually transient
* Orthostatic hypotension
* Syncope

Technique
1. Patient is supine.
2. A 20- or 22-gauge IV catheter is placed in the affected extremity.
3. Another 18- or 20-gauge IV catheter is placed in a nonaffected extremity, for IV access and prehydration.
4. The affected extremity is exsanguinated by elevating it and binding it tightly with an elastic bandage (Esmarch bandage) from fingers to axilla.
5. A pneumatic cuff is applied proximally, at a pressure of 250 mm Hg.
6. Labetalol, 20 to 30 mg, with 100 mg of lidocaine, is made up to 20 mL of solution by adding normal saline, and it is injected into the affected upper extremity, OR.
7. Labetalol, 30 to 40 mg, with 200 mg of lidocaine, is made up to 35 mL with normal saline and is injected into the affected lower extremity.
8. The cuff's pressure is maintained at 250 mm Hg for 20 min, then either deflated slowly or intermittently deflated and re-inflated over 5 to 10 minutes, while monitoring vital signs closely.

Evaluation of procedure
Baseline (prior to procedure) and postprocedure pain evaluations are performed, including obtaining a VAS score. A time course of the pain relief is noted, as relief can range from hours to months.

VII. CONCLUSION
The blocks most commonly utilized in the MGH Pain Center are described. When used in carefully selected patients for specific in-

dications, nerve blocking procedures are extremely helpful. Perhaps their greatest value is in (1) diagnosis, (2) facilitating physical therapy in CRPS, (3) maintaining mobility during episodes of acute back pain, and (4) end-of-life pain management. It is not good practice to offer blocks to patients with no purpose other than short-term pain relief, or to give false hope of a cure. Patients will ultimately become disenchanted with this type of practice, as will health care insurers.

SELECTED READING

1. Bogduk N. Back pain, zygapophysial joint blocks and epidural steroids. In: Cousins MJ, Bridenbaugh PO, eds. *Neural blockade in clinical anesthesia and management of pain*, 2nd ed. Philadelphia: Lippincott, 1988.
2. Bonica JJ. *The management of pain*, vols. 1 and 2, 2nd ed. Philadelphia: Lea & Febiger, 1990.
3. Cousins MJ, Bromage PR, eds. *Neural blockade*, 2nd ed. Philadelphia: JB Lippincott, 1988.
4. Moore DC. *Regional block*, 4th ed. Springfield, IL: Charles C. Thomas, 1965.
5. Raj PP, ed. *Practical management of pain*, 2nd ed. St. Louis: Mosby– Year Book, 1992.
6. RAJA et al. Systematic alpha-adrenergic blockade with phentolamine: a diagnostic test for sympathetically maintained pain. *Anesthesiology* 1991;74:691–698.
7. Wall PD, Melzack R, eds. *Textbook of pain*, 3rd ed. New York: Churchill- Livingstone, 1994.
8. Mixter WJ, Barr JS. Rupture of intervertebral disc with involvement of the spinal cord. *N Engl J Med* 1934;211:210–215.

Interventional Treatment for Chronic Pain

Milan Stojanovic

Divinum est sedare dolorem—"It is divine to allay pain."
—*Galen (A.D. 129–199)*

In recent years, complex interventions for pain control have become part of everyday practice in pain clinics. Although interventions are more invasive than nerve blocks, many of them are not neurodestructive. Unlike nerve ablation, they may be reversible and therefore more appropriate for use in patients with nonmalignant pain. Their clinical efficacy has been widely documented. In carefully selected patients, these interventions can reduce pain and suffering, increase functional status, decrease oral medication intake, and facilitate an early return to work. In comparison with the more conservative measures for pain control, interventional treatments may appear costly, but when a good outcome is achieved, their overall cost can actually be lower (e.g., decreased cost of medications, fewer emergency room visits, less absence from work).

The implementation of these interventions should be integrated into a multidisciplinary team treatment plan. Patient benefit from these procedures can be achieved only by careful evaluation of scientific evidence, good clinical judgment, and excellent technical skills.

I. SPINAL CORD STIMULATION FOR CHRONIC PAIN

Electrical stimulation for treatment of pain was first documented in 600 B.C., utilizing electrical power from the torpedo fish. However, electrical treatment did not find a place in pain medicine until 1967, when spinal cord stimulation (SCS) was introduced by Shealy and associates. Their work was based on the "gate control" theory of pain proposed by Melzack and Wall and published just 2 years earlier. Initially, the SCS implantation involved open laminectomy, performed only by neurosurgeons. With recent advances in technology, the SCS has become a minimally invasive treatment and it is currently performed by physicians from various specialties. Further improvements in hardware design and patient selection criteria have enhanced the efficacy of SCS, and success rates of 50% to 70% have been recently reported. Besides SCS, peripheral nerve stimulation (PNS) can be performed in selected patients with localized neuropathic pain. Today, SCS presents a valuable tool for treatment of many chronic pain conditions.

1. Mechanism of action

The Melzak and Wall gate control theory of pain was a foundation for the first SCS trials. It was based on the idea that stimulation of A-beta fibers closes the dorsal horn "gate" and reduces the nociceptive input from the periphery. However, it seems that other mechanisms play a more significant role in the mechanism of SCS action.

One proposed mechanism involves increased dorsal horn inhibitory action of neurotransmitters, such as γ-aminobutyric acid (GABA) and adenosine A-1, during SCS. The potential activation of descending analgesia pathways by serotonin and norepinephrine is another explanation for SCS action. In patients with peripheral ischemic pain, the SCS may act by a combination of two mechanisms: suppression of sympathetic activity and suppression of a calcitonin gene-related peptide (CGRP)–mediated mechanism. The probable mechanism for pain relief in ischemic heart disease is redistribution of the coronary blood flow from regions with normal perfusion to regions with impaired perfusion. Also, SCS may suppress the excitatory effects of myocardial ischemia on intrinsic cardiac neurons.

2. Indications and patient selection

Patients with **complex regional pain syndrome** (CRPS) or with **neuropathic pain with upper and lower extremity involvement** are the best candidates. Excellent long-term success rates (50% to 91% efficacy and a decrease in analgesic consumption by 50%) have been reported for SCS used in patients with CRPS.

However, the same does not apply to phantom limb pain, stump pain, or spinal cord injury pain. The most likely explanation is that central nervous system (CNS) remapping, which may be critical to the development of these pain syndromes, is not affected by SCS. Diabetic neuropathy may respond well to SCS, but the infection risks in these patients are higher than in the nondiabetic population. The use of SCS in postherpetic neuralgia is controversial.

Patients with **failed back surgery syndrome** (FBSS) may respond well to SCS. It has been documented that patients with FBSS respond better to SCS than to reoperation. This applies in particular to low back pain (LBP) with a radiating component to the leg. In these patients, the chance of long-term success with SCS varies from 12% to 88%, with an average efficacy of 59% as indicated by a systematic review of the literature. In addition, 25% of patients may return to work, 61% show an improvement in activities of daily living, and 40% to 84% decrease their consumption of analgesics. Opinions on axial LBP (pain limited only to the low back area) are divided. Some studies show that the dual-lead system provides better pain relief for axial LBP than single-lead stimulation, but others find the opposite.

Severe peripheral vascular disease is also an indication for SCS. Patients with advanced peripheral vascular disease who are not surgical candidates respond well to SCS, with reported efficacy rates ranging from 60% to 100%. Besides providing pain relief, SCS promotes ulcer healing and potentially contributes to limb salvage.

Ischemic heart disease refractory to pharmacologic and surgical treatments may respond well to SCS, with reported efficacy rates of 60% to 80% several years after implantation. These patients have demonstrated a reduction in anginal pain, decreased use of short-acting nitrates, and increased exercise capacity. SCS does not completely abolish anginal pain, but it raises the anginal threshold. Fear of a potential increase in myocardial damage does not seem to be justified.

New indications and techniques for PNS have emerged recently. Some patients with occipital neuralgia seem to respond well to PNS. In those cases, the SCS lead is placed subcutaneously around the C1-2 spinous process. In patients with pelvic pain (e.g., interstitial cystitis, pain of unknown origin), sacral placement of two to four SCS leads may provide adequate analgesia. Sacral placement can also be helpful in patients with impaired bladder control. Some cases of lumbar radiculopathy may respond better to SCS leads placed directly through neural foramina (retrograde lead placement).

Infection, drug abuse, and severe psychiatric disease are major contraindications for SCS implantation. Before SCS implantation, a psychological evaluation of patient is recommended.

3. Stimulator trials

Before proceeding with permanent SCS implantation, a stimulation trial is warranted. The trial allows patients to evaluate the SCS analgesic activity in their everyday surroundings. The criteria for a successful trial include at least a 50% pain reduction, a decrease in analgesic intake, and a significant functional improvement. The SCS trial is a minimally invasive procedure (similar to placing an epidural catheter), and it can positively predict a long-term outcome in 50% to 70% of cases.

There is no consensus on the length of an SCS trial. Minimal trial time should be 24 hours, although many centers perform 3- to 5-day trials. The trial begins in the hospital with proper SCS adjustment, after which the patient is discharged for several days of home trial. In cases of equivocal results, the trial time can be extended.

There are two technical approaches for an SCS trial. In the first approach, the SCS lead is placed percutaneously. This has the advantage of minimal invasiveness. At trial completion, the lead is removed, and a new lead and internal pulse generator (IPG) are placed (on a separate occasion). The other approach is to tunnel in and anchor the trial lead via a surgical incision. This approach simplifies the final procedure and ensures that stimulation coverage remains the same during both the trial period and the permanent implantation. The major disadvantage of the second approach is the need for a second visit to the operating room for lead removal in the case of an unsuccessful trial.

A percutaneous trial followed by lead placement via a laminotomy is another, less frequently utilized approach for SCS. In this case, a lead with wider electrodes is placed via laminotomy during permanent implantation. Wider electrodes might provide better coverage in certain patients, and they are less prone to migration than standard SCS leads.

4. Choice of hardware

The permanent SCS hardware consists of the SCS lead, an extension cable, a power source, and a pulse generator.

The number of electrodes in the lead varies from four (Medtronic and ANS) to eight (ANS). The distance between the electrodes and the length of the leads also can differ. It is not clear whether an increased number of electrodes provides better coverage, but it might be beneficial in case of lead migration. The leads with minimal space between electrodes (such as the Medtronic Quad compact lead) are better suited for localized pain (such as foot pain) or cases of isolated axial LBP. Many leads contain a removable stylet, which eases lead steering during implantation.

There are two types of pulse generators: (a) the completely implantable pulse generator containing a battery, and (b) an IPG supplied by external power through the radiofrequency antenna applied to the skin. The implanted pulse generator is more convenient to use and can be easily adjusted by the patient using a small telemetry device. Patients can turn the stimulator on and off, and they can control the stimulation amplitude, frequency, and pulse width. A separate external programmer allows more complex IPG reprogramming by the physician. In case of inadequate stimulation, the physician can change the polarity and the number of functioning electrodes to provide better stimulation coverage. The batteries have to be changed every 3 to 6 years, which requires a brief visit to the operating room. The battery life depends on the time the stimulator is used and the stimulation amplitude. The externally powered IPG, therefore, has an advantage over the implanted one in patients requiring higher amplitudes of stimulation, which deplete implanted batteries in a short time.

5. Implantation techniques

For lumbar lead placement, the patient is placed in the prone position, and for cervical placement both prone and lateral decubitus positions are used. The patient is prepared and draped in usual fashion. Both trial and permanent implantations are performed under local anesthesia with light intravenous (IV) sedation. The most common entry sites are the T12-L1 and L1–L2 spinal interspaces for the lumbar area and C7-T1 for the cervical area. These interspaces are first identified with fluoroscopic guidance, making sure to obtain a true anteroposterior (AP) view. The true AP view is achieved by C-arm rotation until the spinous process is placed on the midline in relation to the spinal pedicles.

For the percutaneous SCS trial, the Tuohy needle entry site is at the level of the spinous process below the desired interspace. It is important to achieve a shallow entry angle or to use the alternate Piles needle. The needle tip should stay close to midline during insertion. As the needle is advanced, lateral fluoroscopic view can be obtained to assess needle depth. Once adequate depth is achieved, the loss-of-resistance technique is used to identify the epidural space. At this point, the SCS lead is inserted into the epidural space under continuous fluoroscopic guidance. The curved stylet, or curved lead tip, allows lead steering. The lead tip during insertion and at final position should lie at the lateral border of the spinous process on the ipsilateral side of the pain.

Once adequate lead position is obtained, the trial stimulation is performed. It is important that stimulation paresthesias provide 70% to 80% overlap with the patient's pain location. Adequate patient feedback during this stage is important. Maximal effort should be used to provide adequate pain coverage, since this optimizes the trial. Frequent lead repositioning might be needed during this stage. Once adequate coverage is achieved, the needle is removed under continuous fluoroscopy, ensuring no change in lead position. The lead is then taped to the skin.

Permanent stimulator placement technique is similar to the trial. Although the trial is usually done in the pain clinic setting, permanent SCS placement is performed in the operating room. Under local anesthesia and IV sedation, a skin incision is made along the cervical or lumbar insertion site. Tissue dissection is performed until lumbar fascia is encountered. At that point, the Tuohy needle and the stimulator lead are inserted as done in the SCS trial. Once adequate coverage is obtained, the Tuohy needle is removed under continuous fluoroscopic guidance and the SCS lead is anchored with sutures to the fascia and supraspinous ligament. The pocket for the IPG is made in the gluteal or abdominal area. The SCS lead is then connected to the IPG through an extension cable tunneled through the skin. The skin and subcutaneous tissues are closed in layers.

Patients should avoid any extreme activity for the first 6 to 8 weeks following permanent SCS implantation to prevent lead migration and allow for epidural scar tissue formation.

Lead positioning

The SCS topographic coverage depends on the spinal level at which the SCS lead tip is positioned. The following landmarks are for orientation only; the variance can be very high in individual patients. Careful intraoperative mapping is needed for optimal coverage ("sweet spot placement").

Upper extremity: SCS tip at a level between C2 and C5. The shoulder area can be difficult to cover (Fig. 1).

Foot: SCS lead tip at a level between T11 and L1 (Fig. 2).

Lower extremity: SCS lead tip at the T9–10 level

Low back: SCS lead tip at a level between T8 and T10; two parallel leads can be used.

Chest: SCS lead tip at the T1–2 level.

Occipital neuralgia: SCS lead placed around C1–2 subcutaneously.

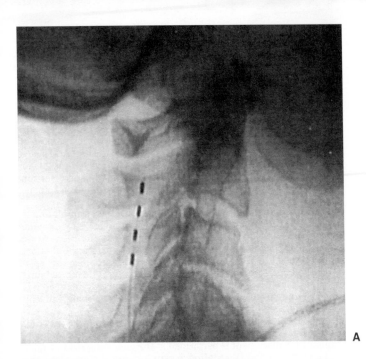

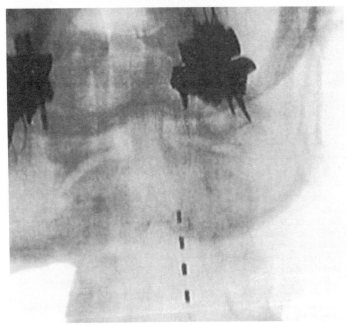

Figure 1. Spinal cord stimulation (SCS) lead at the C2-3 level as seen on lateral fluoroscopic view (A) and anteroposterior (AP) view (B). Note the alignment of the SCS lead with a lateral margin of the odontoid process in the AP view.

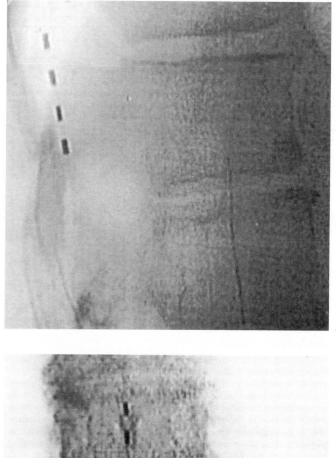

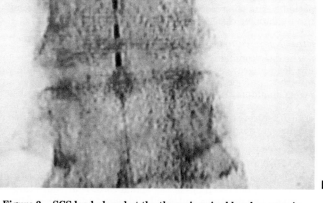

Figure 2. SCS lead placed at the thoracic spinal level as seen in lateral (A) and AP fluoroscopic view (B).

Pelvic pain: multiple SCS leads placed retrogradely within the sacrum or through foramina at S2 to S4.

6. Troubleshooting and complications

SCS Not Functioning or Inadequate Coverage

1. Obtain AP and lateral fluoroscopic images of SCS lead tip to rule out lead migration.
2. Image the IPG and all connections, and search for disconnection or breakage.
3. Using programmer, check the batteries.
4. Change amplitude and pulse width.
5. Reverse electrode polarity, and change electrodes activated if there is no response to prior measures.
6. If adequate pain coverage cannot be obtained, measure impedance of each electrode in relation to the IPG. Exactly the same impedance on two electrodes raises the possibility of a short circuit between the two electrodes. Some mechanical failures might require surgical revision and replacement of affected SCS components.

Progressive decrease in stimulation threshold

Consider intrathecal migration of the SCS lead. If it stays unnoticed, it can lead to serious complications such as spinal cord injury. Intrathecal migration is most common in patients with significant spinal canal stenosis. If this condition is suspected, a magnetic resonance imaging (MRI) scan of the targeted spinal level should be obtained before anticipated SCS placement.

SCS and pacemakers

The SCS can cause interference and inhibition of a cardiac pacemaker if they are used simultaneously. However, both devices can be used in the same patient if these guidelines are followed: (a) both devices should be programmed in bipolar mode, (b) the SCS frequency should be set at 20Hz, and (c) each SCS programming should be performed using continuous electrocardiographic (ECG) monitoring. A cardiology consult should be obtained in these patients, and the recommendations of the pacemaker's manufacturer should be closely followed.

Other complications

The most common other complications of SCS are hardware failure, lead migration, infection, skin irritation at the IPG site, and failure to provide pain relief. Bleeding at the IPG site (subcutaneous hematoma) is usually self-limiting and gradually reabsorbs in a few weeks. If infection occurs at the IPG insertion site, make sure to aspirate the site before initiating antibiotic coverage and removing the hardware.

II. CHRONIC INTRATHECAL THERAPY FOR CANCER AND NONMALIGNANT PAIN

Intrathecal drug delivery has gained its popularity since the discovery of opioid receptors in the spinal cord. It provides targeted delivery of medications and avoids side effects encountered by systemic administration of drugs. Opioids are delivered to the intrathecal space via a surgically implanted subcutaneous pump containing a reservoir for the medication. The pump is easily refilled with medication every 2 to 4 months depending on the infusion rate.

Medications other than opioids have been used recently for intrathecal delivery. This includes local anesthetics, clonidine, and baclofen, given alone or in combination with opioids. Because numerous receptors involved in nociceptive transmission are located in the spinal cord, this approach seems to be very promising. The efficacy of intrathecal drug delivery has been shown in patients with malignant and nonmalignant pain.

The completely implanted intrathecal system has many advantages over the epidural drug delivery via an external catheter. The epidural route is more costly because of the maintenance needed for the external system, and it is frequently more inconvenient for the patient; therefore, it should be reserved for short-term use only (less than 3 months). The completely implanted intrathecal delivery is preferred when treatment is expected to last longer than 3 to 6 months. Patients with implanted intrathecal pumps may safely undergo an MRI procedure for other purposes.

1. Patient selection

Cancer pain responds well to intrathecal therapy in carefully selected patients. The following cancer patients might be considered for intrathecal trial:

- Patients who have failed oral or IV opioids as a result of severe side effects (nausea, vomiting, sedation, constipation)
- Patients who have a life expectancy of more than 3 months
- Patients who have no obstruction in CSF flow
- Patients who have neuropathic cancer pain that does not respond to oral regimen and nerve blocks.

The main contraindication for intrathecal therapy is infection.

Nonmalignant pain may respond to intrathecal therapy but it should be considered as a last resort. In general, patients with cancer pain tend to respond better to intrathecal therapy than patients with nonmalignant pain. Therefore, the selection criteria for intrathecal therapy for nonmalignant pain should be very strict. Only patients who have failed nerve blocks, oral medications, physical therapy, and cognitive-behavioral programs and who have passed psychological evaluation should be considered for intrathecal trial.

2. Screening

Before considering implantation of intrathecal hardware, patients should undergo a trial procedure to better assess the odds of a favorable outcome. The actual trial procedure varies, and no consensus has been made on the best procedure. Preceding the trial, oral opioids are either discontinued or decreased substantially. It is important to monitor the patient for signs of respiratory depression during the trial. The most common screening methods are the following:

An **intrathecal trial** is performed by implanting the temporary intrathecal catheter. Pediatric or standard epidural catheters can be used for this purpose. After intrathecal placement, the catheter is taped to the skin. The medication bolus is given first, followed by continuous infusion via an external infusion pump. The intrathecal opioid dose starts at 1/300th of the usual oral daily dose. The patient is kept in a hospital, for several days up to 3 weeks, during which time the infusion rate is gradually increased. The longer the trial time is, the smaller the likelihood of a placebo response. The patient pain intensity score, functional status, and use of medications for breakthrough pain are monitored during the trial period.

An **epidural trial** is performed in the same way as the intrathecal trial, except that the catheter is placed in the epidural space. The administered epidural opioid daily dose is higher than the intrathecal one, representing 1/30th of the usual daily oral dose.

A **one-time bolus** is the simplest screening method. The intrathecal bolus of medication is given and the patient is monitored for 24 hours. The patient pain intensity score, functional status, and use of medications for breakthrough pain are monitored. This method does not allow dose titration, as the other methods do, but it can provide information on patient response to intrathecal opioids.

A **side-port catheter** can be surgically implanted for a trial. Its advantages include the ease of adding an implanted infusion pump in case the trial is successful. However, the added risk of infection, and the need to surgically remove the catheter in the case of a failed trial, are disadvantages of using this approach.

3. Hardware selection

Two kinds of pumps exist: (a) battery powered externally programmable pumps and (b) nonprogrammable pumps, many of them gas driven. The amount of medication delivered by nonprogrammable pumps is dependent on drug concentration. Although externally programmable pumps offer the great advantage of an adjustable infusion rate, continuous-rate pumps can be used in patients requiring less frequent rate adjustments.

4. Medication selection and dosage

All intrathecally administered medications should be preservative free. The most commonly administered intrathecal medication is morphine. Other opioids include fentanyl, sufentanil, hydromorphone, and meperidine.

To convert intrathecal doses to other routes of administration, the following ratios are used: (a) intrathecal to epidural, 1:10; (b) intrathecal to IV, 1:100; (c) intrathecal to oral, 1:300. In opioid-naive patients, morphine should be started at 0.2 mg/day and gradually increased. In opioid-tolerant patients, the initial intrathecal dose should be less than the conversion dose, and oral opioids should be used for breakthrough pain. Gradually, the intrathecal dose should be increased and breakthrough pain medications discontinued.

The addition of local anesthetics to intrathecal opioids may be used for cancer and nonmalignant pain, with particular benefit to patients with a neuropathic component of pain. A typical bupivacaine dose range is from 2 to 30 mg/day, although dosages of over 100 mg/day have been reported. Alpha-adrenergic agonists (clonidine, epinephrine) can be used in conjunction with opioids. Clonidine is now approved by the U.S. Food and Drug Administration (FDA) for epidural administration, and its intrathecal-equivalent dosage is 50 to 900 μg/day. It should be carefully titrated since it can cause significant hypotension (most severe in dosage range of 400 to 570 μg/day).

Other investigational drugs are used intrathecally, and their use is supported by excellent results in clinical trials. Somatostatin seems to be particularly beneficial for the treatment of cancer pain. For neuropathic and nociceptive pain, the new investigational drugs include: calcium channel blockers (SNX-111), acetylcholinesterase (neostigmine), N-methyl-D-aspartate (NMDA) receptor antagonist (ketamine), GABA-A receptor agonists (midazolam), and GABA-B receptor agonist (baclofen). Many other intrathecally administered analgesics have proven their efficacy in animal research and await final testing in human clinical trials.

5. Complications and side effects

Medication-Related Complications

Medication-related side effects and complications of neuraxial opiates include respiratory depression, pruritus, nausea, vomiting, urinary retention, reduced libido, edema with weight gain, and constipation.

Respiratory depression can occur immediately after opioid administration or with several hours' delay. It is much more frequent in opioid-naive patients. The factors increasing the risk for respiratory depression are advanced age, high opioid dose, and concomitant use of baclofen, benzodiazepines, and sedatives. Monitoring the vital signs and pulse oximetry is mandatory following initiation of an intrathecal opioid infusion.

The treatment of respiratory depression depends on its severity. The intrathecal infusion should be discontinued or reduced. If the patient cannot be aroused, IV naloxone should be administered. In severe cases, intrathecal naloxone can be administered in conjunction with airway protection and assisted ventilation.

Pruritus, nausea, and vomiting usually occur with initiation of intrathecal opioid bolus administration and can precede the onset of pain relief. These side effects can be prevented by more gradual opioid dose increase.

The incidence of *urinary retention* ranges from 40% to 80% and is not dose dependent. It occurs most often in men with an already-enlarged prostate. Cholinomimetic drugs (terazosin and carbachol) can be effective in treating urinary retention.

Hormonal abnormalities are reported with intrathecal opioid administration. Serum lipids, estrogens, androgens, insulin-like growth factor (IGF-1), and 24-hour urinary cortisol should be monitored in these patients. There is a 3% to 5% incidence of *decreased libido* in patients receiving intrathecal opioid therapy, because of hormonal abnormalities. Persistent decreased libido may require hormonal replacement. Approximately 5% to 10% of patients may experience weight gain and edema, which is not dose dependent.

Surgical complications

Infection at the pump insertion site may require complete hardware removal. Symptoms of infection are pain at the insertion site, local increase in temperature, and edema. Antibiotics should be started after wound cultures (by aspiration) are obtained. *Seroma* at the insertion site is usually benign and does not require revision. Necrosis and skin perforations can also occur and should be surgically treated.

Meningitis presents with stiff neck, fever, and meningeal signs. The CSF can be obtained from the pump for cultures and cell count.

Granuloma formation at the catheter tip is a very rare complication, potentially leading to cord compression. MRI of the spinal cord is indicated if neurologic symptoms occur in these patients.

Bleeding at the pump site usually spontaneously resolves, although it can increase the incidence of infection. *Epidural hematoma* can lead to spinal cord compression.

A *CSF leak* occurs after almost any intrathecal pump placement and if significant can lead to severe *postdural puncture headache*. If conservative therapy fails, headache can be treated with an epidural blood patch. However, the patch should be performed under fluoroscopic guidance to avoid risk of intrathecal catheter damage.

Hardware complications

Hardware complications usually involve the catheter and rarely the pump. *Catheter* kinking, disconnection, dislodgement, breaks, and migration can occur. Withdrawal symptoms and loss of analgesia are signs of inadequate drug delivery and warrant further investigation. Although the catheter is radiopaque and can be seen on fluoroscopy, it should be tested with a nonionic-contrast bolus. Before administering the bolus, medication should be aspirated from the catheter dead-space to avoid overdose. This can be accomplished through the pump side port. If the pump does not have a side port, it should be emptied, filled with radiolabeled tracer, and imaged.

Pump failures can also occur. Torsion of the pump within the pocket, and subsequent catheter kinking, can be prevented by adequate pump anchoring. The most serious technique-related complication is drug overdose caused by filling the pump through the side port. If this occurs, the CSF should be partially replaced with saline and the patient immediately transferred to the intensive care unit. Intrathecal naloxone should be administered.

Other mechanical pump failures include battery depletion and internal pump failure. The manufacturer's recommendations and testing protocols should be followed meticulously to rule out internal pump failure.

III. DISCOGRAPHY

Discography is a diagnostic procedure and has no therapeutic value. It is best suited for diagnosis of discogenic low back pain caused by internal disc disruption. The term *discogenic pain* should not be confused with disc herniation or protrusion. The pathology of and treatment options in these two conditions differ significantly.

1. Brief overview of disc anatomy and pathophysiology

Each disc consists of a central mass, the nucleus pulposus, and an outer ring, the annulus fibrosus. The annulus fibrosus is connected by Sharpey's fibers to the articular surface of vertebral bodies. The inner structure of the annulus is formed of concentric lamellae of collagen fibrils. There are 10 to 12 overlapping concentric lamellae in each annulus. The lamellae are thinner and less numerous at the posterior portion of the disc. Many studies suggest that the annulus is a well-innervated structure. Degenerated discs lose nuclear hydrostatic pressure, which leads to buckling of the annular lamellae. With progressive degeneration of the disc, the annulus undergoes delamination and develops fissures. "Microfractures" of the annular collagen fibrils have been demonstrated using electron microscopy. The annular nociceptors become sensitized with the decrease in their firing thresholds. The increased stimulation of the dorsal root ganglion by sensitized nociceptors may cause a referred pain pattern to the lower extremities. Furthermore, the damaged disc promotes the growth of nerve fibers along radial tears into the inner annulus.

2. Discogenic low back pain: diagnostic studies

Most patients with discogenic LBP have increased pain with prolonged sitting. The pain can be limited to the back area (axial pain), or it can radiate to one or both lower extremities. The physical exam, including the straight leg raising test, can be normal.

Normal diagnostic imaging findings (e.g., by MRI) do not rule out internal disc derangement pathology. However, certain MRI findings are highly suggestive of discogenic disease:

- Decreased disc signal intensity on T2-weighted MRI images is suggestive of disc dehydration.
- High T2-weighted signal intensity within the annulus of a disc has been termed the high intensity zone (HIZ) and is associated with annular tears. Patients with an HIZ are more likely to suffer from LBP than patients without it.
- A "bulging" or "protruding" disc on MRI is more likely associated with disc disruption and pain than a "normal" disc.
- Even a disc that is completely normal on MRI can be associated with discogenic pain. The decrease in disc height is often seen when internal disc derangement has taken place.

Provocation discography remains the gold standard for the diagnosis of discogenic pain. The key feature of discography is the reproduction of the patient's pain. Discography is performed at three or four lumbar levels, using unaffected discs as controls. Morphologically, a normal disc presents as a unilocular, bilocular, spherical, or rectangular shape. A degenerated disc loses its water content and may have tears and fissures in the annulus fibrosus. The most common types of annular tears are concentric, radial, and transverse tears. Although the pattern of the spread of contrast material is important, the concordant pain with low pressure or low volume discography is the most important diagnostic finding.

3. Technical aspects of lumbar discography

The patient is placed in the prone position and the lower back area is adequately prepared and draped. An AP fluoroscopic image is obtained first, providing good visualization of the selected disc. The end plates of adjacent vertebral bodies are aligned. The C-arm is then rotated to the oblique view, maintaining alignment of the vertebral bodies. The optimal endpoint of the rotation angle is when the superior articular process (SAP) image reaches the midline of the corresponding vertebral end plate. At this point, the skin entry site is determined by the radiopaque pointer overlapping the SAP projection.

After anesthetizing the skin with 1% lidocaine, an 18-gauge, 3-inch needle is inserted in a "tunneled view" toward the SAP. The needle tip should be advanced approximately 2 inches. A 22-gauge, 6-inch needle with a slightly bent tip is then inserted through the 18-gauge needle. Under tunneled fluoroscopic guidance, the needle is steered just lateral to the SAP, making sure that it is approaching the disc at midline. A slightly caudally placed needle can help to avoid contact with the nerve root. Once the needle has entered into the disc, a "spongy" feeling is encountered. From that point, several AP and lateral fluoroscopic views should be obtained to ensure that the needle tip is in the center of the disc.

The L5-S1 disc level can be more difficult to approach because of the iliac crest. Maneuvering the needle bend at its distal tip around the iliac crest usually helps.

Discography is performed once the needles are placed at all desirable levels (Fig. 3). Nonionic contrast (Omnipaque-240) is appropriate for discography, and it should be mixed with 5 to 10 mg/cc of antibiotic such as cefazolin.

The concordant pain is sought at less than 30 pounds per square inch above opening pressure, or with less than 1.25 mL of contrast material administered into the disc. The reproduced LBP (or pain referred to the lower extremity) under these conditions is considered to be discogenic in origin. Disc disruption and leakage of dye through an annular tear is usually seen with the onset of pain. Disc disruption alone, without reproduction of the patient's pain, is an insufficient finding for the diagnosis of discogenic pain.

Postdiscography computed tomography (CT) is not an absolutely necessary diagnostic tool, but it can be helpful in planning further treatments. The CT should be performed within 2 hours of discography. The most serious complication of discography is discitis. Although rare, it is very resistant to treatment because of the limited blood supply to the disc. Intradiscal administration of antibiotic minimizes its occurrence. Discography has been shown to be a generally safe procedure and has not been found to produce damage to the disc.

4. Discogenic low back pain: treatment options

There are several treatment options in a patient presenting with discogenic pain. Conservative therapy such as McKenzie exercises or dynamic lumbar stabilization exercises can be helpful in some patients.

Radiofrequency (RF) denervation of the annulus appears to be of limited value since RF requires a fluid environment to adequately disperse RF energy. In the case of discogenic pain, disc and annular tissues are often dehydrated. Also, current RF probes seem to be too small to treat large surface areas of annular tissue. Alternatively, the technique of annular denervation can be used. For this purpose, the RF lesioning of gray rami has been used with mixed results. Intradiscal steroid injections have also been used but with

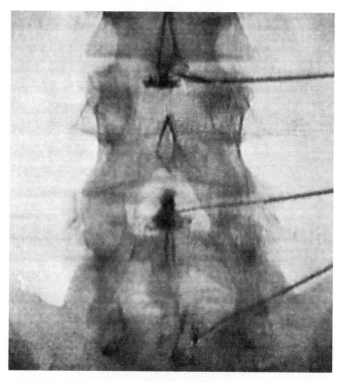

Figure 3. Appropriate needle position for lumbar discography at L4, L5, and S1 levels as seen in AP fluoroscopic view. Note contrast spread, down the annular fissure at the L4 level to the right.

mostly unsatisfactory results. Laser disc lesioning has a high risk of complications.

Surgical approaches (anterior and posterior lumbar fusion, titanium cages) are the most commonly used treatments for discogenic LBP, with success rates in the range of 50% to 85%. Drawbacks of surgery are its expense and potential complications. Surgery may be reserved for severe morphologic disc damage, when regeneration of annulus fibrosus is unlikely.

IV. INTRADISCAL ELECTROTHERMAL THERAPY

Intradiscal electrothermal therapy (IDET) is a new, minimally invasive approach for the treatment of discogenic LBP. Initial results with this treatment are encouraging, but more clinical studies are needed to prove its efficacy. It involves percutaneously threading a flexible catheter (SpineCath) into the disc tissue with fluoroscopic guidance. The catheter is composed of thermal-resistive coil, enabling heating its distal part to the desired temperature.

The technique for approaching the disc for the IDET procedure is similar to that of discography. After the skin is infiltrated with local anesthetic, a 17-gauge introducer needle is inserted in the disc tissue guided by oblique fluoroscopic imaging. Once appropriate needle position is established by AP and lateral fluoroscopic views, the catheter is inserted through the needle. The SpineCath is designed to be easily navigated through the disc tissue. The final position of the electrode is such that the end of the catheter is placed circumferentially around the inner surface of the posterior annulus (Fig. 4). The best approach to the disc is from the side opposite the symptoms; however, some patients require ipsilateral approach if catheter navigation from the opposite side fails. IV sedation can be administered, but IV anesthesia is contraindicated during IDET procedure to ensure appropriate patient feedback.

Once the catheter is in a satisfactory position, as confirmed by AP and lateral fluoroscopy, the distal part of the catheter is heated gradually with the ORATEC ElectroThermal Spine System Generator. Increments in temperature are achieved automatically, and the target temperature is 80° to 90°C, which must be maintained for 4 to 6 minutes to achieve optimal results. The actual annular

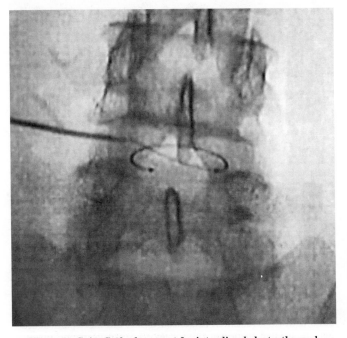

Figure 4.   SpineCath placement for intradiscal electrothermal therapy (IDET) procedure at the L4 spinal level as seen on AP fluoroscopic view. The thermal-resistive coil is placed along the inner surface of the posterior disc annulus.

tissue temperature is up to 15°C lower than the temperature of the catheter tip. Comprehensive patient and cadaver temperature-mapping studies have shown the safety of reaching this high target temperature as long as the catheter tip is located within the disc tissue. The simultaneous epidural space temperatures remain within the normal range, reaching a maximum of 39.3°C even if the catheter tip is heated to 90°C. A slight increase in concordant pain during heating is normal. Patients can be discharged home 1 hour after the procedure.

The putative mechanisms of IDET action are thermal modification of collagen fibers and destruction of sensitized nociceptors in the annular wall. Besides the usual risks such as infection and bleeding, a possible serious complication of IDET is catheter tip shearing due to forceful manipulation. Inappropriate catheter handling can result in more serious complications, such as nerve damage or cauda equina injury.

Patients with discogenic pain for more than 6 months who have failed conservative treatment are considered appropriate candidates for IDET. However, patients with severe radicular symptoms due to a herniated disc or those with severe spinal stenosis are not good candidates. Also, a severely collapsed disc (>50% of disc height) or a disrupted disc might not respond well to IDET. In patients over 50 years of age, there may be an adverse effect on the disc healing process and therefore lower success rates with treatment. Multilevel disc disease and a history of prior spinal fusion are not contraindications for IDET.

Considering its potential advantages over surgery, IDET might become the treatment of choice for discogenic pain. It could potentially fill the large gap between conservative treatment and surgical options.

V. VERTEBROPLASTY

Percutaneous vertebroplasty is a relatively new procedure consisting of percutaneously injecting polymethylmethacrylate cement into vertebral bodies destabilized by osseous lesions and causing intractable pain. By reinforcing vertebral lesions, injected cement provides analgesia in these patients. The major indications for vertebroplasty are osteoporotic vertebral compression fractures, vertebral angiomas, and osteoporotic vertebral tumors.

The procedure is performed under fluoroscopic or CT guidance. With the patient in the prone position and under local anesthesia, an 11-gauge bone marrow biopsy needle is directed through the transpedicular approach into the vertebral body. The depth of the needle is ensured in lateral fluoroscopic views. An intraosseous venogram is then performed to ensure that the needle tip is not within a blood vessel. The cement is than injected under continuous fluoroscopic guidance.

Recent clinical studies have shown good efficacy of vertebroplasty. Potential complications include leakage of cement into adjacent structures with neural damage caused by mechanical compression and thermal necrosis. Therefore, high technical expertise is needed to perform this procedure. Current research efforts are focused on designing improved bone cement that does not leak into unwanted areas and that minimizes tissue damage.

SELECTED READINGS

1. Barr JD, Barr MS, Lemley TJ, McCann RM. Percutaneous vertebroplasty for pain relief and spinal stabilization. *Spine* 2000;25: 923–928.

2. Carey C, Lee H, Schaff RA, eds. *The Washington manual of medical therapeutics*, 29th ed. New York: Lippincott Williams & Wilkins, 1998.

3. Cousins M, Bridenbaugh P, eds. *Neural blockade in clinical anesthesia and management of pain*, 3rd ed. Philadelphia: Lippincott, 1998.

4. Deer T, Winkelmuller W, Erdine S, et al. Intrathecal therapy for cancer and non-malignant pain: Patient selection and patient management. *Neuromodulation* 1999;2:55–66.

5. Kay J, Findling JW, Ralf H. Epidural triamcinolone suppresses the pituitary-adrenal axis in human subjects. *Anesth Analg* 1994; 79:501–505.

6. Kemler MA, Barendse GA, van Kleef M, et al. Spinal cord stimulation in patients with chronic reflex sympathetic dystrophy. *N Engl J Med* 2000;343:618–624.

7. Krames E, Bucher E, Hassenbuch S, Levy R. Future trends in the development of local drug delivery systems: Intraspinal, intracerebral and intraparenchymal therapies. *Neuromodulation* 1999; 2:133–148.

8. North RB, Kidd DH, Zahurak M, et al. Spinal cord stimulation for chronic intractable pain: Two decades' experience. *Neurosurgery* 1993;32:384–395.

9. Parry SW, Kenny RA. The management of vasovagal syncope. *Q J Med* 1999;92:697–705.

10. Saal SS, Saal AS. Management of chronic discogenic low back pain with a thermal intradiscal catheter. *Spine* 2000;25:382–388.

11. Stanton-Hicks M. Spinal cord stimulation for the management of complex regional pain syndromes. *Neurostimulation* 1999;2: 193–201.

12. Stojanovic M. Stimulation methods for neuropathic pain control. *Curr Pain Headache Rep* (in press).

13. Tehranzadeh J. Discography 2000. *Radiol Clin North Am* 1998; 36:463–495.

14. Waldman SD, Winnie AP, eds. *Interventional pain management*. Philadelphia: WB Saunders, 1996.

15. Weissberg D, Refaely Y. Pneumothorax. *Chest* 2000;117: 1279–1285.

Neurosurgical Interventions for Chronic Pain

G. Rees Cosgrove and Emad Eskandar

Pain is the psychic adjunct of an imperative protective reflex.
—*Sir Charles Sherrington*

A multidisciplinary approach to patients with chronic pain is the best way to individualize treatment plans and optimize clinical results. Neurosurgical participation in the management plan is variable. In general, neurosurgical consultation is sought only after the patient's pain has been proven refractory to all appropriate medical therapies. However, in some clinical situations, it is appropriate that neurosurgery be considered during the initial evaluation of the patient with chronic pain.

I. GENERAL CONSIDERATIONS

1. Timing of neurosurgical interventions

All patients should undergo a reasonable trial of conservative therapy before any neurosurgical intervention is discussed. Specifically, oral analgesics, parenteral agents, and usually short-term anesthetic interventions (e.g., local blocks, temporary spinal infusion catheters) should be tried as preliminary treatments. Enhancing the quality of life of the patient with chronic pain is paramount, and when it is clear that the overall goals of pain management are not being met by less invasive treatment, surgical approaches should be considered. In particular, early neurosurgical intervention can optimize function and greatly improve pain control during the final months of life in patients with terminal cancer. Surgical treatment for only the most debilitated patient reduces its functional benefit and increases the surgical risk. Unfortunately, there are no rules for when neurologic interventions are appropriate, and individual clinical situations must be carefully assessed.

2. Augmentative versus ablative procedures

Neurosurgical approaches to chronic pain can be loosely grouped into two broad categories: **augmentative**, when a device or substance is "added," such as a pump system designed to infuse opiates or electrodes implanted for electrical stimulation, and **ablative**, when nervous input is severed, such as the many spinal cord lesioning techniques for treating chronic pain of malignant origin. Augmentative techniques have the advantage of being reversible: they can be discontinued if they prove ineffective, with no loss of function. Many augmentative procedures, however, suffer technical problems inherent in infusion pumps and chronic stimulator systems. They also require more regular and frequent follow-up visits. Research and development of biologic delivery systems may lead to improvements in this aspect of neuroaugmentation.

Ablative procedures for chronic pain carry with them the finality of neural tissue destruction as well as the potential loss of function that accompanies the destruction of nervous tissue. In addition, chronic pain frequently recurs months to years after an initially successful ablative procedure. In pain of malignant origin, where the patient's life span is limited, this is less a concern than in pain associated with benign causes.

3. Scope of neurosurgical manipulations

Functional neurosurgical interventions for pain are directed at various levels of the nervous system, including the peripheral nerves, spinal cord, and brain. When selecting a surgical intervention, it is important to balance the **potential benefit to the patient against the risk of loss of function**. The technical requirements of the procedure, postoperative management issues, and the general condition of the patient must all be considered. Many pain complaints can be addressed by some neurosurgical intervention, but the important issue is: At what cost?

4. Variability of approach

There is no uniformity of approach in evaluating the pain patient for neurosurgical intervention. Although algorithms exist for choosing specific procedures designed to relieve specific complaints, each patient merits careful evaluation before a surgical procedure is even suggested. This way, unrealistic expectations can be prevented, while flexibility is maintained in designing a course of therapy best suited to the individual patient. Indeed, a given neurosurgical procedure used to treat identical complaints in different patients can produce vastly different results. For these reasons, we caution against a rigid approach to neurosurgical intervention.

II. APPROPRIATE SELECTION AND EVALUATION OF THE NEUROSURGICAL PAIN PATIENT

1. Medical workup and treatment

Before considering any procedure for pain control, it is extremely important to exclude an underlying treatable medical condition. Unrecognized causative pathology or correctable structural lesions must be excluded before any functional neurosurgical procedure is undertaken.

All candidates for neurosurgery require the usual preoperative evaluations for anesthetic management and surgery. Patients at high risk for surgery (e.g., those with end-stage malignancy) may be eager for intervention but may be unable to withstand the physiologic stresses of surgery. Medical optimization of the preoperative status may require manipulations not in accord with a patient's wishes or with the approach of the care team. This situation can be avoided through the neurosurgeon's early involvement with the patient who is difficult to manage on an oral or parenteral analgesic regimen.

2. Malignant versus benign pain

The common differentiation of pain into that of malignant or benign origin is clinically useful. In general, ablative approaches are more suitable for pain of malignant origin, when quality of life may be paramount to functional outcome. Ablative surgery for pain of benign origin, except for some specific conditions such as trigeminal neuralgia, is fraught with difficulties, especially when factors such as disability status, concurrent litigation, and psychosocial status dominate the clinical picture.

A second, more practical consideration is that patients who have benign pain and a normal life expectancy must be managed for decades after their surgical procedure. For example, the maintenance requirements for both the technical and emotional support of every patient can be significant after implantation of chronic stimulators in the spinal canal or drug infusion systems. This is not a major consideration for patients with progressive malignant disease.

3. Multidisciplinary team approach

The comprehensive pain service, with its neurologic, anesthesiologic, psychiatric, nursing, and social service components, remains the best resource for ensuring optimal patient care. Neurosurgeons who elect to treat chronic pain patients without this support network may find that the care of their patients is compromised. Similarly, the treatment of chronic pain is significantly hampered without the neurosurgeon's input. Early involvement of the neurosurgeon with patients who respond poorly to conservative measures, with a careful evaluation of each patient's needs and status, and deliberate review of all nonsurgical and surgical options will generally produce the best results.

III. SPECIFIC NEUROSURGICAL INTERVENTIONS ENCOUNTERED IN PAIN PRACTICE

1. Ablative procedures

(i) *Peripheral ablative procedures*

There is very little published information on peripheral neurotomy other than for the cranial nerves, except in the case of pain related to spinal facet innervation. Peripheral nerve lesions in the extremities can eventually result in a deafferentation pain syndrome. The procedure of choice for appendicular mononeuralgias is currently chronic stimulation, as described later. Results of facet denervation are variable, and although good results for chronic back pain have been reported, these have not been widely reproducible.

Surgical intervention for craniofacial pain syndromes has met with greater success. Trigeminal neuralgia can be treated with peripheral neurectomy with excellent results. Unfortunately, as in all peripheral lesions, nerve regeneration usually recurs, along with the pain syndrome. For these reasons, peripheral neurolytic procedures are generally not performed for chronic pain unless the patient's life expectancy is extremely limited or the medical conditions are severe.

The craniofacial pain caused by trigeminal and glossopharyngeal neuralgia can be treated by percutaneous peripheral nerve or ganglionic ablation in the intracranial space. This is generally done by radiofrequency lesions (RFLs) or by injection of a sclerosing agent such as glycerol. The results of these ablations are variable, but in the case of RFLs for trigeminal neuralgia, initial pain relief followed by several years of comfort can be expected in 70% to 80% of patients. Open craniotomy and microvascular decompression or cranial nerve section is also an option for younger patients with craniofacial pain or for those who have failed percutaneous rhizotomy. The success rates of these interventions are similar but the operative risk is higher for open surgical procedures.

In recent years, focused radiosurgery has been utilized as a noninvasive method for controlling trigeminal neuralgia. A single focused dose of external radiation is directed at the trigeminal nerve root. This has provided encouraging, early control of trigeminal neuralgia, although long-term results have yet to be confirmed.

(ii) *Spinal cord ablative procedures*

The rationale for ablative lesions in and around the spinal cord is based on the anatomy of nociceptive pathways, from the periphery to the spinal cord with its central connections. The approach to spinal cord lesioning can be divided into lesions of the dorsal root ganglia, dorsal rootlets, dorsal root entry zone, crossing fibers of the spinothalamic tracts, and lesions of the ascending tracts (Fig. 1).

The dorsal ganglia can be surgically excised (**ganglionectomy**) in an open or percutaneous procedure, providing relief of pain in a roughly dermatomal distribution. This procedure must be performed at multiple levels but provides pain relief with concurrent loss of sensory input. Attempts have been made, with variable success, to limit the ablation to nociceptive input only. For defined pain of the thoracic or upper lumbar roots, this procedure can be of great benefit. The loss of sensation that accompanies the pain relief in these areas does not typically impart any significant functional difficulties.

Dorsal rhizotomy was one of the first operations used for pain control. Although generally effective, it is accompanied by complete sensory loss in the appropriate dermatomal distribution. Extensive dorsal root sectioning in an extremity leads to a useless limb and is not recommended. Partial or incomplete posterior rhizotomies have therefore been employed for certain chronic pain states and painful spasticity and have been especially useful in occipital neuralgia.

Deafferentation pain related to root avulsion or phantom limb pain has been successfully treated with an open operation to cause

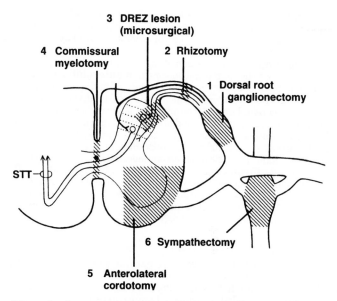

Figure 1. Cross-sectional view of the spinal cord showing approximate sites of common spinal cord ablative interventions—midline myelotomy, cordotomy, sympathectomy, dorsal root entry zone (DREZ) ablation, dorsal root ganglionectomy, and peripheral rhizotomy. STT, spinothalamic tract.

lesions in the dorsal root entry zone (DREZ). Small thermocoagulation lesions are made in the posterior spinal cord in the DREZ at multiple levels, presumably interrupting nociceptive pathways in Lissauer's tract or destroying neurons of the substantia gelatinosa. Significant pain relief lasting several years has been achieved in a variety of chronic pain states, including postherpetic neuralgia. Early results are generally good but the recurrence of pain is common.

A variation on this theme is **open microsurgical rhizidiotomy** or **DREZotomy**, in which small, 2-mm lesions are placed into the ventral aspect of the DREZ under each rootlet. This procedure theoretically destroys the ventrolateral fibers, which are primarily nociceptive, while preserving the dorsal medial fibers ascending into the posterior columns, which are primarily somatosensory. The procedure has been especially useful for painful spasticity and chronic painful states of a single involved extremity.

The spinothalamic tract input from a specific dermatome crosses the midline of the spinal cord over several levels before ascending into the anterolateral aspect of the spinal cord as the lateral spinal thalamic tract. Localized bilateral pain, such as that seen with sacral tumors and pelvic malignant disease, can be addressed by **midline (commissural) myelotomy**. Good bilateral pain relief can be achieved, although the potential for functional loss is great.

The high likelihood of postoperative neurologic deficit restricts this approach to pain of malignant origin in patients who already have functional disturbance (i.e., bladder and bowel dysfunction) preoperatively.

The procedure of interruption of the ascending lateral spinothalamic tract by either percutaneous or **open anterolateral cordotomy** has been used successfully for pain of malignant origin for many years. As with all ablations in the spinal cord, the risk of functional loss is real. Lower extremity pain is most easily approached by open thoracic cordotomy, and bilateral lesions can be performed. Bilateral cordotomy increases the risk of neurologic deficits, especially autonomic disturbance. Cordotomy at the cervical levels above the diaphragmatic input on one side and below it on the other (i.e., C3 and C6) can avoid complex postoperative respiratory difficulties (Ondine's curse). For reasons that are unclear, pain often returns 1 to 2 years after cordotomy of either type. Repeat cordotomy at a higher level can be performed, although this is rarely needed if the procedure is restricted to patients with a limited life expectancy.

(iii) *Central ablative procedures*

Accurate lesioning of nociceptive pathways in the mesencephalon, diencephalon, and cortex has been greatly aided by technical advances in computed tomography (CT)- and magnetic resonance imaging (MRI)-guided stereotaxis. Long-term results, however, are disappointing and for these reasons the use of central nervous system ablative surgery is controversial and generally considered only for pain of malignant origin.

The general approach to deep brain lesioning is similar to that used in deep brain stimulation (see later). An electrode is placed into a stereotactically targeted site. The area is then stimulated as the electrode position is adjusted to achieve the desired effect. At this point, a lesion is created, or in the case of stimulation, the electrode is secured in place.

Lesioning the spinothalamic and secondary ascending trigeminal tracts in the midbrain (**mesencephalotomy**) can provide unilateral relief of head and neck pain. More rostral lesions in the medial thalamus (**thalamotomy**) can also provide unilateral or in some cases bilateral pain relief. A procedure for destroying the cingulate gyrus and bundle in the frontal lobe (**cingulotomy**) has also been used in cases of diffuse chronic pain associated with depression. These approaches should be reserved for the experienced functional neurosurgeon.

For reasons that are unclear, pain from hormonally responsive tumors that produce bony pain (carcinoma of the prostate and breast) is sometimes very amenable to **pituitary ablation**, either stereotactically or via a transsphenoidal approach. The sudden and complete relief of bone pain that is often evident even on emergence from anesthesia makes the procedure worth trying despite the expected postoperative endocrine deficits.

2. Augmentation procedures

(i) *Peripheral nerve stimulation*

Pain arising from a mononeuropathy may be treated by chronic stimulation, particularly when the pain is the result of nerve injury. Cancer pain has also been treated in this way but with less success. The long-term implantation of a stimulating electrode requires a significant investment of time and effort to manage the technical aspects of the device. Newer hardware designed for this purpose has simplified these techniques, but the clinical results are as yet unproven.

(ii) *Spinal cord stimulation*

Spinal cord stimulation (SCS) is frequently used for treating chronic pain, particularly of nonmalignant origin, because of its reversibility. It remains popular despite the high cost of the hardware and its maintenance. Spinal cord stimulators can be inserted percutaneously or during open procedures. The scientific basis for pain relief is unclear, although, as with peripheral nerve stimulation, the stimulation causes paresthesia within the painful area, which somehow modulates pain perception. Unfortunately, no specific markers have emerged of "best responders" to spinal cord stimulation. The best responders to date have been patients with failed back syndrome, lower-extremity pain of vascular origin, and other neurogenic pain syndromes. Published reports predict an approximately 50% long-term success rate overall for patients treated with SCS.

(iii) *Deep brain stimulation*

Deep brain stimulation (DBS) is confined to pain centers where there is significant interest in the procedure and a commitment to the management of patients with implanted stimulators. The two targets include the periaqueductal gray matter areas of the brainstem, and the nuclei ventralis posteromedialis and ventralis posterolateralis within the thalamus. Reports of DBS used for a variety of chronic pain states suggest that initial success is often followed by decremental effectiveness over time. Relief can be expected in 50% to 80% of patients initially, but the long-term results seem to indicate that only about half of DBS patients derive significant benefit. The most appropriate use of this technique appears to be in addressing chronic pain refractory to all other approaches in patients with a long life expectancy.

Finally, in patients with atypical facial pain or phantom limb pain, chronic stimulation of the motor cortex with subdurally implanted electrode arrays has demonstrated some encouraging results in these otherwise treatment-refractory cases.

(iv) *Implantable infusion systems*

The infusion of spinal epidural opiates or local anesthetic solutions is now an accepted and frequently used procedure for extremity and occasional truncal pain. The role of the neurosurgeon in the management of spinal infusion techniques is to offer the long-term surgical implantation of subcutaneously tunneled catheters leading to a reservoir, or the placement of catheters that exit the anterior abdominal wall that can be injected externally. In general, surgically implanted catheters have a longer life and lower complication rate.

Opiate infusion into the spinal intradural space or through the intraventricular route will always involve a neurosurgeon for catheter placement and avoidance of complications. It would appear that these intradural routes provide superior analgesia to epidural routes; however, there is an increased incidence of postoperative deficits and infectious complications and a risk of overdose. A spinal intradural or frontal intraventricular catheter can be adapted to any of several commercially available infusion systems. Since excellent short-term pain relief is achieved after relatively minor surgery, intradural therapy should probably be utilized more frequently.

3. Miscellaneous neurosurgical interventions

(i) *Trigeminal and glossopharyngeal neuralgia*

The neurosurgical approach to trigeminal and glossopharyngeal neuralgia includes percutaneous rhizotomy, open partial cranial rhizotomy, and microvascular decompression. These treatments are described in Chapter 12 (II, 5). For any patient who has a trigeminal pain syndrome that is not controlled well by medication, the likelihood of satisfactory pain relief without medication is approximately 90% for any of these approaches. Recurrent trigeminal neuralgia can also be treated with repeat rhizotomy with good relief. Complication rates are extremely low for these procedures, but the specific procedure recommended must be tailored to each patient's needs and risks.

(ii) *Low back pain*

Low back pain is a problem commonly encountered by the neurologist and the neurosurgeon. In particular, the failed back syndrome is a frequent management problem for the pain service. Most of these patients can be managed with an aggressive medical regimen, but a detailed evaluation of patients with a failed back should be considered, as with any other pain syndrome. In carefully selected patients with continued underlying spinal structural pathology, reasonable success has been achieved with reoperation for recurrent disc disease or continued nerve root compression. In addition, spinal cord stimulation or epidural opiate infusion can be of value in those patients who have failed all other forms of therapy.

(iii) *Sympathectomy*

Sympathectomy for autonomic and visceral pain is now almost exclusively performed by the anesthesiologist via percutaneous approaches. For specific cases of reflex sympathetic dystrophy (RSD), surgical sympathectomy may be necessary because of the difficulty in achieving adequate technical results percutaneously. The advantage of open sympathectomy is the excellent anatomic definition of the lesion. However, pain recurrence is as likely to occur after sympathectomy performed in an open fashion as after percutaneous approaches. Selective peripheral nerve stimulation has also been used for RSD confined to a single nerve distribution or extremity.

IV. CONCLUSION

Although the surgical treatment of chronic pain should always follow a reasonably exhaustive trial of conservative medical approaches, there is a role for surgical intervention in many chronic pain patients. The neurosurgeon's participation in the overall treatment plan of the patient with chronic pain provides an opportunity for early surgical intervention, before worsening of the disease or frustration with lack of progress renders neurosurgical intervention impossible. A judicious approach by the referring pain specialist, as well as frank discussions with the patient, family, and care providers, is likely to yield the best results for a patient who has not responded to medical management. Unfortunately, multiple factors and individual variability still render the surgical outcome for each patient somewhat difficult to predict.

As for all patients with chronic pain, the entire multidisciplinary pain service should take responsibility for preoperative and postoperative care. No one specific neurosurgical intervention will totally relieve persistent pain; it should be considered only as a single therapeutic option in the overall treatment plan. The management of chronic pain can, at times, be greatly improved by timely, selective neurosurgical interventions to provide an excellent quality of life in the face of intercurrent disease and chronic pain.

SELECTED READINGS

1. Burchiel KJ, ed. *Pain surgery*. New York: Thieme, 1999.
2. Gybels JM, Sweet WH. Neurosurgical treatment of persistent pain. In: *Pain and headache*, vol 11. Basel: Karger, 1989.
3. Schmidek HH, Sweet WH. *Operative neurosurgical techniques: Indications, methods, and results*, 3rd ed. Philadelphia: WB Saunders, 1995.
4. Tasker RR. Neurosurgical and neuroaugmentative intervention. In: Patt RB, ed. *Cancer pain*. Philadelphia: Lippincott, 1993.
5. Tasker RR. The recurrence of pain after neurosurgical procedures. *Qual Life Res* 1994;3:S43–49.
6. Wall PD, Melzack R, eds. *Textbook of pain*, 3rd ed. New York: Churchill-Livingstone, 1989.

Psychosocial and Behavioral Approaches

David K. Ahern

The pain of the mind is worse than the pain of the body.
—*Publilius Syrus (1st century BC)*

I. Psychosocial aspects: Depression, anxiety, and fear
II. Clinical interview: behavioral analysis, pain behavior, medication use, and disability
   1. Clinical interview
   2. Paper-and-pencil measures
III. Nonpharmacologic interventions
   1. Modification of verbal behavior or pain behavior
   2. Increased activity level
   3. Somatic therapies
   4. Cognitive interventions

I. PSYCHOSOCIAL ASPECTS: DEPRESSION, ANXIETY, AND FEAR

It is well established that the experience of chronic pain can have serious adverse consequences for the psychological, social, and economic well-being of patients. Pain that becomes persistent following an acute injury places the patient at risk for depression, anxiety and fear, personality changes, and lifestyle disruptions that can be devastating, not only to the patient but to his or her family as well. For example, it has been estimated that 60% or more of patients with chronic pain are at risk for development of clinically significant depression, which complicates medical assessment and treatment of the pain per se. Depression can distort, color, and confound the pain experience such that the patient reports pain as excruciating and overwhelming (often using affect-laden terms to describe the pain), resulting in a nonanatomical presentation of symptoms, diagnostic uncertainty, and frustration for the clinician.

Anxiety and fear are equally common psychological and behavioral disturbances associated with chronic pain. In fact, a fear-avoidance model has been promulgated to help explain the progression from acute to chronic pain syndromes. Figure 1 presents the fear-avoidance model that illustrates the path from initial injury and acute pain to chronic pain and associated psychological disturbance and disability. For most patients, the course is one of relatively short-term pain that resolves. If, however, pain from an initial acute injury is perceived as threatening and a cognitive process of catastrophizing develops, pain-related fear will emerge. Subsequently, this pain-related fear leads to avoidance behaviors, a heightened awareness, and a focus on bodily sensations followed by disability, disuse, and depression.

For the patient, the chronic pain experience, if untreated or managed inappropriately, can lead to substantial and sustained emotional distress, psychological difficulties, and progressive im-

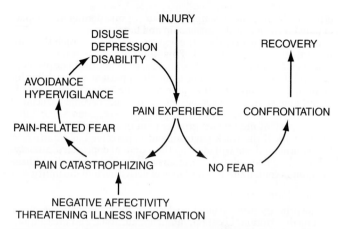

Figure 1. The "fear avoidance" model. If pain, possibly caused by an injury, is interpreted as threatening (pain catastrophizing), pain-related fear evolves. This leads to avoidance behaviors and hyper-vigilance to bodily sensations, followed by disability, disuse, and depression. The latter will maintain the pain experience, thereby fueling the vicious circle of increasing fear and avoidance. In non-catastrophizing patients, no pain-related fear and rapid confrontation with daily activities is likely to occur, leading to fast recovery. Pain catastrophizing is assumed to be influenced also by negative affectivity and threatening illness information. (From Vlaeyen JWS, Linton SJ. Fear-avoidance and its consequences in chronic musculoskeletal pain: A state of the art. *Pain* 2000;85:317–332.)

pairment and disability. The extent of a patient's disability is often greater than the documented medical and physical findings would support. This observation is not so surprising, however, when considering that psychosocial and behavioral factors can help to explain symptom amplification and disability disproportionate to the available medical findings, as predicted by the fear-avoidance model. Thus, in the clinic setting, assessment of psychosocial and behavioral factors are as important to understanding a patient's pain experience and disability as the medical history and physical examination.

II. CLINICAL INTERVIEW: BEHAVIORAL ANALYSIS, PAIN BEHAVIOR, MEDICATION USE, AND DISABILITY

1. Clinical interview

A semistructured clinical interview is conducted to obtain detailed information related to psychosocial and behavioral aspects of the chronic pain problem. Attention is given to relationships between individual aspects of the pain experience, and data obtained are combined with supplementary data from medical chart review and standardized assessment instruments in individualized treatment planning and recommendations. Whenever possible, the interview is conducted with both patient and spouse or significant other to obtain a more complete picture of functioning and impact of pain on the marital relationship and family unit.

Behavioral analysis is the framework within which the clinical interview is conducted. This approach focuses on the contingencies of reinforcement, which serve to maintain or promote pain-related dysfunction. For example, a patient may exhibit increased pain complaints (i.e., pain behavior) in the presence of his or her spouse in part because the spouse has become associated with administration of pain relief procedures (e.g., massage). Likewise, a patient may report greater pain in anticipation of returning to work if the work environment is perceived as punitive. A behavioral analysis will identify the extent of depressive, anxiety-related, and fear-related symptoms and the degree to which these symptoms contribute to avoidance of activities and disability.

(i) *Pain characteristics*

The primary starting point is a focus on the actual pain complaint and its description. Location, intensity, duration, and fluctuations in actual pain patterns are assessed. Subjective descriptors (e.g., "dull," "throbbing," "shooting,") should be noted. The use of affective descriptors, as well, is important in obtaining a more thorough understanding of the patient's emotional response to his or her pain.

Self-report pain scales are another commonly used method of assessing the individual's pain experience. The patient is asked to rate his or her pain on a scale (from 0 to 10, e.g.) for a given time period, either at that moment or for a specified time period such as an hour, a day, or longer. In the initial assessment, pain ratings are usually obtained for current pain level as well as the range of pain experience.

Determining overall parameters of pain leads naturally into elaboration of influencing factors: for example, those activities associated with pain exacerbation, and those activities or factors associated with pain relief, even if only temporary. Close attention is paid to both of these areas, as important information about the extent to which environmental or operant factors may play a part in the pain syndrome can be identified here.

(ii) *Pain behavior*

Paying attention to the patient's verbal and nonverbal behavior is also very informative. Besides the use of pain descriptors, patients may communicate the extent of suffering by grimacing, groaning, or moaning, and by frequent postural shifts during the course of the interview. These behaviors are considered to be reflective of the patient's pain experience; consequently, they are conceptualized as pain behaviors. Frequently, patients call attention to their suffering by pointing out their behavior or excusing themselves for it to the clinician. In other patients, these behaviors have become automatic aspects of their self-presentation and are not acknowledged. Some patients evidence the grimacing, guarding, or verbalizations but do so to a much lesser degree.

Still other individuals evidence very little or no pain behavior. In these patients, particularly, it is important to note any discrepancies between their verbalized reports of pain or distress, and their appearance. Pointing out such discrepancies to the patient can yield useful information about the patient's preferred coping style, as some patients will acknowledge that they have pain but choose not to show it, whereas other individuals sometimes become rather defensive at the perceived questioning of their self-report. Clearly, the clinician must exhibit good judgment as to the appropriate timing and extent of questioning along these lines.

(iii) *Medication use*

Evaluation of medication use patterns can alert the clinician to problematic aspects of medication use that may in turn contribute to a worsening pain problem. These patterns are as follows:

- *Increasing frequency or quantity of medication use* without related improvements in pain level (suggests habituation)
- *Multiple pain prescriptions* from multiple providers; combining use
- *Signs of withdrawal symptoms* with reduced or discontinued use of pain medication
- *Recurrent emergency room visits* with resultant dispensing of medication
- Prior or current history of *alcohol or substance abuse*
- Medication used primarily for *mood—rather than pain-altering* effect (e.g., reduced anxiety, feeling "high")
- Medication use results in *decreased activity or cognitive functioning*
- *Discrepancies between patient-reported use* and other information sources (medical records, spouse report)

(iv) *Functional disability*

Assessment of functional disability consists of determining the activities that the patient avoids or that are limited by pain. A useful technique in helping formulate a picture of the patient's current functional level is to ask him or her to describe a typical day in as much detail as possible. For example, time of awakening, getting dressed, eating breakfast (including type and amount of meal, who prepares it, and kitchen cleanup), and reading the paper might be noted as standard daily routines. The amount of time required to complete each activity is also important to ascertain, as for some patients the general routine might take 45 minutes, whereas for others it could take 2 hours.

When patients with pain lose a sense of structure to their day and have many hours to fill, it is not uncommon to find that a good amount of the day is spent lying down or resting. For these patients, treatment might focus on increasing the range and scope of daily activities in order to increase physical endurance as well as combat depressive syndromes resulting from inactivity and loss of reinforcing activities or social interaction. Alternatively, some individuals have full, if not hectic, schedules with few or no rest periods. Still others exhibit a pattern of prolonged periods of inactivity and "recovery" from sporadic bursts of high activity. Again, the treatment is based on the individual's stated level and pattern of activity.

2. Paper-and-pencil measures

The role of standardized assessment instruments in chronic pain evaluation is crucial. An instrument can provide detailed self-report information about an individual's specific condition (helpful in providing a quick overview of the patient's problem as well as in providing reliability and validity checks on verbal interview data), and in many cases the patient's responses can be compared to existing norms to assess where the individual lies in relation to other patients with the same or similar problems. In addition, previous research can highlight the probability of success or appropriateness of a given treatment protocol or approach.

A number of instruments are commonly used to evaluate psychosocial and behavioral aspects of chronic pain syndromes:

(i) Sickness impact profile

The Sickness Impact Profile (SIP) is one of the most widely used measures of health status in pain clinics. It consists of 136 items, in checklist format, that assess the impact of health problems on 12 areas of functioning: ambulating, mobility, body care and movement, social interaction, communication, alertness, emotional behavior, sleep, eating, work, home management, and recreation. It is scored to form three composite scales: physical, psychosocial, and total (which includes physical, psychosocial, and work and recreational pastime information). Its reliability and validity as a measure of dysfunction in pain patients has been well established.

(ii) Pain and impairment relationship scale

Because attitudes, beliefs, and expectations have been implicated in determining response to pain rehabilitation, the patient's beliefs regarding his or her pain must be assessed. Often, as a result of lengthy and unsuccessful (or unsatisfactory) treatment, patients can develop beliefs and expectations that can complicate further treatment efforts. One such belief is that they are unable to live normal, productive lives as long as they experience pain.

The Pain And Impairment Relationship Scale (PAIRS) was developed to assess the extent to which patients with chronic pain believe that they cannot function normally because of their pain. It is a 15-item measure designed to assess the degree to which patients perceive their functional status as related to their pain level. Each statement measures a given thought, attitude, or opinion about pain. Patients endorse each item along a seven-point Likert-type scale (i.e., strongly disagree to strongly agree). Responses are summed to obtain an overall score. High scores indicate a person's greater tendency to equate pain with impairment, and to restrict functioning when pain is present.

(iii) Multidimensional pain inventory

The Multidimensional Pain Inventory (MPI) is a comprehensive 52-item self-report measure of pain and pain-related characteristics including pain severity, interference with activity, affective distress, and support or concern from significant others. The measure has good reliability and validity and has been used to assess change with pain treatment.

(iv) Coping strategies questionnaire

The Coping Strategies Questionnaire (CSQ) is a 50-item questionnaire that assesses the range of ways that patients cope or deal with their pain. It is designed to assess seven coping strategies:

diverting attention, reinterpreting pain sensation, use of coping self-statements, ignoring pain sensations, praying and hoping, catastrophizing, and increasing activity level. The CSQ helps to identify patients who tend to catastrophize or use fewer adaptive coping strategies for dealing with their pain.

To conclude, it is clearly important to determine the contribution of psychosocial and behavioral factors to a patient's pain complaints in order to conduct an adequate chronic pain evaluation. As important, identifying relevant psychosocial and behavioral factors will very likely increase the potential for a more favorable response to medical management, because these factors have been found to contribute to protracted symptoms and disability and to poor response to interdisciplinary treatment. Indeed, psychosocial and behavioral factors have been shown to be better predictors of treatment outcome than either medical or physical factors. Table 1. presents a summary of potential psychosocial and economic predictors of response to treatment.

III. NONPHARMACOLOGIC INTERVENTIONS

Intervention is predicated, in part, on the patient's willingness to accept learning how to better manage pain and attaining maximal function despite residual pain. Overall goals of treatment are as follows:

1. Reduction of pain behavior and the degree to which pain is a focus
2. Increased activity level and functional capacity
3. Reduction of distress and the attendant emotional suffering
4. Rearranging contingencies to pain behavior by family and significant others

1. Modification of verbal behavior or pain behavior

A primary treatment goal is to decrease pain behavior and related dysfunctional behaviors while increasing functional activities and "well" behaviors. Often, specific pain behaviors targeted for elimination or reduction are enumerated in a treatment contract filled out and signed by both patient and therapist during the sec-

---

Table 1.   Summary of potential psychosocioeconomic predictors of response to treatment

Depression
Somatization
History of childhood abuse
Psychiatric disturbance (presence of Axis I clinical disorders)
MPI subgroup categories
Elevation of the Emotional Vulnerability scale of the MBHI
Poor coping skills/strategies
Unresolved workers' compensation/personal injury cases
Positive attitudes and expectations about path and disability

---

MBHI, Millon Behavioral Health Inventory.
Reprinted, with permission, from Gallagher RM. Treatment planning in pain medicine. Integrating medical, physical, and behavioral therapies. *Med Clin North Am* 1999;83:823–849.

ond session. More adaptive behaviors targeted for increase are likewise specified in the treatment contract.

Most commonly seen is an increase in pain behaviors such as facial grimacing, groaning, guarding, and frequent postural shifts. Concomitant behaviors not apparent on clinical exam are related decreases in previous levels of activity. These include, but are not limited to, reductions in work (either at home, at the office, or on the job site); recreational activities such as hobbies, sports, family interactions, and sex; and broader-based social interactions, such as family and friend involvement. Amount of time spent in or out of bed (up-time) provides another good indicator of current activity level. To the extent that these behaviors have come under the influence of external factors, behavior modification designed to eliminate or reduce their frequency is an initial target of treatment.

Typically, reduction in pain behaviors is achieved through use of learning theory techniques. For example, the therapist and members of the treatment team ignore pain behavior. Moans, pain complaints, grimacing, and guarding are not responded to, nor does treatment staff engage in talk about pain-related behavior or activity except when medically indicated (new symptoms suggestive of objective changes in health status such as neural involvement, for example). Instead, the staff reinforces the patient for gains made in his or her exercise program, time spent walking, or time out of bed, for example. Emphasis is on gains in function, with increased independence despite pain.

2. Increased activity level

The patient is reinforced for meeting functional activity goals, which can include decreasing "down" time as well as increasing repetitions of exercises and engaging in other functional activities such as walking or increasing social interactions. This is accomplished through a variety of techniques, as described in the following sections.

(i) *Self-monitoring, or behavior charting*

Patients are encouraged to keep records of their activities on a daily basis. Such events as relaxation sessions (complete with before-and-after ratings of both pain and tension) are recorded, as are physical therapy exercises. Time spent walking, or engaging in social activities is also noted. Again, emphasis is on noting patterns of behavior, with expected increases in functional and positive activities with concomitant decreases in dysfunctional behaviors (e.g., inordinate bedrest, social isolation). Patients quickly begin to be able to track their own activity patterns and progress once they have become accustomed to self-monitoring. Treatment sessions use the logs, or patient notations, to pinpoint problem areas and find solutions, or to reinforce patient gains and initiative. During later treatment phases, activity logs can be used as a goal-setting aid, with progressive increases in those behaviors leading to goal attainment.

(ii) *Goal setting*

Initially, goal setting serves as a means of preparing the patient for behavior change and as an educational tool. Patients learn the basic principles of taking an activity and breaking it into manageable and achievable behaviors. For example, "going out to dinner" involves building sufficient sitting tolerance to handle a multicourse meal. As skills are acquired, behaviors are shaped to resemble the goal (meeting a friend for coffee). Finally, goals are met, and new ones building on old skills are set to take their place. Not all goals involve purely physical activities—increasing contact with friends or former colleagues, job seeking, and socializing all serve to increase functioning of the patient.

(iii) *Pacing*

Being able not only to regulate the type of activity in which one engages, but also to determine appropriate timelines for doing so is addressed in teaching pacing. Patients learn to engage in certain behaviors for set periods of time to prevent overdoing (i.e., sitting in front of the computer for 25 minutes, then taking a 2- to 5-minute break before returning). Breaking a large task into smaller components is another method of pacing; for example, preparing a meal in phases rather than waiting until dinnertime.

(iv) *Health care utilization*

Treatment also encourages a reduction in the amount of pain-related office and emergency room visits, number of surgeries, and number of pharmacists contacted. This objective is achieved through coordination and communication among all members of the treatment team, so that the patient receives consistent messages and treatment approach from all relevant care providers.

MEDICATION INTAKE. Patients with chronic pain frequently use a variety of pain-relieving medications. Treatment focuses on appropriate medication reduction. Again, medication reduction is usually accomplished within the framework of increased strength, endurance, and physical capacity training, as well as with relaxation, stress management, and pacing skills utilization. After the initial assessment period, the patient's schedule for taking pain-related medications is shifted, if necessary, from an activity- or pain-contingent basis to a time-contingent system. This lays the groundwork for breaking the learned association between the occurrence of pain and automatic medication use.

Concurrently, either the prescribing physician decreases the dosage (the strength or amount prescribed per allotted time period), or the patient is encouraged to decrease dosage within preset limits established in consultation with the physician, the behavioral medicine psychologist, or both. The desired goal of this aspect of treatment is to achieve as great a reduction as reasonably possible in the patient's medical regimen, especially in opiate or narcotic use. Understandably, some patients require some degree of ongoing analgesic use, but others are able to eliminate these drugs entirely or switch to less habit-forming medications.

3. Somatic therapies

Progressive muscle relaxation is a deep relaxation technique that is designed to help teach the patient awareness of overall muscle tension levels and to maintain relaxation baselines at low levels, rather than letting muscle tension build throughout the course of the day or a particular activity and in this way exacerbate the pain.

Additional benefits of engaging in deep muscle relaxation are increases in peripheral circulation and a heightened sense of body awareness that can cue appropriate pacing or coping measures. Finally, some patients report that taking a few seconds out between sets of physical therapy exercises to relax their worked muscles is a helpful pacing technique.

Three basic approaches to muscle relaxation are taught in pain clinics. Although the overall desired result is the same, techniques differ. Basically, the three techniques are progressive muscle relaxation, autogenic muscle relaxation, and diaphragmatic breathing.

(i) *Progressive muscle relaxation*

In this technique, after beginning with several deep breaths, the patient alternately tenses, holds, and then relaxes groups of muscles in his or her body. Attention is paid to the sensations of tightness felt while contracting and tensing the muscles, and this is then compared to the sensations produced by sudden and immediate relaxing of those muscle groups.

Patients are instructed to pay attention to the sensations of warmth, heaviness, and relaxation in their body, and to review each muscle group individually, spending some (but not too much) additional time on problem areas.

Over several weeks (usually 2 to 4, if patients have been compliant with at-home practice sessions), the number of individual muscle groups addressed decreases as patients tense the entire leg instead of upper and lower individual components, the entire arm instead of upper and lower parts, and so forth. Patients will be able to relax just as deeply with this streamlined technique as with more detailed one.

(ii) *Autogenic relaxation*

DIAPHRAGMATIC BREATHING. This technique is similar in many respects to muscle relaxation, but it is favored by some therapists for its relative ease of learning and quickness of implementation, as well as its "portability." The only specific instruction the therapist needs to make to the patient is teaching where the diaphragm is located. The therapist lets the patient practice feeling his or her chest expanding as diaphragmatic breathing takes place. (Some patients find it interesting to hear that this is the type of breathing frequently practiced by professional singers, not just patients who are experiencing stress or in chronic pain.)

4. Cognitive interventions

Cognitive-behavioral treatment typically includes restructuring cognitive schemata that may perpetuate excessive pain and disability. Among these are general beliefs (such as those assessed by the PAIRS) that increased pain levels automatically call for cessation of activity, and that pain is linked invariably with impairment as well as self-defeating and catastrophizing self-statements, such as "Oh, no, here it comes again! Why won't it stop? I can't do anything about it. This is terrible!" Additional emphasis is placed on teaching cognitive techniques directed specifically at coping with the pain. Among these are the following:

(i) *Attention / diversion*

The patient is taught to divert attention away from pain sensations by focusing on activities, behaviors, and thoughts that require redirection of effort. Encouraging physical activities, for example, shifts from somatic preoccupation, provides incompatible behavior, and provides reinforcing activity, all of which enhances coping.

(ii) *Reinterpretation of pain sensations*

Emotion-laden labels are removed from the patient's vocabulary. In addition, patients are taught to recognize an increase in pain as a signal to alter pacing or to modify the activity rather than cease altogether or to engage in catastrophizing thoughts.

(iii) *Problem-solving strategies*

Problem solving requires using not only specific pain reduction techniques but also a host of other cognitive coping strategies. Success in this area depends not only on the patient's awareness of the techniques but also on his or her ability to draw on and use a variety of different approaches to meet specific challenges. The aim of treatment, therefore, is not only to provide the patient with specific techniques but also to be able to recognize and use them together to cope effectively.

Patients should be taught the basic principles of behavioral/ situational analysis. Breaking situations into separate components (e.g., before, during, and after) helps pinpoint problem areas and determine specific strategies. For example, an upcoming wedding poses a challenge to the patient because of the sheer number of tasks to be done. Breaking the event into components helps the patient pace appropriately (shopping for attire, arranging catering, and so on). Learning how to delegate tasks helps reinforce a sense of pacing, as well as being another appropriate coping technique. Successes in these areas enhance self-control and mastery experience, furthering cognitive coping abilities. Finally, the patient learns that by breaking down tasks into component parts and with appropriate planning, required behaviors can be accomplished without undue hardship.

Frequently, as in the preceding case, time-management skills are as important in preventing pain flare-ups as the more pain-focused coping strategies of relaxation or medication intake. This is true of other strategies as well. In addressing problem-solving skills in therapy, therefore, patients should be taught to take stock of all aspects of the situation in planning appropriate pain management strategies. If stress increases pain level, appropriate stress management techniques are crucial components of treatment. Using an abbreviated relaxation method may be helpful in decreasing muscle tension levels as well as in maintaining some degree of emotional calm.

(iv) *Assertiveness training*

This can help not only in stress management itself but in aiding the patient to carry out other components important to pain management: for example, learning to say no, appropriately, to unreasonable requests by others, especially when pacing is important. As important is the ability to graciously decline well-meaning but unhelpful overtures by others to do for the patient what he or she can do alone. In general, the ability to assert oneself is of benefit in all areas of interaction and should be addressed as part of pain treatment.

(v) *Pain-management skills training*

The interventions just described are all potentially beneficial to patients who deal with chronic pain. To facilitate implementation of these approaches, Table 2 presents a list of the tasks and interventions in the order they are introduced in pain-management skills training.

Table 2. Sequential tasks in pain management training

Rationalize pharmacology
Review pain physiology and the specificity of medication for different aspects of the pain cycle
Teach pain/tension cycle and biopsychosocial pain physiology; instruct in use of pain diaries to record daily and hourly fluctuations in pain
This skill assists in planning medication trials and evaluating their outcome and helps plan and implement appropriate physical therapies and behavioral lifestyle changes
Begin psychophysiologic relaxation training
Group training is supplemented by daily home practice with tapes, which can be ordered commercially or made by any behavioral clinician. Relaxation training, particularly in combination with pharmacologic treatment, has been shown to be effective in reducing pain and improving coping in several painful conditions. Biofeedback may enhance learning of the relaxation response but is usually not needed. Portable biofeedback devices are more practical for home use
Continue baseline data collection
Review record-keeping practice and skill with diaries
Introduce pacing skills
Daily diaries help correlate activities, treatments, and symptoms and establish patterns of precipitation and amelioration. Patients learn to pace activities to avoid flare-ups.
Review relaxation training and pacing skills
Frequent review reinforces practice and training principles. Mistakes include using tapes to fall asleep or to reduce pain before the relaxation skills have been learned through regular practice.
Assess environmental, cognitive, biologic, and behavioral precipitants and consequences of pain
Construct dynamic flow charts of interacting factors using BBS treatment to interrupt causal pathways
Plan how to integrate medication use with behavioral and physical therapies
The physician should participate in this session
Introduce stress management and cognitive interventions
Continue stress management—communication skills training, assertion training, cognitive distortions
This task includes learning effective communication skills with the physician and may include the physician for all or part of a session for role playing and problem solving

Table 2. *Continued*

Develop pain management protocols for individual patients
  Include medication, physical therapy techniques (ice, TENS
    stretching, exercise), stress management (relaxation, cognitive-
    emotional-behavioral-pain cycles)
**Reinforce pain management protocol and establish
  maintenance program**
  This session may take place after a 2-week gap to allow patients
    an opportunity to *field test* their pain management protocols;
    maintenance programs for individual patients are discussed
**At regularly scheduled follow-up visits, reevaluate and refine
  pain management protocol**

TENS, Transcutaneous electrical nerve stimulator.
Reprinted, with permission, from Gallagher RM. Treatment planning in pain
medicine. Integrating medical, physical, and behavioral therapies. *Med Clin
North Am* 1999;83:823–849.

ACKNOWLEDGEMENT
  The author would like to express thanks to the former staff, in-
terns, and fellows of the MGH Behavioral Medicine Unit for their
contributions to behavioral chronic pain management.

SELECTED READINGS
  1. Aberger EW, Adams A, Ahern DK, Follick MJ. Clinical assess-
     ment of chronic low back pain. *Clin Rehabilitation* 1987;1:19–46.
  2. Follick MJ, Ahern DK, Aberger EW. Development of an audio-
     visual taxonomy of pain behavior: Reliability and discriminant
     validity. *Health Psychol* 1986;17:445–449.
  3. Follick MJ, Ahern DK, Laser-Wolston N. Evaluation of a daily ac-
     tivity diary for chronic pain patients. *Pain* 1984;19:373–382.
  4. Follick MJ, Smith TW, Ahern DK. The sickness impact profile: A
     global measure of disability in chronic low back pain. *Pain* 1985;
     21:67–76.
  5. Fordyce WE. *Behavioral methods for chronic pain and illness.*
     St. Louis: Mosby, 1976.
  6. Gallagher RM. Chronic pain. *Med Clin North Am* 1999;83:
     823–849.
  7. Gatchel RJ, Turk DC, eds. *Psychosocial factors in pain.* New
     York: Guilford Press, 1999.
  8. Guck TP, Fleischer TD, Willcockson JC, et al. Predictive validity
     of the pain and impairment relationship scale in a chronic non-
     malignant pain population. *Arch Phys Med Rehabil* 1999;80:
     91–95.
  9. Kerns RD, Haythornthwaite JA. Depression among chronic pain
     patients: Cognitive-behavioral analysis and effect on rehabilita-
     tion outcome. *J Clin Consulting Psychol* 1988;56:870–876.
 10. Kerns RD, Turk DC, Rudy TE. The West Haven-Yale Multi-
     dimensional Pain Inventory. *Pain* 1985;21:345–356.
 11. Linton SJ. The socioeconomic impact of chronic back pain: Is any-
     one benefiting? *Pain* 1998;75:163–168.

12. McCracken LM. Learning to live with the pain: Acceptance of pain predicts adjustment in persons with chronic pain. *Pain* 1998;74: 21–27.

13. NIH Technology Assessment Panel on Integration of Behavioral and Relaxation Approaches into the Treatment of Chronic Pain and Insomnia. Integration of behavioral and relaxation approaches into the treatment of chronic pain and insomnia. *JAMA* 1996; 276: 313–318.

14. Rainville J, Ahern DK, Phalen L, et al. The association of pain with physical activities in chronic low back pain. *Spine* 1992;17: 1060–1064.

15. Riley JF, Ahern DK, Follick MJ. Chronic pain and functional impairment: Assessing beliefs about their relationship. *Arch Phys Med Rehabil* 1988;69:579–582.

16. Slater MA, Hall HF, Atkinson JH, Garfin SR. Pain and impairment beliefs in chronic low back pain: validation of the Pain and Impairment Relationship Scale (PAIRS). *Pain* 1991;44:51–56.

17. Vlaeyen JW, Linton SJ. Fear-avoidance and its consequences in chronic musculoskeletal pain: A state of the art. *Pain* 2000;85: 317–332.

Physical Therapy

Harriet M. Wittink and Theresa Hoskins Michel

Life begins on the other side of despair.
—*Jean Paul Sartre (1905–1980)*

The goal of physical therapy is to restore or improve function and prevent disability. Referral to a physical therapist is appropriate when pain impairs a patient's optimal functional ability or inhibits his or her independence in activities of daily living, or when physical rehabilitation is a necessary component for treating the underlying cause of pain. The physician supplies a diagnosis and communicates any precautions, thereby allowing the physical therapist to use clinical judgment in designing an appropriate treatment program. Although it is always appropriate to offer detailed prescriptions for specific functional evaluation and physical therapeutic modalities, an "evaluate and treat" order is also a reasonable means of asking a physical therapist to provide comprehensive assessment and a treatment plan based on this assessment. In either case, the key is collaboration between physician and physical therapist and integration of component therapies.

Physical therapists attempt to identify the relationship between pathology, impairments, functional limitations, and disability to direct treatment appropriately. In acute pain, a clear relationship exists between nociception, perceived pain, and impairments; therefore, treatment focuses on the elimination of pain. As a result, impairments diminish, functional ability is restored, and disability is prevented. In chronic pain patients, however, the relationship between pain, impairments, and disability is unclear. Treatment that solely addresses elimination of pain in patients with chronic pain will very likely fail to alter the illness and disability behavior of the chronic pain patient. Instead, treatment addresses function in spite of pain and promotes independence at a level of tolerance.

I. PHYSICAL THERAPY EVALUATION

Physical therapists are trained to assess physical impairments, such as flexibility, strength, and endurance. Through an interview and physical examination, most of the information needed to develop an appropriate treatment plan should be obtained. Although the physical therapist's interview and examination closely resemble those of other health care providers, specific to the physical therapy examination is the observation of the patient's movement patterns and willingness to move. Transitional movements are observed when the patient sits, stands, walks, or climbs onto a plinth. Important diagnostic features include quality of motion, which can be distorted and erratic, and dysfunctional movement patterns including muscle guarding and pain behaviors.

Functional testing helps to compare the patients' *perception* of what they are able to do versus what they are can actually accomplish. Patients' self-reports of their functional ability have been shown to be influenced by mood. Some functional tests that have been applied to a chronic pain population include the 5-minute walk test (meters walked in 5 minutes), number of stairs climbed in 1 minute, and the stand-up test (number of times a patient can stand up from sitting down in 1 minute).

A functional capacity evaluation (FCE) is usually performed to determine a patient's physical capacity to perform work. Assessment includes the patient's ability to lift weights from the floor to waist level and from the waist to overhead, carry, crawl, squat, sit, stand, walk, climb stairs, and push and pull weights. Aerobic fitness may be determined from a (submaximal) bicycle or treadmill test. Aerobic fitness represents the ability to generate energy and is part of the measure of a person's work capacity. An FCE is always somewhat subjective as it can only document how much a patient is willing to do on a given day.

II. PHYSICAL THERAPY INTERVENTION

Physical therapy treatment should be time-limited and have an observable endpoint associated with the following:

- Restoration of optimal physical functioning
- Reduction of the impact of pain on the patient's life (i.e., reduced disability)
- Resolution of treatable impairments that interfere with normal function
- Prevention of future occurrences
- Improvement of the patient's knowledge of independent pain management

Components of physical therapy intervention for pain include the following:

- Teaching self-management techniques
- Treatment or management of pain by active modalities (exercise) and/or passive modalities (massage, joint mobilization, electrotherapy, heat and cold)

1. Education and self-management

Perhaps the most important goal in educating patients and teaching them self-management techniques is increased self-reliance. Many patients report feeling helpless and hopeless and at a loss at understanding why they have pain. Increased self-reliance increases their participation in the intervention and leads to better outcomes. Educating them about their diagnosis and pathology is helpful in reducing fear and eliminating catastrophizing.

It is important that the patient agrees with the goals of treatment. For example, if a patient feels that the only helpful treatment is medication, the chances of a successful outcome from physical therapy intervention are slim. When patients understand their pathology and agree with the goals of intervention, they are more likely to be compliant with the intervention offered.

It is helpful to instruct patients in self-massage, applying heat or cold as an active pain-control modality whether they have acute or chronic pain. For self-massage, patients can use a cane or umbrella handle to press against a trigger point and apply ischemic pressure, or they can slowly rotate two tennis balls around a painful area. Heat and cold packs in all sizes are commonly available through pharmacies.

2. Pain treatment and/or management

(i) *Active modalities*

Active modalities can be subdivided into three categories: (a) stretching exercise, (b) strengthening, and (c) endurance exercise.

a) Stretching exercise

The purpose of stretching is to regain normal flexibility around joints to allow them to function in their optimal position. Muscle imbalance can be a precipitating factor in the development of both trigger points and joint pain and therefore must be addressed. Certain muscles respond to a given situation (e.g., pain, impaired afferentiation by a joint) with tightness and shortening, whereas others respond by inhibition and weakness. Muscle responses seem to follow some typical rules, thus development of tightness or weakness may be considered a systematic and characteristic deviation in the functional quality of these muscles. The result of this deviation is a general imbalance within the whole muscular system. With an imbalance, a change in the sequence of activation of the muscle in the movement pattern occurs. This can further spiral the patient into a continuous cycle of weakness, tightness, abnormal movement patterns, and pain. As tight muscles are thought to inhibit their antagonists, stretching these muscles indirectly helps to restore strength.

Changes in muscle function play an important role in many painful conditions of the motor system and constitute an integral part of postural defects in general. Postural adjustments are the body's strategy to maintain the center of gravity of the total body. An increase in any one curve must be compensated by a proportionate increase or decrease in the other curves. Fine muscle coordination is needed to prevent damage to a joint, especially during fast movement. Thus, balanced muscle coordination may be the best protection of our osteoarticular system. Treatment consists of stretching the short musculature and strengthening the weak muscles. Normal posture is sought, resulting in normal bony alignment and normalized stresses across the joints. Restoration of normal muscle balance results in the following:

- Decreased repetitive microtrauma through normalization of biomechanical forces
- Normalization of reciprocal action muscles
- Restoration of normal flexibility (normal range of motion)

Passive stretching exercise is used in the treatment of trigger points (TPs). An active TP is associated with spontaneous pain at rest or with motion that stretches or overloads the muscle. Specific to a TP is referred pain and the "jump sign." The pattern of referred pain from TPs and associated phenomena is relatively constant and predictable and does not follow a dermatomal pattern or nerve root distribution. TPs and their referral patterns are described in detail in the classic works by Travell and Simons. Passive stretching is combined with spray-and-stretch techniques, which employ a vapocoolant spray and stretching of the involved muscle to render the TPs inactive. The spraying is thought to reduce the painfulness of the stretch tension by blocking reflex muscle spasm initiated by autogenous stretch reflexes.

b) Strengthening exercise

Directly increasing muscle strength is achieved by high-intensity, short-duration exercise. Neuronal adaptation occurs first by increased efficiency to recruit motor neurons, followed by an increase in myofibrillar protein after about 6 weeks of exercise. Increased muscle strength helps patients perform functional tasks such as lifting and carrying. It may also be helpful in decreasing pain perception. Increasing strength has been shown to decrease pain in patients with back and neck pain.

c) Endurance exercise

Endurance exercise involves two types of exercise:

- Exercise for whole body endurance
- Exercise for specific muscle endurance

Whole body exercise is targeted to increase the patients' maximal aerobic power or cardiovascular capacity by exercising them at 65% to 80% of their maximal heart rate, usually by treadmill walking, biking, or any form of dynamic exercise of large muscle groups. Work and functional tasks such as walking, climbing stairs, repetitive lifting, fighting fires, carrying loads, scaling walls, and running (necessary, e.g., for police or fire-fighting work) have a significant aerobic endurance component. Many tasks are defined by their energy cost as expressed in oxygen consumption or metabolic equivalents (METS). Patients need to have a maximal aerobic power high enough to perform functional tasks (work) without excessive fatigue.

Low-intensity, long-duration exercise is targeted to increase the aerobic capacity of a specific muscle so that it can sustain contraction for prolonged periods of time without fatiguing. This improves neuromotor control and coordination and thus prevents injury to passive structures during prolonged activities. Physical forces provide important stimuli to tissues for the development and maintenance of homeostasis. Endurance exercise of specific muscles is associated not only with increased capillary density of that muscle but also with increased strength of muscle, bone, and tendons. It results in thicker, stronger ligaments that maintain their compliance and flexibility and that are stronger at the bone–ligament–bone complex. This type of treatment is thus essential in the management of sprains and strains of ligaments, and of tendonitis.

Synovial fluid lubricates the ligamentous structures of joints and provides nourishment to cartilage, menisci, and ligaments. Repetitious motion enhances this transsynovial nutrient flow. In the spine, the health of the joints is largely dependent on repeated low-stress movements. The intervertebral joints and the facet joints require movement for the proper transfer of fluid and nutrients across the joint surfaces. In the same way, the intervertebral disc is largely dependent on movement for its nutrition. Endurance exercise thus improves the body's ability to withstand repetitive physical forces and muscle fatigue. As most functional tasks are repetitive in nature, most patients have a greater need of increased endurance than of increased strength. Lack of trunk muscle endurance plays an important role in chronic back pain. Jette and Jette (1996) showed that endurance exercise is associated with better outcomes in the treatment of patients with chronic back pain. Guidelines for the treatment of chronic back pain advocate the use of exercise and the avoidance of passive modalities.

Aerobic exercise is thought to have beneficial effects on pain perception and mood. It appears that pain inhibition through exercise can be mediated through the opioid and the nonopioid systems. Analgesic effects of exercise have been found at submaximal workloads of around 63% of maximum oxygen consumption (VO_{2max}). Rhythmic exercise stimulates the A-δ or group III afferents arising from muscle. Histologically, A-δ or group III afferents are a prominent group of fine myelinated fibers located in skeletal muscle nerves. Recent investigations indicate that these afferents respond to muscle stretch and contraction with low frequency discharge. For this reason, Kniffeki et al. called the endings of these afferents *"ergoreceptors"*. Thoren et al. and Lundeberg hypothesize that rhythmic exercise activates the ergoreceptors, which then activate the descending pain modulating systems.

Moderate aerobic exercise has been shown to be effective in the treatment of mild to moderate forms of depression and anxiety, which can be a powerful aid in the treatment of patients with chronic pain. Exercise in general should be focused on regaining physical functioning. For that reason, exercises should imitate functional movements. Weightbearing exercise helps reduce osteoporosis and is the treatment of choice in chronic complex regional pain syndrome (CRPS). Patients with CRPS are loath to use their affected body segment since any light touch stimulus causes dramatic pain. A hand or a foot held in a protective posture and not put to any use will exhibit shortened muscles and tendons (e.g., foot plantar flexion and inversion). Functional activities are initiated, often beginning with reflexively provoked action, such as catching or kicking a ball, or catching one's balance after perturbation. Functional progress is made through gait training using a mirror to promote symmetrical motion, or correcting improperly used muscles, restoring normal muscle length and postural alignment, and working on strength and endurance to balance muscle groups around major joints. Treatment can be made more tolerable with the assistance of lumbar sympathetic blocks if there is sympathetic mediation of pain present.

(ii) *Passive modalities and physical agents*

Physical agents commonly used in physical therapy are electrical stimulation ranging from low-volt to high-volt, ultrasound, heat, and cold.

Electrical stimulation is most commonly used for reduction of pain, edema, and muscle spasm, and stimulation of muscle contraction. For each type of neural tissue, there is an optimal frequency at which the maximal response is elicited: 0 to 5 Hz for sympathetic nerves, 10 to 150 Hz for parasympathetic nerves, and 10 to 50 Hz for motor nerves. Iontophoresis involves the transmission of medication through the skin by means of electrical stimulation. Commonly used medications are lidocaine and dexamethasone for the treatment of pain and local inflammation such as occurs in any kind of tendonitis. Transcutaneous electrical nerve stimulation (TENS) was developed on the basis of gate control theory by Melzack and Wall. High-frequency stimulation is thought to stimulate Aβ fibers, "closing the gate," whereas low-frequency stimulation is thought to activate the pain-inhibiting descending pathways. TENS, both high and low frequency, was shown to reduce pain and improve range of motion in patients with chronic back pain.

Ultrasound, a form of mechanotherapy, has both thermal and nonthermal effects. The thermal effects include increased blood flow, increased extensibility of collagenous tissues, and decreased pain and muscle spasm. The nonthermal effects of ultrasound include cavitation and microstreaming, which results in mast cell degranulation, altered cell membrane function, increased levels of intracellular calcium, and stimulation of fibroblast activity. This results in an increase in protein synthesis, vascular permeability, angiogenesis, and the tensile strength of collagen. Ultrasound, therefore, may be beneficial when a limitation in range of motion is caused by contractures of ligamentous or capsular tissues, or to accelerate inflammatory processes, thus decreasing associated edema with subsequent pain relief and wound healing.

Local heat causes vasodilatation and local erythema, decreased fast fiber sensation, and, with prolonged exposure, decreased slow nerve fiber sensation. The electrical resistance of the skin is reduced as well. Superficial heat is used to increase circulation, reduce pain, and promote relaxation.

Local cooling produces an intense vasoconstriction followed by periods of vasodilatation. Prolonged cooling decreases nerve fiber conduction. Cold is used in acute injuries to decrease swelling and pain, in chronic forms of musculoskeletal pain for pain relief, and in spastic muscle to reduce muscle tone. From clinical observation, most patients with neuropathic pain have difficulty tolerating cold and report that it increases their pain.

Joint mobilization is a technique used to improve joint mobility when the ligamentous and capsular structures limit passive range of motion. A variety of pathologic mechanisms can be involved in joint contracture development: immobilization, joint trauma, sepsis, degenerative processes, and a variety of disturbances that result in mechanical incongruity of the joint surfaces. A lesion of the capsule gives rise to limitation of capsular mobility, which limits the patient's active and passive range of motion and causes pain with movement. Treatment is directed to restoration of normal capsular mobility and thus normal range of motion. Joint mobilization can restore normal capsular extensibility by applying carefully directed forces across the articular surfaces. All collagenous tissues rely heavily on movement to ensure adequate nutrition, and they respond to loading much as bone does, according to Wolff's law. When not stretching the tissues, joint mobilization can be used to decrease pain by stimulation of types I and II mechanoreceptors. Joint mobilization is usually combined with ultrasound or heat, as this is thought to make the tissue more extensible and treatment thus more effective. Several studies have pointed out the immediate or short-term symptomatic reduction of pain after spinal manipulation or mobilization in patients with low back pain of less than a month's duration. Long-term results, however, were comparable for both the experimental and control groups in most studies.

Soft-tissue mobilization includes massage, passive stretching, and myofascial techniques such as myofascial release and craniosacral therapy. Massage can provide symptomatic relief of pain by increasing local circulation and stimulating Aβ fibers. TP massage in combination with passive stretching is thought to inhibit TPs in muscle, thus reducing muscle pain. A special form of massage, called "desensitization," includes techniques such as tapping, stroking, and massaging the skin and is used in the treatment of patients with CRPS to increase their tolerance of touch to the allodynic area. Patients are instructed to wear gloves or socks with progressively rougher inside surfaces (hair shirt analogy!) in addition.

III. PATIENTS WITH CHRONIC PAIN

Treating patients with nonmalignant chronic pain is a challenge that is ideally accomplished in a team format. These patients often present with pain complaints that seem out of proportion to objective findings, and they are completely disabled due to their pain, often in their work life as well as in their social and recreational lives. Patients with chronic pain usually present with primary as well as secondary impairments.

The primary impairments are the result of the original injury and may or may not be treatable by physical therapy. The secondary impairments are the consequence of the patients' response to the initial injury with self-immobilization. Lack of exercise, poor body alignment, shortening and weakening of the joint structures, and overguarding of the injured part of the body result in a weakened physical condition that can make normal daily activities more difficult, uncomfortable, and stressful. As a result, pain and suffering increase. These patients are commonly depressed as well, thus further spiraling into a cycle of disuse, pain, and impairment. The impairments resulting from disuse are readily addressed by an aggressive exercise program composed of stretching, cardiovascular conditioning, strength and endurance training, and behavioral modification tailored to the patient's individual needs.

Behavioral modification approaches are an important part of treatment and include ignoring pain behavior, education on the "hurt not harm" principle, and quota-based exercise. Patients are often afraid they will harm themselves as they get more active. To address this, a quota-based exercise approach is used. The patient is made to progress systematically, thus learning that increased activity does not equal increase in pain. Strong emphasis is placed on self-management techniques of pain, as chronic pain is a long-term condition that patients need to be able to manage on their own.

Although exercise programs are tailored to patients' individual needs, they commonly include the following:

- Aerobic exercise: such as bike or treadmill, at 65% to 80% of predicted maximal heart rate
- Stretching exercises for shortened musculature
- Endurance exercise for the major postural muscles
- Coordination/stabilization exercises
- Mobilizing exercise, if needed

Physical therapy goals for these patients are to increase function, decrease disability, establish effective pain coping and management skills, and decrease health care utilization in the long term. To achieve these goals, it is best that the physical therapist works within a team, including behavioral therapists, occupational therapists, social workers, and physicians. More detailed information on the treatment of patients with chronic pain can be found in Chapter 19.

IV. CONCLUSION

The key to the success of physical therapy in the treatment of pain is the incorporation of physical therapy into a comprehensive treatment plan. Although physical therapy helps to restore function, the therapy may be less effective if the pain is not optimally controlled by medical or interventional treatment (thus impeding any improvement in physical function). Equally, attention to psychological well-being is important, since physical therapy may not be successful if the patient approaches it with a negative state of mind or in a state of severe depression. Physical therapy is a vital component of multimodal pain management, and the physical therapist is an important members of the pain team.

SELECTED READINGS

1. Gurevich M, Kohn P, Davis C. Exercise-induced analgesia and the role of reactivity in pain sensitivity. *J Sports Sci* 1994;12:549–559.
2. Harding VR, Williams AC, Richardson PH, et al. The development of a battery of measures for assessing physical functioning of chronic pain patients. *Pain* 1994;25:367–375.
3. Hays KF. *Working it out: Using exercise in psychotherapy*. Washington, DC: American Psychological Association, 1999.
4. Lundeberg T. Pain physiology and principles of treatment. *Scand J Rehabil Med* 1995;Suppl 32:13–41.
5. Shutty MS, DeGood DE, Tuttle DH. Chronic pain patients' beliefs about their pain and treatment outcomes. *Arch Phys Med Rehabil* 1990;71:128–132.
6. Thoren P, Floras J, Hoffman P, Seals D. Endorphins and exercise: Physiological mechanisms and clinical implications. *Med Sci Sports Exerc* 1990;22:417–428.
7. Travell JG, Simons DG, eds. *Myofascial pain and dysfunction: The trigger point manuals*. Baltimore: Williams and Wilkins, 1983.
8. Wittink H, Michel TH, eds. *Chronic pain management for physical therapists*. Boston: Butterworth Heinemann, 1997.
9. Wittink H, Michel T. Physical therapy: Evaluation and treatment of chronic pain patients. In: Aronoff GM, ed. *Evaluation and treatment of chronic pain*, 3rd ed. Baltimore: Lippincott Williams and Wilkins, 1999.

Physical Medicine in the Treatment of Pain

Joseph F. Audette

What is needed most in architecture today is the very thing that is needed most in life—integrity. Just as it is needed in a human being, so integrity is the deepest quality in a building. . . . Integrity is not something to be put on and taken off like a garment. Integrity is a quality within and of the man himself. . . . It cannot be changed by any other person either, nor by the exterior pressures of any outward circumstances; integrity cannot change except from within because it is that in you which is you—and due to which you will try to live your life. . .in the best possible way. To build a man or building from within is always difficult.
—*From The Natural House, Frank Lloyd Wright (1954)*

Physical medicine and rehabilitation (PM&R) is one of the medical specialties that evaluates and treats patients with chronic pain conditions. The primary focus of the physiatrist's treatment approach is to restore structural integrity and maximize function rather than focusing solely on eliminating pain. To initiate a successful treatment plan, the physical and psychological obstacles to functional normalization must be identified and treated with the same aggressiveness that would be used to identify and treat the cause of nociception. As a corollary, the extent to which our patients have learned to be passive in the face of their chronic condition is a vitally important part of the chronic pain syndrome. Through this approach, we are able to help patients regain an internal locus of control in order to become active in the rehabilitation of their painful condition.

PM&R referrals should be made when a determination of a patient's residual functional capacity and potential for further functional restoration is needed. In particular, pain conditions with an industrial or work-related cause are often best treated with such a functional focus. In addition, physiatrists typically work in a team with physical and occupational therapists, mental health providers, and others to manage complex pain patients in an interdisciplinary setting.

I. PHYSIATRIC ASSESSMENT

1. History

Medical / surgical history

In addition to obtaining a standard medical and surgical history, the physiatrist gives special attention to determining the extent to which these historical factors may have an impact on future function. For example, the fact that a patient has had multiple prior surgical or other procedures may indicate a poor prognosis. This can suggest passive participation in the therapeutic process and dependence on multiple external sources for a "cure" despite repeated failures.

Internal fixation with hardware or implantation of devices such as pumps or stimulators may have a structural impact on rehabilitation. In the vast majority of cases, however, erroneous, limiting beliefs about the functional implications of the hardware or devices should be explored with the patient and eliminated. For instance, a history of spinal fusion does not mean a patient is permanently disabled.

Pharmacologic history

The way a patient takes medication is just as important as what they take. Frequent use of short-acting analgesics can indicate an overdependence on medications and poorly developed internal resources to cope with normal fluctuations in pain intensity. Determine if nonpharmacologic approaches for pain management such as distraction, relaxation, ice, heat, and stretching are used.

Assess whether analgesics are being used to treat emotional distress more than nociception. Does the patient *do more* if he or she is in less pain?

Psychosocial history

Psychosocial issues relevant to a detailed pain assessment are discussed elsewhere (see Chapter 15). Two especially important issues to elucidate are (a) a family history of disability (which can be a negative prognostic indicator), and (b) readiness to change (the patient's comfort with the current level of disability is revealing; ongoing litigation can interfere with a patient's readiness to change).

History of prior and present function

An accurate assessment of a patient's functional status can be difficult to acquire in a medical interview. Ask specifically "What can't you do?" rather than "What can you do?" Determining the level of function prior to the onset of the pain syndrome helps set the goals of treatment. Do not assume that, just because other physicians, including surgeons, have reinforced the patient's disability, they are correct. Numerous studies have shown that even after spinal surgery, patients can return to their former work capacity if motivated to do so.

History of prior treatments

The nature of prior physical rehabilitation should be determined. There are two broad categories: **passive**, or modality- and hands-on-driven treatments, and **active**, or patient-participation-driven treatments. If patients have failed an active rehabilitation program, it is important to determine the cause. Fear of increased pain during treatment or belief that they are at risk for harm with movement requires active psychological treatment in conjunction with continued active therapy. Some increase in pain, initially, is unavoidable in rehabilitation. Appropriate use of therapeutic injections and medications can ameliorate this.

2. Physical examination

Pain, and in particular chronic pain, causes significant alteration in body mechanics and can lead to pain perpetuation and continued disability despite appropriate treatment of the principal nociceptor involved. Addressing these structural factors and the resultant biomechanical perpetuators of pain and disability are a critical part of a comprehensive treatment plan.

GAIT.   Antalgic gaits are common with chronic pain. Use of assistive devices, except in the elderly, is usually a sign of illness behavior and is rarely necessary for safety.

A compensated Trendelenburg gait is a sign of hip abductor weakness, caused either by true neurologic weakness (rare) or by reflex inhibition of the hip abductor as a result of sacroiliac (SI) joint dysfunction or hip joint disease.

SPINE.   Congenital scoliosis can be distinguished from a functional or acquired scoliosis by forward flexion of the spine, bringing out the rotatory component of congenital scoliosis (the Adams test).

Apparent short leg syndrome (ASLS), best seen with patient lying supine, is caused by muscle shortening of the hip rotators such as the gluteus medius and piriformis, and it is commonly associated with SI joint dysfunction. The short leg in this syndrome is more externally rotated while supine because of the contraction of the hip external rotators. Use of a lift in the shoe is contraindicated, as it could exacerbate the problem.

Thoracic kyphosis with a thrust-forward head, extended cervical spine, and internally rotated shoulders is common with pain syndromes of the mid back, head, and neck. This puts the patient at risk for myofascial pain and muscular nerve entrapment syndromes at the occipitocervical junction and the anatomic thoracic inlet.

II. PHYSIATRIC TREATMENT OF PAIN

1. Physical and occupational therapy referral

The type of physical therapy referral depends on the conditions found in the assessment phase of the evaluation. This topic is discussed in further detail in Chapter 16. Brief guidelines for establishing physical therapy should include determination of any contraindications or limitations to a full functional restoration treatment plan. Special consideration is warranted if there is a cardiopulmonary impairment that may impact therapeutic conditioning and medication trials. Severe psychological or motivational impairments should be identified and treated by mental health professionals before any pain rehabilitation is initiated.

Referral options should be considered for patients with chronic pain who exhibit the following characteristics:

a) *Chronic pain with moderate functional limitations but without major psychological impairments*

If motivational issues are not predominant, and there are no return-to-work issues, refer the patient to physical therapy, with goals of correcting structural deviations seen on examination, improving strength, and increasing aerobic conditioning. Emphasize an active program rather than a passive, modality-based treatment. Desensitization techniques, including transcutaneous electrical nerve stimulation (TENS), thermal modalities, and self-massage, can be taught.

If motivational issues are more predominant or there are return-to-work issues, refer the patient to a quota-based rehabilitation program (Table 1).

b) *Chronic pain with major functional and psychological impairments.*

Refer the patient to a multidisciplinary functional restoration program. This treatment team is more robust, usually involving medical, psychological, and rehabilitative (both physical therapy and occupational therapy) services. Treatment is still goal based but can be more individualized and is not limited to treatment of spine pathology (Table 2).

Occupational therapy referrals can be useful when work dynamic issues are influencing the pain. Ergonomic factors can be assessed and corrected, and issues of pacing and functional adaptations to various tasks can be addressed. Upper extremity pain and cervical pain with headaches are special areas of expertise of occupational therapy, which can complement a good physical therapy program.

2. Therapeutic injections

When used by a physiatrist, an invasive technique (see Chapter 12) is never the sole method of treatment for a painful condition but rather an adjunct to allow better participation of the patient in the

Table 1.   Goals of quota base system

Rehabilitation Task	Goal
Flexibility	
	100 degrees of lumbar flexion
	25 degrees of lumbar extension
	Straight leg raise of 75 degrees
Strength	
	Trunk extension and flexion strength 100%–120% of ideal body weight
	Functional lift from floor 40%–50% of ideal body weight
Conditioning	
	Heart rate 80% of age-determined target
	Work load greater than 6,000 Kg-m/9 min

Modified from Rainville, J, Sobel JB, Banco RJ, et al. Low back and cervical spine disorders. *Orthop Clin North Am* 1996;27:729–746, with permission.

Table 2. Details of services offered in functional restoration program

Rehabilitation Tasks	Detail
Physical	
	Treatment approach not specific to spinal pathology, more flexible
	Goals set in conjunction with patient's input, not imposed by quotas
	Emphasis placed on education and self-management of pain
	Work simulation activities individualized to patient's return-to-work goals
Cognitive	
	Counseling on sleep hygiene
	Counseling on social, environmental, and psychological barriers
	Behavioral approach applied to address fears, passivity, kinesiophobia
	Relaxation, muscle tension reduction, reduction of physiologic arousal
Medical	
	Pharmacologic management of sleep disturbance and mood disorder
	Medication education and optimization of pharmacologic regimen
	Overseeing of goal accomplishment; medical limitations addressed
	Therapeutic injections given to assist in reaching functional goals

process of functional restoration. Many physiatrists have training in spinal injections as well as other techniques such as joint injections for the knee, shoulder, ankle, wrist, and digits (Table 3).

Injection techniques for myofascial pain vary widely. Typically, a 25- to 27-gauge needle $1\frac{1}{2}$ to 2 inches long is adequate. The local anesthetic varies, but generally 0.5 to 10 mL of either 0.5% to 1% lidocaine or 0.25% bupivacaine is used, depending on the size of the muscle and the technique used. Dry needling either with a standard needle (as just described) or with an acupuncture needle (32 to 34 gauge) is also effective.

Botulinum toxin (Botox or Myobloc) injections into trigger points are being studied in many centers. Botulinum toxin binds irreversibly to the presynaptic motor endplate and prevents the release of acetylcholine, leading to chemical denervation. This technique essentially inactivates the muscle for up to 2 to 4 months. Some people advocate its use in myofascial trigger point injections, using anywhere from 20 to 100 units (Botox) depending on muscle size.

3. Pharmacologic management

Certain patients with chronic pain are unlikely to benefit greatly from invasive measures. In these cases, the appropriate use of

Table 3.   Common sites of injection[a]

Injection Sites	Needle	Volume	Comments
Joints			
Ulnocarpal	#25, 1.5 in	1–3 mL	Steroid-volume-to-anesthetic ratio, 1:1
Radiocarpal			
Carpometacarpal			
Elbow	#25, 1.5 in	2–3 mL	Steroid-volume-to-anesthetic ratio, 1:2
Ankle			
Shoulder	#25, 1.5 in	7–10 mL	Steroid-volume-to-anesthetic ratio, 1:6 to 9
Knee			
Sacroiliac joint			
Bone-tendon			
Med/lat epicondyle	#27, 1.25 in	2–3 mL	Steroid-volume-to-anesthetic ratio, 1:1
Plantar fascia			
Patellar tendon			
Achilles tendon			
Pubic symphysis	#25, 1.5 in	3–5 mL	Steroid-volume-to-anesthetic ratio, 1:2 to 4
Hamstrings			
Adductors			
Tendon sheaths			
Thumb extensor	#27, 1.25 in	1–3 mL	Steroid-volume-to-anesthetic ratio, 1:1
Finger flexors			
Posterior tibial	#27, 1.25 in	3–5 mL	Steroid-volume-to-anesthetic ratio, 1:2 to 4
Biceps (long head)			
Bursae			If aspirating, will need 18–20-gauge needle first.
Prepatellar	#25, 1.5 in	2–3 mL	Steroid-volume-to-anesthetic ratio, 1:1
Pes anserine			
Olecranon			

Table 3. *Continued*

Injection Sites	Needle	Volume	Comments
Subacromial	#25, 1.5 in	7–10 mL	Steroid-volume-to-anesthetic ratio, 1:6 to 9
Greater trochanter			
Perineural			
Carpal tunnel	#27, 1.25 in	2–5 mL	Steroid-volume-to-anesthetic ratio, 2:1
Tarsal tunnel			
Suprascapular notch			
Cubital tunnel			

a Use 1% lidocaine or 0.25% bupivicaine with insoluble steroid salts such as triamcinolone acetate or betamethasone acetate.

medication can help achieve the functional goals of rehabilitation. The goals of medication are to restore sleep, to modulate pain without causing excessive dependence or dysfunction, and to stabilize mood. Often, psychopharmacologic assessment is needed to optimize treatment. In general, short-acting opioids (see Chapter 9) are avoided so that the patient recognizes the value of nonpharmacologic approaches to managing pain.

III. PHYSIATRIC ASSESSMENT AND TREATMENT OF SPECIFIC PAIN SYNDROMES

1. Back and neck pain

Spinal pain syndromes are among the most common presenting problems in pain clinics and can be complicated by issues of secondary gain and excessive illness behavior (Table 4). The Waddell signs are not evidence of malingering but rather signs of disease affirmation, conviction, and psychological distress.

Selected syndromes

CERVICAL FACET SYNDROME. Often associated with trigger points in specific zones of occipital region (C2-3), neck (C4-5, C5-6), and scapular region (C6-7, T1-2, T2-3, and down). Positive local pain with Spurling test (extension and rotation of neck with compression).

LUMBAR FACET SYNDROME. Increased pain with extension, less with flexion, or increased pain with extension together with rotation. Occasional referred pain to buttocks and anterior thigh.

SI JOINT DYSFUNCTION. Pain can radiate to groin or in sciatic nerve distribution. Lying supine, patient may have shortened and externally rotated leg. Pain on palpation over the joint when lying prone.

Table 4.   Characteristics of abnormal illness behavior

Assessment Methods	Normal Illness Behavior	Abnormal Illness Behavior
Pain drawing	Localized with appropriate neuroanatomic features	Magnified, covering diffuse regions of body
Pain adjectives	Sensory	Affective, evaluative
Symptoms		
Pain	Localized	Whole leg pain
Numbness	Dermatomal	Whole leg
Weakness	Myotomal	Whole leg giving away
Time pattern	Varies with time	Never free of pain
Response to treatment	Variable benefit	Intolerance of treatments
		Frequent emergency department visits
Signs		
Tenderness	Localized	Superficial, nonanatomic
Axial loading	No lumbar pain	Lumbar pain
Straight leg raise	Limited on distraction	Improves with distraction
Sensory	Dermatomal	Regional
Motor	Myotomal	Jerky, give-away weakness
Tenderness	Appropriate pain	Overreaction

Modified from Waddell G, Pilowsky I, Bond MR. Clinical assessment and interpretation of abnormal illness behavior in low back pain. *Pain* 1989;39:41–53, with permission.

2. Myofascial pain

Myofascial pain syndrome (MPS) can mimic a number of clinical conditions, making diagnosis by history alone difficult (Table 5). Physical examination of myofascial trigger points should include more than identification of point tenderness over a muscle, which can be seen in many conditions (e.g., myositis, polymyalgia rheumatica, fibromyalgia, muscle spasm, and focal dystonias). *Spot tenderness*, the presence of a *taut band*, and *pain recognition* by the patient are the most reliable indicators.

Successful treatment demands an identification of the underlying cause. This can include anything from overuse syndromes, to prolonged structural deviations in body mechanics, to facet syn-

Table 5.   Clinical presentation of myofascial pain

Clinical Condition	Muscles Involved with Myofascial Trigger Points
Tension headaches	Upper trapezius, splenius capitus, semispinalis, scalenes, sternocleidomastoid
Temporomandibular joint pain	Masseter, temporalis, sternocleidomastoid
Cervical radiculopathy	Upper trapezius, scalenes, levator scapula, teres minor
Thoracic back pain	Lower trapezius, rhomboids, serratus anterior and posterior
Lumbar back pain	Quadratus lumborum, gluteus medius, ileopsoas
Lumbar radiculopathy	Gluteus medius and piriformis
Greater trochanter bursitis	Gluteus medius and piriformis without sciatic entrapment
Coccygodynia	Piriformis and gemelli without sciatic entrapment
Biceps tendinitis	Pectoralis minor, biceps, subscapularis
Rotator cuff tendinitis	Supra- and infraspinatus, teres minor, latissimus dorsi

drome and underlying radiculopathies. Initial treatment should not be directed at the trigger point but at the identified cause, either with appropriate rehabilitation or injections. If there continues to be local muscle irritability, trigger point injections will have a sustained effect. Low-dose tricyclic antidepressants are particularly useful to correct associated sleep disorders and modulate the pain. Once adequate release of muscle tension is achieved, an aggressive strengthening program should be initiated to harden the muscle.

3. Fibromyalgia

Fibromyalgia can be distinguished from MPS by the diffuseness of the tender points that may or may not be trigger points. These points are symmetrically distributed and affect both upper and lower parts of the body in fibromyalgia but not in MPS. In addition, historical factors, such as sleep disturbance, depression, chronic fatigue, irritable bowel, dysmenorrhea, cystitis, and chronic sinusitis, are more commonly found in fibromyalgia. Fibromyalgia is a systemic not a localized disease.

Treatment should focus exclusively on functional restoration, as pain elimination is generally not possible. Use of both low-dose tricyclic antidepressants at night and the newer antidepressants such as the serotonin uptake inhibitors during the day may be helpful. Pharmacologic treatment should be combined with skilled relaxation training and other cognitive and behavioral techniques to modulate pain. Although the use of opioids in fibromyalgia has some proponents, in general there is a risk of poor functional outcome and worsening depression and fatigue.

Physical rehabilitation should focus on flexibility and conditioning rather than aggressive strengthening to avoid pain exacerbation. Invasive procedures should be avoided unless there is a comorbid condition such as a radiculopathy or joint effusion that would have a reasonable probability of responding.

IV. CONCLUSION

Physiatrists have a very broad understanding of the physical and psychological factors contributing to pain and are therefore in a strong position to evaluate pain patients, to determine if specialist treatment is indicated, and to treat patients whose pain is not amenable to, or has been failed by, other specialist treatment. Their role and that of physical treatments in the management of chronic pain patients are invaluable.

SELECTED READING

1. Chesire WP, et al. Botulinum toxin in the treatment of myofascial pain syndrome. *Pain* 1994;59:65–69.
2. Chu J. Dry needling in myofascial pain related to lumbosacral radiculopathy. *Eur J Phys Med Rehabil* 1995;5:106.
3. Fishbain DA, et al. Male and female chronic pain patients categorized by DSM-III psychiatric diagnostic criteria. *Pain* 1986;26:181–197.
4. Fricton JR, et al. Myofascial pain syndrome: Electromyographic changes associated with local twitch response. *Arch Phys Med Rehabil* 1985;66:314–317.
5. Fukui S, et al. Referred pain distribution of the cervical zygapophyseal joints and cervical dorsal rami. *Pain* 1996;68:79–83.
6. Gerwin RD, et al. Interrater reliability in myofascial trigger point examination. *Pain* 1997;69:65–73.
7. Han S, et al. Myofascial pain syndrome and trigger-point management. *Reg Anesth* 1997;22:89–99.
8. Hong CZ, et al. Lidocaine injection vs dry needling to myofascial trigger points. *Am J Phys Med Rehabil* 1994;74:256.
9. Hong CZ. Current research on myofascial trigger points—pathophysiological studies. *J Musculoskeletal Pain* 1999;7:121–129.
10. Mense S. Nociception from skeletal muscle in relation to clinical muscle pain [review]. *Pain* 1993;54:241–289.
11. Rainville J, et al. Low back and cervical spine disorders. *Orthop Clin North Am* 1996;27:729–746.
12. Simons D, Travell J. *Myofascial pain and dysfunction: The trigger point manual*, vol. 1, 2nd ed. Philadelphia: Williams & Wilkins, 1999.
13. Waddell G, et al. Clinical assessment and interpretation of abnormal illness behaviour in low back pain. *Pain* 1989;39:41–53.

Acupuncture

May C. M. Pian-Smith

In any path of study, knowledge never comes entirely at once but piece-meal. Truth presents herself in fragmentary form, and we put pieces together.
—*R. Abbe*

I. THE GROWING SIGNIFICANCE OF COMPLEMENTARY THERAPIES

There is increasing patient demand for, and acceptance of, "unconventional" therapies. It is now incumbent on healthcare practitioners to have knowledge of complementary therapies and to understand their clinical implications. In a national survey published in the Journal of the American Medical Association in 1998, Eisenberg and colleagues found that 42% of American adults use some form of "unconventional" therapy. The number of visits for alternative therapy was 629 million in 1997, which far exceeded the number of visits to all primary care physicians that year, totaling 386 million. That year, the total expenditure for complementary therapy was estimated to be $27 billion, compared to out-of-pocket expenditures for conventional care of $29 billion. Back pain, headache, depression, and anxiety were the main clinical entities for which people were interested in pursuing unconventional therapies. The survey also revealed that most patients do not inform their regular physicians when they seek help outside the realm of standard medical care.

The United States government has made several initiatives in response to the evolving acceptance of unconventional therapies in Western medical practice. In 1996, the U.S. Food and Drug Administration relabeled acupuncture needles as medical equipment rather than experimental equipment. The marketing and use of acupuncture needles is therefore now under the same strict quality control standards that are demanded for medical needles, syringes, or surgical scalpels. In 1997, the National Institutes of Health (NIH) convened a consensus conference on acupuncture. The NIH Consensus Statement on Acupuncture concluded that sufficient evidence exists to support the efficacy of acupuncture for postoperative and chemotherapy-induced nausea and vomiting, nausea of pregnancy, and postoperative dental pain. The conference panel also determined that acupuncture may be an effective adjunctive therapy for other conditions, including addiction, headache, low back pain, asthma, and carpal tunnel syndrome. The NIH Office of Alternative Medicine has since been expanded to the Center for Complementary and Alternative Medicine.

A 1998 survey revealed that alternative medicine coursework is now offered at 75 American medical schools. As an indication of how complementary therapies are being integrated into regular medical practices, there has been reevaluation of third-party reimbursements for these alternative therapies, and more insurance plans are covering these services.

II. CLASSICAL AND MODERN MECHANISMS OF ACUPUNCTURE

Acupuncture is a medical practice that has been used for about 3,000 years. Acupuncture methods promote natural healing and functional restoration. This is achieved by inserting very thin needles, and sometimes applying manual stimulation, heat, or electrical stimulation, at very precise acupuncture points.

There are many hundreds of acupuncture points located over the entire body. Some of the points are theoretically connected with one another energetically. According to classical Chinese teachings, channels of energy ("qi") run in regular patterns through the body and over its surface. These energy channels are called meridians and are analogous to rivers that irrigate and nourish the body's tissues. Disease and pain are thought to reflect imbalances in the flow of energy, with energy deficiencies occurring in some areas and energy excesses in others. The principal meridians are named after organ systems and are often linked to one another on the basis of having either complementary or opposing effects. The meridians can be influenced by needling of acupuncture points; the needles can unblock obstructions and/or allow excess energy to be dissipated and thus correct imbalances.

Different acupuncture traditions trace roots back to various regions in Asia as well as Europe. On the basis of the traditions or beliefs of a particular acupuncture school (e.g., Traditional Chinese Medicine, Five-Elements theory, Korean Hand acupuncture, scalp or ear acupuncture, Japanese acupuncture, and the French energetics system), various acupuncture points are selected and manipulated in different ways. Points might be selected on the basis of the clinical symptoms to be treated, because of intrinsic properties or the "spirit" of the points, or because of their location in a theoretical energy pathway or network. Once needled, the points can be stimulated to either add energy to a depleted system or to dissipate excess energy. Heat or electrical (electroacupuncture) stimulation can be used to tonify, or add energy to, acupuncture needles; alternatively, heat energy, from a heat lamp or from burning herbs (moxa), can be applied over acupuncture points even in the absence of needling. In many acupuncture traditions, the elicitation of "deqi" sensation, an achy, warm, tingly, or swollen feeling at the needle insertion site, is thought to be necessary for therapeutic effect.

III. THE SCIENTIFIC BASIS OF THE ACUPUNCTURE EFFECT

Since the 1970s there has been a great deal of laboratory research to elucidate a more "scientific" basis for acupuncture's effects. Neurophysiologic data support the efficacy of acupuncture for painful syndromes. In summary, the central nervous system, peripheral nerves, various endorphins, and monoamine neurotransmitters have all been implicated in the process. Different types of acupuncture stimulation (depending on the location of the needle and its relationship to the site of pain, and depending on the electrical frequency with which the acupuncture needles are stimulated) elicit different mechanisms of pain inhibition.

In the most widely accepted acupuncture model, needling of nerve fibers in the muscle sends impulses to the spinal cord and then activates three centers: (1) areas of spinal cord, (2) the midbrain, and (3) the hypothalamus-pituitary system. The spinal cord site uses enkephalin and dynorphin to block incoming messages during electroacupuncture at low frequency (2 to 4 Hz). Other neurotransmitters (e.g., gamma-aminobutyric acid, or GABA) are stimulated with high-frequency acupuncture stimulation (on the order of 50 to 500 Hz).

The midbrain uses enkephalin to activate the raphe descending system, which inhibits spinal cord pain transmission by a synergistic effect of monoamines, serotonin, and norepinephrine. The midbrain also has a circuit that bypasses the endorphin steps during high-frequency electroacupuncture. At the hypothalamus-pituitary level, the pituitary releases B-endorphin into the blood and cerebrospinal fluid (CSF) to cause analgesia at a distance. The hypothalamus also sends long axons to the midbrain, and via B-endorphin, it activates the descending analgesia system. This center is not activated at high frequency but with low-frequency electroacupuncture stimulation.

The following findings (coming from several laboratories) support the role of endorphins during some forms of electroacupuncture:

The acupuncture effect is not immediate; rather, analgesia occurs after a 20- to 30-minute induction period, as might be expected with a humorally mediated mechanism.

Analgesia persists 1 to 2 hours after the cessation of acupuncture.

Naloxone and other opiate antagonists inhibit acupuncture analgesia.

Animals genetically deficient in opiate receptors or deficient in endorphins show poor acupuncture analgesia.

Endorphin levels rise in the blood and in the CSF during acupuncture.

Acupuncture effects are enhanced by inhibitors of endorphin enzymatic degradation.

Acupuncture analgesia can be transferred to a second animal via CSF transfer or blood cross-circulation between two animals, and this effect is blocked by naloxone given to either animal.

On the other hand, during high-frequency electroacupuncture, it seems that other neurotransmitters (e.g., serotonin and norepinephrine) mediate the effects. This is supported by the following findings:

Under these conditions, there is a rapid onset of analgesia, without a long induction period.

When lesions are made in parts of the brain that are rich in serotonin-releasing cells (e.g., in the raphe magnus of the brainstem and the medial medulla oblongata), acupuncture-induced analgesia is abolished.

Agents that block biosynthesis of serotonin (e.g., parachlorophenylalanine) block acupuncture analgesia.

Agents that block serotonin receptors also block acupuncture. Analgesia is enhanced when serotonin levels are increased. Norepinephrine has also been implicated in studies showing inhibition of acupuncture's effects with yohimbine and phentolamine.

A recent study from Massachusetts General Hospital reported the use of functional magnetic resonance imaging (fMRI) to investigate the effects of acupuncture in the brain. This study provides a foundation for future studies on mechanisms of acupuncture as a therapeutic intervention. Functional MRI signals are thought to reflect changes in metabolic activity or blood flow. The results of this study suggest that acupuncture needling modulates the activity of the limbic system and subcortical structures. Further studies are underway to correlate signal changes with changes in pain thresholds.

IV. SUITABILITY, EFFICACY, AND SAFETY OF ACUPUNCTURE

Diehl and colleagues recently conducted a survey of American physicians who use acupuncture as well as conventional therapies in their practice. The study estimated that there are about 3,000 physician acupuncturists in the United States. These physicians choose acupuncture over conventional therapy most often for low back pain, myofascial pain, simple headache, sciatica, and shoulder pain. Reasons for using acupuncture in these settings included efficacy of acupuncture and failed or inadequate standard medical therapy.

Many benefits of acupuncture are reported in the literature; the World Health Organization (WHO) has published a list of clinical indications for which acupuncture may be helpful that includes illnesses involving virtually every organ system. Despite these reports, there is little support from randomized controlled trials (RCTs), and there are several impediments to conducting RCTs of acupuncture. True blinding of either the patient or the treating acupuncturist is clearly impossible. At the same time, controversy surrounds the development of appropriate controls for acupuncture studies, as even nonspecific needling (i.e., not at recognized acupuncture sites, or not site specific for the disease in question) can elicit responses that may be similar to the response to active treatment. Most of the published reports about clinical applications of acupuncture are case reports or case series. In many cases, individual subjects have served as their own historical controls. Very few studies include long-term follow-up data. It has been difficult to make generalized conclusions based on the results of different studies because of the variation in acupuncture points used for a given clinical condition, the mode of needle stimulation, variations in treatment duration and intervals between treatments, and variations in electrical frequency where electroacupuncture was employed.

The effectiveness of acupuncture for managing the pain of primary dysmenorrhea was demonstrated in a randomized clinical study by Helms in 1987. Forty-three women were followed for a year, and they were allocated to receive weekly acupuncture for three menstrual cycles (n = 11), weekly sham acupuncture (at random points; n = 11), weekly visitations but no acupuncture (n = 11), or no intervention (n = 10). There was an improvement in dysmenorrhea in 10 patients in the real acupuncture group (90.0%), 4 in the sham acupuncture group (36.4%), 2 in the visitation control group (18.2%), and 1 in the no care group (10%). The improvement in the group receiving real acupuncture was significantly better than all other groups combined ($p < .001$) and there was a 41% reduction in analgesic medication used by the women who received acupuncture.

The efficacy of electroacupuncture for low back pain was described by Ghoname in 1999. Sixty adults with chronic low back pain associated with degenerative disc disease were studied in a randomized, single-blind, sham-controlled cross-over study. Four therapeutic modalities, percutaneous electrical nerve stimulation (PENS, a form of electroacupuncture), sham PENS, transcutaneous electrical nerve stimulation (TENS), and physical therapy were each given for a period of 30 minutes three times per week for 3 weeks. PENS was significantly more effective in decreasing pain scores after each treatment than sham PENS, TENS, or physical therapy. The average daily oral intake of nonopioid analgesics was decreased by PENS significantly more than by sham-PENS, TENS, or physical therapy ($p < .008$). The majority of study patients (91%) reported that PENS was most effective in decreasing their low back pain. The PENS therapy was also significantly more effective in improving physical activity, quality of sleep, and sense of well-being ($p < .05$ for each).

Several notable studies have been done on acupuncture that do not relate directly to pain, but they are so beautifully designed and controlled that they warrant mention. For example, Dundee and colleagues have published many reports of studies in which acupuncture was effective for management of chemotherapy-induced nausea and vomiting. In one illustrative study, statistically significant differences were found in a small sample of 10 men undergoing cisplatin therapy for testicular cancer. Patients were treated with electroacupuncture stimulation at MH-6 (on the ventral wrist) or with electroacupuncture at a dummy point on the arm. The patients were then asked to rate their nausea on a scale of 0 to 4 (4 being maximal relief of symptoms). The group receiving real electroacupuncture gave a mean score of 3.76, compared to 1.6 for the control group ($p < .001$).

Cardini and colleagues reported in 1998 the results of a study carried out in the People's Republic of China in which moxibustion (burning of herbs near the skin) over an acupuncture point on the fifth toe resulted in version of breech fetus presentation. Specifically, 260 healthy primigravida women at 33 weeks gestation and with breech fetuses were randomized to two groups. One group received daily moxibustion therapy and the other group received no special intervention. Two weeks later, at 35 weeks gestation, 75% of those who had received moxibustion had fetuses that had flipped to the head-down position, compared to 48% in the control group ($p < .001$). The results correlated with an increased number of fetal movements perceived by the mothers (48 movements per hour in the treatment group versus 35 movements per hour in the control group; $p < .001$). Although the subjects were not blinded to the treatment, the level of significance of the results, and the potential impact on rates of cesarean sections and birth complications, makes this an important study.

Acupuncture, properly performed, is a procedure that is rarely associated with complications. The most common include minor bruising or a transient vasovagal response that responds quickly and completely to body repositioning. When sterile, disposable needles are placed carefully and skillfully, complications such as transmission of infection, nerve injury, and pneumothorax are avoided.

V. CONCLUSION

Acupuncture therapy can play an important role as part of a multidisciplinary approach to the management of chronic and acute pain. Analgesia is thought to be mediated by the activation of several pathways involving neurotransmitters and hormones. Alterations in neurotransmitter handling, or "balancing of energy," are thought to also affect associated symptoms of fatigue and depression, and to improve the overall sense of well-being. Physician acupuncturists cite the following reasons for choosing acupuncture:

- Good efficacy
- Useful adjunct to standard care
- Use as part of a multidimensional, holistic, mind–body–spirit approach
- Preferred by some patients
- Safety
- Avoidance of side effects and complications of standard treatments
- Cost effectiveness
- Worth trying when standard therapies have failed

Acupuncture has become increasingly popular in the West as people of Western culture become more familiar with the customs and cultures of the East, and as the healing qualities of acupuncture and other Eastern therapies are recognized. Acupuncture has a very long history of success in the East, but we are still learning the scientific basis of its effects, how it interacts with conventional therapies, and how effective it is in Western patients.

SELECTED READINGS

1. Cardini F, Weixin H. Moxibustion for correction of breech presentation: a randomized controlled trial. *JAMA* 1998;280:1580–1584.
2. Diehl DL, Kaplan G, Coulter I, et al. Use of acupuncture by American physicians. *J Altern Complement Med* 1997;3:119–126.
3. Dundee JW, Ghaly RG, Fitzpatrick T, et al. Acupuncture to prevent cisplatin-associated vomiting. *Lancet* 1987;1:1083.
4. Eisenberg DM, Davis RB, Ettner SL, et al. Trends in alternative medicine use in the United States, 1990–1997. Results of a Follow-up National Survey. *JAMA* 1998;280:246–252.
5. Ghoname EA, Craig WF, White PF, et al. Percutaneous electrical nerve stimulation for low back pain: A randomized crossover study. *JAMA* 1999; 281:818–823.
6. Helms JM. Acupuncture for the management of primary dysmenorrhea. *Obstet Gynecol* 1987;69:51–56.
7. Helms JM. An overview of medical acupuncture. *Altern Ther* 1998;4:35–45.

8. Hui KKS, Liu J, Makris N, et al. Acupuncture modulates the limbic system and subcortical gray structures of the human brain: Evidence from fMRI studies in normal subjects. *Hum Brain Mapp* 2000;9:13–25.
9. Lewis L, Kaplan G, LaRiccia PJ, et al. Acupuncture: Another therapeutic choice? *Patient Care* 1999;33:149–176.
10. NIH Consensus Conference Report on Acupuncture. *JAMA* 1999; 280:1518–1524.
11. Pian-Smith MCM et al. Neurophysiologic basis of acupuncture. In: Gellman H, ed. *Acupuncture for orthopaedics and rehabilitation*. Langhorne, PA: Gordon and Breach Science (in press).
12. Pomeranz B. Scientific research into acupuncture for the relief of pain. *J Altern Complement Med* 1996;2:53–60.

Chronic Pain Rehabilitation

Elizabeth Loder, Penelope Herbert, and
Patricia McAlary

Like an alarm bell stuck in the "on" position . . . such is chronic benign pain.
—*Bruce Smoller and Brian Schulman*

I. THE SCOPE OF THE PROBLEM

Despite steady improvements in the treatment of pain, a group
of patients remains whose recovery is minimal despite concerted
attempts at appropriate therapy. Unrelieved pain is associated with
dramatic impairment of physical, psychological, and social well-
being. Unemployment, reduced physical activity, and sleep disruption associated with chronic pain may lead to a downward spiral
of physical inactivity, decreased socialization, altered sleep/wake
cycles, and medication overuse. Once entrenched, these maladaptive behavior patterns are difficult to reverse. Secondary depression
and medication overuse may develop, along with family dysfunction and poor work performance. Patients with chronic pain are five
times more likely than the general population to use medical services, and 58% of patients with chronic pain have anxiety or depression that can further complicate their management.

The development of **chronic pain syndrome** (Table 1), in
which patients develop disability out of proportion to the underlying disease, with associated behavioral abnormalities, requires
multidisciplinary treatment. The treatment philosophy, which
must be accepted by the patient and the family, shifts from cure to
management. Medication reduction, increased "up" time and regular physical exercise, involvement in hobbies or return to work,
and psychological intervention all help return the patient to some
semblance of normal living, despite the persistence of pain.

Optimal management of chronic pain must address not only the
initiating physical pathology but also the social and psychological
sequelae that accompany the pain and contribute to poor quality of
life. Specialized outpatient pain rehabilitation programs that provide coordinated, multidisciplinary care can be helpful. Inpatient

Table 1. Characteristics of patients with chronic pain syndrome

Demanding, angry, skeptical (of help)
Doctor shopping ("fix me")
Somatizing; dependency on health care system—often for multiple medical problems
Preoccupation with pain
Significant pain behavior
Passive-dependent personality traits
Caretaker—meets needs of others at own expense
Denial of emotional or family conflicts
Significant life disruption in multiple areas
Feelings of isolation and loneliness
Lack of insight into self-defeating behavior patterns
Use of pain as a symbolic means of communication
May be conscious or unconscious of secondary gain

Adapted from Aronoff GM. Psychological aspects of nonmalignant chronic pain: A multidisciplinary approach. *Resid Staff Physician* 1984;3, with permission.

treatment may be necessary for patients with impaired mobility or advanced debilitation, severe medication overuse (requiring special tapering from opioid or barbiturate drugs), or associated medical or psychiatric morbidity that precludes outpatient treatment.

The Pathologic Nature of Chronic Pain

Chronic pain differs from acute pain in that it is a pathologic state that is of no benefit to the individual, unlike acute (physiologic) pain, which arises in response to injury or inflammation and protects the individual from further injury. Acute pain is time limited and resolves as healing takes place. Chronic pain, on the other hand, is caused by changes in the nervous system that are not reversible (e.g., nerve injury, sensitization, new fiber growth, reorganization), and it is unremitting and extremely difficult to treat. Standard acute pain treatments (nonsteroidal anti-inflammatory drugs and opioids) have only limited efficacy in treating chronic pain. Moreover, the pain, muscle guarding, and decreased activity that serve a useful purpose in acute pain become counterproductive in chronic pain. Avoiding activity no longer serves the purpose of protecting healing tissues from further injury but instead leads to deconditioning. Patients tend to respond to chronic pain in the same way that they respond to acute pain, but the response is dysfunctional and paradoxically promotes worsening rather than improvement.

II. GENERAL PRINCIPLES OF CHRONIC PAIN TREATMENT

In nearly all cases, multidisciplinary treatment rather than medical treatment alone is required to reverse the complex behavior patterns that develop as a result of chronic pain. When it is not possible to eliminate pain, emphasis shifts from efforts directed solely at pain relief, whatever the cost, toward efforts to maximize the patient's ability to function.

It is important that this change in philosophy be accepted and understood by patient, physician, and family.

It is often hard for patients (or families) to reach the point at which they are ready to embrace a treatment model that emphasizes management and coping but does not promise a cure. They feel compelled to seek further medical opinions or treatment options before accepting the rehabilitation approach. Physicians may contribute to the problem when they focus only on the specialty treatments they are trained to provide. Prolonged searches for a "cure" can be counterproductive and expose the patient to further harm from aggressive surgical, medical, or alternative treatments. Tactful discussion can help make clear that rehabilitation does not mean giving up on efforts to improve the underlying problem, or simply learning to live with the pain.

III. EVALUATION OF THE PATIENT

1. History and examination

A thorough physical examination is essential to identify sources of pain and reassure the patient that the pain problem is taken seriously. A history of the pain problem and a detailed review of previous medical records documenting treatment trials, reasons for treatment failures, and the timing of interventions are helpful. Information about specific dosages and length of pharmacologic treatment trials helps to assess the adequacy of previous treatments. Whenever possible, original test results (computed tomography and magnetic resonance imaging scans) should be reviewed rather than relying on summary information in medical records. Access to comprehensive records may be difficult to obtain, in which case patients or family members can participate by obtaining and organizing this information.

During the initial evaluation, special attention should be paid to the emotional context of the pain problem and its meaning in the patient's life. For example, pain resulting from an accident in which others were killed or injured, or from what is perceived as a botched surgical procedure, will be difficult to treat without attention to the psychologic aspects. Likewise, a history of repeated adversarial or unsatisfactory interactions with multiple health professionals should prompt consideration of the presence of personality or other psychiatric disorders that could complicate treatment. Speaking directly with previous or current caregivers can provide invaluable insight into patterns of self-defeating behavior or other reasons for treatment failure.

2. Pain intensity and impact

Patient complaints of pain, functional disability, medication use or overuse, and comorbid psychiatric and medical illnesses must be taken into account to develop an appropriate, individualized treatment plan. In the treatment of chronic pain, ratings of functional ability are more useful than conventional 0-to-10 pain rating scales in gauging the impact of pain and judging treatment. A 0-to-3 scale is often employed, with 0 indicating no impact of pain on ability to function, and 1, 2, and 3 representing minimal, moderate, and severe impairment of function by pain. The use of obsessive or overly detailed pain charts is discouraged (unless they are needed to judge specific interventions), because it encourages somatic preoccupation and attention to pain. In most chronic pain treatment plans, pain behaviors such as grimacing, sighing, or rubbing affected body parts are discouraged because they draw the attention to the pain rather than reinforcing productive "well" behaviors (Table 2).

Information should be obtained on the impact of pain and pain treatment on the patient's social, family, and occupational or school function. It helps to ask patients to describe a typical day's schedule and activities, and what would be different if they were not in pain. Disability and financial status and involvement with Worker's Compensation or the legal system are factors that can influence pain presentation and may also have a bearing on treatment. Education and work history can be important, especially if the pain results from a work-related injury.

Detailed information on sleep disturbance, alterations in sleep/wake cycles, and depression or anxiety should be obtained. Psychiatric or personality disorders exacerbate chronic pain and should be identified and treated. A family history of psychiatric illness or disability may be contributory. Finally, family beliefs about the patient's condition and the family's role in the pain problem ("enabling" or overly solicitous behavior, anger, or neglect) should be determined.

3. Attitudes toward pain

Patients who believe that they can help control or manage their pain are often referred to as having an **internal locus of control.** In contrast, patients who feel dependent on physicians, the healthcare system, or medications to control their pain are often referred to as having an **external locus of control.** Successful adaptation

Table 2. Pain and well behaviors

Pain behaviors
    Pain talk, focus, and verbal complaints
    Facial grimacing
    Moaning, groaning, and crying
    Shifting position, guarded movement, limp
    Quiet and withdrawn
    Self-neglect and self-denial
    Blaming attitude
    Avoids self-help groups

Well behaviors
    Takes responsibility for own actions
    Understands own limits and strengths
    Sets realistic goals
    Exercises regularly
    Practices pain-reducing techniques
    Appropriate assertive behavior
    Positive attitude
    Seeks out group support

Adapted from Hayes MA, McAlary PW, Popovsky J, Zapporo NA. Alteration in comfort: A nursing challenge. In: Aronoff G, ed. *Evaluation and treatment of chronic pain*, 2nd ed. Baltimore: Williams and Wilkins, 1992, with permission.

to chronic pain is more likely in patients with an internal locus of control. Treatment efforts should aim to reinforce a patient's belief in his or her ability to affect pain levels. Efforts to involve the patient in treatment and create a sense of control should be a part of all aspects of chronic pain treatment. Self-management strategies, such as those outlined in Table 3, help to de-emphasize the pattern of reliance on medications, procedures, and other passive treatments.

IV. TREATMENT

The effects of unrelieved pain are pervasive, and rehabilitation demands coordinated, multidisciplinary treatment. Patients are encouraged to set functional goals during the initial evaluation, and regular meetings of the treatment team should occur to assess progress toward these goals, to share information, and to refine treatment plans. Appropriate functional goals should be realistic, achievable, and under the control of the patient.

A specialized inpatient or outpatient treatment program provides a team of appropriately trained personnel to coordinate an intensive, synergistic treatment plan. Early targeted intervention for patients whose pain is not improving is helpful and ultimately cost effective. All too often, however, early intensive intervention for chronic pain is precluded by factors such as lack of insurance coverage, so that only the most refractory patients (whose outcomes are actually substantially poorer) receive such treatment.

1. Group therapy

A variety of topics and skills can be effectively taught to chronic pain patients in a group setting. Group meetings offer support and reinforcement of adaptive behaviors through group feedback and discussion. In all cases, the group must be carefully supervised to ensure positive educational experiences. Family education, postural reeducation and movement, stress management skills, substance abuse information, life skills training, and other topics are appropriate for group teaching. The therapeutic milieu is an es-

Table 3.   Examples of independent pain control techniques

Ice massage/cold packs
Hot packs
Transcutaneous electrical nerve stimulation (TENS)
Acupressure
Self-massage, use of theracane
Whirlpool baths/showers
Exercise
Distraction
Meditation/relaxation/biofeedback
Self-hypnosis/imagery
Music therapy
Humor
Therapeutic touch
Pain diaries and journals
Rest periods

sential component of both outpatient and inpatient pain programs and is helpful in reducing the isolation and lack of social understanding encountered by patients with chronic pain.

2. Individual components of a chronic pain treatment program

The following components of chronic pain treatment are useful in nearly every case. Certain patients with less complicated presentations may require only some of these interventions.

(i) *Medication reduction and optimization*

The use of medication in chronic pain is best viewed as one component of the patient's overall management plan. Medication alone is unlikely to be effective in dealing with the problem, and its importance should be placed in perspective. An important aspect of treatment is a thorough, thoughtful review of medications, with the dual goal of eliminating unnecessary medications and ensuring that the patient has had an adequate trial of disease-specific treatments. Since the causes of chronic pain are heterogeneous, it is important to carefully ascertain, through repeat trials of treatments if necessary, that patients have had appropriate trials of treatments known to be helpful for their particular condition.

Many medications that provide short-term relief of symptoms can cause long-term complications that interfere with successful treatment. Medications prescribed for sleep, muscle spasm, or anxiety are in this category. Their use over a prolonged period can cause sedation, poor concentration, and emotional detachment that impede the ability to function. Patients also come to rely on the sedative and psychoactive effects of medications in modulating emotional as well as physical pain. In many cases, medications are no longer helping, yet patients and physicians are reluctant to discontinue them, fearing that things might get worse if they are stopped.

The decision to use long-acting or maintenance opioids must be made on an individual basis. Many patients with chronic pain show improved function and decreased pain on these medications. Unfortunately, a subset of patients do poorly, requiring increasing doses without satisfactory pain relief, deteriorating functionally, and possibly displaying drug-seeking or addictive behavior. As a general principle, chronic pain patients are offered only long-acting opioids. Short-acting opioids are more likely to produce a "high" and have a higher addictive risk. Patients who come to associate an altered sensorium with pain relief may regard alternative therapies (including long-acting opioids) as less than optimally effective. An insistence on only short-acting opioids is a marker of possible addiction.

(ii) *Physical reconditioning*

As a result of avoiding activities that aggravate or produce pain, nearly all patients with chronic, unrelieved pain develop some measure of physical deconditioning. This decreased activity generally results in a downward spiral of physical inactivity and reduced capacity for exercise that exacerbates, rather than improves, pain. Physical therapy supervision of a gradual program of reconditioning and therapeutic exercise is the cornerstone of successful rehabilitation. The roles and contributions of therapists in a multidisciplinary pain team vary according to the needs of the patient and the interests and expertise of the therapists. A system that allows therapists to have a flexible role and the ability to treat in conjunction with other disciplines provides optimal results.

Physical therapy is aimed at increasing patients' use of independent pain-management modalities such as self-massage, heat and cold, and transcutaneous electrical nerve stimulation (TENS). Physical therapy modalities such as massage and ultrasound, which are passive and do not foster independence, are less useful in chronic pain treatment.

An important focus of physical therapy is on improved aerobic and functional capacities. Chronic pain patients may have failed prior physical therapy regimens when they were encouraged to discontinue activity with the onset of pain. A major challenge for the physical therapist working with these patients is to educate them that hurt does not always mean harm. It is advisable to begin in small increments and to use a realistic, quota-based program that encourages a gradual increase in exercise tolerance. With this approach, patients quickly come to understand that some of their pain may be caused by previous inappropriate use of assistive devices, muscle weakness, and muscle guarding. A physical therapist with experience in the treatment of chronic pain can develop an appropriate program for chronic pain patients.

Not only does exercise improve physical functioning, it also improves pain levels, has a beneficial impact on depression and feelings of self-worth, and aids in restoration of a normal sleep/wake cycle. Exercises aimed at improving postural tension, body mechanics, and muscle imbalance can also have a beneficial impact on pain and function.

(iii) *Occupational therapy*

The impact of pain on daily life can be severe. Patients may be limited in their ability to perform basic self-care activities such as bathing and dressing, or find it difficult to prepare meals, perform housekeeping chores, or shop for groceries. Occupational therapists help patients incorporate effective pain control strategies into activities of everyday life. Specific strategies can include goal setting, group programs, pacing techniques, assertive communication, the use of appropriate body mechanics during everyday activities, and the use of assistive devices or environmental modifications to support independent function.

Activity levels in chronic pain patients often closely mirror pain levels; patients remain in bed or do very little on days when their pain is particularly severe, then compensate with intense overactivity on days when their pain is better. This leads to a sense of frustration on the part of the patient and makes it difficult to participate reliably in work, social, and school activities. Occupational therapists can work with patients to identify such patterns and concentrate on pacing techniques. These emphasize avoidance of large swings in activity levels and encourage the use of frequent breaks in activity regardless of pain level. They also involve the incorporation of active pain control techniques on a regular basis to prevent pain escalation. These techniques include the development of a schedule that incorporates such things as the use of heat, ice, and relaxation strategies into the daily routine. Scheduled use of ice massage, theracanes, TENS, or hot packs can enhance the effectiveness of other therapeutic and pharmacologic interventions.

(iv) *Nonpharmacologic pain control techniques*

Biofeedback, self-hypnosis, and other relaxation strategies are useful adjuncts to chronic pain treatments. They often reduce, although they may not eliminate, the use of pain medication, and they improve a patient's sense of control over pain. These strategies are most effective when used preemptively on a regular basis; they work less well once pain is established. Many of these techniques are taught by psychologists, who can at the same time identify counterproductive and maladaptive behavior patterns. Patients often benefit from cognitive-behavioral therapy aimed at altering beliefs and ideas about pain and improving coping mechanisms.

(v) *Psychiatric and psychological intervention*

Psychiatric disorders can complicate the management of chronic pain. Patients with premorbid psychiatric disorders cope less well with chronic pain, and unrelieved chronic pain can trigger the development of psychiatric disorders, particularly depression. Psychiatric evaluation is therefore essential in all patients with debilitating chronic pain. Appropriate management of identified disorders will improve the patient's ability to cope with chronic pain and to comply with treatment. Psychiatric oversite of the many psychoactive medications used in the chronic pain population is also important.

A history of prior physical, sexual, or emotional abuse or trauma is common in patients with chronic pain. Recent work suggests that early trauma may produce permanent changes in the functioning of the hypothalamic–pituitary axis and response to later painful events. The identification of a history of trauma has important treatment implications and should be sought in all patients with disabling chronic pain. Patients with a history of a traumatic childhood with unmet dependence needs, early adult responsibilities, or physical, emotional, or sexual abuse are often less able to cope with pain. These patients may have coped well prior to the onset of pain but the development of a pain problem can provide an unconscious but socially acceptable way to ask to be taken care of.

Patients with chronic pain may deny family or relationship stressors, blaming all life disruption on their pain and consciously or unconsciously using pain as a way to avoid unpleasant or unwanted obligations in many areas. For this reason, a careful review of social and family relationships is helpful. An assessment of mood and suicidal potential is also important, as chronic pain is a risk factor for both suicide attempts and completed suicide.

(vi) *Family intervention*

Perhaps the most neglected aspect of chronic pain is its impact on family members and other elements of a patient's social support network. Chronic pain in one member of a family commonly causes shifts in family roles and functions. Spouses or children may take over aspects of the patient's role, such as housework, shopping, or wage-earning. Family and friends may inadvertently support or encourage further disability and dependency through enabling, over-solicitous behavior. Alternatively, they may gradually become impatient with the patient's disability and withdraw from the relationship, further isolating the patient from emotional and social support.

It is important to recognize that in many cases, the patient's family and social network gradually adapts to the presence of an ill member, and the patient may be relegated to the designated sick role in the family. Family dynamics then act to perpetuate and reinforce pain behavior and illness roles. Once established, these maladaptive family behaviors can be difficult to change. Inattention to these family patterns places patients at high risk for relapse after rehabilitation. Family-treatment team meetings or groups aimed at teaching family and social supporters the principles and philosophy of pain management, improve outcomes and reduce relapse.

(vii) *Return to productive activities*

Many patients believe that the presence of chronic pain means that they cannot or should not participate in occupational, social, or academic activities. They fear aggravation of their pain, or worry that overexertion will cause permanent physical harm. In fact, participation in appropriate work, school, and social activities is generally therapeutic for patients with chronic illness. In the majority of patients with chronic pain, the benefits of social interaction, regular sleep/wake cycles, and improved self-esteem that productive activities promote far exceed any drawbacks. In general, patients should be encouraged to remain as active as possible. Decisions by the treatment team to support disability status, withdrawal from school, or the avoidance of social activities or hobbies should be very carefully considered. Although the intention—relieving the patient of an activity that seems to aggravate pain—is laudable, very often, discontinuation of such activities does not improve the pain and leads to further isolation, depression, and reinforcement of the sick role. In most cases, it is preferable to have a vocational counselor or other treatment team member help the patient develop realistic plans for return to activity that can be implemented over time. Job descriptions should be carefully reviewed, and genuine medical contraindications to certain activities or work demands should be incorporated into any return-to-work or other plan.

(viii) *Follow-up*

Chronic pain can be managed but not cured; the majority of patients will require careful and regular multidisciplinary follow-up indefinitely. Unfortunately, this is often not understood by insurers, and treatment resources are limited. Periodic review of medication regimens, attention to psychosocial aspects of the patient's situation, and careful evaluation of the progression of any underlying disease are all important in chronic pain. A solid physician–patient relationship is therapeutic and can help keep the patient from further iatrogenic harm. A physician whom the patient has come to know and trust, and who shows sincere interest in the patient's well-being over time, is in the best position to help the patient consider the advantages and disadvantages of any new or alternative treatment options.

V. MEASURING THE BENEFITS OF TREATMENT

The benefits of chronic pain treatment are reflected by a patient's return to a more normal, less pain-focused life, rather than by an improvement in pain level. This can be assessed by measuring decreased use of the healthcare system (fewer emergency department visits, acute medical and psychiatric admissions, decreased physician office visits, decreased polypharmacy), return to productive activities (not just paid work), decreased pain-related depression, improved sleep, and resumption of normal family and social relationships. A tool frequently used to measure pain program outcomes is the SF-36, a standardized measure of health-related quality of life, which produces measures of physical, role, and social well-being.

VI. CONCLUSION

Chronic pain rehabilitation programs provide an opportunity for chronic pain patients to take a completely different approach to their pain problem. Most of these patients have had multiple treatments, sometimes from many different treatment centers, in an attempt to relieve their pain. The rehabilitation approach will, for the first time, take a broad look at the patient's situation (physical, medical, psychological, social, educational, and so on) and set up an intensive program that will address all aspects of the pain. The program will teach the patient how to manage and live with pain and how to live as normal a life as possible.

A list of rehabilitation programs can be obtained from the Commission of the Accreditation of Rehabilitation Facilities (CARF) (see Appendix 3).

SELECTED READINGS

1. Allen M, Giles G. Occupational therapy in the treatment of patients with chronic pain. *Br J Occup Ther* 1986.
2. Bogduk N, Mersey H, eds. *Classification of chronic pain: descriptors of chronic pain syndromes and definitions of pain terms*. Seattle: IASP [International Association for Study of Pain] Press, 1994.
3. CARF [Commission on Accreditation of Rehabilitation Facilities]. *Standard Manual and Interpretive Guidelines for Medical Rehabilitation*. Tucson, AZ, 1997.
4. Jamison R. Psychological factors in chronic pain. *J Back Musculoskel Rehabil* 1996.
5. Michel T, Wittink H, eds. *Chronic pain management for physical therapists*. Boston: Butterworth-Heinmann, 1997.

Radiotherapy and Radiopharmaceuticals for Cancer Pain

Thomas F. DeLaney

The report of my death was an exaggeration.
—*Note to London Correspondent of the New York Journal, June 1897,*
Mark Twain (1835–1920)

I. GENERAL PRINCIPLES

Pain is a frequent complication of cancer. It can be a presenting symptom of the disease, a sign of local recurrence of tumor after prior treatment, or a symptom of metastatic disease. Palliative radiation therapy has been a mainstay of nonsurgical cancer treatment since soon after the discovery of x-rays. Radiation, delivered either by external beam, implantation (placement of radioactive sources within the tumor), or systemic radiopharmaceutical, can be effective in the management of cancer pain. Radiation therapy can relieve pain related to either metastatic disease or symptoms from local extension of primary disease. This chapter will focus on the treatment of pain related to metastatic disease. It is worth emphasizing that radiation therapy can complement analgesic drug or other therapies and may enhance their effectiveness *because it directly targets the cause of pain.*

In principle, ionizing radiation is delivered to the tumor with the intent of reducing or eliminating viable cancer cells while maintaining normal tissue integrity. It is most commonly given as megavoltage external beam photons produced by a linear accelerator. Electrons, which have a more limited range in tissue defined by their energy, can also be produced by linear accelerators and can be very useful in the treatment of superficial tumors with the additional benefit of sparing normal tissues below the tumor. Systemically administered radiopharmaceuticals such as strontium-89 (^{89}Sr) and samarium-153 (^{153}Sm) have a role in the treatment of patients with symptomatic metastatic disease involving multiple bones, whereas iodine-131 (^{131}I) is appropriate treatment for patients with metastatic thyroid cancers that are iodine avid.

Brachytherapy (implantation of radioactive sources into tumor) is a useful mode of radiation delivery because of the physical advantage of very high radiation doses given to the tumor compared to surrounding normal tissue and the biologic advantage of a low dose rate (which differentially spares normal tissue). Brachytherapy is usually used in the management of the primary tumor; it is less commonly used for palliation of metastatic disease.

External beam radiation is prescribed by absorbed radiation dose (the SI unit is the gray, 1 Gy is equal to 100 rads) per unit volume in a selected field. The total dose, the number of fractions given daily, and the volume of tissue irradiated are determined by considering the needs and likely benefit for each patient.

II. INDICATIONS FOR RADIATION THERAPY

The primary indications for radiotherapy in the management of cancer pain are listed in Table 1. These include bone pain due to metastases (with or without pathologic fracture), spinal cord compression, tumor infiltration of nerve plexus, blockage of hollow viscera, and reduction in space-occupying lesions (particularly cerebral metastases). Radiotherapy can also be very useful in palliation of bleeding from tumors, cough or dyspnea secondary to tumor invading the bronchus, and superior vena cava syndrome.

The decision to use radiation therapy includes consideration of the type of neoplasm, relative effectiveness of available treatment modalities, prior treatment, extent of disease (single or limited versus multiple metastatic sites), the patient's performance status and length of expected survival, and bone marrow reserve. The efforts of the radiation oncologist should be closely coordinated with those of other physicians and healthcare personnel. Patients with particularly difficult pain problems may benefit from presentation at a tumor board or other appropriate multidisciplinary conference to allow for input and discussion among the varying specialists with expertise in the management of cancer pain.

Table 1.   Indications for palliative radiation therapy

Pain relief
  Bone pain
  Nerve root and soft-tissue infiltration

Control of bleeding
  Hemoptysis
  Vaginal bleeding
  Hematuria
  Rectal bleeding

Control of fungation and ulceration

Dyspnea
  Tumor obstructing trachea or bronchus

Oncologic emergencies
  Spinal cord compression
  Cerebral metastases causing raised intracranial pressure
  Superior vena cava syndrome

Relief of blockage of hollow viscera

Shrinkage of tumor masses
  Causing symptoms by virtue of site or space occupancy

Adapted from Ashby, M. The role of radiotherapy in palliative care. *J Pain Symptom Manage* 1991;6:383, with permission.

III. GOALS OF PALLIATIVE TREATMENT

The intent of palliative treatment is *rapid* and *durable* pain relief, ideally maintaining symptom control for the remainder of the patient's life, with minimal associated morbidity. Radiation therapy can arrest local tumor growth that might otherwise lead to intractable pain, cord compression, airway obstruction, uncontrolled bleeding, or pathologic fracture. For some patients, the resultant elimination of or reduction in the need for narcotic pain medications can improve quality of life. Reduction in pain can also result in improvement in ambulation.

Treatment should be tailored to the patient's clinical condition and overall prognosis. Patients with good performance status and a limited burden of metastatic disease near critical structures such as the spinal cord or brachial plexus may benefit by radiation treatment programs that give a higher total radiation dose delivered in multiple fractions. Although such a program may require more initial visits to the radiotherapy clinic, it is likely to result in more durable palliation in the patient with a longer life expectancy. In contrast, patients with widely metastatic disease and limited life expectancy should be considered for rapid, limited-fraction treatment courses.

IV. RADIATION THERAPY FOR TREATMENT OF BONE METASTASES

For a single site or a limited number of sites of bony metastatic disease, external beam radiation therapy is appropriate and may relieve symptoms for an extended period of time. For patients with symptomatic bony disease at multiple sites, it is more appropriate to institute analgesics along with available systemic chemotherapy or endocrine therapy and bisphosphonates. If symptoms persist, consider systemic radiopharmaceuticals, localized external radiotherapy to the most symptomatic areas, or hemibody irradiation.

Most patients referred for palliation of metastatic bone pain have primary tumors of the highest overall incidence—namely, breast, prostate, or lung. Eighty percent to 90% of these patients experience pain relief, and it is complete in 50%. The majority of patients experience some pain relief within 10 to 14 days after the start of therapy. Seventy percent of patients have pain relief by 2 weeks after the completion of treatment. Ninety percent have relief within 1 to 3 months. Pain relief after radiation therapy is durable in 55% to 70% of patients.

Although it has been supposed that tumor shrinkage is responsible for this pain relief, the exact mechanism is poorly understood. Patients often experience pain relief at radiation doses that are well below that necessary to induce a complete regression of tumor.

Several small studies did not report any clear differences in overall response rates among patients with different tumor tissue types. A large, randomized study by the Radiation Therapy Oncology Group (RTOG), however, that examined different radiation fractionation schemes reported a higher percentage of complete pain relief in patients with breast and prostate primary tumors compared to patients with lung and other primary tumors. Sites of metastases do not correlate with the degree of pain relief. Severe and frequent pain is a poor prognostic feature. A sudden increase in pain during treatment should raise concern about a pathologic fracture, and appropriate radiographs and orthopedic evaluation should be performed.

Radiation affects both tumor cell and adjacent normal osteo-clasts and osteoblasts. The presence of tumor, however, is a greater threat to the structural integrity of bone than the adverse effects of radiation on bone healing. Bone reossification often occurs fol-lowing tumor eradication. Seventy-eight percent of osteolytic le-sions treated in one study recalcified, and another 16% showed no further progression after radiation therapy.

Evaluation of patients with bone metastases includes the use of bone scintigraphy, which is more sensitive than skeletal radiog-raphy except in patients with purely lytic (osteoclastic) disease such as myeloma. Bone scintigraphy also detects many initially asymptomatic metastases, some of which may subsequently be-come symptomatic. Abnormal areas on a bone scan of long bones should be examined by skeletal radiographs to determine if there are areas of significant lytic disease that should be radiated or or-thopedically stabilized to prevent pathologic fracture. Lytic lesions that are 2.5 cm or more in weight-bearing bones or have lysis of at least 50% of cortical bone may require orthopedic fixation. Mag-netic resonance imaging (MRI) should be used in patients with bone pain and normal bone scans and radiographs. MRI of the spine is appropriate in patients with suspected spinal cord com-pression. In such patients, at least a sagittal midline scout view of the entire spine should also be obtained to rule out the occasional second site of spinal cord compression.

The radiation therapy ports are planned using data from the his-tory and physical examination, bone scan, skeletal films, computed tomography and MRI scans, and a review of any prior radiation therapy fields. Soft-tissue masses, most often associated with bony metastases to the vertebral bodies or pelvis, must be included in the radiotherapy fields. The distribution of bone marrow must be considered, especially in patients receiving chemotherapy.

There is considerable debate about the optimal total dose, frac-tion size, and duration of treatment for metastatic lesions in bone. In patients with metastatic cancer in whom life expectancy is lim-ited, quick and effective treatment with minimal morbidity is de-sired. One of the most commonly employed fractionation schemes, 3000 cGy in 10 fractions over 2 weeks, has been compared in a number of recent studies to shorter treatment schedules. An RTOG study randomized 759 patients to one of five treatment schedules that ranged from 4 days to 3 weeks in overall duration: 2000 cGy in four fractions, 1500 cGy in five fractions, 2000 cGy in five frac-tions, 3000 cGy in 10 fractions, or 4050 cGy in 15 fractions. No significant difference in response was seen. An independent re-analysis of the data, however, noted that the protracted fraction-ation schemes were more likely to provide complete relief and cessation of opioids. In other randomized trials, there is no clear advantage for the longer, multiple-fraction regimens when com-pared to shorter or single-course regimens. Three large European randomized studies compared 800 cGy in one fraction with 3,000 cGy in 10 fractions (Royal Marsden Hospital, 288 patients), with 2,000 cGy in five fractions or 3,000 cGy in 10 fractions (Bone Pain Trial Working Party, 765 patients), or with 2,400 cGy in six frac-tions (Dutch Bone Metastasis Study, 1,171 patients). No difference was seen with respect to pain relief, time to its achievement, duration of relief, or toxicity. Re-treatment was given more frequently in the single-fraction arms, which may in part be related to physician willingness to re-irradiate an area that had received the lower prior radiation dose. An ongoing trial in the United States is underway to validate these results.

The following are guidelines for treatment fractionation. It is expedient to give single-fraction irradiation to the debilitated patient with a very short life expectancy. Single large fractions, however, to some sites such as the abdomen and brain may not be well tolerated acutely. Hence, each radiation oncologist must consider the site of disease, the patient's performance status and social situation, and any normal tissue in the treatment field when deciding on a treatment regimen. Patients with one or few sites of metastases who have a good performance status and a primary disease that responds well to systemic therapy may live for many years after irradiation for bony pain. Large fractions that are known to produce more late effects in normal tissue must be used with considerable caution in these patients, especially when radiation fields include the brain, spinal cord, kidneys, or significant portions of the liver or bowel.

At the same time, these patients may survive long enough to have problems with recurrent tumor in involved bony sites that have not been radiated to sufficiently high doses. Patients with bony metastases producing spinal cord compression are not suitable for single-fraction treatment because of the obvious neurologic risks of recurrent tumor in this site.

It has been difficult to demonstrate a clear dose–response relationship in treatment of bone metastases, often because the groups studied have been heterogeneous, with different tissue types and survival times after treatment. Arcangeli from Italy reported a higher frequency of complete pain relief when doses of 4,000 cGy or more were employed.

Hence, in patients with good performance status, limited metastatic disease, and long expected survival after palliative irradiation, doses of at least 4,000 cGy with conventional fractionation are recommended. For patients whose expected survival is short, a high dose is less important, as they will not live long enough to manifest recurrent tumor.

V. HEMIBODY IRRADIATION

Sequential hemibody irradiation has been utilized for patients with diffuse, widely disseminated bony metastases. It is designed to avoid repeated trips to the hospital for multiple courses of irradiation. It results in complete relief of pain in 21% and partial relief in 77% of patients; most of those treated have had breast, prostate, or lung cancer. Pain control is achieved rapidly, with improvement noted within 2 days among half of the patients experiencing pain relief. Kuban reported good palliation with hemibody irradiation in patients with disseminated prostate cancer. Palliative effects were maintained until death in 82% of the patients treated to the upper half of the body and 67% of patients treated to the lower half.

For hemibody radiation, 600 cGy of irradiation is delivered to upper body and 800 cGy to lower body. Patients treated for metastases of the upper body are usually hospitalized for a day, hydrated, and premedicated with antiemetics and corticosteroids. Mid- and lower-body therapy patients are premedicated as outpatients to minimize nausea and vomiting.

In one large study of hemibody irradiation by the RTOG, there were no fatalities related to treatment. Treatment to the lower and mid body were well tolerated, with severe nausea and vomiting, diarrhea, or hematologic toxicity occurring in 2%, 6%, and 8% of patients, respectively. Upper-body treatment with partial lung shielding induced severe nausea and vomiting, fever, or hematologic toxicity in 15%, 4%, and 32% of the patients, respectively. Hematologic complications are worse in patients who have received prior chemotherapy or who receive the treatment with low peripheral blood counts. Fractionated hemibody irradiation (2,500 to 3,000 cGy in 9 to 10 fractions) has been reported to yield more durable pain relief by a group from Memorial Sloan-Kettering without any increase in complications.

VI. SYSTEMIC RADIOISOTOPES

Several systemically administered radiopharmaceuticals have been used to palliate pain caused by multiple osseous metastases. [131]I can provide pain relief in patients with well-differentiated thyroid carcinoma, with bone scan evidence of response in 53% of patients. [89]Sr and [153]Sm-ethylenediaminetetramethylenephosphonate ([153]Sm-EDTMP) are used to treat patients with sclerotic metastases (metastatic prostate cancer and other selected cases).

Patient selection is important. Relative indications include bone metastases causing pain that is not controlled by analgesics or arising in a narcotic-intolerant patient, absence of soft-tissue masses, osteoblastic lesions, multiple metastatic sites, and tumor that is refractory to hormonal treatment or chemotherapy. Because of the limited penetration of the beta emissions delivered by systemic radioisotopes, radioisotope therapy is not appropriate for patients with spinal cord compression, who instead should be treated with external beam radiation. As radioisotopes can depress the marrow and are cleared by the kidneys, significant thrombocytopenia, neutropenia, or renal impairment are also relative contraindications. Urinary incontinence, which presents a radiation safety hazard, is also a contraindication.

[89]Sr is a bone-seeking calcium analog incorporated by osteoblasts into new bone. It is a beta (electron) emitter with a 1.46-megavolt (MeV) maximum energy, a physical half-life of 50.6 days, and a penetration range in tissue of 4 to 6 mm. It has no significant gamma emissions, so it cannot be imaged. Patients give off very little radioactivity into the environment and most can thus be treated as outpatients. Unbound ^{89}Sr is eliminated in the urine within 2 days. [89]Sr has been well studied in prostate and breast cancer, but it can be used for osteoblastic metastases from other primary tumors. Moderate or greater pain relief has been documented in approximately 80% of patients with prostate or breast cancer, with complete relief in approximately 10% to 30%. Pain relief is not usually seen until 2 to 3 weeks after injection. The recommended dose of ^{89}Sr is approximately 4.0 mCi (60 to 80 μCi/kg). Strontium can be retained in metastatic bone for up to 90 days. The dose delivered to tumor depends on disease burden; it is estimated to be 800 to

2,000 cGy in patients with diffuse disease, or 3,000 to 10,000 cGy with a limited or moderate tumor burden.

When evaluated in a placebo-controlled phase III trial as an adjuvant therapy in patients treated with external beam radiation, ^{89}Sr did not affect the degree of pain relief at the index lesion, but a greater proportion of patients in the ^{89}Sr group were able to discontinue analgesics (17.1% versus 2.4%), remained free of new painful bone metastases at 3 months (58.7% versus 34%), and had a longer time to further radiation therapy (35.3 versus 20.3 weeks).

Toxicities that can result from ^{89}Sr include thrombocytopenia, neutropenia, and, hemorrhage. In the adjuvant trial cited earlier, grade 3 thrombocytopenia was seen in 22.4% and grade 4 in 10.4% of the ^{89}Sr group, resulting in the need for platelet transfusions in 5.2%. This compares with 1.7% patients with grade 3 and 1.7% with grade 4 thrombocytopenia in the placebo group who did not require any platelet transfusions. Hemorrhage occurred in 14.9% of the ^{89}Sr patients and in 5.2% of the control patients. Grade 3 neutropenia was seen in 10.4% and grade 4 in 1.5% of the patients in the ^{89}Sr arm and in none of the control patients. Occasional patients have a pain flare several days after administration. This may be a good prognostic indicator according to some investigators. Some patients have reported a flushing sensation, often facial, but this is self-limited.

[153]Sm-EDTMP is a therapeutic agent composed of radioactive [153]Sm and the tetraphosphonate chelator EDTMP. It has recently been approved for use as a systemic radiopharmaceutical. The recommended dose is 1 mCi/kg. The agent has an affinity for bone and accumulates in osteoblastic regions of bone. Its physical half-life of 1.9 days results in higher rates of dose delivery than ^{89}Sr, which typically translates into a more rapid onset of action and more rapidly reversible toxicity. Its 0.81-MeV maximum energy beta emission is lower than that of ^{89}Sr, yielding a lower penetration in tissue of 2 to 3 mm and theoretically less marrow toxicity. It also has a gamma emission, which allows imaging with a gamma camera to document accumulation of isotope at affected sites. Treatment efficacy seems similar to that of ^{89}Sr, with a risk of marrow toxicity that is approximately half that reported for [89]Sr.

VI. CONCLUSION

It is easy for pain specialists treating patients with pain due to cancer to forget the powerful effects of radiation therapy in reducing pain and treating various other symptoms (see Table 1). Radiation is effective not only to shrink the primary tumor but also for soft-tissue metastases and for widespread bone metastases. Radiation therapy can be palliative as well as curative. The building of a good working relationship between pain physicians and radiation oncologists contributes greatly to the effective management of cancer pain.

SELECTED READINGS

1. Anderson PR, Coia L. Fractionation and outcomes with palliative radiation therapy. *Semin Radiat Oncol* 2000;10:191–199.
2. Ashby M. The role of radiotherapy in palliative care. *J Pain Symptom Manage* 1991;6:380–388.

3. McEwan AJB. Use of radionuclides for the palliation of bone metastases. *Semin Radiat Oncol* 2000;10:103–114.

4. McQuay HJ, Collins SL, Carroll D, Moore RA. Radiotherapy for the palliation of painful bone metastases. *Cochrane Database Syst Rev* 2000;2:CD001793.

5. Ratanatharathorn V, Powers WE, Moss W, Perez CA. Bone metastasis: Review and critical analysis of random allocation trials of local field treatment. *Int J Radiat Oncol Biol Phys* 1999;44:1–18.

6. Rose CM, Kagan AR. The final report of the expert panel for the Radiation Oncology Bone Metastasis Work Group of The American College of Radiation Oncology. *Int J Radiat Oncol Biol Phys* 1998; 40:1117–1124.

7. Arcangeli G, Giovinazzo G, Saracino B, et al. Radiation therapy in the management of symptomatic bone metastases: the effect of total dose and histology on pain relief and response duration. *Int J Radiat Oncol Biol Phys* 1998;42(5):1119–26.

8. Kuban DA, Delbridge T, el-Mahdi AM, Schellhammer PF. Half-body irradiation for treatment of widely metastatic adenocarcinoma of the prostate. *J Urol* 1989;141(3):572–4.

Acute Pain

Postoperative Pain in Adults

Elizabeth Ryder and Jane Ballantyne

Rich the treasure, Sweet the pleasure
Sweet is pleasure after pain
For all the happiness man can gain
Is not in pleasure, but in rest from pain.
—*John Dryden (1631–1700)*

Few Americans will go through life without having surgery. Those who undergo surgery will experience varying degrees of pain, and in many cases this postoperative pain will be the worst pain of their lives. Postoperative pain is one of the most feared and is probably the most prevalent of all pain conditions, yet in many cases it continues to be inadequately controlled. Physicians, nurses, and patients alike fear opioids, even though they remain the mainstay of acute pain treatment. Furthermore, because of the acute and finite nature of postoperative pain, a degree of complacency in treating it sometimes prevails. Patients who have received exemplary pain management rate their surgical and hospital experience highly, and it may be important to optimize postoperative pain treatment for that reason alone. Research findings over the last several years have shown that the sequelae of undertreated pain are far reaching and often have a deleterious effect on patients, which provides a greater impetus to improve pain treatment in postoperative patients. This chapter outlines the principles of postoperative pain management and briefly describes the treatments used at the Massachusetts General Hospital (MGH).

I. RATIONALE FOR ACTIVE TREATMENT

1. Conventional versus active treatment

Conventionally, postoperative pain has been managed with intramuscular opioids given intermittently, as needed. "Active" pain management implies a greater effort to optimize pain control, and it entails preoperative preparation, patient choice of treatment, regular pain assessments, and the use of newer treatment modalities such as patient-controlled analgesia (PCA), epidural anesthesia and analgesia, and continuous nerve blocks. It will become clear later in this chapter that active pain management offers better pain relief than conventional treatment. First, we explore other reasons to support the use of active pain management.

2. Ethical and humanitarian issues

No one would argue against the ethical and humanitarian need to treat postoperative pain. But can the ethical and humanitarian argument be used to support active pain management? Do conventional methods satisfy the ethical need to treat pain, or should we improve on conventional methods? Perhaps the answer to these questions lies with the individual physicians, who weigh the risks and benefits of each treatment and, rightly or wrongly, use personal experience as well as scientific evidence to decide whether to use a specific treatment. But in weighing the risks and benefits, physicians should also assume the ethical responsibility of relieving pain and suffering. When treating pain, ethical and humanitarian issues are particularly important, since relief of suffering is the chief and the only undisputed benefit of pain treatment.

3. Barriers to effective pain management

There are, unfortunately, some barriers to effective pain management, usually in the form of prejudice on the part of caregivers, or even on the part of patients themselves. Perhaps most prominent is the fear of opioids. Addiction is a well-known and disastrous side effect of chronic opioid treatment, and its association with opioids places a stigma on the use of these drugs. In the case of acute pain, the fear of addiction is unfounded, and addiction does not seem to occur when the drugs are used short term. Nevertheless, many caregivers and patients are afraid of addiction and need to be reassured that opioid treatment is entirely appropriate in the acute pain setting. Other prejudices include fears of delayed recovery because of overuse of analgesics, and religious and cultural prejudices against removing the "natural phenomenon" of pain.

4. Patient comfort and satisfaction

Nothing satisfies operative patients more than having sailed through surgery with a minimum of pain and discomfort. Producing such a state of satisfaction is not, however, simply a matter of providing adequate doses of pain medication. Patients are more satisfied if their therapy is properly tailored to their needs, with side effects titrated against efficacy. They are also more likely to be satisfied if they have been adequately prepared for the experience of postoperative pain, if they understand that they will need to tolerate a certain degree of pain at times but that over the days the pain will abate, if they have been offered choices of methods of achieving pain relief, and if they know that their doctors and nurses are working with them to achieve the greatest possible relief.

5. Decreased morbidity and recovery time

Although some trials have demonstrated reduced recovery times and a shorter length of hospital stay associated with the use of the more aggressive pain treatments (such as epidural therapy and IV PCA), other trials have not shown significant improvement. There is no true consensus on whether aggressive pain treatment can speed recovery after surgery, although careful analysis of the evidence leads to the conclusion that there are advantages to aggressive pain management in certain patients and certain surgical groups.

For example, pulmonary function is undoubtedly improved by epidural therapy after thoracotomy and laparotomy; early results of a big multicenter trial confirm this and point to an increased magnitude of this effect in patients with preexisting lung disease. Bowel mobility recovers more rapidly in patients treated with epidural analgesia after bowel surgery, allowing an early return home. Cardiac ischemia occurs less frequently in the postoperative period when pain is adequately controlled, especially in patients with preexisting ischemic heart disease. After joint surgery, regional anesthesia/analgesia (via epidural catheters, femoral sheath catheters, and brachial plexus catheters) allows aggressive mobilization during the early recovery phase and can hasten postoperative rehabilitation, even months after surgery. On the other hand, inappropriate use or overuse of opioids and nonsteroidal anti-inflammatory drugs (NSAIDs) can be deleterious, resulting in respiratory depression, slowing of the bowel, oversedation, gastric ulceration, bleeding, and so on. Clearly, the key is to choose the right treatment for each clinical situation, and to use it appropriately.

There may also be harmful sequelae of undertreated pain. The fact that pain treatment can alter physiologic stress responses to surgery and trauma is well established. Whether these changes are desirable is less clear. Pain treatment can modulate immune responsiveness, thus lessening immune suppression (presumably a desirable effect); on the other hand, high-dose opioid therapy can suppress immune responses (presumably an undesirable effect). At the level of the spinal cord, genetic alterations in neurons in response to unmodulated sensory stimuli have been observed, which may account for long-term problems such as trauma-related chronic pain syndromes and phantom limb pain. Of particular interest was one study's finding that preoperative lumbar epidural blockade before lower limb amputation can lessen phantom limb pain.

II. PRINCIPLES OF POSTOPERATIVE PAIN MANAGEMENT

1. Psychological preparation

Patients who are well prepared psychologically for the experience of surgery and postoperative pain are markedly less anxious and easier to treat during their perioperative period than unprepared patients. Patients need reassurance from their surgeon, anesthesiologist, nurses, and others. If they have never had surgery before, they should be told about the operative process and about postoperative pain. They should be aware that some degree of postoperative pain is inevitable, and that their doctors and nurses will work with them to treat it. Patients should also be familiar with the concept of pain assessment and the need to assess pain on a regular basis in order to modify treatments. They should be told about the choices for postoperative pain management, and they should discuss these options with their surgeon and anesthesiologist during their preoperative visit.

2. Assessing pain

Regular pain assessment is fundamental to good pain management; it is also essential to act on the assessments when necessary. Assessments of pain severity, analgesic side effects, and markers of recovery are the tools by which analgesic regimens can be tailored to meet patients' needs. The method chosen does not need to be elaborate; in fact, it is inappropriate to use complicated analog scales in the setting of acute or postoperative pain. Simple questions such as "How bad is your pain?" "Do you have any nausea?" and "Do you feel like getting out of bed?" will provide important clues to the patient's comfort.

It is also necessary, however, to have some means of quantifying pain, since physicians and nurses change shifts and are not always able to communicate with each other. For this reason, rudimentary pain scales are used, such as a 0 to 10 verbal analog scale (VAS). It is now standard practice at MGH to record pain scales on the vital signs chart (the so-called fifth vital sign) as well as in the patient's chart. A policy of regular assessment is important because it draws attention to the existence of pain and forces improved treatment.

The assessment of pain has become a part of standard care in hospitals and other healthcare facilities throughout the United States. In fact, the Joint Commission on Accreditation of Healthcare Organizations (JCAHO) has developed new standards for both pain assessment and pain management (see web address, Appendix III). These standards apply to any organization involved in the direct provision of patient care wishing to receive accreditation from this organization.

3. Preemptive analgesia

It is well known that established pain is more difficult to treat than new pain. People with recurring pain, such as headache, know that if they treat their pain early, it is easier to abolish than if they allow it to mount. The same is true of postoperative pain. Patients who wake from anesthesia in pain appear to be more resistant to pain medication than those who are comfortable on awakening. Recently, a scientific basis for the "preemptive" effect of analgesia has been established. Using animal models of pain, researchers have convincingly demonstrated that changes occur in the spinal cord and brain in response to painful stimulation that result in enhanced pain transmission, and ultimately enhanced pain perception. These changes can be modified or abolished by opioid analgesics or by neural blockade. The importance of the phenomena of "wind-up" and "central sensitization," both occurring in the spinal cord and both resulting in pain enhancement, is well established. Clinically, these changes may result in a worsening of postoperative pain, or even in establishment of a chronic pain syndrome.

The concept of preemptive analgesia grew from these observations. It was once surmised that if a good level of analgesia were established *before* a surgical incision, this would minimize postoperative pain. Unfortunately, treating the pain of an incision is only part of the story, and it is now clear that although the concept still applies, it applies to the preemption of spinal cord changes, not the preemption of a surgical incision per se. Trials of "preemptive analgesia" treating only incisional pain were remarkably unsuccessful. However, analgesia maintained throughout the surgical and postoperative phases of surgery, including pre-incision, is effective. This is illustrated in an important paper published in 1998 by Gottschalk and colleagues, who demonstrated clearly that good perioperative analgesia when compared to no intraoperative analgesia resulted in improved pain and mobility for up to 9.5 weeks after surgery.

The concept of preemptive analgesia was further confused by the publication in 1988 of a paper by Bach and colleagues who demonstrated that epidural analgesia maintained for 72 hours before limb amputation effectively prevented postamputation phantom limb pain. This was hailed as a convincing demonstration of preemptive analgesia, at a time when preemptive analgesia concepts were being developed. However, it now seems that the benefit Bach and colleagues achieved was not so much a preemptive analgesic effect but rather a manipulation of a preexisting pain memory. It is becoming clear that central mapping in the cerebral cortex is a key factor in the establishment of phantom limb pain, and that merely "preempting" the surgical incision is not sufficient to alter the postamputation pain experience.

III. SPECIAL POPULATIONS

1. The elderly

The elderly often appear to be stoical and it is not clear whether they have a different threshold for pain, whether past experience has altered their attitude toward pain, or whether they truly do not feel pain to the same extent as younger adults. It is tempting to undertreat pain in the elderly because these patients do not always communicate pain very clearly. Moreover, the elderly may not metabolize drugs efficiently, so this is an additional concern, especially when using opioids. The elderly are more likely to become sedated and confused when given opioids, and they are at increased risk of sedation and confusion when sleep deprived and taken out of their normal environment. The best approach is to offer structured treatment. For severe pain, small, intermittent doses of morphine (2 to 6 mg every 4 hours), or other opioids, are suitable.

Epidural therapy can be helpful and circumvents the use of systemic opioids, although even epidural fentanyl can cause confusion in these patients.

2. Patients with mental or physical handicaps

Patients with mental or physical handicaps present a challenge because they may be unable to communicate pain in a normal way. As with the very young and the very old, effective pain management may involve time and patience in an effort to learn what patients are experiencing and how best to help them. Vital signs, behavioral cues, positioning, muscle guarding, and facial grimacing may be the only guiding factors. The cooperation of those who normally care for these patients is indispensable. Although drugs are metabolized normally in most of these patients, individuals with baseline breathing difficulties may be more sensitive to the respiratory depressant effects of opioids.

3. Substance abusers and drug addicts

Patients who have actively abused drugs and other substances before surgery (or injury) are often difficult to manage in the postoperative or post-trauma phase. At the MGH, we believe this population, like all others, should be given the benefit of optimal pain control, and that treating their addiction should be postponed until the acute pain phase subsides. During patients' hospitalization, we work closely with addiction specialists in preparing patients for discharge and possible rehabilitation.

Several factors should be considered when treating addicts. Always obtain a history of recreational substances used in both the past and the present; although this information may be unreliable, it should at least be sought. Ascertain if the patient is in a withdrawal state, and if so, treat the withdrawal. In cases of narcotic abuse, opioid drugs are a good choice for treating pain, but withdrawal symptoms may still be manifest if the patient has been consuming large quantities for recreation. PCA is an effective modality for drug abusers, since it provides an element of control and lessens the anxiety associated with trying to obtain additional medication. Adding a clonidine patch may be useful in this situation. Never use an opioid antagonist (naloxone) in narcotic addicts, as this could result in an immediate and extreme withdrawal response with a sympathetic outpouring, cardiac dysrhythmias, or even cardiac arrest and death.

It may be advantageous to minimize opioid requirements by supplementing treatment with opioid-sparing therapies (NSAIDs, epidurals, local nerve blocks, or anxiolytics). On the other hand, total reliance on these therapies and total withdrawal of opioids from a narcotic abuser are ill advised, partly because they will result in an unnecessarily severe withdrawal syndrome, and partly because pain will be very difficult to control without opioids.

Patients in methadone programs should continue with their preadmission doses, and additional medication should be prescribed to treat nociceptive pain as needed. Patients who have been abusing other substances such as alcohol, cocaine, and marijuana may exhibit some degree of cross-tolerance with the opioid, thus requiring higher than normal doses. At the same time, they may present with a withdrawal syndrome requiring treatment with neuroleptics, or various supportive measures. Medications should be titrated to effect (be it analgesia or side effects).

4. Intensive care patients

Patients admitted to intensive care form a special population because, in many cases, they are unable to communicate, either because of severe illness or because they are ventilated, sedated, and sometimes even paralyzed. It is important to treat pain in these patients to reduce the extreme anxiety associated with pain and inability to communicate it, and to attenuate stress responses. When it is impossible to assess pain, as in heavily sedated or unconscious patients, it is reasonable to assess analgesic requirements on the basis of the amount of surgical or other trauma the patient has undergone.

Ventilated patients can be treated with higher than normal doses of opioids (if desired) because there is no risk of respiratory depression. Continuous infusions of opioids can be used in the intensive care unit (ICU) to sedate ventilated patients, independent of their use as analgesics. Morphine is the drug of choice for opioid infusions at the MGH, starting at 0.1 mg/kg per hour. Fentanyl at a starting dose of 1 μg/kg per hour is a useful alternative in patients with renal insufficiency who have impaired excretion of the active morphine metabolite morphine-6-glucuronide. In normal patients, fentanyl has a greater tendency to accumulate than morphine because of its long elimination half-life. Alert or unventilated ICU patients can be treated as normal patients, with the proviso that sick patients may handle drugs inefficiently. Epidurals are useful even in ventilated patients and may actually aid weaning from ventilation.

IV. TREATMENT OPTIONS

1. Nonsteroidal anti-inflammatory drugs

NSAIDs are useful as sole analgesics for mild to moderate pain, and they are useful alternatives or adjuncts to opioid therapy and regional analgesia. Since they act by a unique mechanism, mostly in the periphery [i.e., not in the central nervous system (CNS)], their action complements that of other analgesic therapies. Their analgesic effect is secondary to their anti-inflammatory effect, which in turn is the result of prostaglandin inhibition. Prostaglandin inhibition is also responsible for their chief side effects—namely gastritis, platelet dysfunction, and renal damage. NSAIDs are contraindicated in patients with a history of peptic ulcer disease, gastritis, or NSAID intolerance, and in those with renal dysfunction (creatinine >1.5) or bleeding diatheses. Many of our surgeons prefer not to use NSAIDs in the immediate postoperative period for patients who have undergone renal or liver surgery, grafts, muscle flaps, or bone fusions, as the drugs may either increase bleeding or decrease healing time.

Only one NSAID, ketorolac, is available in a parenteral form. This medication is extremely potent (equipotent with morphine) and has become a popular alternative to opioid therapy in postoperative patients. There are a few drawbacks to its use, however. Ketorolac is expensive (about 20 times more costly than morphine) and, because of its potency, applying equally to side effects and efficacy, it may be safely used for only up to 5 days (manufacturer's recommendation). The newer selective prostaglandin antagonists [cyclooxygenase (COX)-2 inhibitors], celecoxib and rofecoxib, are associated with fewer side effects (notably a lower incidence of gastrointestinal symptoms) but are only available in an oral formulation. (See Chapter 8 and Appendix VIII for full descriptions of these drugs.)

2. Systemic opioids

Systemic opioid therapy has long been the conventional treatment for postoperative pain, and it is the standard by which other treatments are measured. This does not, in any way, make it inferior to other pain treatments. In fact, systemic opioid therapy (either oral or parenteral) remains the primary treatment for patients experiencing moderate to severe acute pain.

When administering systemic opioids, the treatment goal is to maintain plasma levels within the therapeutic window. This ranges between the level at which satisfactory analgesia is reached and the level at which toxic effects are noted. The most challenging patients are those who have a narrow therapeutic window—that is, a limited dose range—in which useful analgesia without side effects is provided. The best principle of successful opioid therapy is to first administer enough drug to reach the patient's threshold for analgesia and to then maintain a constant plasma level by administering low doses on a regular schedule.

Routes of opioid administration and their indications are summarized in Table 1. Conventionally, the intramuscular route was chosen for use in postoperative patients because the intravenous route was believed to be unsafe (because of the risk of respiratory depression), the subcutaneous route less reliable, and the per rectum route undesirable. The oral route is, of course, unusable in nil per os patients, and the sublingual route is limited by lack of

Table 1.   Methods for achieving pain control

Intervention	Comments
NSAIDs	
Oral (alone)	Effective for mild to moderate pain. Begin pre-op. Relatively contraindicated in patients with history of peptic ulcer or renal disease & risk of, or actual, coagulopathy. May mask fever.
Oral (adjunct to opioid)	Potentiating effect resulting in opioid sparing. Cautions as above.
Parenteral (ketorolac)	Effective for moderate to severe pain. Expensive. Useful where opioids contraindicated, especially to avoid respiratory depression & sedation. Cautions as above.
Opioids	
Oral	As effective as parenteral in appropriate doses. Use as soon as oral medication tolerated.

Table 1. *Continued*

Intervention	Comments
IM	Has been the standard parenteral route, but injections painful & absorption unreliable. Hence, avoid this route when possible.
SQ	Preferable to IM for low-volume continuous infusion. Injections painful & absorption unreliable. Avoid this route for long-term repetitive dosing.
IV	Parenteral route of choice after major surgery. Suitable for titrated bolus or continuous administration (including PCA), but requires monitoring. Significant risk of respiratory depression with inappropriate dosing.
PCA	IV or SC routes recommended. Good, steady level of analgesia. Popular with patients but requires special infusion pumps and staff education. Cautions as for IV opioids (above).
Epidural & intrathecal	When suitable, provides good analgesia. Expensive if infusion pumps employed. Significant risk of respiratory depression, sometimes delayed in onset. Requires careful monitoring.
Local anesthetics	
Epidural & intrathecal	Limited indications. Expensive if infusion pumps employed. Effective regional analgesia. Opioid sparing. Addition of opioid to local anesthetic may improve analgesia. Risks of hypotension, weakness, numbness.
Peripheral block	Limited indications. Limited duration unless catheters employed. Effective regional analgesia. Opioid sparing.
TENS	Effective in reducing pain and improving physical function. Requires skilled personnel and special equipment. Useful as an adjunct to drug therapy.
Education/ instruction	Effective for reduction of pain. Should include procedural information and instruction aimed at reducing activity-related pain. Requires staff time.

NSAID, nonsteroidal anti-inflammatory drug; TENS, transcutaneous electrical nerve stimulation; IM, intramuscular; IV, intravenous; SQ, subcutaneous; PCA, patient-controlled analgesia.

availability of sublingual preparations. It is unnecessary to subject patients to painful intramuscular injections, as judiciously administered intravenous opioids (i.e., given as small boluses while monitoring pain level, respiratory effort, and alertness) are just as safe and preferable.

The intravenous route is also ideal for PCA, which is discussed later. Most postoperative patients receive bolus administration of opioids, which allows ready titration of dose according to need. Continuous intravenous or subcutaneous therapy may sometimes be useful—for example, in ventilated patients in whom there is no danger of respiratory depression. The oral route should be used as soon as patients are able to tolerate tablets. The short-term use of long-acting opioids is sometimes helpful.

Commonly used opioids and their doses are summarized in Table 2. Morphine is the opioid of choice at the MGH. Dose ranges are usually prescribed so that nurses can select specific doses that best meet the patients' needs. Morphine is a naturally occurring

Table 2.   Analgesics and related drugs:
Dosage examples for adults

Generic name	Proprietary Name	Oral Dose (mg)	Parenteral Dose (mg)
Nonsteroidal anti-inflammatory agents			
Acetaminophen*†	Tylenol	500–1,000 q 3–4 h	—
Ibuprofen†	Motrin, Advil	200–800 q 6 h	—
Ketorolac	Toradol	10 mg q 4–6h	30 (load) + 15–30 q 6 h
Naproxen	Naprosyn	250–500 q 12 h	—
Opioids			
Butorphanol	Stadol	—	2–4 q 3–4 h
Codeine	—	15–60 q 4–6 h	30–60 q 4–6 h
Hydromorphone	Dilaudid	2–4 q 4–6 h	2–4 q 4–6 h
Meperidine	Demerol	50–150 q 3–4 h	100–150 q 2–3 h
Methadone	Dolophine	2.5–10 q 6–8 h	2.5–10 q 6–8 h
Morphine†	—	10–20 q 2–3 h	5–10 q 3–4 h
Morphine SR	MS Contin, Oramorph, Kadian	15–30 q 6–8 h	

Table 2. *Continued*

Generic name	Proprietary Name	Oral Dose (mg)	Parenteral Dose (mg)
Nalbuphine	Nubain	—	5–10 q 4–6 h
Naloxone (antagonist)	Narcan	—	0.2–1.2 bolus
Oxycodone	(Also in Percocet, Percodan)	5–10 q 3–4 h	—
Oxycodone SR	OxyContin	10–20 q 12 h	—
Antiemetics, major tranquilizers			
Droperidol	Inapsine	5–15 q 8 h	1.25–5 q 6 h
Metoclopramide	Reglan	10 tid	10 q 6 h
Ondansetron	Zofran	4 q 4–8 h	4 q 4–8 h
Prochlorperazine	Compazine	5–10 tid	5–10 q 4–6 h
Antihistamines, anxiolytics			
Diphenhydramine	Benadryl	25–50 q 4 h	25–50 q 4 h
Hydroxyzine	Vistaril	50–100 qid	25–100 qid
Lorazepam	Ativan	0.5–2 q 6–8 h	0.5–2 q 6–8 h
Laxatives			
Senna	Senokot	1–2 tab tid	—
Docusate	Colace	100 tid	—

[†]Also available as suppository.
[*]Acetaminophen is not anti-inflammatory but is efficacious in acute pain.
Dosages and intervals are initial estimates for an average 70-kg adult and may need to be adjusted according to the individual patient's weight, preference, or tolerance.
This list is not comprehensive. Other classes of drugs, not listed, may be beneficial in postoperative pain for individual cases.

opioid and is the oldest, best tried, and least expensive of all the opioid drugs. It is a simple agonist at mu, kappa, and delta receptors, and its actions are not complicated by partial agonism or mixed agonism/antagonism. Its effects and side effects are well known and understood. Morphine may be contraindicated in patients with biliary spasm because it is believed that it can worsen the spasm, but this issue is still under debate.

Other opioids are used when patients express a preference for another drug, when they are either "allergic to" or report significant side effects to morphine, or when morphine does not appear to be effective. For many years, meperidine was popular for treating acute pain. We discourage the use of this drug as a first-line treatment because of its known toxicity (excitatory effects in the CNS due to the metabolite normeperidine), which may be especially marked in patients with renal dysfunction. Meperidine has traditionally been used in woefully deficient doses. A 50-mg bolus is inadequate for severe pain in most adults, and 100 to 150 mg should be considered the standard adult dose. Bolus administration should be given every 2 to 3 hours, not every 4 hours, to avoid reemergence of pain, as meperidine is a relatively short-acting drug. Hydromorphone is a useful alternative to morphine, and some patients who express an intolerance for morphine, particularly when this is a sense of dizziness, nausea, and light-headedness, do better on hydromorphone.

The side effects of opioid drugs occasionally limit their use. Respiratory depression is a true risk of opioid treatment, and patients receiving opioids should always be closely watched. Monitoring for adequacy of ventilation includes observing the patient's state of arousal, respiratory rate, including depth and pattern of breathing, and color (skin and mucous membranes). Monitors such as the pulse oximeter are useful in the immediate postoperative period and in patients with known risk (e.g., baseline ventilatory compromise), but they are not necessary or even useful later in the postoperative phase.

Severe respiratory depression should be treated with small intravenous boluses of naloxone (Narcan). If naloxone is given too quickly, severe agitation, and in extreme cases, flash pulmonary edema secondary to aggressive respiratory effort, may result. We recommend diluting an ampule of naloxone (0.4 mg) into a 10-mL syringe of normal saline and administering 2 to 3 mL every minute or so. After naloxone reversal, patients should continue to be closely monitored, as naloxone's duration of action is only approximately 20 minutes, and the effects of the agonist may outlast this. Naloxone reverses opioid effects quite rapidly, so if the patient does not respond, one should think about alternative causes of the respiratory compromise.

Other opioid-related side effects are more of a nuisance than a barrier to treatment and can most often be treated—nausea with antiemetics, pruritus with antihistamines, constipation with laxatives (see Table 2). Decreasing the opioid dose, changing the opioid, or even stopping opioid treatment may also decrease side effects. Other causes of side effects should always be considered— for example, nausea could be caused by anesthetics, antibiotics, or the surgery itself. The opioids are also described in Chapter 9 and Appendix VIII.

3. Patient-controlled analgesia

In many institutions, including MGH, PCA is the standard therapy for postoperative pain management. PCA is defined as the self-administration of analgesics (usually via the IV route) by patients instructed in the use of a device specifically designed for that purpose. The goal of PCA is to provide doses of analgesic immediately on the demand of the patient. The use of portable microcomputer-controlled infusion pumps allows this dosing to be achieved quickly and easily (literally at the touch of a button), so that small, frequent, and easily titratable doses can be given. This avoids the extreme swings in plasma levels and efficacy, and the side effects associated with the larger, less frequent doses associated with conventional analgesia (see earlier discussion). Other advantages of PCA are its inherent safety because of the small doses used and the fact that obtunded patients do not press for additional doses, and patients' preference for the technique associated with the sense of control it offers.

An exception to the general safety of PCA is its use by elderly and confused individuals, who, despite confusion and early obtundation (or maybe because of it), sometimes overdose themselves. Studies show that patients vary widely in their physical need for opioids, and PCA accommodates a wide range of analgesic needs; with standard PCA orders, patients can receive anywhere between 0 and 10 mg of IV morphine each hour.

Carefully monitored, nurse-controlled boluses may be needed at the start of treatment, as patients may be too sedated by residual anesthesia to use PCA properly in the early postoperative period. It is tempting to think that once patients are connected to PCA pumps, they do not need further pain assessment or treatment, but if pain is neglected in the early postoperative period, it may be more difficult to treat later. Individualizing the PCA settings and frequently assessing patients' analgesia levels are critical during the first 24 hours following surgery. The MGH PCA orders are shown in Figure 1. They include an alternative treatment should the intravenous route fail, as well as general guidelines for dosing and monitoring. Morphine continues to be the drug of choice for PCA, with hydromorphone used when morphine has failed or is contraindicated. Meperidine can also be used, but, as discussed previously, it has limited indications.

The success of PCA depends first on patient selection. Patients who are too old, too confused, too young, or unable to control the button, and those who do not want the treatment, are not suitable candidates. Ideally, patients should be educated before surgery about PCA and the concept of self-dosing. Teaching points include expectations for pain relief, informing patients of their active role in pain management (both in pain reports and medication management), and elimination of fears and misconceptions about opioids, including fear of addiction and fear of overmedication.

4. Epidural analgesia

For certain well-chosen indications, a functioning epidural catheter produces superior pain relief, and is known to improve surgical outcome (Table 3). However, a considerable degree of technical expertise is needed to place epidural catheters and, even in the best hands, the treatment can fail. Thus, a promise of superb pain relief is not always fulfilled. Since it involves carefully and blindly locating the epidural space (Fig. 2), epidural placement and management is time consuming and labor intensive. Nevertheless, both surgeons and anesthesiologists at MGH are sufficiently convinced of the positive benefits of epidural analgesia to offer the treatment to all our patients in whom it is indicated, being careful to explain both its risks and its benefits. A description of the technique of epidural catheter placement can be found in Chapter 12 (II, 2, iii).

Massachusetts General Hospital
PCA Order Sheet

DOCTORS' ORDER SHEET

Date	Req Area
	PATIENT IDENTIFICATION AREA

	Monitoring
1. Date: Time:	1. Record baseline HR, BP, RR.
2. Drug: (check one) ☐ Morphine 1mg/ml ☐ Hydromorphone (Dilaudid) 0.5mg/ml	2. Record HR, BP, RR 15 minutes after ending
3. Orders for Pump Settings (May refer to guideline - below right)	initial bolus infusion loading dose.
Demand Dose from _____ ml to _____ ml	3. Record RR, analgesia, and sedation levels every 4
Start Dose at _____ ml	hours (refer to Scoring Guide below).
Delay Time _____ minutes	If vital signs, mental status, or sedation problems appear,
Basal Rate _____ ml/hr 7A-11P	record RR and BP every 1 hour or more often until stable.
_____ ml/hr 11P-7A, prn	4. Discontinue PCA and call House Officer for:
Hour Limit ≤ _____ ml/hr	HR < _____ SBP < _____ RR < _____
4. Bolus Loading Dose:	Increasing lethargy.
_____ ml every 5 minutes until patient	5. Prior to pump availability, if patient reports a pain level
comfortable. Maximum total loading dose	≥ 5 (on the 0-10 scale), initiate orders in #6 (in left column)
_____ ml. Notify HO if patient remains	until PCA pump started.
uncomfortable after completing maximum bolus dose.	6. Call floor pharmacist for special problems.

Guidelines for standard starting doses:

	Morphine	Hydromorphone
Demand Dose	0.5 - 2ml	0.2 - 1ml
Delay	6 min.	10 min.
Basal	0 - 0.5ml	0ml
Hour Limit	≤ 20ml	≤ 6ml
Start with: Dose/Delay time/Basal Rate	1/6/0	0.5/10/0

5. Infuse D5W at KVO via Y set if no maintenance
IV solution ordered.

6. In the event of pump failure or nonpatent IV,
administer drug _____ , _____ mg,
IM every _____ hr., prn, pain.

Doctor's Signature _____

PATIENT-CONTROLLED ANALGESIA SCORING GUIDE

PAIN LEVEL:	Use a range from 0 - 10 where: 0 = "no pain" 10 = "worst pain imaginable"
SEDATION LEVEL:	1 = wide awake 2 = drowsy 3 = dozing 4 = awakens when aroused 5 = asleep
VERBAL RESPONSE:	5 = oriented and converses 4 = disoriented and converses 3 = inappropriate words 2 = incomprehensible sounds 1 = no response

Figure 1. PCA order sheet.

Table 3. Known benefits of postoperative epidural analgesia

Superior analgesia
Improved pulmonary function
Better graft survival after lower limb vascular procedures
Increased bowel mobility, associated with shorter hospital stay
Fewer cardiac ischemic events
Shorter recuperation after joint surgery, associated with early
   aggressive mobilization

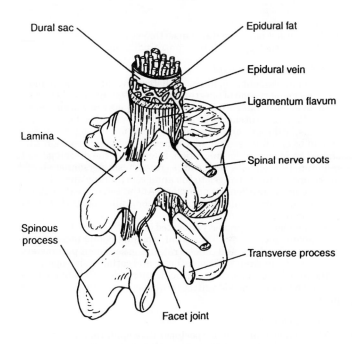

Anatomy of the epidural space.

Figure 2.   Anatomy of the epidural space.

(i) *Indications*

We recommend epidurals for postoperative pain, primarily in the following situations (a discussion of when to use intraoperative epidurals is beyond the scope of this chapter):

- Patients having thoracic or abdominal surgery
- Patients having lower limb surgery, in whom early mobilization is important (early active or passive mobilization)
- Patients having lower body vascular procedures, in whom a sympathetic block is desirable
- Patients who are not anticoagulated, or for whom anticoagulation is not planned in the immediate postoperative period
- Especially patients with compromised cardiac or pulmonary function

(ii) *Contraindications*

Contraindications to epidural placement are the following:

- Patient refusal
- Coagulopathy
- Concurrent or planned treatment with low-molecular-weight heparin (LMWH)

- Bacteremia
- Local infection at epidural insertion site
- Spine pathology (a relative contraindication)

(iii) *Management principles*

The management of epidural catheters should always be under the direct supervision of anesthesiologists. Patients should be seen daily to ensure that catheters and medications are working effectively. Pain reports should be satisfactory, and side effects such as pruritus, sedation, and changes in sensation or motor function should be carefully evaluated. Catheters and their insertion sites should be inspected for migration, integrity of the dressings, and inflammation or back tenderness. Anesthesia personnel should make prescription changes to the analgesic therapy and administer specific medications as necessary. At the end of treatment, the anesthesia team should be responsible for pulling the catheter and ensuring that it is removed intact.

Nurses should be properly educated before they care for patients with epidural catheters. Important teaching points include typical medication doses and concentrations, assessment parameters, the normal appearance of the catheter and catheter site, operation of the infusion pumps, common medication side effects that can be treated by them, and side effects requiring a call to the physician in charge.

(iv) *Drug choices*

The standard infusion for postoperative epidural therapy at the MGH is a mixture of 0.1% bupivacaine with 20 μg/mL of hydromorphone. A synergistic effect occurs when local anesthetic is combined with opioid, rendering this mixture optimally effective. However, there may be reasons to remove one or the other component (e.g., a local anesthetic causing hypotension, or an opioid causing pruritus), in which case, dose adjustments need to be made to the remaining drug. In the case of sole local anesthetic treatment, it may be necessary to add a systemic analgesic (opioid or NSAID).

Continuous epidural infusions vary between 4 and 8 mL/hr depending on the catheter location, with possible infusion rates of up to 20 mL/hr. Fentanyl is the second choice of epidural opioid, reserved for patients who might be particularly sensitive to opioid effects (e.g., the very young and the very old). Because it is lipophilic, fentanyl tends to bind locally to spinal cord receptors rather than spread with cerebrospinal fluid (CSF) movement. The result is an analgesic effect localized around the level of insertion of the epidural catheter, in contrast to hydromorphone and particularly morphine (the least lipophilic of the opioids), which produce a better spread of analgesia but a greater risk of delayed respiratory depression resulting from the spread of drug to higher centers in the CNS. Standard epidural orders include infusion dose ranges for nurses to titrate based on the patient's report, orders for alternative treatments should the epidural fail, and orders for the treatment of adverse side effects.

(v) *Management of inadequate analgesia*

The best way to ensure that an epidural catheter is well positioned to provide analgesia is to establish an anesthetic level using local anesthetic. Optimally, if a patient undergoes surgery under combined epidural or general anesthesia, catheter function should be tested preoperatively. Testing catheter function by establishing a level can be achieved at any stage, but (a) this is less specific in a patient who is in the early stages of recovery after anesthesia, and (b) it will be necessary to monitor for possible hypotension and to be prepared to treat hypotension. Another, less time-consuming and surprisingly helpful test is to inject 5 to 7 mL of the analgesic infusion (i.e., a low dose of local anesthetic). If the catheter is well positioned, analgesia should be noticeably improved by the injection, and this injection is unlikely to produce hypotension.

Once good catheter function is established, several approaches to improve analgesia can be taken. A bolus injection can be given (as described) if it has not already been given. The infusion rate can be titrated upward, as tolerated. Systemic analgesics can be given. NSAIDs are useful adjuncts to epidural analgesia, especially when the epidural level does not cover the area of surgical pain, as when the incision is high, or when pain is referred outside the epidural area (as in shoulder pain associated with chest tubes and diaphragmatic irritation). Systemic opioids (including PCA) can also be added, but in this case, the opioid should be removed from the epidural mix to avoid possible overdose.

(vi) *Patient-controlled epidural analgesia*

Patient-controlled epidural analgesia (PCEA) has become a standard of care in many institutions around the country. Although the MGH has not begun this modality yet, plans are underway to start this in the near future. Allowing patients to gain control over their own pain medication (as stated before) is one great advantage to PCEA.

When demand doses and lockout intervals are prescribed, several aspects of the opioid must be considered: how lipophilic it is, its onset of action, and the duration of pain relief that can be expected. The PCEA dosing for the standard MGH epidural mix (0.1% bupivacaine with 20 μg/mL hydromorphone) is a 2-mL bolus every 20 minutes (lockout), with a basal infusion of 4 to 6 mL/hr.

(viii) *Side effects*

Most side effects (Table 4) are alleviated by either lowering the infusion rate or changing the drug or dose. Pruritus is a common side effect of neuraxial opioid that usually responds well to anti-

Table 4. Common side effects of epidural analgesia

Opioid
  Pruritus
  Sedation
  Dizziness
  Urinary retention
Local anesthetic
  Hypotension
  Mild sensory changes
  Urinary retention

histamine treatment. The mixed agonist/antagonist nalbuphine (Nubaine) (5 to 10 mg IV, 4 to 6 times per hour) also works well, as does a low-dose naloxone infusion. Contrary to popular belief, nausea rarely occurs with epidural opioids, as doses used are extremely small. Gut mobility is in fact improved by epidural therapy, not the contrary.

Urinary retention may be a problem, especially when lumbar catheters are used, so indwelling Foley catheters are kept in patients receiving epidural analgesia. Unilateral lower extremity numbness with occasional weakness or motor block is a side effect of the local anesthetic. This usually occurs when the epidural catheter tip has migrated along a nerve root, and pulling the catheter back or lowering the infusion rate tends to rectify the problem. However, one should always maintain vigilance and continue to watch for possible complications.

(ix) *Complications*

Although most complications are rare, when they do occur they can be devastating; an integral part of epidural management is the avoidance of serious complications (Table 5). Postdural puncture headache (PDPH) is a recognized and relatively common complication that is thought to be the result of a small CSF leak secondary to accidental dural puncture. Typically, there is a delay in onset of the headache (approximately 24 hours), so that the complication tends to manifest on the first postoperative day. Because PDPH tends to worsen on sitting up, and particularly on walking, and to improve on lying down, it may not appear until the patient gets out of bed for the first time after surgery. Other characteristics of the headache are that it tends to occur at the back of the head (occiput) and neck, and it produces a tight, pulling, and throbbing sensation. Conservative management consists of bed rest (up to bathroom only), plenty of fluids (IV or oral), and headache medication (NSAIDs, acetaminophen, caffeine, and theophylline all work well).

If there is no resolution, or if conservative measures are contraindicated, a blood patch is recommended. This consists of an epidural injection of 20 mL of the patient's own blood (drawn under sterile conditions), which is thought to close the dural puncture. The exact mechanism by which an epidural blood patch works is uncertain, but it is probably either a pressure effect or a laying down of clot or fibrosis onto the puncture site.

Much more serious are complications caused by the development of space-occupying lesions within the spinal canal—hematomas and abscesses—the former being the more common. If there is any

Table 5. Epidural complications arising postoperatively

Common	Post–dural puncture headache
Rare	Skin infection
	Epidural hematoma or abscess
Extremely rare	Anterior spinal artery syndrome
	Transverse myelitis
	Meningitis

reason for concern, the first response should be to discontinue the epidural infusion, and possibly to remove the epidural catheter, the latter especially if there is evidence of infection at the skin. (If there are coagulation issues, it may be better to leave the catheter until they are resolved—see below). As long as these lesions are recognized, they can be surgically decompressed without consequent permanent neurologic damage. Failing this, spinal cord compression, and later paraplegia, may develop.

Cardinal signs of impending spinal cord compression are sensory and motor changes in the lower extremity (often bilateral) and pain in the back. Although minimal sensory changes are common and may be benign, prolonged motor changes that do not resolve with discontinuation of the epidural infusion are always worrisome, as is back pain. In the case of lesions in the sacral canal, cardinal signs are changes in bladder and bowel function, and pain may be absent. If there is any concern, magnetic resonance imaging should be ordered and the involvement of neurology is always helpful. Early intervention is key to preventing disastrous complications. Other serious complications such as anterior spinal artery syndrome, transverse myelitis, and meningitis have been reported but are extremely rare.

(x) *Anticoagulation and epidurals*

Some patients are placed on anticoagulants while receiving epidural analgesia. Because there is a small but real risk of starting an epidural bleed when removing an epidural catheter in an anticoagulated patient (best estimate, between 0.01% and 0.1%), it is prudent to develop a protocol for catheter removal in these patients. The policy for removing epidural catheters at the MGH is based on a consensus statement from the American Society of Regional Anesthesia, entitled *Neuraxial Anesthesia and Anticoagulation* (available on the web from address listed in Appendix III).

If a patient is receiving a high-dose heparin infusion and the epidural catheter must be removed, the primary service is notified to coordinate an appropriate plan of care. Heparin is stopped for 2 to 3 hours before removing the epidural catheter and then resumed without a bolus dose approximately 2 hours after epidural catheter removal. Low-dose heparin (prophylaxis) is not a contraindication to catheter removal.

Patients on Coumadin should have the catheter removed within 48 hours of the first dose of Coumadin. Any time thereafter, prothrombin times (PTs) should be obtained to ensure that the range is appropriate. The acceptable range for PT is below 17, for International Normalized Ratio (INR) is below 1.9, and for partial thromboplastin time (PTT) is below 35.

LMWH should be held for at least 12 hours prior to catheter removal. It can be started or restarted 8–12 hours (or later) after the epidural catheter is pulled. There is no practical test for LMWH activity (the anti-Xa level is not a reliable predictor of the risk of bleeding, and the test is available on only a limited basis); PT, INR, and PTT values do not reflect LMWH activity. Administering fresh frozen plasma to restore coagulation factors is rarely indicated and entails many risks (fluid overload, cardiac failure, transfusion reaction, immunological changes, transmission of infection), some more common than others and some unpredictable and/or irreversible. Patients with a known risk of coagulopathy who have a catheter removed should be monitored for at least 24 hours to rule out hematoma development.

5. Single-shot neuraxial morphine

Neuraxial morphine can be safely used provided that large bolus doses and repeat bolus doses are avoided, and that patients are appropriately monitored. In general, infusions are safer than bolus doses; however, epidural morphine infusions are not used routinely at the MGH. A single shot of morphine into the epidural or intrathecal space can provide prolonged analgesia (up to 24 hours), but it carries a risk of delayed respiratory depression. As discussed, morphine is poorly lipophilic, tends to stay in CSF once there, and is subject to CSF flow with passage to higher centers including the respiratory center.

At the same time, the fact that morphine tends to remain in CSF is the reason that it produces excellent selective spinal analgesia (i.e., good spread to spinal cord receptors). Thus single-shot neuraxial morphine is an excellent means of providing analgesia when single-shot spinal (intrathecal injection) or epidural (epidural injection) anesthesia is used for surgery, provided the risk of delayed respiratory depression is recognized. At the MGH, we monitor patients who have been given neuraxial morphine in exactly the same way we monitor those with epidural opioid infusions, which we feel is an adequate level of monitoring for these patients (Fig. 3). We provide supplementary analgesia with PCA opioid, but for safety we rely solely on demand doses and do not use continuous opioid infusions.

6. Intraoperative neural blockade

Nerve blocks performed before or during surgery provide excellent pain control during the early postoperative period. Infiltration of wounds with local anesthetics by surgeons can also contribute significantly to the control of early postoperative pain. Intraoperative neural blockade can reduce postoperative analgesic requirements and, in some cases, negate the need for postoperative analgesia. Intraoperative nerve blocks are particularly useful in children, who tolerate analgesics poorly and in whom pain is particularly distressing.

7. Prolonged neural blockade: use of catheters

Neural blockade can be prolonged beyond the life of the chosen local anesthetic only by using continuous infusions of local anesthetic via catheters. Neural cryotherapy and direct severance of nerves used to be performed for prolonged nerve blockade, but these practices are no longer recommended as they are known to result in an unacceptably high incidence of chronic pain. Continuous infusions of local anesthetics can be administered at various sites. For example, local anesthetic infusion into the pleural space via an intrapleural catheter provides effective pain relief following thoracotomy and upper abdominal procedures, but this has yet to prove its worth in comparison to thoracic epidural therapy.

Local anesthetic infusion into the brachial plexus is useful after shoulder or hand surgery, especially when physical therapy is needed. Bupivacaine 0.1% at 10 to 15 mL/hr is used while the pa-

Massachusetts General Hospital

Epidural Order Sheet

DOCTORS' ORDER SHEET

UNIT NO.
NAME

Date:
Patient's age:
Patient's weight:
Drug allergies:

Pain service page number is 27246 (PAIN)

(See guide on the back of this sheet for scales of pain level, sedation level, verbal response and motor strength)

1. **Prepared epidural mixture:**
   - ☐ bupivacaine 0.1%, dilaudid 0.02 mg/cc
   - ☐ bupivacaine 0.25%, dilaudid 0.02 mg/cc
   - ☐ bupivacaine 0.1%, morphine 0.05 mg/cc
   - ☐ bupivacaine 0.1%, fentanyl 2 μg/cc
   - ☐ bupivacaine 0.1%
   - ☐ bupivacaine 0.25%

2. **Rate and range**
   initial rate ________ cc/hr
   titrate within the range ________ – ________ cc/hr

3. **Backup orders**
   For respiratory depression give Narcan 0.1 mg, repeated q 5 mins to a maximum of 0.4 mg if necessary

   If epidural fails for any reason, stop the epidural infusion, call the Pain Service, and give:
   DRUG: ________
   DOSE: ________ mg IV q 5 minutes until comfortable
   MAXIMUM DOSE: ________ mg
   Monitor vital signs q 5 mins x 3 after bolus doses

For PCA (use only when directed to by the Pain Service):

DRUG/CONCENTRATION ________ / ________ mg/cc
BOLUS DOSE ________ cc
BOLUS LOCK-OUT ________ minutes
RATE 7am - 11pm ________ cc
11pm - 7am ________ cc
HOURLY LIMIT ________ cc

Signature: ______________________ MD

82658 8/98

1. **Epidural management**
   - A. 15 minutes after a bolus dose, initiation of infusion, or an increase in rate:
     - record HR and BP
     - record verbal response and motor strength
     - record RR q 1° x 4
     - record pain and sedation levels q 1° x 4 if patient is awake
   - B. At steady state (ie > 4 hrs after a bolus dose, initiation of infusion, or an increase in rate:
     - record RR q 2°
     - record HR and BP q 4°
     - record pain and sedation levels, verbal and motor responses q 4° if patient is awake

2. **For the following side effects, call the Pain Service:**
   RR < 10, HR < 50, SBP < 90
   nausea, vomiting, itching, urinary retention

3. **For RR < 8, call the Pain Service, and:**
   1. if the patient is obtunded, give O_2
   2. stop the epidural infusion
   3. give Narcan 0.1 mg q 5 mins, to a maximum of 0.4 mg, if necessary
   4. monitor O_2 saturation, if necessary

NO SYSTEMIC OPIATES OR SEDATIVES UNLESS ORDERED BY THE PAIN SERVICE

IN THE CASE OF PROBLEMS CALL THE PAIN SERVICE, PAGE # 27246 (PAIN)

In an emergency, if unable to contact the Pain Service, call anesthesia in the operating room, 6-8995 or 6-8910

Figure 3. Epidural order sheet.

tient is hospitalized (approximately 2 days). If that is not effective, the concentration can be increased to 0.25% or a bolus of 20 mL of 0.25 to 0.375% bupivacaine can be added to the catheter prior to physical therapy. Patients may also take oral analgesics as needed.

8. Transcutaneous electrical nerve stimulation

Transcutaneous electrical nerve stimulation (TENS) is useful for postoperative pain in selected patients. The device consists of a series of electrodes that are placed on the site of the pain (either side of the surgical incision in the case of postoperative pain), through which a low-voltage electrical stimulus is passed. The treatment is based on the gate-control theory of pain by Melzack and Wall. Randomized, controlled trials have confirmed its efficacy in postoperative pain compared with controls (no TENS), but they have not shown it to be better than sham TENS (electrodes with no current); likewise, sham TENS is also better than no TENS. It is likely, therefore, to have predominant a placebo effect. It does not stand up against drug therapies as a sole treatment for anything other than mild postoperative pain, but it may be useful in reducing analgesic requirements and possibly improving pulmonary function in selected patients. At the MGH, TENS is not offered routinely for postoperative pain, but a few patients do request it and can obtain it through our physical therapy department.

9. Behavioral therapy

The goal of behavioral therapy is to provide patients with a sense of control over their pain. All patients benefit from being well prepared psychologically for the experience of surgery and postoperative pain. Simple relaxation strategies and imagery techniques can help those patients who find such interventions appealing. Relaxation strategies and imagery techniques do not need to be complex to be effective. Simple strategies, such as brief jaw relaxation, music-assisted relaxation, and recall of peaceful images, have been found to be effective in reducing anxiety and analgesic requirements. They take only a few minutes to teach, although they may require continual practice and reinforcement at times. Patients who wish to learn simple relaxation exercises can be given information and recommended techniques.

Therapeutic touch is becoming another popular mode of therapy and is particularly helpful when postoperative pain is refractory to other modalities. Elaborate behavioral therapy techniques (i.e., biofeedback or counseling) have no place in the treatment of acute postoperative pain, unless the pain is likely to be prolonged or to recur.

V. CONCLUSION

Effective postoperative pain management involves adherence to certain basic principles. First, pain must be assessed on an ongoing and systematic basis, with data documented in the medical records, so that pain treatment can be modified according to the patient's needs and communicated throughout the healthcare disciplines. Pain that is treated preemptively or controlled early is easier to manage than established or severe pain, so treatment during the intraoperative and early postoperative period is essential. Patients should be involved with their treatment and be educated about their surgery and the options available for treating postoperative pain. The actual choice of treatment is of secondary importance, as long as the principles of postoperative pain management are adhered to.

Postoperative pain has often been inadequately treated in the past, partly because of complacency, and partly because of fear of analgesic side effects. But today's patients expect better pain control and are better educated in their healthcare needs. The provision of exemplary pain management goes a long way toward improving patient satisfaction with hospital care. For this reason, and because good pain control is humane and reduces morbidity, we should endeavor to treat postoperative pain to the best of our ability.

SELECTED READING

1. Bach S, Noreng MF, Tjellden NU. Phantom limb pain in amputees during the first 12 months following limb amputation, after preoperative lumbar epidural blockade. *Pain* 1988;33:297–301.

2. Ballantyne JC. Does regional anesthesia improve outcome after surgery? *Curr Opin Anesthesiol* 1999;12:545–549.

3. Ballantyne JC, Carr DB, DeFerranti S, et al. The comparative effects of postoperative analgesic therapies on pulmonary outcome: Cumulative meta-analyses of randomized, controlled trials. *Anesth Analg* 1998;86:598–612.

4. Carr DB. Acute pain management: Operative or medical procedures and trauma. In: *Clinical practice guideline.* AHCPR pub no 92-0032. Rockville, MD: Agency for Health Care Policy and Research, Public Health Service, US Department of Health and Human Services, 1992.

5. Cousins M, Power I. Acute and postoperative pain. In: Wall PD, Melzak R, eds. *Textbook of pain,* 4th ed. Philadelphia: Churchill Livingstone, 1999:447–491.

6. de Leon-Casasola OA, Parker B, Lema MJ, et al. Postoperative epidural bupivacaine-morphine therapy: Experience with 4,227 surgical cancer patients. *Anesthesiology* 1994;81:368–375.

7. Gottschalk A, Smith DS, Jobes DR, et al. Preemptive epidural analgesia and recovery from radical prostatectomy: A randomized controlled trial. *JAMA* 1998;279:1076–1082.

8. Horlocker TT, Wedel DJ. Spinal and epidural blockade and perioperative low molecular weight heparin: Smooth sailing on the Titanic. *Anesth Analg* 1998;86:1153–1156.

9. Liu S, Carpenter R, Neal JM. Epidural anesthesia and analgesia: Their role in postoperative outcome. *Anesthesiology* 1995;82:1474–1506.

10. Ready LB, Loper KA, Nessly M, Wild L. Postoperative epidural morphine is safe in the surgical ward. *Anesthesiology* 1991;75:452–456.

11. Melzack R, Wall PD. Pain mechanisms: a new theory. *Science* 1965;150:971–979.

Postoperative Pain in Children

William T. Denman and Jane Ballantyne

Charm ache with air and agony with words.
—*William Shakespeare (1564–1616)*

It has been only over the last two decades that pain relief in children has become an area of major concern. As an example of this, in a paper published in 1976, the anesthesia technique for ligation of patent ductus arteriosus was oxygen and muscle relaxants. Major strides have been made over the last 10 years in assessment, monitoring, and therapy. Pain services have been developed to deal with the special issues surrounding postoperative analgesia in infants and children. Why has pain relief been denied to children for so long? The reasons are multifactorial: neonates and young infants were presumed to be insensitive to pain, children heal quickly, caregivers have had a fear of prescribing opioid analgesia to children for a variety of reasons.

Recent research shows clearly that neonates and infants are in fact sensitive to pain and mount physiologic, sometimes deleterious, responses in much the same way as adults. Moreover, it shows that traumatic pain experiences can scar young children and make them fearful for a long time because they are not mature enough to be able to rationalize their experience.

There are many differences between adults and children that make pain treatment in children a particular challenge. It is not as easy to assess pain in children. Children, particularly neonates and infants, do not handle drugs as well as adults. Children hate needles. Epidurals are technically more difficult to place and more difficult to maintain. And the sight of a child in pain is particularly distressing, especially to the parents.

I. PLANNING FOR POSTOPERATIVE ANALGESIA

The intraoperative and postoperative courses and the postoperative analgesia plan cannot be viewed separately. Planning for postoperative analgesia should begin prior to surgery and involves choosing an anesthetic that provides postoperative as well as intraoperative analgesia, and preparing the child and parents for the surgical experience.

Children should be told honestly what to expect, and they should be reassured that they will be cared for and everything will be done to alleviate any pain or discomfort. This reassurance is also of great importance to parents.

It is often helpful to ask how the child copes with pain and distress, and how he or she communicates pain. For example, what words are used to describe pain (e.g., "boo-boo," "hurt," "sore"), and does the child rely on special blankets or toys? If the child has had surgery before, the parents and child should be questioned about the previous experience:

- What medications were used in the past and did they work well?
- What was the past pain experience of the child?
- Were nonpharmacologic techniques used?
- What has worked well in the past?
- What coping techniques were beneficial?

Choosing an assessment tool and preoperatively teaching the child how to use it will ensure the best results from the assessment process. If patient-controlled analgesia (PCA) is to be used, it is helpful to teach children and their parents the principles of PCA. Similarly, explain regional anesthetic techniques if these are chosen.

II. ASSESSING ACUTE PAIN IN INFANTS AND CHILDREN

Pain assessment is the key to effective pain management. Consistent assessment must occur regularly and the same scale and format must be used for each assessment so as not to confuse the child or the parents, and so that the process is as objective as possible and comparisons can be made between nursing shifts. The parent and child should be intimately involved in the evaluation, management, and decision making whenever possible.

The assessment of pain in children is challenging because they may be nonverbal (very young) or they may communicate pain in ways we do not always understand (e.g., by withdrawing, or by telling us they do not have pain in case we inflict more). In neonates and infants, clinical judgment alone is used, whereas simple assessment tools are useful in older children. Appropriate methods of pain assessment in children differ at different ages. Broadly, there are three stages of a child's development when different means of pain assessment are suitable.

1. Infants, neonates, and very young children (0 to 4 years)

Infants and neonates clearly cannot report their pain. However, children as young as 18 months can indicate their pain and give a location, although they cannot give a self-report of pain intensity before about 3 years of age. At 3, they can give a gross indication, such as "no pain," "a little pain," and "a lot of pain," but this is not always reliable. The mother's or father's impression is often the best indicator in these very young patients. Nurses and doctors need to listen to the parents in addition to using objective measures of pain. Behavioral and physiologic responses can be used as a measure of pain in young children, particularly in noncommunicating ones. These signs, which may not be specific to pain, include the following:

- Crying, screaming, moaning, whimpering
- Facial expression, grimacing, furrowed brow

- Posture, tone, guarding, thrashing, touching painful area
- Palmar sweating
- Sleep pattern
- Respiratory rate and pattern
- Heart rate and blood pressure

Hospitals may choose to use one of several systematic and validated measurement tools [e.g., CRIES (Krecehel and Bildner)] that utilize various combinations of these physiological and behavioral indicators of pain, although their use is not often warranted in the acute pain setting. The principles of pain assessment in very young children, and issues of nervous system and cognitive development are described in Chapter 33.

2. Young children (4 to 7 or 8 years)

Assuming developmental normality, older children (from 4 years to 7 or 8 years old) can provide reliable self-reports of pain by using assessment tools designed for young children, such as the faces scale (see Chapter 6, Fig. 1), by communicating via their parents, and often by direct communication with their doctors and nurses. Simple numeric scales using childish language may be helpful at the upper end of this age range. For example, "If 0 means no hurt and 10 means the biggest pain you've ever had, what is your pain now?"

3. Older children (>7 or 8 years)

Older children who understand the concept of numeric order can use verbal or visual numeric scales such as those used in adults (see Chapter 6).

III. TREATMENT CHOICES

Treatment of both procedural and postoperative pain has improved greatly over the last 20 years. This has come about with the development of pain centers, protocols, and a realization that pain treatment and prevention is important. Children now are benefiting from improved analgesia in the form of topical analgesics, opioids, patient controlled analgesia (PCA), and regional anesthesia and analgesia. There has also been an increase in the provision of sedation and general anesthesia for children undergoing painful procedures.

When children are being prescribed for, the following guidelines should be kept in mind:

- Liver conjugation is the predominate method of metabolism for most analgesics.
- Neonates, having an immature cytochrome P450 system, conjugate drugs slowly.
- Renal function in the first few weeks of life is decreased compared to adults. Usually, clearance of drugs and metabolites is adequate within 2 weeks of birth. Prior to this, the half-life of many drugs may be increased, necessitating an increase in dosing intervals.
- Because of the increase in total body water in neonates, drugs that are water soluble have a larger volume of distribution.
- Neonates have less plasma protein binding, resulting in increased free drug.

Massachusetts General Hospital

Pediatric Continuous Intravenous Analgesia

DOCTORS' ORDER SHEET

UNIT NO.
NAME

Date:
Patient's age:
Patient's weight:
Drug allergies:

Pain Service page number is 27246 (2-PAIN)

(See guide on the back of this sheet for scales of pain level and sedation level)

---

1. **Discontinue previous pain medications.**

2. **No systemic narcotics to be given except by order of the Pain Service.**

3. **Drug (check one):**

   ☐   morphine 0.2 mg/cc

   ☐   morphine 1 mg/cc

   ☐   _____

4. **Initial bolus loading does (if needed):**

   _____ cc (_____ mg) every _____ minutes, prn until patient is comfortable.
   Maximum total loading dose:
   _____ cc (_____ mg)

5. **Infusion rate:**

   (a) For Abbott (APMII) pump, select PCA mode 1: "Continuous Only"

   (b) Range _____ - _____ cc/hr (_____ - _____ mg/hr)

   (c) Start at: _____ cc/hr (_____ mg/hr)

6. **For respiratory depression:**

   (a) Discontinue infusion

   (b) Narcan 2μ g/kg, repeated q 5 mins x 2 if necessary, maximum 6 μ g/kg

   (c) Administer oxygen by facemask (4L/min), if necessary

8. **In the event of pump failure or non-patent IV:**

   _____, _____ mg SQ/IM q _____ hr prn
   for pain

Signature: _____ MD

83418 2/99

MONITORING

1. Record baseline HR, BP and RA (respiratory assessment of rate and depth) 15 and 30 minutes after initial bolus loading dose.

2. Record RA q 2 hrly and analgesic and sedation scores q 4 hrly

3. Page the Pain Service for:

   (a) Inadequate analgesia
   (b) Respiratory depression (RR < _____)
   (c) Excessive sedation
   (d) Mental status change
   (e) Change in vital signs
       HR <
       SBP < _____

IN THE CASE OF PROBLEMS CALL THE PAIN SERVICE, PAGE # 27246 (2-PAIN)

In an emergency, if unable to contact the Pain Service, call anesthesia in the operating room, 6-8995 or 6-8910

Figure 1.   Continuous IV morphine order sheet.

In general, these pharmacokinetic factors mean that lower doses per kilogram are needed in neonates and infants, sometimes at increased dosing intervals. However, the effects of immaturity are complex, and some drugs may actually be needed in greater doses because of differences in drug sensitivity and distribution. There is no substitute for using pediatric drug tables when prescribing drugs for young children.

1. Acetaminophen and the nonsteroidal anti-inflammatory drugs

Acetaminophen and the nonsteroidal anti-inflammatory drugs (NSAIDs) are cyclooxygenase/prostaglandin inhibitors. They are effective for mild to moderate pain, or as adjuncts to opioid and regional analgesia. They have the great advantage in children of not being associated with respiratory depression. However, although acetaminophen is relatively free of side effects, the NSAIDs have several potentially dangerous side effects that limit their use. These drugs (including acetaminophen) are described in Chapter 8. Pediatric dosing for the more commonly used of these drugs is presented in Table 1.

(i) *Acetaminophen*

Acetaminophen is the most widely used analgesic and antipyretic, both in the home and in hospitals. It has only minimal anti-inflammatory effects since its effects are mainly central. This accounts for its lack of adverse effects on the renal and gastrointestinal (GI) systems and on platelet function. It is probably the most useful adjunct and analgesic for mild pain in the management of pediatric pain. Acetaminophen is available in many formulations, including tablets, capsules, syrups, suspensions, and suppositories. It is also included in many commercially available combination analgesics. Doses of 10 to 15 mg/kg every 4 hours up to a daily maximum of 100 mg/kg are useful for the treatment of mild to moderate pain, and a single dose of 30 to 40 mg/kg may be given either

Table 1.   Pediatric dosing of commonly used NSAIDs and acetaminophen

Drug	Dose	Comments
Acetaminophen (PO and PR)	10–15 mg/kg q 4 hr	Lacks the peripheral anti-inflammatory activity of other NSAIDs. Doses up to 30–40 mg/kg can be given PO or PR for severe pain; maximum daily dose is 100 mg/kg
Aspirin	10–15 mg/kg q 4 hr	Limited usage in children because of its association with Reye's disease
Ibuprofen	4–10 mg/kg q 6–8 hr	Available under several brand names and as generic; also available as oral suspension
Naproxen	5 mg/kg q 12 hr	Also available as oral liquid
Ketorolac (IV)	0.5 mg/kg q 6–8 hr	Potent and injectable; usage limited by side effects; should not be used for more than 5 days

NSAID, nonsteroidal anti-inflammatory drug; PO, by mouth; PR, by way of the rectum; IV, intravenous.
Note: Doses are oral unless otherwise stated.

orally or rectally to aid in the management of acute postoperative pain. The rectal route is useful in children and used frequently for acetaminophen. Usually, children do not mind rectal drug administration, preferring it to injection by needle. Rapid absorption occurs because there is no first-pass liver metabolism from the distal rectum. Occasionally, drugs are rapidly expelled from the rectum (before absorption can take place), which precludes the use of this route.

(ii) *Nonsteroidal anti-inflammatory drugs*

Because currently used NSAIDs do not cross the blood–brain barrier in appreciable amounts, their effects are mainly peripheral. This contributes to their value as adjunctive analgesics, as their mechanism of action is completely different from that of centrally acting analgesics such as the opioids. NSAID use is associated with well-recognized side effects, including gastritis, possible GI bleeding, and platelet and renal dysfunction. These side effects limit the use of NSAIDs after major surgery and in certain patients (e.g., those with renal disease or coagulopathies). However, when used with care, these are useful analgesics for children undergoing surgery, as they are free of the respiratory depressant and mood altering effects of opioids.

Aspirin (acetylsalicylic acid), the most utilized NSAID for over 100 years, currently has very limited use in pediatrics because of its recently recognized association with Reye's syndrome. The most widely used NSAID is ibuprofen, available in a number of formulations including an oral suspension and chewable tablets appropriate for pediatric use. Doses of 5 to 10 mg/kg every 4 hours, up to a daily maximum of 40 mg/kg, may be used either as needed, or preferably around the clock for 48 to 72 hours. With refractory pain, ibuprofen and acetaminophen doses can be alternated every 3 hours, allowing the maintenance of a steady-state inhibition of prostaglandin synthesis while minimizing side effects and staying below maximum dosage guidelines.

Other NSAIDs used in the treatment of children include naproxen, tolmetin, diclofenac, and ketorolac. Of these, only ketorolac, at doses up to 0.5 mg/kg, is approved for parenteral as well as oral administration for the treatment of pain. Ketorolac can be very useful for treating postoperative pain when the oral route cannot be used, when opioids are poorly tolerated, or when additional analgesia is needed. Intravenous (IV) indomethacin is used to treat patent ductus arteriosus, but it has virtually no application in the treatment of pain. Indomethacin suppositories may be useful occasionally.

The newer selective COX-2 inhibitors (rofecoxib and celecoxib) are less likely to cause side effects because they selectively inhibit the inducible cyclooxygenase (COX-2), sparing the constitutive enzyme (COX-I), particularly in the GI tract. They may be useful as an alternative to standard NSAIDs when there is a concern about the GI effects of the latter, although studies of the use of these drugs in the pediatric population have not yet been completed.

2. Opioids

Opioids (see Chapter 9) are the most commonly prescribed analgesics in the treatment of moderate to severe pain; they are the only analgesics that do not have a ceiling effect and the only analgesics that are effective for severe pain. Opioids can be used safely in children with appropriate monitoring, dosing regimens, and techniques of administration. Traditionally, opioids have been underused in children for a variety of reasons, including misconceptions about children's ability to feel pain, a lack of familiarity with dosing, and fear of side effects.

(i) *Pharmacokinetics*

Children handle opioids differently at different ages, and it is necessary to understand these differences to prescribe opioids safely to pediatric patients. In newborns and infants, the pharmacokinetic factors described earlier mean that lower per kilogram doses are needed than in older children, although opioids' larger volume of distribution may mean that a relatively large loading dose (given under controlled conditions) may be needed.

Neonates and premature infants are extremely sensitive to the respiratory depressant effects of opioids, and respiratory depression may occur at doses that are not even analgesic. Infants are also at an increased risk for the development of apnea following a rapid bolus dose because of the rapidity at which the circulation delivers the peak dose to the brain. The half-life of morphine in neonates is 6 to 8 hours and about 10 hours in the premature (compared to 2 hours in adults), necessitating markedly lower infusion rates than in older individuals. However, higher plasma levels of morphine are needed for equal analgesia, possibly because the production of morphine-6-glucuronide (an active metabolite of morphine) is greatly reduced. As children grow, morphine clearance rapidly approaches adult levels, and in adolescence it is actually greater than in adults. Young children appear to be less likely to vomit after opioids. Recommended opioid dosages for children are presented in Table 2.

(ii) *Choice of opioid*

For IV use, morphine is the drug of choice in the pediatric population because it is well tolerated, caregivers are familiar with its use, and it has been widely used in children. Because of its associated histamine release, morphine may be contraindicated in asthmatics, but most asthmatics actually tolerate morphine infusions well. Hydromorphone or fentanyl may be used instead. Codeine, oxycodone, and morphine are the opioids most commonly chosen for oral administration in children.

Table 2.   Recommended starting doses for opioids in children weighing under 50 kg

Drug	Oral	Parenteral
Morphine	0.3 mg/kg q 3–4 hr	0.05–0.1 mg/kg q 3–4 hr
Codeine	1 mg/kg q 3–4 hr	Not used
Hydromorphone (Dilaudid)	0.06 mg/kg q 3–4 hr	0.015 mg/kg q 3–4 hr
Oxycodone	0.2 mg/kg q 3–4 hr	Not available

Note: Equianalgesic doses are listed Appendix VIII.

(iii) *Routes of administration*

Opioids can be given parenterally, orally, rectally, or neuraxially. In the immediate postoperative period, since the oral route may not be available, the IV route (via an indwelling catheter) is most commonly chosen for ease of titration and avoidance of needles. If there is no IV in place, the rectal route may be useful. Pain after minor surgery can often be satisfactorily treated with nonopioid analgesics, so that oral opioids usually follow an IV regimen only in the case of major surgery. Neuraxial opioids may be given by the spinal and epidural routes.

a) **Parenteral**

Intramuscular and subcutaneous injections are avoided because they are distressing (especially to young children), and unnecessary and unpredictable in their effects. An indwelling subcutaneous needle is occasionally used when there is difficulty with IV access. The IV route is the parenteral route of choice. Drugs can be given either intermittently or by continuous infusion. Continuous infusions are the standard at MGH for small children who cannot use PCA. Intermittent boluses are used as a backup if pain gets out of control. PCA is used as soon as children are old enough to use this technique.

To provide effective and safe analgesia using IV opioids in children, it is necessary to understand a very basic principle of opioid dosing in young patients. As already stated, when children are too young to communicate their pain, judgments about pain are derived from signs such as screaming and crying, but these signs are not at all specific to pain. Thus, it is quite possible to assume pain exists when a child is simply fed up and exhausted.

The correct response is for an experienced physician or nurse to stay with the child and give monitored intermittent bolus injections (morphine at 0.025 to 0.1 mg/kg) every 5 minutes, while the child is soothed, until the child settles. If a continuous infusion of opioid is being used, the rate may be increased slightly in response to uncontrolled pain but *it should not be repeatedly and rapidly increased.* When the child finally settles, the increased infusion rate can result in overdose and respiratory depression—often well after medical personnel have left the room. This inappropriate reaction to a child's distress is such a common error, and a regular cause of potentially dangerous respiratory depression, that it is worth emphasizing.

Continuous IV infusion

In young children (<5 to 7 years) with moderate to severe pain, continuous IV infusions are used to maintain steady plasma drug levels and stable analgesia. Prior to starting the infusion, a loading dose is given to achieve a steady state, after which the infusion maintains effective analgesia. Careful monitoring, using regular vital sign assessments and sometimes special monitors, is necessary to prevent excessive sedation and respiratory depression. This is particularly important in neonates and all spontaneously breathing children.

Morphine is the most commonly used opioid for continuous infusions. It has been extensively studied in all age groups. Analgesic levels are usually obtained after a loading dose of 25 to 100 µg/kg of morphine and then starting an infusion at 2 to 5 µg/kg/hr. Recommended infusion rates vary according to age and pain severity

(Table 3). In some circumstances, it may be desirable to use an alternative opioid (see Chapter 9). However, as a general principle, it is wise to use and become familiar with a single opioid in pediatric practice because correct dosing is so critical. The MGH standard orders for continuous opioids infusions are shown in Figure 1.

Patient controlled analgesia

PCA is used in older children (>5 to 7 years) at MGH as soon as they understand how to use it. Unfortunately, PCA is not available in all hospitals, and if it is not, continuous IV infusions should be substituted, with bolus injections for breakthrough pain. For children, it is sometimes appropriate to allow parents or nurses to control PCA, but caution should be exercised. Before allowing parents to participate, the prescribing physician should be absolutely certain that the parents understand the principles of PCA (see Chapter 21), and in particular that they should not press the button unless the child is awake and requesting analgesia, or obviously in pain. Standard MGH PCA orders are shown in Figure 1 of Chapter 21. Table 4 presents dosage guidelines for morphine and hydromorphone.

b) Oral

The oral route is used when pain is subsiding and when it is mild to moderate. Clearly, this route cannot be used if the child is nil per os (NPO) or vomiting. Either pure opioid or opioid combinations can be chosen. Codeine, oxycodone, morphine elixir, Tylenol #3 (acetaminophen with codeine), and Percocet (oxycodone with acetaminophen) are all useful in children. Recommended doses can be found in Table 2. Tylenol #3 and Percocet are reserved for children over 20 kg; one to two tablets are used every 4 hours, according to weight and pain severity.

c) Rectal

Morphine and hydromorphone are available as suppositories and may be useful when the oral and IV routes are not available. Rectal doses are the same as oral doses (see Table 2).

d) Neuraxial

Opioids given intrathecally or epidurally provide selective spinal analgesia that is both effective and relatively free of side effects be-

Table 3. Guidelines for continuous intravenous infusion of morphine

Population	Pain level	Morphine (µg/kg/hr)
Pre-term neonate	Severe	5–10
	Moderate	2–5
	Mild	0–2
Term neonate	Severe	10–20
	Moderate	5–10
	Mild	0–5
Older infant	Severe	15–30
	Moderate	10–20
	Mild	0–10

Adapted from Yaster M, Krane EJ, Kaplan RF, eds. *Pediatric pain management and sedation handbook.* St. Louis: Mosby, 1997:199, with permission.

Table 4. Guidelines for patient-controlled analgesia (PCA) dosing

Drug	Bolus dose (µg/kg)	Lockout (min)	Basal rate (µg/kg/hr)	Hourly limit (mg/kg)
Morphine	10–30	6–10	10–30	0.1–0.15
Hydromorphone	3–5	6–10	3–5	0.015–0.02

Adapted from Yaster M, Krane EJ, Kaplan RF, eds. *Pediatric pain management and sedation handbook.* St. Louis: Mosby, 1997:100, with permission.

cause much smaller doses are used. Hydromorphone and fentanyl are used at MGH. Differences between opioids when administered neuraxially are described in Chapter 21 (IV, 4, iv). As a general principle, epidural doses are one-tenth IV doses, whereas intrathecal (spinal) doses are one–one hundredth IV doses.

3. Regional anesthesia and analgesia

Regional and local anesthetic techniques, which are often used in children, have the great advantages of providing prolonged analgesia that extends into the postoperative period, reducing distress, and reducing the need for opioids. Infants and young children appear to be relatively resistant to the hemodynamic and respiratory effects of epidural or spinal blockade, so the techniques are generally safe. Catheters may be utilized to prolong the effects of regional anesthesia even further, and to provide analgesia. The most common catheter therapy used in children is epidural therapy. For epidural analgesia, low-dose local anesthetics are used (blocking C-fibers specifically, and sparing sensory and motor nerves so that patients can move normally) with or without opioids. Opioids have a selective spinal effect because of their preferential absorption onto spinal cord receptors from the proximal site of administration.

(i) Epidural analgesia

Many of the principles of epidural analgesia use in adults (see Chapter 21) apply also to children and are not repeated here. In small children, epidural catheters are technically more difficult to place (although with experience this difference disappears), and once placed, it is more difficult to keep them in, to protect them from the diaper area, and to maintain their patency because of their smaller size. As in adults, epidural catheter maintenance is time consuming, labor intensive, and not without complications, so catheters should be reserved for cases where the benefit outweighs these considerations (e.g., major abdominal and thoracic surgery). Many hospitals choose not to offer epidural catheter treatments to their pediatric patients on regular floors because of the difficulty of providing appropriate staffing to manage these catheters.

Single-shot epidural injections, including caudal injections, are very useful in children and provide excellent analgesia during the early postoperative phase. For a single-shot caudal injection, we give 1 mL/kg of 0.125% to 0.25% bupivacaine, sometimes with the addition of 2 to 4 μg/kg clonidine, which provides additional analgesia with minimal risk of hypotension (see Appendix VIII).

a) *Indications*

At MGH, postoperative epidural catheter treatments in children are reserved for thoracic, abdominal, and lower limb procedures that are expected to produce severe pain. Single-shot techniques are much simpler and provide useful analgesia after many surgical procedures of the torso, pelvis, and lower limb, including hernia repair, circumcision, tendon lengthening, and club foot release. The caudal route is most commonly selected for single-shot epidural injections.

b) *Contraindications*

Contraindications to epidural placement are the following:

- Patient or parent refusal
- Coagulopathy
- Bacteremia
- Local infection at epidural insertion site
- Spine pathology, neurologic deficit, raised intracranial pressure (relative contraindications)

c) *Benefits*

The benefits of epidural analgesia that apply particularly to children are superior analgesia, opioid sparing with clear sensorium and decreased risk of respiratory depression, increase in bowel mobility, and decrease in bladder spasms after urologic surgery.

d) *Disadvantages and risks*

- Risk of local anesthetic toxicity
- Respiratory depression if central neuraxial opioids are used
- Urinary retention (common)
- Pruritus (in up to 30% of patients)
- Nausea (rare in this population)
- Catheter migration, resulting in intrathecal, intravascular, or extradural placement (indicators: sudden increase in block density, blood in catheter, or failure to provide analgesia)
- Epidural hematomas and abscesses (rare)

e) *Epidural placement in children*

ANATOMIC DIFFERENCES. In infants, the level of the spinal cord and dural sac are continuously changing up to 1 year of age. In the full-term neonate, the dural sac extends to S3-4, with the spinal cord ending at L4. By 6 months, the dural sac ends at S2 and the spinal cord at about L2-3. At 1 year, the dural sac terminates at about S1, with the cord reaching L1 (adult levels). The line drawn between the iliac crest changes relative to the spine: the line crosses L5-S1 in the neonate, L5 in the older child, and L4-5 in adults.

It is useful to have an idea about the depth of the epidural space in children, especially because the ligaments are less dense and provide a feel that is different from that of the adult ligaments. A useful formula to approximate depth (in millimeters) of the epidural space in children is as follows:

Infant: depth (mm) = 1.5 × weight (kg)
Child: depth (mm) = 1 × weight (kg)

TECHNIQUES. The epidural space is located outside the dural sac. A needle or catheter may be placed in this space at the appropriate dermatomal level to inject or infuse local anesthetics, opioids, or other medications. Epidural catheters may be placed via several routes. It is possible to position the catheter either by inserting it at the appropriate dermatomal level without threading or, in small children, by threading the catheter up the epidural space to the desired location.

For caudal epidural injections, the needle is inserted between the sacral cornua at the base of the sacrum, and if a catheter is used, this is threaded into the caudal canal. The caudal epidural space is contiguous with the lumbar epidural space, and catheters can usually be threaded upward in the epidural space. In infants and young children, catheters can usually be threaded to any level desired. In older children, it still may be possible to thread epidural catheter several vertebral levels above the insertion site. In fact, it is common practice to place all epidurals in young children at the caudal or lumbar (not the thoracic) level, threading upward if necessary. This is because epidural catheters are usually placed under general anesthesia (or deep sedation) in young children and asleep thoracic epidural placement is considered unsafe because of the proximity of the spinal cord to the epidural space at this level.

f) *Managing epidural infusions*

CHOICE OF MEDICATION. The selection of dosage and drug used in epidural infusions depends on the surgery, the site of the surgery, the age of the child, and comorbidity, although standard infusions work well in most cases. Epidural opioids are avoided or used with caution in infants and children at risk (e.g., those with pulmonary dysfunction or developmental delay).

The infusion is normally started at a standard rate (0.2 to 0.3 mL/kg if the catheter tip is below T10; 0.1 to 0.2 mL/kg if the catheter tip is above T10), and titrated upward as needed. The standard infusion for use in infants and young children (3 months to 5 years) at MGH consists of 0.1% bupivacaine with 2 µg/mL fentanyl. We use plain 0.1% bupivacaine in neonates (<3 months) and 0.1% bupivacaine with 20 µg/mL hydromorphone in older children (>5 years). Figure 3 in Chapter 21 shows the standard epidural order sheet used at MGH. Occasionally, if analgesia is inadequate, the concentration and/or volume of infusate may need to be adjusted.

If a child leaves the operating room with inadequate analgesia, a bolus injection will be needed before beginning the infusion. The bolus can be a local anesthetic or a standard epidural mix. If this initial bolus is needed, it is acceptable to give either lidocaine or bupivacaine at 0.05 mL/kg per spinal segment. It is important not to exceed a dose of 5 mg/kg of lidocaine or 2.5 mg/kg of bupivacaine. If the analgesia is expected to cover a large range of dermatomes, a more dilute solution may be needed to ensure that the local anesthetic fills the epidural space without toxicity.

GENERAL CARE. The standard of care when providing epidural analgesia for children is similar to that given to adults:

- 24-hour anesthesia coverage for patients receiving epidural analgesia
- Ventilatory status monitored and recorded hourly
- Vital signs monitored and recorded every 4 hours
- Pain service evaluation daily, including check of neurologic status

- Daily examination of the catheter site for signs of inflammation or infection
- Low threshold for more intensive monitoring in children less than 6 months old (considered at risk of ventilatory depression)
- Heels padded to prevent pressure sores
- No systemic opioids given while receiving epidural opioids

g) *Treatment of side effects and complications*

Local anesthetic toxicity is rare in the postoperative setting. If it occurs, it should be treated as described in Chapter 37. Sensory or motor changes are common after injection of local anesthetics but are not expected when low-dose (0.1%) bupivacaine is used. The abnormal neurologic examination may indicate residual block from surgery, migration of the catheter to one side or one nerve root, catheter irritation, or, more sinisterly, impending epidural hematoma or abscess. In most cases, recovery occurs when the dose of infusate is reduced, the catheter is pulled back, or the treatment is stopped.

The cardinal signs of epidural hematoma or abscess are back pain and sensory or motor weakness. These symptoms and signs should always prompt withdrawal of treatment, close monitoring, and possible investigation with magnetic resonance imaging. Surgical decompression is the only way to prevent permanent neurologic damage.

Epidural opioid side effects include pruritus, nausea and vomiting, urinary retention, and respiratory depression. Treatment is summarized in Table 5. Respiratory depression is the most serious of these complications. Lipophilic agents such as fentanyl are less likely to cause respiratory depression than the more hydrophilic opioids (especially morphine), but vigilance is still required (see Chapter 21).

Treatment is the administration of oxygen, ventilatory support if necessary, stopping of the epidural infusion, and naloxone (2 μg/kg IV). It is also possible that catheter migration could have occurred, resulting in an intrathecal infusion. Pruritus is treated with diphenhydramine (Benadryl), 0.5 mg/kg, or low-dose naloxone (Narcan), 0.5 to 1 μg/kg. Nausea is treated with ondansetron, 0.1 mg/kg, or droperidol, 0.01 to 0.025 mg/kg 6 hourly.

(ii) Spinals

Spinal anesthesia is capable of providing good postoperative analgesia for several hours after surgery. This can be prolonged by injecting a bolus dose of opioid with the local anesthetic. Spinal anesthesia and analgesia are most commonly used in neonates, in

Table 5.   Adjuncts in pediatric acute pain management

Drug	Indication	Dose
Naloxone	Respiratory depression	2 μg/kg
Naloxone	Pruritus	0.5–1 μg/kg
Benadryl	Pruritus	0.5 mg/kg
Ondansetron	Nausea	0.1 mg/kg
Droperidol	Nausea	0.01–0.025 mg/kg

whom the risk of apnea and bradycardia after general anesthesia is highest. The space chosen is L4-5, since there is a risk of injuring the spinal cord if a higher space is used. In the neonate, the doses of local anesthetic are higher than they would be for an older child or adult, and the duration of action is shorter than in the older patient.

Hyperbaric bupivacaine and tetracaine are the most commonly used agents. A single injection of an opioid (most commonly preservative-free morphine, Duramorph) into the spinal fluid prolongs the analgesia (12 to 24 hours or more) despite the small dose (2 to 10 µg/kg), but this is reserved for older children (>5 years). There is little or negligible systemic absorption, but respiratory depression is liable to occur because of the passage of morphine to higher centers in the cerebrospinal fluid.

(iii) Other techniques

Peripheral nerve blocks provide anesthesia and analgesia in the early postoperative period and are often chosen for this reason. Useful blocks in children include ilioinguinal, femoral, penile, brachial plexus, and lumbar plexus blocks. Occasionally, catheters are inserted so that the block can be prolonged further. EMLA cream (a eutectic mixture of local anesthetic, lidocaine, and prilocaine) has proved very useful in children to numb the skin before needling, and even to provide postoperative pain relief (e.g., after circumcision). Other topical local anesthetic preparations are occasionally useful (e.g., lidocaine gel for mucus membranes).

4. Nonpharmacologic techniques

Nonpharmacologic techniques are adjuncts to analgesic medications that can be used to help ease a child's discomfort or anxiety level associated with pain or painful procedures. They work best when the patient and family are introduced to the particular technique and are offered the opportunity to actively participate.

Cognitive approaches

Education has been shown to be effective in children, especially when preoperative teaching has been conducted. Children are also excellent at developing pain-controlling strategies that involve imagination.

Distraction may be useful in all age groups but needs to be age specific. Attention is focused on stimuli other than the pain sensation. Distraction can be very effective with children for brief episodic pain such as that associated with drain removal. To be effective, the distraction must be interesting to the patient and consistent with the developmental level, energy level, and capability of the child, and it must stimulate major sensory modalities (hearing, vision, touch, movements). Some examples for specific ages are as follows:

- Toddler/preschooler: blowing bubbles, singing, music cassettes, pop-up books, "I Spy" books
- School age/adolescent: music or story via headset, singing or tapping rhythm, conversation

Cutaneous stimulation

Massage or rubbing the skin may be very soothing but is generally not recommended for premature or full-term neonates. The application of heat or cold is often useful for localized pain. Transcutaneous electric nerve stimulation (TENS) can also be used (see Chapter 16).

Guided imagery

This uses the patient's own imagination to develop sensory images to decrease the pain, make it more acceptable, or change it into a different sensation that is less intense—for example, throwing pain away like a snowball, blowing pain away, or imagining the medication traveling through the body to relieve the pain.

Distraction

For example, tell a story in which the child can be actively involved. Utilize the child's favorite place or fictional character and include the child as part of the story. Ask questions to keep the child engaged.

Relaxation

These techniques are used to decrease anxiety and skeletal muscle tension, potentially relieving some of the mental and physical effects of pain. Techniques include breathing exercises, progressive relaxation, remembering past peaceful experiences, and, in infant and toddlers, the use of pacifiers and stroking.

IV. CONCLUSION

The increase in concern and improvement in pain therapies for children is a welcome and much-needed improvement in the medical care of children. Further advances in education, research, and knowledge will allow us to apply the lessons learned in adults to the benefit of our pediatric patients. It is incumbent on all anesthesiologists and other caregivers to consider pain and analgesia at every juncture in the process of caring for children.

ACKNOWLEDGEMENT

The authors gratefully acknowledge the help of Dr. Michael Girshin and Dr. David B. Kaplan, Fellows in pediatric anesthesia at New England Medical Center.

SELECTED READING

1. Ashburn M, Rice L, eds. *Management of pain.* New York: Churchill Livingstone, 1998.
2. Berde CB, Sethna NF, Levin L, et al. Regional analgesia on pediatric medial and surgical wards. *Intensive Care Med* 1989;15 (suppl 1):S40–43.
3. Carr DB. Acute pain management: Operative or medical procedures and trauma. In: *Clinical practice guideline.* AHCPR Pub No 92-0032. Rockville, MD: Agency for Health Care Policy and Research, Public Health Service, U.S. Department of Health and Human Services, 1992.
4. Dalens B, ed. *Regional anesthesia in infants, children and adolescents.* London: Williams & Wilkins, 1995.
5. Krechel SW, Bildner J. CRIES: A new neonatal postoperative pain measurement score. Initial testing of validity and reliability. *Paediatr Anaesth* 1995;5:53–61.
6. Lloyd-Thomas AR. Pain management in paediatric patients. *Br J Anaesth* 1990;64:85–104.

7. McKenzie IM, Gaukroger PB, Ragg PG, Brown TCK, eds. *Manual of acute pain management in children*. Melbourne: Churchill Livingstone, 1997.
8. Yaster M, ed. Acute pain in children. *Pediatr Clin North Am* 2000;47:487–755.
9. Zwass M, Polaner D, Berde C. Postoperative pain management. In: Cote CJ, Todres ID, Ryan JF, Goudsouzian NG, eds. *A practice of anesthesia for infants and children*. Philadelphia: WB Saunders, 2001:675–697.

Pain in Burn Patients

Salahadin Abdi and Bucknam J. McPeek

There is physical pain, there is mental pain and scarring. You can see the outside, but what a lot of people don't see is that we are truly burned on the inside as well.
—*Burn survivor*

More than 2 million burn injuries occur annually in the United States: thermal burns are the most prevalent, and chemical and electrical burns occur less commonly. Approximately 1 in 20 burn patients requires extended hospitalization. Burn injury results in both physical and psychological distress, and pain is a major component of both. In fact, burns are among the most painful of all injuries. Pain evaluation and treatment is an important aspect of the care of patients inflicted with burn injuries.

The management of acute and chronic burn pain is challenging and may require input from an experienced pain specialist. A careful pain management plan helps circumvent potential hazards in these often critically ill and psychologically disturbed patients. It is important to be attentive to the specific type of pain the patient is experiencing, as well as to the risks of pain treatment in relation to the pathophysiology of the injured patient. The likelihood of the development of chronic pain and life-long suffering (e.g., chronic pain, post-traumatic stress disorder) can be reduced by appropriate and aggressive acute pain management, with meticulous attention to psychological and social factors. The purpose of this chapter is to outline the essential issues so that proper planning and care can be provided.

I. TYPES OF BURN INJURY

The extent of a burn injury is measured as the percentage of body surface area burned. Burns vary in depth from superficial to full thickness, with a possibility of massive destruction of muscle and bone in the latter.

In **first-degree burns,** the injury is superficial, characterized by erythema, and it involves only the epidermis. There is usually only mild to moderate discomfort, and healing occurs within a week.

Second-degree burns are deeper, partial-thickness injuries that destroy the epidermis and variable amounts of dermis as well as epidermal appendages. Second-degree burns are extremely painful. Most of the pain is the result of the damage of sensory nociceptive receptors that are preferentially sensitive to tissue damage. In addition to direct damage from the burn, second-degree burns leave the protective layer of skin damaged, and the normally protected nerve endings exposed. These lesions heal slowly with some tissue contraction, nerve regeneration, and the occasional need for skin grafting.

Third-degree burns destroy the skin completely. They are, by definition, full-thickness injuries. Regions of third-degree burns may be painless after the initial injury for a period because of the destruction of cutaneous nociceptors. Although the central part of the initial wound may be analgesic, painful areas of second-degree injury surround almost every third-degree burn. These areas heal by epidermal regeneration, since some of the epidermal appendages remain intact, and this healing process can be painful. With inadequate cleansing and debridement, a surface pseudomembrane composed of wound exudate and necrotic eschar accumulates. As long as the eschar and pseudomembrane exist, the center of a third-degree burn is painless. The eschar is usually removed surgically since the unremoved eschar and membrane serve as a nidus for infection (the major life-threatening factor in burn injury). It is important to emphasize that patients with third degree burns suffer severe pain needing treatment despite some areas of the burn being analgesic.

II. TYPES OF BURN PAIN

There are two categories of pain:

First, **procedural pain (incidental or evoked)** is pain experienced during or after wound care, stent removal, dressing change, physical therapy, or other treatments. This type of pain is usually acute and short lasting but of great intensity. Debridement usually requires general anesthesia. It is helpful to administer an adequate and appropriately timed dose of narcotic and/or benzodiazepine before beginning any procedure.

Second, **background pain (spontaneous or resting or constant)** is pain experienced by the patient while at rest. This type of pain is usually dull, continuous, and of lower intensity. Nevertheless, this low-intensity pain should be controlled or it may prime patients to experience more pain, as well as increasing their anxiety, particularly about procedures. Background pain is best treated with regularly administered opioids (or alternative analgesics), not on an as-needed basis.

In addition, there are two temporal components of burn pain, acute and chronic. Immediately after the burn, the most severe pain results from therapeutic procedures such as dressing changes. Background pain may persist for weeks to months or even years. Pain related to burn injury might worsen with time as a result of several factors, including increased anxiety and depression, continuing sleep disturbance, and deconditioning and regeneration of nerves endings (possible neuroma formation, known as post-burn neuralgia). Chronic pain may result from contractures, nerve injury (neuropathic pain), or subsequent nerve and tissue damage following surgical procedures.

III. ACUTE TREATMENT FOR BURN PAIN

The main treatment goal for serious burns is to clean the burn area by debridement or surgical excision, thus removing necrotic tissue and other sources of infection. Microorganisms that release exotoxins and endotoxins exacerbate the inflammation already present in burns and quickly colonize retained necrotic tissue. After removal of necrotic tissue by cleaning or surgical excision, the next step is to promote coverage of the open wound wherever possible by a skin graft from unburned areas of the patient's own body. In large burns, allografts, xenografts, or artificial skin can provide temporary coverage.

Patients suffer continual shifts, from mild to moderate background discomfort to excruciating pain associated with treatments such as burn dressing changes, manual debridement of open wounds, and physical therapy. In addition, there are frequent surgical operations, excisions of eschar, and harvesting of large areas of normal skin for grafting (also a source of pain). Burn dressing changes and debridements may occur twice a day, physical therapy once or twice a day, and surgical interventions several times a week. Because of the variation in the intensity of pain from hour to hour or even minute to minute, burn pain treatment for patients suffering from acute burns requires repeated assessments and titration of analgesic drugs for treatment. Patients typically require increasing amounts of opioid medication for the control of pain during these procedures as they become tolerant to the opioid (Chapter 30).

The interpretation and assessment of pain behavior in these patients can be very difficult. The pain is often superimposed by anxiety. Giving the patient a role in the pain management helps to alleviate the anxiety. An honest explanation about procedure-related pain and how it can be relieved is a necessary prerequisite to being able to develop a plan with the patient. The following are treatment options for burn-related pain.

1. Acetaminophen

Acetaminophen is a weak analgesic and antipyretic. It is a useful first-line treatment for minor burns, but it can also be used as an adjunct to opioids for major burns. Because this drug acts mainly centrally, it is not associated with the typical nonsteroidal anti-inflammatory (NSAID) side effects that are produced by prostaglandin inhibition in the periphery. Acetaminophen is not useful for long-term pain management because of its toxic and cumulative effects on the liver (see Chapter 8).

2. Nonsteroidal anti-inflammatory drugs

NSAIDs reduce inflammation and pain. They may be used as sole analgesics for mild to moderate pain or as adjuncts to more potent analgesics. Side effects, specifically gastrointestinal (GI) bleeding, may limit their use in seriously burned patients, who are particularly susceptible to GI bleeding. If used, prophylaxis should be given with a prostaglandin analog (e.g., misoprostol) or H_2 blockers (e.g., ranitidine). (Cave: DO NOT give a high dose of an NSAID as a substitution for opioids in the management of procedural pain.) A full description of the NSAIDs and their uses is provided in Chapter 8.

3. Opioids

Opioids (see Chapter 9) are the mainstay of treatment for severe acute pain, and various routes of administration have been described and tested for burn patients. Morphine is the most widely used drug in burn centers. Hydromorphone (Dilaudid) is useful in patients who have intolerable side effects to morphine, or who are morphine sensitive. Meperidine is not recommended because of the toxicity of its metabolite normeperidine. Continuous fentanyl infusion tends to cause the rapid development of tolerance with a resultant need for high dosage, but bolus fentanyl administration is sometimes useful for procedures such as burn dressing changes. High-dose fentanyl, however, can produce chest wall rigidity and should not be used in self-ventilating patients in whom muscle relaxants cannot be used to overcome the rigidity. Methadone can also be used, and it has the advantage of having *N*-**methyl**-D-**aspartate** (NMDA) receptor antagonist activity, which, theoretically at least, could be important in the prevention of neuropathic pain. In patients who are fed by mouth, a bowel regimen should be initiated with the initiation of opioids.

For most burn patients, probably the best mode of administration of opioids is intravenous patient-controlled analgesia (PCA) (see Chapter 21). This technique allows patients to self-administer the drug, usually morphine or hydromorphone. This eliminates the dependency of patients on nurses, and it provides a means of receiving immediate relief when needed. Most patients, even children as young as 6 or 7 years, can learn to control pain using PCA. Younger children, or adults who cannot push a button, may require a continuous infusion of opioid, at least during the acute phase. The onset of analgesia after an intravenous morphine bolus is approximately 6 to 10 minutes, so patients can pretreat themselves or be pretreated by a physician or nurse before painful therapeutic procedures. When patients have significant background pain, they may require a basal infusion in addition to demand doses.

4. Ketamine

Ketamine is an atypical anesthetic and a potent analgesic that is an NMDA receptor antagonist. It induces a dissociative anesthetic state. It can be used for both anesthesia and analgesia in burn patients. The main advantages of ketamine over the opioids are that spontaneous ventilation and airway reflexes are preserved, and the cardiovascular system is stimulated secondary to induced catecholamine release. Ketamine anesthesia is commonly associated with unpleasant postanesthesia phenomena such as vivid nightmares and hallucinations, which can be minimized by the concomitant use of a benzodiazepine. These effects are rarely associated with the subanesthetic doses that are used for analgesia. Ketamine should be used with an antisialagogue such as atropine or glycopyrrolate.

5. Antihistamines

Antihistamines are used in the burn center for the management of anxiety, itch, and pain (adjunctive effect). These drugs potentiate opioid analgesia and have a useful antipruritic effect, as the pruritus in burn patients is sometimes worse than the pain, especially in the healing phase of the injury. They are also useful to promote sleep and relieve anxiety.

6. Regional anesthesia

Regional anesthesia can be used for analgesia or even anesthesia if the burn wound is limited and accessible for a regional anesthesia technique. Epidural and spinal anesthesia and analgesia are relatively contraindicated in seriously ill patients with hypotension or sepsis.

7. General anesthesia

General anesthesia is sometimes needed for minor procedures if pain is severe and cannot be adequately and safely controlled in the awake patient.

IV. CHRONIC TREATMENT OF BURN PAIN

Unfortunately, the pain experience for burn patients often does not end after the acute phase, and many patients continue to have chronic pain even after complete wound healing. It is sometimes necessary to use chronic opioid therapy to maintain a reasonable level of comfort for these unfortunate patients, and it may be necessary to add adjuvant pain medications for the specific treatment of neuropathic pain. As already stated, the NSAIDs and acetaminophen are less suitable for long-term pain therapy. Issues of opioid therapy in chronic nonmalignant pain (CNMP) are discussed in Chapter 30. A description of neuropathic pain and its treatment can be found in Chapter 25. The most intractable cases should be referred to a pain clinic. Many of these patients need nonpharmacologic as well as pharmacologic treatment, and a multidisciplinary approach (including behavioral therapy, physical therapy, and occupational therapy) is optimal.

V. NONPHARMACOLOGIC TREATMENTS FOR BURN PAIN

Burn patients need psychological support in both the acute and chronic phases of burn treatment. Burn survivors frequently suffer fear, depression, nightmares, and hallucinations. Psychosocial support is as necessary as pharmacologic intervention (e.g., anxiolytic and antidepressants). Burn injury results not only in short-term changes and severe acute pain but also in chronic pain, long-term changes in health status, and often distressing permanent disfigurement. There are many psychological interventions that can be helpful to burn patients, including hypnosis, relaxation, and biofeedback. These techniques are described in Chapter 15.

VI. CONCLUSION

In summary, the pain experienced by burn patients is often excruciating and unrelenting, an unwelcome accompaniment to an already devastating injury. The management of these patients' pain can be extremely challenging and demands expertise and experience. It is important to choose the right modality (or combination of modalities) with the aim of adequately controlling background as well as procedural pain. It is equally important to consider the psychological aspects of the pain, and to provide psychosocial as well as pharmacologic support. An interdisciplinary team approach is the key to successful pain management.

SELECTED READINGS

1. Atchison NE, Osgood PF, Carr DB, Szyfelbein SK. Pain during burn dressing change in children: Relationship to burn area, depth, and analgesic regimens. *Pain* 1991;47;41–45.
2. Carr DB, Osgood PF, Szyfelbein SK. Treatment of pain in acutely burned children. In: Schechter NL, Berde CB, Yaster M, eds. *Pain in infants, children, and adolescents.* Baltimore: Williams & Wilkins, 1993.
3. Choiniere M, Auger FA, Latarjet J. Visual analogue thermometer: A valid and useful instrument for measuring pain in burned patients. *Burns* 1994;20:229–235.
4. Choiniere M, Grenier R, Paquette C. Patient-controlled analgesia: A double-blind study in burn patients. *Anesthesia* 1992;47;467–472.
5. Dauber A, Carr DB, Breslau A. Burn survivors' pain experiences: A questionnaire-based survey. Presented at the 7th World Congress on Pain, International Association for the Study of Pain, Paris, 1993.
6. Herman RA, Veng-Pederson P, Miotto J, Komorowski J. Pharmacokinetics of morphine sulfate in patients with burns. *Burn Care Rehabil* 1994;15:95–103.
7. Osgood PF, Szyfelbein SK. Management of pain. In: Martyn JAJ. ed. *Acute management of the burned patient.* Philadelphia: WB Saunders, 1990.
8. Perry S, Heidrich G. Management of pain during debridement: A survey of U.S. burn units. *Pain* 1982;13;267–280.

Pain Management in Sickle Cell Disease

Jatinder S. Gill

Pain is not just a symptom demanding our compassion; it can be an aggressive disease that damages the nervous system.
—*Gary Bennett*

Sickle cell disease is an inherited hemoglobinopathy primarily affecting individuals descending from equatorial Africa, around the Mediterranean Sea, Saudi Arabia, and some parts of India. It is a multisystem, chronic, debilitating disease with variable phenotypic expression. Acute pain is often the first symptom and the most common reason patients seek medical attention.

One third of the patients enjoy a benign course, one third have two to six hospital admissions for pain per year, and one third have more than six pain-related hospitalizations per year. Hospital personnel often develop biased views about the genuine nature of painful crises in the latter group, especially since pain is a subjective sensation. It is, however, this group that is most in need of medical help. The extreme variability in severity of clinical phenotype remains unexplained and probably relates to genetic, microvascular, rheologic, and hematologic factors.

I. PATHOPHYSIOLOGY

Hemoglobin S (HbS) has a tendency to polymerize when deoxygenated but rapidly reverts with oxygenation. Repeated cycles of polymerization cause oxidative damage to the red cell membrane and lead to irreversibly sickled cells, adhesion to the endothelium of the vessel, and vascular occlusion. The resultant hypoxia causes further sickling and starts a vicious cycle leading to tissue infarction and pain. Increased intramedullary pressure secondary to inflammation and necrosis within the bone is an important cause of the pain. Sickling seems to correlate directly with high hemoglobin levels and neutrophil counts, and indirectly with fetal hemoglobin (HbF) values.

II. CLINICAL FEATURES AND CONTEMPORARY MANAGEMENT

Sickle cell disease is a multisystem disease. Infants and children are at risk for overwhelming infection from encapsulated bacteria such as *Pneumococcus*. The function of the spleen, and therefore immune function, is deficient even before the eventual autoinfarction. Penicillin prophylaxis, vaccination, and a high index of suspicion are advocated. Meningitis, bacterial pneumonias, cholecystitis, and osteomyelitis are common in adults.

Sickle cell patients are chronically anemic, and profound anemia may occur in the setting of splenic sequestration, exaggerated hemolysis, or aplastic crisis requiring transfusion. Folic acid supplementation is required to support high turnover rates.

Neurologic complications resulting from cerebrovascular occlusion occur in up to 25% of patients. A schedule of monthly transfusions is recommended for children to prevent recurrent stroke. Primary prevention using magnetic resonance imaging and transcranial Doppler screening and initiation of transfusion programs for at-risk patients have been suggested.

These patients often have restrictive lung disease, hypoxemia, and pulmonary hypertension, probably secondary to past pulmonary occlusions and infarctions. They are at risk for acute chest syndrome, with infection usually due to atypical agents. Acute chest syndrome has a high mortality and requires treatment in the intensive care setting. A high index of suspicion is required in patients presenting with chest pain and fever, especially in the presence of hypoxemia.

Hepatobiliary complications are common, with up to 70% of patients demonstrating gallstones. Many patients eventually need a cholecystectomy. Hepatic dysfunction may relate to transfusion-associated iron overload or infection. Hyperbilirubinemia secondary to benign cholestasis (no fever or pain) should be differentiated from hepatic crisis presenting with fever, pain, abnormal liver function tests, and hepatic failure.

Poor medullary flow in the kidneys leads to papillary infarctions, hematuria, and renal tubular acidosis. In addition, patients may develop glomerular dysfunction. Proximal tubular dysfunction may lead to hyperuricemia especially in the setting of heavy analgesic use. These patients eventually develop chronic renal failure.

Proliferative sickle cell retinopathy with the potential of bleeding leading to blindness should be appropriately treated with laser photocoagulation.

Priapism develops in many individuals, and if prolonged it may lead to impotence. If this is poorly responsive to conservative treatment for 12 hours, exchange transfusions, corporal aspiration, the use of alpha-adrenergic agents, and even surgical creation of fistula may be required to prevent impotence.

Osteonecrosis, leading to vertebral fractures or necrosis of the femoral head, can be acutely painful. In patients with advanced disease of the joints who fail to rehabilitate, major reconstructive surgery may be required. Bone marrow infarction may be differentiated from osteomyelitis by scans. Arthritis may result from periarticular infarction or from gout. Nonsteroidal anti-inflammatory drugs (NSAIDs) are useful adjuncts in patients with bone pain.

Chronic bilateral leg ulcers are common over the shins. In addition to causing chronic pain, these may also lead to osteomyelitis and septicemia. Subdermal vascular occlusions can lead to chronic myofascial pain.

Mean life expectancy is about 42 years in men and 48 years in women. Patients with severe disease and multiple crises tend to have a shorter lifespan.

III. ACUTE PAIN CRISIS

Despite the multiple problems associated with sickle cell disease, the most common reason for these patients to be hospitalized is for an acute pain crisis requiring aggressive inpatient management. The usual precipitants are exposure to cold, dehydration, alcohol intake, infections, stress, and menstruation. In more than half the cases, there is no clear cause of the pain.

About 5% of patients account for one third of hospital admissions, and regrettably, caregiver hostility toward this group of patients is common. It is important to remember that these are the patients who tend to die young, and pain is a direct marker for mortality. The incidence of pain is highest in young male adults.

Pain typically affects one region of the body. Common sites of pain include the back, bilateral large joints, chest, sternum, ribs, and abdomen. In children, the smaller joints of the hand and feet may be involved. In about half the patients, fever is present. Patients are usually able to tell whether a new crisis feels like their typical crisis.

The cause of the pain is probably related to ischemia of the tissue undergoing infarction and an increase in intramedullary pressure due to inflammation. The pain of sickle cell disease is often described as excruciating, commonly rating more than nine on the visual analog scale. It is important to rule out any catastrophic events, being alert for acute chest syndrome in a patient with acute chest pain, osteomyelitis or septic arthritis in a patient with bone or joint pain, or acute abdomen in a patient with abdominal pain. Further workup may be needed (e.g., chest films in a dyspneic patient with chest pain, diagnostic aspiration of an acutely tender joint). A good history and a physical, together with a review of previous admissions, are indispensable.

1. Management of mild vaso-occlusive crisis

Old admissions records, previous treatments, complications of the disease, and baseline pain medications are very helpful in directing treatment. Once it has been established that the patient does not require emergent investigation or intervention, aggressive hydration and pain treatment should be instituted. Fluids may be taken by mouth or given intravenously. Opioid medication may be given by mouth if tolerated, but the intravenous (IV) route is usually preferable at least in the initial period. For oral use, oxycodone, hydromorphone, and morphine are good choices. NSAIDs are very useful for bone pain and should be freely used if no contraindications exist. For the latter, a fixed dose regime is preferable to an as-needed regimen.

If the patient can be stabilized, he or she may be discharged home with a tapering supply of oral opioids. Failure to adequately manage pain is likely to result in readmission, so it is important that the patient be provided with an adequate supply of analgesics. If the pain does not improve, or if the patient has other symptoms (e.g., fever or severe nausea), a longer hospital admission may be required.

2. Hospital management of painful sickle cell crisis

(i) Opioids

The pain of sickle cell crisis is described as excruciating, and narcotics are often the first-line treatment. There is no benefit to trying alternative analgesics before opioids in the acute situation. Adjuncts may, however, be used simultaneously.

The care team must take patient reports of pain seriously and administer medications in a timely manner. This fosters trust in the patient and prevents undue suffering.

a) *Route of administration*

Opioids may be given orally if tolerated, but in most situations parenteral narcotics are needed in the initial stages. In patients with chronic pain using opioids on a long-term basis, the baseline (chronically used) medications can be continued to provide continuous background analgesia, supplemented with the regimen chosen to treat the acute episode. Alternatively, the chronic analgesic requirement can be given intravenously after calculating the equivalent IV dose, further supplemented with additional medication to cover the acute pain. Transdermal fentanyl can be used in the later stages of the crisis, but in the initial acute setting, slow onset and difficulty with titration make this a poor choice.

Traditionally, these patients have been treated with intramuscular injections of meperidine and hydroxyzine (Vistaril). However, in light of the improved understanding of meperidine toxicity, and the ease with which IV therapy can be used, there is very little rationale for continuing to recommend this treatment. Intramuscular injections should probably be reserved for situations where there is no IV access, or before IV access is obtained. Intramuscular injections are painful and may lead to myositis and abscesses; in addition, the rate of drug absorption is unpredictable.

Intravenous narcotics can be given by continuous infusion, by nurse-administered bolus injection, or by using a patient-controlled analgesia (PCA) pump. Patient-controlled analgesia is a very attractive option in the acute management of sickle cell crisis, and it is probably the treatment of choice. Unfortunately, it is not widely available and may not be an option in some settings. Patients can be maintained on a safe low basal rate of opioid, especially at night, and demand doses titrated to comfort and safety.

b) *Choice of opioid*

Morphine and hydromorphone are the first-line narcotic agents. Hydromorphone may be preferred in patients with renal dysfunction because morphine-6-glucuronide, an active metabolite of morphine, may accumulate in renal failure. Formerly, meperidine was considered the opioid of choice in sickle cell patients, but it should no longer be used as a first-line opioid (see Chapter 9). However, some patients tolerate other opioids poorly and prefer meperidine. In these patients, it is reasonable to consider meperidine but with due caution for its potential toxicity (especially in patients with renal involvement and seizure disorder) and its potential for producing addiction.

Narcotics often give rise to adverse side effects such as nausea, itching, and sedation. Different medications and dosing intervals may be tried to get the best match in terms of side-effect profile. Side effects should be treated with appropriate medications such antiemetics and psychostimulants.

c) *Weaning*

The typical crisis last for about 4 to 7 days and its course is often unpredictable. However, some patients with a typical crisis may repeat the course of their last crisis. As pain improves, the demand for analgesics and reports of pain decrease. At this point, the patient may be switched to an oral regimen. The total IV dose used by the patient over the last 24 hours is measured, then converted to an equivalent oral dose (using an approximately 1:3 ratio; see Table 2, Appendix VIII). Other routes could also be chosen at this point, including rectal and transdermal. The dose is gradually reduced, as tolerated.

For a successful change from parenteral to oral narcotics, it is critical (a) that a plan be individualized for the patient and (b) that an adequate amount of medication be prescribed. Prompt attention to the patient's reports of pain at this juncture will go a long way toward achieving a successful weaning.

d) *Tolerance and addiction*

Tolerance to narcotics is a well-known and poorly understood phenomenon. It usually develops over weeks, but acute tolerance in the setting of high doses can also occur. The analgesic effects as well as the sedative and respiratory depressant effects of these medications are decreased. Thus these patients may require high doses of narcotics to achieve adequate pain control. This phenomenon should not be interpreted as addictive behavior.

Sickle cell patients are also at risk of withdrawal if their narcotic regimen is abruptly discontinued. Reducing opioid dose by no more than 20% per day prevents withdrawal in most individuals. If a withdrawal syndrome does occur, it can be reversed by reintroducing the opioid at 25% to 40% of the original dose.

The term *addiction* is employed when medication is used primarily for its mind-altering effects and not for its intended analgesic effect. Addiction is a behavioral problem, and addicted patients always display compulsive drug-seeking behavior that is distinct from the drug-seeking behavior of patients in pain (see Chapter 35). Sickle cell patients are not more prone to addiction than any other group of patients. The incidence of addiction in the opioid-treated population as a whole, and in the sickle cell population, ranges from 2% to 3%. Wrongly assuming addiction in sickle cell patients plays a negative role in effectively treating their pain.

The occasional addicted patient provides a challenge in pain management. On one hand, the need for the opioid medication is clear, but on the other hand the patient is likely to abuse his medication. Management is greatly helped by clear communication, avoiding conflict, a reasonable amount of limit setting, and the involvement of a person who has known the patient for a long time. Acute pain crisis is not the time for initiating detoxification measures.

(ii) Anti-inflammatory drugs

NSAIDs are useful in the treatment of acute crisis, as well as for chronic bone pain. They supplement the opioid analgesia by attacking a different mechanism of pain—that is, by inhibiting prostaglandins at the peripheral level.

Important side effects include decreased platelet adhesiveness (risk of bleeding), renal dysfunction, and gastritis. Ketorolac is available for short-term IV use. These medications are more effective if prescribed as fixed doses and not on an as-needed basis.

The use of steroids is controversial. These drugs may decrease the duration of the episode but can also lead to rebound. Furthermore, their use is complicated by several severe side effects. Hence steroids are not among the first line of drugs in the management of acute crisis.

(iii) Epidural analgesia

Epidural analgesia is a very effective modality for the treatment of pain below the mid-thoracic region. Although it provides excellent regional analgesia, it is not commonly used because adequate analgesia can often be provided by noninterventional techniques. If the pain is widespread, it may not be covered by epidural medication. In a patient with severe pain not responding to parenteral analgesics, epidural anesthesia can be an excellent alternative. Epidural analgesia may also be beneficial in a patient at risk of acute chest syndrome by minimizing systemic medication, respiratory depression, and sedation. Ventilation may be aided with the provision of better analgesia.

(iv) Adjunctive medications

Antihistamines such as hydroxyzine and diphenhydramine (Benadryl) are commonly used in sickle cell patients experiencing pruritus. These medications have been shown to potentiate the analgesic effects of opioids and to increase their sedating effects.

Overall, nausea and vomiting is less a problem in sickle cell patients than in cancer patients. It is often treated with medications such as droperidol, metoclopramide, prochlorperazine, scopolamine, and ondansetron. Ondansetron is a very good choice in a sedated patient because it is free of sedating effects.

Benzodiazepines are used for multiple reasons in sickle cell patients: anxiolysis, sleep induction, myoclonus and muscle spasm, and seizure disorders. Judicious use of these adjuncts is appropriate during an acute episode. They may lead to excessive sedation and inability to properly use PCA. The sedation also limits the amount of opioid that can safely be administered. Alprazolam may induce episodes of mania, hypomania, hostility, and anger.

Analeptics such as methylphenidate (Ritalin) may occasionally be useful in patients experiencing excessive sedation from opioid use.

(v) Other measures

Analgesia and fluid replacement form the cornerstone of the management of acute sickle cell crisis. Fluids may be repleted parenterally or enterally. Although fever is not uncommon during an acute cell crisis, its presence should nevertheless prompt a search for an infective source. These patients remain very vulnerable to infection, and cultures should be done as appropriate. Antibiotics may be used where clinical suspicion of infection is high or in the presence of objective data.

Blood transfusion is restricted to complicated situations such as an acute chest syndrome, a stroke, or a severe and prolonged attack, or if there are frequent recurrent episodes. A hemoglobin level of less than 5 g/dL or a fall of more than 2 g/dL below the baseline may be a rough indication for transfusion. High hematocrit may itself predispose these patients to an acute crisis. Exchange transfusions may be required in the setting of severe, prolonged attack in a patient with a stable hematocrit.

Supplemental oxygen has not been shown to be of any benefit in reducing the pain or the duration of the crisis. This is probably because sickle cell crisis is a vaso-occlusive crisis that has already occurred. Oxygen is, however, essential in a hypoxemic patient.

(vi) Prevention of recurrent crises

Advice on lifestyle (e.g., avoiding extremes of temperature, exercise, and alcohol) may decrease the frequency of these episodes. Patients should be advised to decrease or abstain from smoking, to drink enough fluids on warm days, to wear warm clothing on a cold day, and to obtain early treatment of infections. Medical treatments such as hydroxyurea can significantly lower the incidence of painful crises (see section V, below).

IV. MANAGEMENT OF CHRONIC PAIN

1. Etiology

Some patients with sickle cell experience chronic pain secondary to multiple causes. Their lives revolve around this all-pervasive pain as they go from physician to physician in search of more successful pain relief. Constant pain eventually leads to psychopathology and they are at greater risk for depression. In addition, they have poor prospects for fruitful employment because of the disease-induced physical and emotional impediments. In general, their socioeconomic status is poor at baseline and further complicates their successful rehabilitation.

These patients are too often labeled as drug seekers and difficult patients. It is not difficult to appreciate the reasons for chronic pain in these patients. In the vast majority the pain is of nociceptive origin with diverse causes such as chronic leg ulcers, avascular necrosis of the femur and the humerus, vertebral fractures, chronic osteomyelitis, arthropathies, and constant vaso-occlusive crises.

Neuropathic pain has been very rarely reported in sickle cell patients. Perhaps there is a low incidence of this type of pain in these patients, or more likely, the nociceptive pain is so obvious and the reason so clear that the neuropathic component goes unrecognized. The rich and complex interconnecting blood supply of the nerves may protect them from infarction during a vaso-occlusive crisis. Mental nerve involvement with numbness of the cheek has been most often described in sickle cell patients.

Myofascial pain and fibromyalgia are similarly rarely reported in this group. This may again represent the fact that the predominant nociceptive component overshadows other components.

2. Medications

Since most of the pain in these patients is of nociceptive origin, NSAIDs and opioids are the mainstay of treatment. The medications are preferably prescribed by a single clinic where care is consolidated. Long-term narcotics should be administered using the same principles as for other nonmalignant chronic pain conditions (see Chapter 30). Titration of medications, changes in choice of opioid, and concerns with tolerance and dependence are issues that are best addressed by a single physician or group of physicians. Many sickle cell patients are successfully managed with nonopioid analgesics or with minimal or weak opioids.

Literature regarding the utility of neuropathic pain medications in sickle cell patients is lacking. Anecdotal reports of beneficial effects of tricyclic antidepressants and anticonvulsants warrant trials of these medications in selected patients in combination with other medications. Some conditions such as priapism, seizure disorder, and urine retention in sickle cell patients may contraindicate the use of tricyclics.

Laxatives, antihistaminics, and antiemetics may be required to manage the side effects of medications.

3. Nonpharmacologic interventions

Education goes a long way in helping patients cope with their disease, and in having a compliant patient. Reasonable expectations, knowledge of medications and therapeutic goals, and what to expect from the provider should be clearly explained. Counterirritant measures, such as transcutaneous electrical nerve stimulation (TENS), massage, and heat may be beneficial in selected patients. Intensive physical therapy in a patient with a painful degenerative joint disease helps to ameliorate pain. Biofeedback, coping mechanisms, distraction, and motivation are all valuable adjuncts. Sickle cell patients are poor candidates for interventional pain therapies.

V. NEW THERAPIES

Hydroxyurea is a promising drug that has been shown to reduce the incidence of acute crises by 50%, and it is likely to be more commonly used in the future. Its long-term effects are not clear and therefore warrant close monitoring. Although stem cell transplantation has been used successfully, it carries a 10% risk of periprocedure mortality, and it is largely experimental at present. Gene therapy holds promise but is still elusive. Nitric oxide, by changing the threshold for oxygen dissociation from hemoglobin, can lead to a reversal of sickling during a crisis and is currently being tested.

VI. CONCLUSION

Sickle cell disease is a chronic multisystem disease that subjects a patient to a life of misery and pain. Most patients are socioeconomically disadvantaged, lack good health insurance coverage, and have poor support systems.

Appreciation of the excruciating pain that these patients experience, and prompt treatment based on the patient report are the essence of their pain management. These patients do not have a higher potential for addiction, and pain medications should not be withheld for such concerns. Management of a difficult patient requires tolerance and clear communication. Contact should be established with a physician who knows the patient well.

At the very least, these unfortunate individuals need to be treated with respect, compassion, and extreme patience.

SELECTED READINGS

1. Ballas SK. *Sickle cell pain.* Seattle: IASP Press, 1998.
2. Serjeant GR. Sickle cell disease. *Lancet* 1997;350:725–730.
3. Vijay V, Cavenagh JD, Yate P. The anaesthetist's role in acute sickle cell crisis. *Br J Anaesth* 1998;80:820–828.
4. Yale SH, Nagib N, Guthrie T. Approach to the vaso-occlusive crisis in adults with sickle cell disease. *Am Family Phys* 2000;61: 1349–1356.
5. Yaster M, Kost-Byerly S, Maxwell LG. The management of pain in sickle cell disease. *Pediatr Clin North Am* 2000;47:699–710.

Chronic Pain

IV

Chronic Pain

Neuropathic Pain Syndromes

John D. Markman and
Anne Louise Oaklander

It is evidently impossible to transmit the impression of pain by teaching, since it is only known to those who have experienced it. Moreover, we are ignorant of each type of pain before we have felt it.
—*Galen* (A.D. 129–199)

Neuropathic pain arises from injury to the sensory nervous system. In contrast to acute pain, a beneficial response that safeguards tissue integrity, neuropathic pain is pathologic and can produce devastating disability. It occurs when an abnormal somatosensory system chronically transmits pain signals in the absence of tissue injury. Neuropathic pain syndromes can originate at any point or points along the somatosensory pathways, from the most distal nerve endings in the skin to the somatosensory cortex of the parietal lobe. The cardinal clinical feature of neuropathic pain syndromes is chronic pain associated with abnormalities of sensation.

The causes of neuropathic pain are diverse. In clinical practice, these syndromes are defined by their common symptom pattern, by their neuroanatomic localization, and sometimes by etiology.

The discrepancy between the severity of the pain and the lack of objective evidence of injury or neurologic damage can make these syndromes uniquely disabling. Neuropathic syndromes are perhaps the most formidable treatment challenge for pain specialists.

I. DEFINITIONS AND NOSOLOGY

Acute pain is an adaptive response necessary for the preservation of tissue integrity. The reflexes and emotions induced make it almost impossible *not* to withdraw one's finger from the flame. Loss of normal pain sensation through disease results in potentially life-threatening tissue injuries. *Chronic pain* is different. It is pain that has outlived its usefulness. When pain stems from ongoing tissue damage, as in the arthritides or with tumor-related pain, it is called *nociceptive pain.* The persistent pain is from an intact sensory system that is registering ongoing stimulation.

In *neuropathic pain,* there is sustained transmission of pain signals in the absence of ongoing tissue injury. The primary injury is to the sensory nervous system. Neuropathic pain is *pathologic pain.* This definition is based on the location of the primary pathology, and is independent of its cause. The presence of perturbations of somatosensory function (Fig. 1) hints at the presence of neuropathic pain. Of these, by far the most common is the presence of *numbness,* or hypoesthesia. Patients comment that they paradoxically feel numbness, or decreased sensation, in their area of maximum pain. Pain thresholds can be lowered—*hypoalgesia*—or raised—*hyperalgesia. Paresthesias,* or a pins-and-needles sensation, are a positive sensory phenomenon suggestive of neuropathic

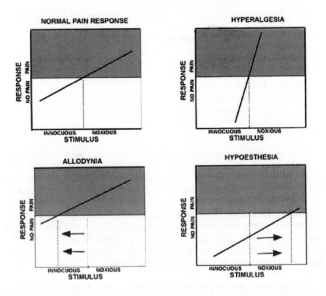

Figure 1. Graphic representation of perturbations of somatosensory function associated with pathologic pain states.

pain. Patients sometimes use the word numbness to describe paresthesias, so the terminology can require discussion.

Some neuropathic pain patients perceive pain from an innocuous stimulus, such as light touch. This aberrant response is *allodynia*. Mechanical allodynia is the greatest handicap, and some patients go to extreme lengths to avoid having their neuropathic area touched (Fig. 2). Pain may be experienced from contact with clothing, bed sheet, or even a breeze. Patients with trigeminal neuralgia may not be able to shave areas of their face, and intraoral allodynic areas can interfere with eating and cause potentially dangerous weight loss or malnutrition. Some women with postherpetic neuralgia (PHN) on the torso are unable to wear a brassiere, and some patients are unable to tolerate wearing clothes over the affected area. Patients with distal painful neuropathies sometimes hang their feet over the edge of their bed to avoid the bedclothes. Many patients describe worsening of their pain in cold weather. This may reflect a component of *cold allodynia*. Cold allodynia interferes with walking barefoot for some, and *warmth allodynia* prompts some patients to carry ice bags or fans to continually cool the painful area.

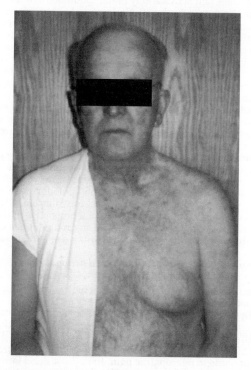

Figure 2.   Some patients go to extreme lengths to avoid having their neuropathic area touched. This man has postherpetic neuralgia and has cut his T-shirt in half because of allodynia.

II. MECHANISMS OF NEUROPATHIC PAIN

Neuropathic pain is associated with abnormalities in the nociceptive neurons that transmit and process pain messages. Identical symptoms can be produced by lesions at different levels of the neuraxis, ranging from the peripheral sensory neurons to the highest levels of cortical processing. It is unequivocal that ongoing neuropathic pain is generated by electrical hyperactivity of neurons along the pain pathways. Unfortunately, it is still unclear where the major site(s) of the electrogenesis are located in the different types of pain syndromes. The impetus for unraveling the complex mechanisms of neuropathic pain is the hope of enabling the development of new classes of medications with greater effectiveness and fewer side effects than those currently available. The following is a brief list of the mechanisms currently thought to contribute to clinical neuropathic pain syndromes. As this is an area of active research, the list is sure to be quickly outdated.

1. Mechanisms involving peripheral neurons

(i) *Primary sensitization of nociceptive nerve endings*

Many (if not most) nociceptors are electrically silent under normal conditions and activate only under conditions of local injury or inflammation (e.g., after burn). Nociceptors have receptors for protons, histamine, bradykinin, and many other inflammatory mediators. Activation of these receptors makes the nociceptor electrically hyperexcitable and induces it to fire after stimuli that would not normally trigger an action potential. Primary sensitization plays a critical role in acute pain by motivating individuals to protect an injured area from further use and potential worsening. It has been conjectured that sustained primary sensitization also contributes to neuropathic pain, but the experimental evidence is weak. It appears likely that peripheral sensitization is much less important for neuropathic than for nociceptive/inflammatory pain.

One area of active investigation is whether sensitivity to molecules released by effector axons contributes to neuropathic pain syndromes. For instance, injured nociceptive nerve endings can develop sensitivity to epinephrine and norepinephrine released by nearby autonomic neurons. The clinical contribution of this phenomenon to pain is not yet clear. Loss of a proportion of the axons innervating a target may alter the local environment in a way that favors abnormal signal transduction by the axons that remain.

(ii) *Ectopically generated or propagated action potentials within damaged nerves*

Normally, the mid axon is insensitive to the stimuli that trigger action potentials in the periphery. In the event that axons are transected by illness or injury, the molecules that transduce sensory action potentials are still inserted into the distal-most portion of the axon, which is now no longer at the periphery. Thus, damaged nerves can acquire the ability to generate ectopic action potentials that contribute to neuropathic pain. In its most florid form, palpable neuromas form. These consist of tangles of axonal sprouts that have not been able to find a distal nerve stump through which to reinnervate their target and are entrapped in connective tissue.

Neuromas can be extremely sensitive to mechanical stimuli. Thus, any pressure or movement can trigger paroxysms of pain. Although some neuromas can be treated medically, some require surgical resection, with burial of the new proximal nerve stump deep in muscle, or in a deeper tissue less likely to be jostled. Occasionally, several surgeries must be performed as new painful neuromas reform.

Even in the absence of a palpable neuroma, injured painful nerves can contain distal ends of axons attempting to regenerate. Neurosurgeons trace the rate of progression of axonal regrowth after a nerve injury by mapping the location of Tinel's sign (painful paresthesias elicited with percussion over the hypersensitive ends of regenerating axons). Occasionally, a pain syndrome that develops after a nerve injury may remit as the hypersensitive axon sprouts finally reach their end-organ target. This can take months or longer because of the slow rate of axonal growth (about 1 mm/day at best). Axonal sprouting varies by disease pathophysiology, so this mechanism does not always play a significant role. Nonneuronal cells such as Schwann cells, macrophages, and mast cells secrete cytokines and other inflammatory mediators that may damage or sensitize axons and contribute to aberrant firing.

(iii) *Abnormal electrogenesis within the sensory ganglia*

The cell bodies of most sensory neurons are another site where it is possible to generate action potentials. Spontaneous potentials have been recorded from healthy neurons, and the frequency of these action potentials increases under conditions of illness and injury. Sensory neuronal cell bodies are exposed to the extraneural environment since most ganglia lack a blood–nerve barrier. Normally, they are protected from mechanical stimuli by their proximal location between the vertebrae. However, it is easy to imagine that they might get compressed under conditions of spinal osteoarthritis or other degenerative conditions.

2. Mechanisms involving central neurons

(i) *Loss of input from peripheral nociceptors into the dorsal horn of the spinal cord*

Some conditions cause frank death of sensory neurons, with degeneration of both the central and the peripheral axons. The most common such condition is shingles, but sensory neuronopathies also occur in autoimmune disease. These conditions eliminate or reduce electrical input from the peripheral sensory neurons into the central nervous system (CNS). Peripheral input can also be lost in diseases that result in truncation of sensory axons (sensory neuropathies). Most distal axonopathies affect the central axon as well as the peripheral one and result in disconnection of the peripheral afferent neuron from its central target. A decrease in peripheral input has a marked impact on the second-order sensory neurons within the spinal and trigeminal dorsal horn, and probably on higher-order neurons as well. Trophic molecules such as nerve growth factor are synthesized in the peripheral tissues, internalized into sensory axons, and transported into the spinal cord, where they profoundly influence the gene expression of these target neurons.

In general, dorsal horn neurons that are deprived of peripheral input become electrically hyperexcitable. They fire spontaneously, and at maximal rates in response to submaximal stimuli. These mechanisms probably evolved to maintain homeostasis under circumstances of mild or moderate loss of peripheral input, but under severe conditions, they contribute to the problem rather than the solution. In its most extreme form, spontaneous activity in deafferented central sensory neurons contributes to phantom limb pain.

(ii) *Ephaptic sprouting within the dorsal horn*

Since neurons abhor a vacuum, when presynaptic inputs from the periphery are lost, other nearby neurons send in sprouts and begin to influence the behavior of the injured central neuron. As remaining peripheral neurons send sprouts into areas vacated by the degenerating axons, the receptive fields of these postsynaptic dorsal horn neurons expand. Stimuli from areas outside the zone of the original injury become capable of eliciting pain. A related mechanism that has been described in animals is the sprouting of peripheral neurons that normally transmit messages of light touch, onto second-order neurons that transmit pain messages. This "mixing" of signals may explain the allodynia (pain triggered by light touch) that is common in neuropathic pain. Since allodynia has also been described after lesions wholly within the brain, this aberrant sprouting may also be possible at centers higher than the dorsal horn.

(iii) *Central sensitization*

Prolonged pain signals arriving from peripheral nociceptors induce molecular changes within even normal dorsal horn projection neurons. There is even some evidence that these "pain memories" can last for years. The contribution of central sensitization to neuropathic pain is hard to assess, since electrical hyperexcitability is also induced by loss of peripheral neurons.

(iv) *Loss of inhibitory interneurons*

Primary sensory neurons influence second-order neurons not only by direct synapses but also indirectly via inhibitory interneurons. These interneurons, which often use gamma-aminobutyric acid (GABA) or glycine as neurotransmitters, are excited by synapses from peripheral sensory neurons, and then form pre- and post-synaptic inhibitory synapses on second-order projection neurons. Since the indirect synaptic pathway involving interneurons is slightly slower than the direct synaptic pathway, the indirect pathway helps bring action potentials of the second-order neurons to a rapid halt. These inhibitory circuits also limit the number of second-order neurons excited by a single primary afferent. There is evidence that these interneurons preferentially die under conditions associated with the development of neuropathic pain. Administration of oral or intrathecal baclofen is an attempt to restore a more normal "inhibitory tone" within the dorsal horn (and potentially higher centers as well).

(iv) *Mechanisms at higher centers*

Much less is known about the more rostral mechanisms of pain. Functional imaging studies have shown that pain is processed in widespread areas of the brain. Ascending pathways from the lateral spinothalamic tract send collaterals to the periacqueductal nuclei of the brain stem before synapsing within the thalamus. Thalamic output radiates widely to the post-central gyrus and anterior cingulate gyrus, as well as other areas of the brain. Central neuropathic pain, originally associated exclusively with the thalamus, has been demonstrated after lesions affecting any part of the central nociceptive pathways. The ventral and posterior portions of the thalamus are particularly involved in pain processing, and electrical hyperexcitability has been demonstrated during recordings from patients with neuropathic pain.

Functional imaging has confirmed that sprouting of neighboring intact neurons into areas vacated by the death of neurons accounts for some of the bizarre features observed in some patients with neuropathic pain. This has best been studied in patients with phantom pain after loss of an innervated body part. For instance, some patients can induce pain in an amputated arm by stroking around their mouth. On the cortical somatosensory homunculus, the mouth area is immediately adjacent to the region that normally receives input from the hand. When innervation from the hand is lost, incoming sensory axons that normally subserve the mouth may sprout into empty synapses within the hand cortex. The finding of these types of phenomena early after injury has suggested that there may be unmasking of normally present but functionally silent synapses.

III. CLINICAL PRESENTATIONS AND SYNDROMES

1. Cardinal clinical features

The clinical spectrum of neuropathic pain ranges from barely noticeable to severely disabling. Certain clinical features are present in many neuropathic pain patients regardless of etiology, mechanism of injury, and location of nerve injury. These features are:

- Ongoing (or stimulus-independent) pain described as "burning," "aching," "crushing," or "gnawing"
- Stimulus-evoked pain (allodynia), especially to mechanical stimuli
- Lancinating pains described as brief severe jolts of pain, sometimes called electrical or lightning pains, which can be spontaneous or stimulus evoked

To some extent, these features are common to almost every clinical pain syndrome. Patients with painful neuropathies may complain most of ongoing pain in the feet, whereas allodynia may be the major concern of a patient with PHN. Trigeminal neuralgia is known for severe lancinating pains, which can be provoked by an allodynic stimulus to a trigger zone on the face. However, questioning will reveal that most patients have also experienced the other cardinal features of neuropathic pain at some time during their illness.

Most of us have transiently experienced mechanical and thermal allodynia after sunburn. Patients with mechanical allodynia go to great lengths to avoid having the affected area touched by other people, bedclothes, or clothing. The allodynia might be so severe as to result in disuse of the affected area. Severe sensory abnormalities frequently occur without visible signs of damage, so patients often find it difficult to convince others of the severity of their disability.

2. Associated clinical features

Although they are not always present, other types of neural damage can occur in these patients. Since different types of neurons are mingled together within the central and peripheral nervous systems, damage the nociceptive pathway can affect other systems as well. Patients with damage to motor pathways can have abnormalities of muscle tone, bulk, and strength. The presence of objective motor signs can be helpful in making the diagnosis of neuropathic, rather than nociceptive, pain. It can be helpful to look for occult motor involvement, for instance, with electromyographic (EMG) examination, if the cause of a patient's pain remains obscure. Increased tone in the affected area is suggestive of a central lesion, such as from stroke, whereas peripheral lesions, such as compressive radiculopathies or nerve injuries, can reduce tone. Sometimes, only minor motor symptoms, such as a tendency to muscle cramps, are present. Of course, disuse of a painful limb can lead to secondary motor changes as well. Occasionally, the motor damage is primary, and the pain is produced by abnormal muscle tone, as in the focal, segmental, or generalized dystonic syndromes.

Autonomic abnormalities are not rare in neuropathic pain syndromes, and they have inspired much confusion and speculation as to their role in the primary pathogenesis of the pain [e.g., sympathetically maintained pain, complex regional pain syndrome I (CRPS-I)]. Fortunately, it is now better appreciated that most neural structures contain autonomic as well as somatic neurons, and that these autonomic fibers are vulnerable to damage by the same lesions that damage the somatic pathways. For instance, a nerve injury that produces CRPS is likely to disrupt the sympathetic fibers that regulate vascular tone that course within the same nerve. Damage to these axons produces changes in color and temperature in the affected tissues, and it can cause swelling due to abnormal leakage of intravascular fluid. Similarly, the growth of skin, hair, nails, and other cutaneous structures can become abnormal if innervation is disrupted.

Patients with painful neuropathies frequently have autonomic damage as well. All such patients should be queried about symptoms such as orthostatic hypotension, impotence, delayed gastric emptying, abnormal sweating and/or thermoregulation, and difficulties with elimination. Occasionally, cardiac arrhythmias are present that require medical or surgical treatment.

IV. SPECIFIC NEUROPATHIC PAIN SYNDROMES

1. Peripheral neuropathic pain syndromes

(i) *Painful polyneuropathies*

The majority of neuropathic pain syndromes affect the peripheral nerves, at least at their onset. Because peripheral nerves contain motor and autonomic fibers, pain is often accompanied by changes in the functions subserved by these components during the course of the syndrome. Motor symptoms typically include weakness and affect the distal muscles, often the extensor groups. Sensory disturbance is confirmed on examination by loss of pinprick, temperature, and vibratory perception. Painful peripheral neuropathies may be classified by etiology, distribution, and pathology. The diagnostic workup includes a thorough history to ascertain the cause, including questions regarding systemic illnesses, nutritional deficiencies, family history, and potential injury.

Painful sensory neuropathies can be associated with systemic disorders such as diabetes mellitus, alcohol abuse, amyloidosis, rheumatoid arthritis, malignant cancers such as oat cell carcinoma, and benign monoclonal gammopathies (IgG, IgA, and IgM). The chronicity of the specific disease process is an important factor. Most inherited neuropathies, such as the hereditary motor and sensory neuropathies, and neurofibromatosis are less commonly associated with neuropathic pain because of their predilection for non-nociceptive neurons. Fabry's disease is a painful inherited sensory neuropathy associated with loss of almost all nociceptive nerve endings in the skin. Some painful small-fiber neuropathies of unknown cause (idiopathic) are present in multiple family members and undoubtedly have genetic causes that await investigation. Other acquired neuropathies are those related to toxin and drug exposure, some of which produce painful neuropathies.

The distribution of neuropathies can be generalized and symmetrical, asymmetrical, multifocal, or focal. The symmetrical generalized polyneuropathies commonly affect sensory and motor modalities in a distal-to-proximal gradient. Neuronal dysfunction is first reported in the extremities, the distal portions of the longest axons. So the earliest symptoms of axonal neuropathy are those of the autonomic and small-fiber sensory modalities. Loss or alteration of pain and temperature perception due to injury to the unmyelinated or thinly myelinated axons can herald more global deficits.

Diabetic neuropathy affects up to 15% of the 5 million patients with diabetes mellitus. It may be the most common peripheral polyneuropathy in the United States. Pain can be due to damage at many levels of the nervous system, but the small nerve fibers are disproportionately affected. The symmetrical, small-fiber neuropathy associated with diabetes mellitus presents with "burning feet" and autonomic features of impaired thermoregulation and sweat production. Neuropathy and vascular insufficiency are the main risk factors for diabetic foot ulcers and amputation.

In patients with painful diabetic polyneuropathy, pathologic studies demonstrate loss of both myelinated and unmyelinated fibers. Demyelination can be present as well. Endoneurial vascular damage, insufficient neurotrophic support, and autoimmune inflammation may all contribute. Diabetes mellitus is associated with other types of peripheral neuropathies, including proximal motor neuropathies (diabetic amyotrophy), autonomic neuropathies, vulnerability to compressive lesions, acute painful neuropathies from nerve ischemia, hypoglycemic neuropathy, treatment-induced neuropathy, and distal motor neuropathies.

Patients with multifocal neuropathies (mononeuropathy multiplex) usually develop focal loss of function in several peripheral nerves. The pathologic basis of these syndromes is usually ischemic with infarction of the vasa nervorum. Prognosis for recovery is favorable if the underlying cause of the infarction can be addressed. Systemic lupus erythematosus, rheumatoid arthritis, cholesterol emboli, and polyarteritis nodosa as well as diabetes mellitus can cause this pattern.

(ii) *Painful mononeuropathies*

Isolated focal peripheral nerve lesions are most commonly caused by trauma. Although accidents are the most common cause, iatrogenic injuries due to surgery or needlestick are a close second. Since a proportion of accidents occur on the job, or from participation in sports, these patients are likely to be young, in their most productive years, and they are often male. Nerve injuries may not be diagnosed at the time of the initial accident, since they are not visible on radiographs, and medical attention usually focuses on more obvious injuries. Nerve lesions affecting predominantly sensory neurons and producing pain as the major symptom are less likely to be diagnosed than those that produce frank motor deficit as well. Such delays in diagnosis are unfortunate, as some peripheral nerve injuries benefit from early surgical nerve repair. Furthermore, failure to diagnose a nerve injury can result in repeated surgeries if the pain is erroneously attributed to other causes.

Patients without a history of trauma or surgery usually have internal entrapment, compression, or nerve ischemia. Chronic nerve entrapment injury can be associated with rheumatic disease, diabetes mellitus, uremia, repetitive use, or malnutrition, or can occur in otherwise healthy individuals.

The hallmark of nerve injuries is that the pain is primarily in the distribution of a particular peripheral nerve or branch. The most useful aid to diagnosis is to ask the patient to outline on their body the area of worst pain. Often, this corresponds to the innervation territory of a specific nerve or branch. However, the clinical picture can be confusing since the pain can spread widely, outside traditional nerve territories. Most often, this is because C fibers trifurcate within the substantia gelatinosa on entry to the spinal cord. They send collateral axons approximately two segments up and down the cord, so that lesions of single nerves can be expected to produce more-widespread effects. Additionally, loss of afferent input into the spinal cord causes ectopic axonal sprouting that serves to enlarge the receptive fields of spinal pain-processing neurons. Interestingly, a few of these patients develop bilateral pain with contralateral pain in the area immediately opposite the nerve injury.

A common focal neuropathy is carpal tunnel syndrome. This causes pain, and in severe cases weakness, of the median-innervated thumb and forefinger. Another common entrapment lesion is meralgia paresthetica. This presents as intermittent pain along the anterior thigh. It is caused by entrapment of branches of the lateral femoral cutaneous nerve as they pass beneath the inguinal ligament. It can be worsened by obesity or pregnancy. Saphenous nerve injury may produce pain in the knee joint and/or medial surface of the lower leg in the setting of prior knee surgery or arthroscopy. Virtually any nerve, branch, or twig containing sensory neurons can be entrapped with resultant neuropathic pain.

Clinicians should evaluate these patients with the aid of a handbook that demonstrates the individual nerve territories. Stewart's textbook *Focal Peripheral Neuropathies* is an invaluable resource for diagnosing these syndromes. Occasionally, it is helpful to refer patients with difficult-to-diagnose syndromes for evaluation by a neurologist or neurosurgeon with subspecialty training in peripheral nerve injury.

(iii) *Painful neuronopathies*

Painful neuronopathies are injuries that are centered on the neuronal cell body. For somatosensory neurons, these are in the dorsal root ganglia, and in the trigeminal (Gasserian) ganglion for axons innervating the face. Sensory neuronopathies can occur from shingles, as paraneoplastic syndromes, and as part of Sjögren's syndrome. In two thirds of patients with paraneoplastic syndromes, the sensory neuronopathy precedes the discovery of the malignancy. An important clue that points to a neuronal rather than an axonal process is that the first manifestations may not involve the neurons with the longest axons (in the feet) as is usual with axonopathies. The onset is usually rapid and associated with burning dysesthesias or paresthesias. Areflexia may ultimately result from this syndrome because of loss of the afferent limb of the monosynaptic reflex.

With over 850,000 cases in the United States annually, acute herpes zoster is by far the most common sensory neuronopathy. Both herpes zoster and PHN disproportionately affect the elderly. Fifty percent of patients over age 60 with zoster will experience PHN. Suppression of cell-mediated immunity often associated with advancing age or concurrent medical illness permits latent varicella-zoster virus (VZV) to erupt into shingles. The dermatomal distribution and vesicular rash are the clinical signatures of VZV reactivation in the dorsal root ganglia. The thoracic segments are the most commonly affected. The next most common site is the ophthalmic division of the trigeminal nerve. The pain is described as burning, often associated with itching and volleys of lancinating pain. The diagnosis of PHN requires the persistence of pain 3 months after the initial rash. Over time, the distribution of pain symptoms can widen to involve adjacent dermatomes.

Shingles causes neuropathic pain syndromes affecting every area of the body including the limbs and genitals. These areas are vulnerable to motor and autonomic abnormalities as well, and adjunctive therapies may be needed. PHN is rarely present after shingles with an absent or inapparent rash (*zoster sin herpete*).

Acute zoster produces a mixed inflammatory/nociceptive and neuropathic pain syndrome that is present in the peripheral nerves, dorsal root ganglia, and spinal cord. Early treatment with antiviral medications (acyclovir, famciclovir, or valacyclovir) shortens and lessens the symptoms of zoster and decreases by about one half the likelihood of progressing to PHN. Antiviral therapy should be used in virtually all shingles patients, and it should be instituted as soon as possible. Early and aggressive pain control with tricyclics and opiates is also helpful in decreasing the likelihood of long-term PHN.

Clearance of myelin debris can take more than 1 year within the CNS, but the inflammation of acute zoster eventually subsides in most patients. Those left with PHN experience neuropathic pain. PHN is an excellent model of neuropathic pain and has been the subject of many research studies. Evidence from psychophysical studies and examination of nerve endings within skin biopsies suggests that in many cases there is severe loss of cutaneous innervation, especially nociceptive innervation, in PHN-affected skin.

(iv) *Amputation*

Pain often remains a major problem following amputation. Although best described after limb amputation, these syndromes can occur after a wide variety of amputations, including mastectomy and removal of visceral organs such as the rectum. Several different mechanisms can cause pain in these patients. Stump pain is pain perceived proximal to the site of amputation. It can have several causes, including skin breakdown or infection, vascular insufficiency, excess pressure by a prosthesis, or mechanical causes. Sectioned nerves can form painful neuromas.

Phantom pain, in contrast, is perceived distal to the site of the amputation. The most important initial question to ask amputees complaining of pain is whether the pain is proximal or distal to the amputation. Pain is only one of many phantom sensations that can be experienced by amputees. Patients in pain before their amputation (e.g., from infection or injury) may experience precise "memories" of their earlier pain. Although incompletely understood, these phantom sensations are thought to result from spontaneous electrical activity in central sensory neurons that are deprived of their normal afferent input.

2. Central pain syndromes

Neuropathic pain of central origin was originally described after thalamic injury, but these syndromes may occur from lesions in various locations throughout the CNS. Virtually any type of lesion including demyelinating, vascular, infectious, inflammatory, and trauma can produce pain. With central lesions, the onset of pain can be delayed by weeks, months, and occasionally years after a temporally well-defined insult such as a stroke. This may reflect the slower rate of degeneration within the CNS than the peripheral nervous system.

The painful somatic territory typically localizes to the corresponding central pain pathway, as in the thalamic pain syndrome characterized by Dejerine and Roussey. In those cases, the entire contralateral hemibody may be involved in the pain syndrome, or merely a portion of it. In virtually every case of central pain, the spinothalamic pathways are implicated. Out of the absence or disruption of sensory input to the CNS, pain attributable to "deafferentation" emerges. The challenging aspect of central pain syndromes is not usually diagnosis, since these patients often have a constellation of neurologic symptoms associated with their primary disorder. Management seems to be even more difficult than for patients with peripheral neuropathic pain syndromes. Phantom sensations in numb regions are described.

(i) *Post-stroke pain*

Up to 6% of all strokes are associated with chronic pain that limits rehabilitation and contributes to the development of post-stroke depression. The most common description is that of "burning," which is remarkably similar to accounts by patients with multiple sclerosis, post-cordotomy dysesthesia, and syringomyelia. The neuropathic features of pain in post-stroke syndromes have several characteristic features:

- The region of most intense pain encompasses only a portion of the total territory of sensory deficits.
- Functional recovery is poorest in the regions of most severe pain.
- The modalities of thermal perception and sensation to pinprick are more commonly affected than light touch.

(ii) *Trigeminal neuralgia*

Most commonly, neuralgias arise from lesions of the peripheral nerve; however, clinically similar syndromes develop with lesions of the cranial nerve nuclei and outflow tracts as a result of ischemic lesions. The peak onset of trigeminal neuralgia is in patients over 50 years old. The syndrome is marked by brief paroxysms of lancinating pain, usually in the territory of the second and third divisions of the trigeminal nerve. Light mechanical stimuli often trigger the pain. New onset of this syndrome in a younger adult (under 30 years) suggests multiple sclerosis. Older adults should be imaged to screen for compression by tumors or aneurysms. Glossopharyngeal neuralgia, which is caused by lesions affecting the somatosensory component of the IXth cranial nerve, shares similar jolts of pain but in the region of the throat or behind the angle of the jaw. These syndromes are also described in Chapter 29.

(iii) *Spinal cord syndromes*

Spinal cord syndromes are most often associated with trauma and demyelinating diseases such as multiple sclerosis. Chronic pain due to dysesthetic phantom limb, and visceral sensations occur in more than one third of patients with spinal cord injury, and 10% of these patients characterize their pain as severely disabling. The pain is classified as (a) peripheral segmental, (b) central cord, (c) visceral, and (d) mechanical. Spinal fractures can also produce pain by compressing the remaining neural structures.

In more than half of the patients, the onset is within 6 months of the initial injury. It is variously described as "burning," "shooting," and "crushing." The most common level of injury associated with pain is the cauda equina, followed by central cord injuries. Syringomyelia and syringobulbia as a delayed consequence of trauma or congenital malformation can interrupt central nociceptive afferents and produce neuropathic symptoms that affect a segment of the body. Since the spinothalamic pathways cross in the midline of the spinal cord near the site of entry to the cord, pain is the most common and earliest symptom of these syndromes.

(iv) *Multiple sclerosis*

Neuropathic pain is frequently associated with multiple sclerosis and is a significant cause of disability. The locations of plaques most commonly implicated are in the cervical spinal cord involving nociceptive afferents. Demyelination of the cervical and thoracic cords is common in multiple sclerosis and can produce lancinating pain in radicular distribution, or episodes of burning pain. Other sites where plaques produce neuropathic symptoms are in the radicular region at the dorsal root entry zone and the cranial nerves (see section IV, 2, ii).

V. DIAGNOSTIC EVALUATION OF PATIENTS WITH NEUROPATHIC PAIN

1. History

Neuropathic pain is a clinical syndrome, *not* a specific diagnosis. For this reason, the history is the most helpful diagnostic tool. The success of the evaluation rests on the clinician's ability and willingness to validate and evaluate the patient's pain. It is paramount to establish the underlying cause of the neuropathic pain at the outset of treatment, since the cause of some syndromes is reversible and further progression of disability can be prevented. The pain assessment integrates the following pain data points: onset, location, temporal profile, pain quality, pace of progression, severity and associated disability, aggravating and alleviating factors, response to past treatments, habits, and coping skills.

2. Examination

The general medical examination and the musculoskeletal examination provide important information about the pain condition. Features such as skin integrity, temperature, and the presence of edema or discoloration are important clues about the level of nervous system involvement and the severity of the condition. The positioning of an extremity or use of clothing to protect a limb from physical contact reveals much about the patient's complaint. As with all components of the examination, the absence of findings does not disprove the presence of a pain condition.

The neurologic sensory examination can be normal or abnormal in the context of chronic pain. The abnormalities of sensory nervous system dysfunction do not usually fit neatly into discrete modalities such as pinprick or temperature sensation. One defining feature of neuropathic pain is the concurrence of distinct abnormal sensory perceptions. For this reason, it is critical to test several different modalities in a given territory.

A second important consideration is specific testing for positive sensory phenomena such as allodynia and hyperalgesia. Allow patients to describe the sensory experience using their own terms. It is often useful to have the patient use markers to map the region of abnormality or discomfort. The sensory exam must be clearly explained to the patient. Normal areas should be examined first to establish a baseline, and to educate the patient about the testing process. The patient should be queried first as to whether the sensation is normal or abnormal. Subsequent questions are used to establish the presence and characteristics of the pain. As always, the behavior accompanying the patient's answers provides helpful context in which to interpret any findings. Sensory losses such as diminished pinprick sensation are routinely noted in patients with painful lesions of the sensory nervous system.

When the pain history suggests neuropathic features, it is important to also evaluate positive sensory signs including allodynia, hyperpathia, and hyperalgesia. These findings are the most specific for neuropathic pain syndromes. Allodynia can be tested mechanically by brushing the affected area with a cotton swab and with a thermal stimulus such as a cool metal reflex hammer or tuning fork. In contrast, to test hyperalgesia, a normally painful stimulus is applied, and an exaggerated pain response is consistent with a positive result. Motor deficits are often associated with neuropathic findings. Specifically, alterations in tone, strength, and endurance should be documented. In the case of central pain syndromes, these signs can be dramatic.

As with the evaluation of any patient with chronic pain, psychological assessment is important. Unrelieved pain often contributes to or unmasks psychiatric disorders such as depression, anxiety, panic disorder, and post-traumatic stress disorder. History taking should include an inventory of mood symptoms and consideration of affective signs of a behavioral problem. Many patients with chronic neuropathic pain need evaluation and treatment for depression at some time during the disease.

3. Imaging

Magnetic resonance (MR) or computed tomographic (CT) imaging is the gold standard for localization of cranial and spinal cord lesions causing central pain syndromes. Increased T2-weighted signal persists in the thalamus of a patient who has a neuropathic pain syndrome from a stroke. Computed axial tomography (CAT) of the head often reveals a hypodense neuroanatomic correlate. For radicular syndromes, CT myelography is the most sensitive imaging modality for bone impingement on nerve roots. MR imaging of the spinal cord is valuable when the examination and history are suggestive of a sensory level and an inflammatory cord lesion is likely or edema, secondary to compression, is suspected.

4. Diagnostic local anesthetic nerve blocks

Nerve blocks are useful diagnostic tools although only rarely indicated for management of chronic neuropathic pain. Temporary relief of pain from a local anesthetic injection near a particular nerve often helps to localize injury to a particular nerve or nerve segment in mononeuropathies and entrapments. Nerve block therapy is not curative and should not be used with this intent.

5. Electrophysiologic studies

Nerve conduction studies and EMG provide physiologic information about the sensory and motor components of peripheral nerves. Most neuropathic pain syndromes are mediated by small-diameter C fibers, which are not evaluated by these tests so their value in the evaluation of neuropathic pain syndromes is limited. It is important to note that the sensory nerve action potentials (SNAP) can have normal amplitudes in patients with neuropathic syndromes of radicular origin, because the causative lesion is proximal to the dorsal root ganglion. The neuropathic features of acute radicular pain in patients with acute inflammatory demyelinating polyneuropathy (Guillain-Barré) produce the characteristic pattern of demyelination in the compound muscle action potential (CMAP)—namely, slowing of conduction velocities, prolongation of the distal motor latencies, conduction block, and temporal dispersion.

Comprehensive evaluation of sensory function can be performed by administering well-characterized stimuli of known intensity and recording the patient's perceptions. This type of testing, termed quantitative sensory testing, is described in Chapter 7. These psychophysical evaluations are commonly used in research labs studying pain and analgesia in humans and animals. Although of some use in clinical practice, considerable expertise, as well as computerized thermal stimulators, are required for a full evaluation. Screening with a pin or nylon von Frey probes can be useful to screen for loss of protective sensation in a diabetes clinic, for instance.

6. Histologic evaluation of sensory nerves by biopsies of skin or sural nerves

Modern histologic examination, especially with quantitation, joins electrophysiologic recording as the most comprehensive way of investigating neuropathic pain. Removal of a segment of the sural nerve for light and electron microscopic analysis has shown loss of all types of axons in patients with painful polyneuropathies of varying causes. However, sural nerve biopsies cannot be repeated, are not useful for lesions that spare the sural nerve, and are quite invasive (occasionally causing neuromas, infections, and other clinical problems). For these reasons, they are largely being replaced by histologic examination of sensory nerve endings by punch biopsies of skin from the affected area, or the removal of epidermis only from induced skin blisters.

Immunohistochemical markers against PGP9.5 allow preferential visualization of the nerve endings as they course through the skin. In the epidermis, which is exclusively innervated by free nociceptive nerve endings, quantitation of the density of nerve endings is feasible. Skin biopsy studies have almost universally shown that chronic neuropathic pain is associated with profound loss of nociceptive nerve endings from painful areas of the skin.

7. Laboratory markers of neuropathic pain

There are currently no diagnostic tests specific and sensitive for neuropathic pain. At present, equivalence between symptoms and cellular mechanisms has not been established. Diagnostic evaluation is important to identify potentially reversible causes of neuropathic pain syndromes. For some of these entities, prevention of ongoing injury is paramount, as in the case of diabetic polyneuropathy, where tight glucose control can minimize disease progression. There is a role for serum titers of VZV in cases of suspected PHN in which the presentation is uncharacteristic. In the case of mononeuropathy multiplex, evaluation of markers for connective tissue disease may be helpful. In polyradiculopathy, where sensory symptoms are accompanied by weakness and areflexia at multiple levels, cerebrospinal fluid (CSF) protein and lymphocyte counts contribute to the diagnosis of acute inflammatory demyelinating polyneuropathy (Guillain-Barré). In chronic sensory neuronopathies without a clear diagnosis, evaluation for paraneoplastic antibodies and basic screening for evidence of tumor may be indicated. Where a sensory level is detected on neurologic examination, CSF samples may show evidence of inflammation and may be cultured to help identify an organism.

VI. TREATMENT OF NEUROPATHIC PAIN

Medical treatment is first-line therapy for neuropathic pain syndromes. It is the character of the prominent pain symptoms that drives therapeutic decision making, and the efficacy of drugs against neuropathic pain has been discovered serendipitously through clinical observation, usually after the drugs have been marketed for other indications. While pain researchers and pharmaceutical companies search for new ligands with molecular specificity, most of the effective treatments in current clinical use have activity at multiple sites within the pain pathways.

The good news is that multiple medications have proven effective against neuropathic pain in blinded, placebo-controlled clinical trials. The bad news is that none of these medications is effective in all patients, and we do not yet know how to predict who will be improved by which medication. Because of these limitations, it is often necessary to try several different medications before identifying the optimal agent and dosage for a particular patient. This sequential process should be explained to the patient to ensure that expectations for the extent and timing of relief are appropriate.

In general, the medication, or class of medications, judged most likely to be effective should be tried first, raised to an adequate level, and monitored for efficacy and side effects. Only if the primary analgesic is ineffective at the maximally tolerated dose should it be discontinued and replaced with a second agent. The four major classes of medications for treating neuropathic pain syndromes are tricyclic antidepressants (TCAs), anticonvulsants, opioid analgesics, and topical agents.

1. Tricyclic antidepressants

Historically, the TCAs have been the mainstay of medical therapy for neuropathic pain. They are well studied and widely prescribed. There is strong evidence of efficacy in diabetic neuropathy and PHN. Initially, the tricyclic antidepressants were thought to be most effective for persistent ongoing pain. More recent studies demonstrate their efficacy for lancinating pain and allodynia as well. Despite this, patients rarely obtain complete relief and frequently are unable to tolerate the side effects of TCAs.

The TCAs increase serotonergic and noradrenergic activity by interfering with their removal from the synaptic cleft. They have substantial sodium channel blocking activity and affect many other transmitters and receptors as well. Imipramine, amitriptyline, nortriptyline, and clomipramine are balanced in their reuptake of serotonin and norepinephrine, whereas desipramine is more selective for norepinephrine and tends to be associated with fewer side effects (see Chapter 11, table 1). In fact, affinity for histaminergic, cholinergic, and adrenergic receptors varies with each agent. This spectrum of receptor affinities accounts for the variability of analgesia and side effects described by patients. Caution is needed in patients with cardiovascular disease and closed-angle glaucoma. A full description of these drugs can be found in Chapter 11 and in Appendix VIII.

Starting doses range from 10 to 25 mg, usually given at bedtime. Choosing the initial dose depends on the patient's age and concerns about side effects. Elderly patients or those on complicated regimens should begin at the lowest dose. Tolerability and degree of relief guide the process of weekly dose escalation in 10- to 25-mg increments. It is important to proceed slowly in the early phase of titration as the anticholinergic side effects (constipation and dry mouth) may prompt susceptible patients to discontinue the medication prematurely. Most patients experience pain relief in the range of 30 to 100 mg/day. If at the upper end of this range significant relief is not attained, other therapies should be tried. Occasional patients require doses from 150 to 250 mg/day.

2. Anticonvulsants

A full description of these drugs can be found in Chapter 10.

(i) *Sodium channel blockers*

First-generation sodium channel blocking anticonvulsant drugs, such as carbamazepine and phenytoin, have long been the preferred drugs for the treatment of lancinating pain. This parsing of treatment by symptom has not been supported by more recent trials. The most effective use of these first-generation agents is in trigeminal neuralgia where carbamazepine markedly reduces pain in approximately 75% of patients. Significant pain relief for patients with diabetic neuropathy has been demonstrated in controlled trials, but second-generation anticonvulsants (e.g., gabapentin) are favored because their side effects are more tolerable. Regardless of the diagnosis, the analgesic dose response varies greatly among patients.

The initial dosage for sustained-release carbamazepine in adults is 200 mg once daily. After a 1-week period to allow induction of hepatic enzymes, slow titration to a daily dose of approximately 400 mg twice daily should follow. The therapeutic range is usually between 800 and 1200 mg/day. For the central syndromes, carbamazepine has been more extensively studied. If effective, it is usually in the dosage range used for treatment of seizures. Blood count and liver and renal function must be monitored.

(ii) *Gabapentin*

The relatively benign side-effect profile of gabapentin (Neurontin) is propelling it to a first-option treatment for neuropathic pain in spite of the fact that it is not approved by the U.S. Food and Drug Administration for this indication. Unlike earlier anticonvulsants, gabapentin causes few drug–drug interactions and less CNS dysfunction. Tolerability allows for the high-dose therapy that is often necessary for significant pain relief. With no need to monitor levels or enzymes, this drug is relatively easy to use. Gabapentin has a broad range of effectiveness for sensory and affective pain qualities in the treatment of PHN and diabetic neuropathy.

The starting dose for gabapentin is 300 mg nightly, or 100 mg nightly in older patients. The regimen is gradually increased every 3 to 7 days to approach a dose of approximately 900 mg three times daily. Most responders report significant relief in the dose range of 2,100 mg to 3,600 mg daily. Dizziness and mild sedation are common. Edema of the extremities is the most frequent specific side effect.

3. Opioids

Although traditionally opioids have been avoided in the treatment of neuropathic pain, in patients who do not respond to non-opioid adjuvant therapy, opioids are an important alternative. These agents may offer the most disabled patients relief when all other drugs and modalities have been ineffective. The basis of the traditional avoidance of opioids was twofold: (a) the belief that they were not effective and (b) the fear of addiction. The efficacy of opioids in chronic neuropathic pain has been demonstrated prospectively in several blinded placebo-controlled trials. Unfortunately, they are not helpful for all patients, and often a trial is necessary to determine efficacy. The risk of addiction is a real though exaggerated concern. Patients with chronic pain rarely develop opiate addiction, except when there is a prior history. The use of opioids in chronic nonmalignant pain is discussed in detail in Chapter 30.

4. Topical agents

The introduction of topical therapies in the form of patches, creams, and gels is a promising advance in the treatment of peripheral polyneuropathies and PHN. These are applied to painful skin and act locally at the peripheral sites of pain generation. The absence of systemic side effects and drug interactions make these treatments an important option. Capsaicin, a substance P depleter occurring in chili peppers, has had limited adoption because of its intolerable side effect, a local burning sensation. Lidoderm, a topical formulation of 5% lidocaine, has proved safe and effective in early, well-designed trials in patients with neuropathic pain. Lidocaine gels, ointments, or sprays can be helpful for patients with pain affecting mucous membranes, allowing them to engage in specific activities such as chewing, defecation, sexual activity, or use of tampons or pads during menstrual periods. Because systemic absorption can occur, serum levels may need to be monitored.

5. Adjunctive treatments

The chronicity of neuropathic pain states creates significant disability. An interdisciplinary approach to the care of these patients should address the psychosocial burdens and functional impact of living with chronic pain. Supportive psychotherapy can be helpful to patient and family alike. Behavioral therapy encourages safely increasing physical activity. Cognitive approaches foster ways of thinking about pain that are less negative and self-defeating. Physical and occupational therapies address the loss of strength, decreased range of motion, and abnormal muscle tone. Physical and occupational therapies maximize functional gains and minimize secondary problems associated with disuse. For example, interventions such as placing a cardboard box under the covers of a patient with allodynia of the feet can prevent a secondary sleep disorder.

6. Invasive options

(i) *Neuraxial catheter treatments and stimulators*

Invasive methods of pain treatment should be considered for the management of neuropathic pain states refractory to medical therapy. The most common interventions are epidural and intrathecal drug delivery systems and dorsal column spinal cord stimulators. In general, these techniques require a long-term commitment on the part of the patient and pain specialist and consideration of possible, but infrequent, surgical complications. Infusion pumps of morphine, hydromorphone, and baclofen have all shown analgesic benefit in several case series, but the variety and range of implantation techniques, drugs, and protocols for infusions have precluded conclusive validation with outcome studies. In patients with opioid-responsive pain, infusion pumps may offer a long-term, alternative route of administration that minimizes dose-limiting side effects.

Spinal cord stimulation over the dorsal pathways has been shown to be effective for diverse chronic pain states over the past 30 years. The evidence supporting the use of dorsal column stimulators is not limited to neuropathic pain states and the mechanism of pain relief is not well understood. Chronic precentral and central motor cortex electrical stimulation, for post-stroke pain and deafferentation syndromes are used in the most advanced centers. Recent technical advances have been promising, but further clinical studies are needed. Peripheral stimulation of individual injured peripheral nerves is a technique with success rates significantly higher than most other medical and surgical options.

(ii) *Decompressive neurosurgery*

Select patients with well-defined lesions may benefit from surgical exploration and decompression. This is well accepted for patients with carpal tunnel syndrome, but unfortunately underutilized for patients with similar problems elsewhere in the body. The relatively benign nature of these procedures, which do not involve cutting or injuring the involved nerves, must be emphasized. Pain relief after lysis of connective tissue bands compressing peripheral nerves has been described at multiple locations in the body.

(iii) *Ablative neurosurgery*

These procedures are performed far less frequently now than in the past. In most cases, this is good, because cutting nerves does not usually relieve the pain, but in a very few instances, these options ought to be considered. These procedures should be performed only by those with subspecialty training in neurosurgical management of pain. Patients in whom these procedures are probably underutilized include those with advanced disease and limited life expectancy. For them, the risks of inadvertent damage to motor or autonomic pathways may be acceptable to achieve good pain control for their remaining time. Transection of the pain pathways of the spinal cord can be performed by a skilled neurosurgeon percutaneously under fluoroscopic guidance. Cutting nerves that innervate areas of neuropathic pain, while a seemingly attractive option, has been shown through a century of clinical practice to be generally ineffective, and it can in fact worsen neuropathic pain. Unfortunately, one still sees patients treated with neurectomies who present with severe and complex neuropathic pain syndromes.

VII. CONCLUSION

Whereas neuropathic pain was considered a distinct entity associated with specific diagnoses such as diabetic peripheral neuropathy, PHN, and trigeminal neuralgia, it is now considered an integral part of many chronic pain syndromes, including CRPS, cancer pain, and even low back pain (under certain conditions). It is certainly the most challenging type of pain we treat in the pain clinic, and the most difficult to understand. It is a prominent focus of attention for clinicians and researchers who together are attempting to unravel its mechanisms and improve the specificity and efficacy of its treatments. Neuropathic pain is ubiquitous in pain practice and worthy of an intensive effort to help its unfortunate victims and to overcome the shortcomings in its treatment.

SELECTED READINGS

1. Backonja MM, Galer BS. Pain assessment and evaluation of patients who have neuropathic pain. *Neurol Clin* 1998;16:775–790.
2. Devinsky O, Feldmann E. *Examination of the cranial and peripheral nerves.* New York: Churchill Livingstone, 1988.
3. Galer BS. Painful polyneuropathy. *Neurol Clin* 1998;16:791–812.
4. Hans G, Davar G. Recent advances in the pharmacology of nerve-injury pain. *Neurol Clin* 1998;16:951–966.
5. Stewart JD, ed. *Focal peripheral neuropathies,* 3rd ed. Philadelphia: Lippincott Williams & Wilkins, 2000.
6. Dejerine J, Roussey G. Le syndrome thalamique. *Rev Neurol* 1906; 14:521–532.

Complex Regional Pain Syndromes

Katharine H. Fleischmann
and Edward Lubin

Pain, whose unchecked and familiar speed
Is howling, and keen shrieks day after day.
—*Percy Bysshe Shelley (1792–1822)*

The term *complex regional pain syndrome* (CRPS) was coined to describe pain syndromes that are often characterized by evidence of sympathetic nervous system dysfunction. This new terminology was suggested in order to break away from traditional concepts of the pain being mediated by the sympathetic nervous system, especially in view of the likely primary neuropathic cause of the pain and in view of the complexity of its cause, which is probably not simply related to the sympathetic nervous system. CRPS I and CRPS II are the two classic neuropathic pain syndromes previously known as reflex sympathetic dystrophy and causalgia.

CRPS I has been recognized as a clinical entity for many years. It is most often initiated by trauma, which can be mild or severe, chronic and repetitive, or a single event. The inciting event may be a minor or major fracture, a crush or amputation injury, or merely a sprain of the affected limb. Other examples stem from chronic repetitive movement trauma ranging from the use of computer or piano keyboards to heavy drilling equipment. Iatrogenic causes include surgery and poorly fitted casts. Up to one quarter of all cases of CRPS I have no clear cause.

The International Association for the Study of Pain (IASP) defines CRPS I as "a syndrome that usually develops after an initiating noxious event, is not limited to the distribution of a single peripheral nerve, and is apparently disproportional to the inciting event. It is associated at some point with evidence of edema, changes in skin blood flow, abnormal sudomotor activity in the region of the pain, or allodynia or hyperalgesia." The patient generally complains of diffuse limb pain associated with a burning or stabbing sensation.

CRPS II involves a similar pattern of symptoms. The IASP definition is "burning pain, allodynia, and hyperpathia usually in the hand or foot after partial injury of a nerve or one of its major branches in the region of the limb innervated by the damaged nerve." The symptoms of CRPS II may not occur immediately after nerve injury. As with CRPS I, they may be more insidious in their onset, occurring days, weeks, or even months after the injury. Concomitant vascular injury is common and exacerbates the sympathetic hyperactivity that often occurs in this syndrome. Essential elements of this syndrome are nerve injury, burning pain, and cutaneous hypersensitivity.

The clinical course of CRPS is divided into three stages. The first stage is the acute or hyperemic stage. The second is the dystrophic or ischemic stage. The third stage is atrophic. Radiography, scintigraphy, thermography, electromyography, and nerve conduction studies provide useful information, but the diagnosis of CRPS remains a clinical one.

I. HISTORY

The clinical syndrome we refer to as CRPS was scarcely mentioned in medical literature prior to 1864. In that year, Silas Weir Mitchell and his colleagues published "Gunshot Wounds and Other Injuries of Nerves." This paper was reissued in its entirety in the orthopedic literature in 1982. Mitchell was a physician during the Civil War and frequently saw nerve injuries caused by low-velocity gunshot wounds. In this context, he described a syndrome in which severe burning pain was seen following peripheral nerve injury. He later introduced the term causalgia, meaning burning pain, to describe the syndrome we now call CRPS II.

Similar pain states were later documented in postsurgical patients, as well as in those with no clear inciting cause. In the 1920s, René Leriche, a French surgeon, was the first to establish a common link between the sympathetic nervous system and causalgia by demonstrating that sympathetic blockade or sympathectomy could relieve the symptoms of many of his patients. Patients with no clear-cut peripheral nerve injury or those with pain in more than one peripheral nerve distribution had what became known as reflex sympathetic dystrophy, now called CRPS I.

II. BASIC MECHANISMS

Numerous theories have been offered to explain the pathophysiology of CRPS I and CRPS II, but the exact mechanisms remain unknown. Most theories, however, postulate that sympathetic dysfunction plays a significant role in the development and maintenance of the syndromes. Indeed, the concepts of CRPS and sympathetically maintained pain are integrally related to one another. However, we now know that there are syndromes in which part or all of the pain appears to be sympathetically independent pain. CRPS most likely involves both peripheral and central mechanisms.

Peripherally, events after nerve injury herald long-term changes in neural processing. In animal models, persistent afferent small-fiber activity begins days to weeks after peripheral nerve ligation or section, and it can be measured at the site of a developing neuroma as well as in the dorsal root ganglia. The neural sprouts at these sites have growth cones that have mechanical and chemical sensitivities not possessed by the original neurons. These neural sprouts may also have increased numbers of sodium channels, leading to increased ionic conductance and hence increased spontaneous activity. There is also evidence of increased innervation by sympathetic terminals on the cell bodies of A-δ and, to a lesser extent, C nociceptor fibers within the dorsal root ganglia, following injury to their axons. It is also hypothesized that a partial nerve lesion induces an up-regulation of functional alpha-2 adrenoceptors at the plasma membrane of intact nociceptive fibers.

Centrally, changes in the morphology of the spinal dorsal horn ipsilateral to a peripheral nerve injury may be secondary to intrinsic mechanisms arising in response to a chronic barrage of impulses, or in response to retrograde transport of chemical factors from the area of the lesion. The role of glutamate release in the spinal cord after peripheral nerve injury is being evaluated with increased interest. Increased spontaneous activity in the primary afferent neuron may be a factor leading to spinal cord glutamate release.

Although some studies suggest alternative neural and excitatory amino acid mechanisms of CRPS, the majority of animal studies point to a key role for the sympathetic nervous system in the maintenance of pain. Many models of sympathetically maintained pain in animals have been developed. Pretreatment with chemical or surgical sympathectomy blunts or abolishes the persistent tactile allodynia that arises in neuropathic pain models after experimental ligation or damage to nerves at sites adjacent to the spinal cord. Subsequent electrophysiologic studies demonstrate that some A-δ and C fibers acquire sensitivity to norepinephrine applied to the nerve injury site. Clinical evidence in patients with CRPS also suggests that the pain is maintained by sympathetic activity, either through the sympathetic nervous system itself or by other mechanisms. Chemical or surgical sympathectomy may transiently alleviate or eliminate the pain, whereas peripherally administered norepinephrine rekindles the pain.

III. CLINICAL PRESENTATION

CRPSs are characterized by pain, changes in cutaneous sensitivity, vasomotor and sudomotor disturbances, and increased muscular tone. These are often followed by weakness, atrophy, and ultimately irreversible trophic changes involving the skin and underlying muscles, bone, and joints. CRPS I and II are divided into grades, which characterize the severity, and into stages, which chart the course over a period of days to several months. In addition, it is now widely accepted that in CRPS there is a component of pain attributable to sympathetic efferent function referred to as sympathetically maintained pain. Interruption of sympathetic pathways early in the disease often provides significant pain relief. Generally, there is also a component of pain that is not influenced by sympathetic activity and is therefore referred to as sympathetically independent pain.

1. Acute stage

The initial signs and symptoms of CRPS may appear at the time of injury or may be delayed for weeks. The acute stage is characterized by constant pain, usually of a burning quality, localized to a specific area of injury but not necessarily following a specific dermatomal or nerve distribution. This pain is aggravated by movement and is associated with abnormal cutaneous sensitivity, including hyperesthesia, hyperpathia, allodynia, and changes in sympathetic tone. The result is often a tender, edematous limb, reduced in functional capacity, with overlying skin that is warm, red, dry, and tense. Later in the acute stage, increasing sympathetic tone is manifested as increasing edema, hyperhidrosis, and decreased limb temperature. Nails become thickened. Hair growth increases and the hair becomes coarser. During the acute phase, the symptoms of CRPS can often be reversed to a significant degree by treatment.

2. Dystrophic stage

CRPS often proceeds to a second stage, which is the dystrophic or ischemic phase, especially if the acute phase is left untreated. This can occur in a couple of months or longer. During this stage, the pain may radiate proximally or distally from the site of injury to involve the entire limb. Burning remains the principal symptom. Joint stiffness may appear along with decreased hair growth, thinning hair, and brittle and ridged nails. The skin over the limb becomes moist, cyanotic, and cold. The muscles may still exhibit spasm, but atrophy is more prominent at this time. Bony changes may start to appear on radiographs, reflecting diffuse bony reabsorption and erosion. Most cases of CRPS are diagnosed at this stage. A sympathetic blockade may still be helpful in treating the disease. However, the response is likely to be less than complete.

3. Atrophic stage

If untreated or unresponsive to treatment, CRPS progresses to the third or atrophic phase, which is characterized by trophic changes that are essentially irreversible. Pain, although quite severe, is not always the most prominent feature of this stage. The entire limb is involved and the process may even extend proximally to the torso or even to the contralateral limb. The skin is smooth, glossy, tight, and cool, the overlying hair has often fallen out, and the nails are severely brittle. The digits become thin and tapered (Fig. 1). Muscle wasting becomes more pronounced. Flexion contractures are likely to be present and the joints are usually ankylosed (Fig. 2). Radiography reveals more diffuse osteoporosis, with marked medullary space widening and cortical thinning.

Treatment is largely palliative, and somatic and sympathetic blockade are likely to provide only transient relief. Physical therapy is aimed principally at increasing range of motion and providing some pain relief. Functional restoration cannot generally be expected. Psychological counseling is an integral part of therapy in treating CRPS, particularly at this stage.

IV. DIAGNOSIS

CRPS includes a number of features that may or may not coexist: sympathetically maintained pain, autonomic dysfunction, and neuropathy resistant to traditional pharmacologic agents. Pain is the cardinal feature of CRPS, but there are also sensory changes,

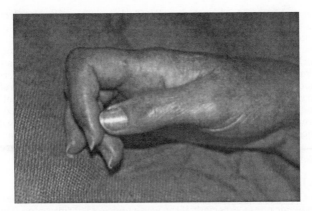

Figure 1.   The appearance of the hand in CRPS. The skin is smooth, glossy, tight and cool, the overlying hair has fallen out, and the nails are severely brittle. The digits are thin and tapered. The joints are ankylosed.

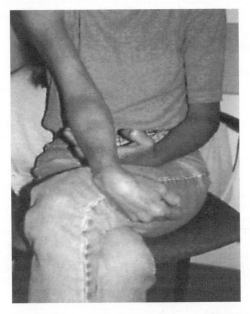

Figure 2.   Woman with severely affected right arm. Muscle wasting is pronounced and there are flexion contractures.

autonomic dysfunction, trophic changes, motor impairment, and psychological changes.

The diagnosis is based on the whole clinical picture, with additional information provided by carefully performed and interpreted confirmatory tests to ascertain the presence or absence of sympathetically maintained pain and autonomic dysfunction. These include sympathetic blockade (i.e., stellate ganglion block, lumbar sympathetic block) performed using local anesthetic and tests such as the quantitative pseudomotor axon reflex test, which allows a continuous hygrometric assessment of pseudomotor activity, felt to be a good indicator of C-fiber function. Clinical experience suggests that early intervention with sympatholytic procedures (pharmacologic or nerve block techniques) may be helpful therapeutically as well. Further data are required to confirm the appropriate timing and relative efficacy of different procedures and medications. Nevertheless, the importance of early diagnosis cannot be overemphasized. Table 1 lists the common clinical features of CRPS that may be useful in its differential diagnosis. Diagnostic criteria are listed in Table 2.

The diagnosis of CRPS is purely clinical and requires the exclusion of confounding medical problems, as well as the evaluation of diagnostic criteria. The IASP continues to clarify and refine the diagnostic criteria for CRPS in an attempt to eliminate the diagnostic and therapeutic dilemmas.

V. TREATMENT

Progress has been slow in refining treatment for CRPS. Because the condition is complex and incompletely understood, the treatment has been varied and formulated to address presumed pathophysiologic causes and to ameliorate specific symptoms. The common goal in the treatment of CRPS is functional restoration. Pharmacologic therapy as well as regional anesthetics and surgical interventions should be seen principally as adjuncts to physical therapy.

1. Physical therapy

Physical therapy should be started as soon as a diagnosis is made, even if the diagnosis is presumptive. Indeed, when physical therapy has already been started (e.g., after surgery on the hand or foot, or after casting for a fracture), the pain may worsen with

Table 1.   Common clinical features of complex regional pain syndrome

A recent or remote history of accidental or iatrogenic trauma

Pain that is burning, aching, or throbbing

The presence of one or more of the following:
    Vasomotor/sudomotor disturbances
    Trophic changes
    Limb edema
    Cold sensitivity
    Muscle weakness or atrophy
    Pain relief after regional sympathetic blockade

Table 2. Diagnostic criteria of complex regional pain syndrome

Allodynia/hyperalgesia
Burning pain
Edema
Nondermatomal distribution of the signs and symptoms
Color changes
Hair growth alterations
Changes in sweating
Temperature differences between involved and uninvolved limbs
Radiographic demineralization
A positive response to sympatholytic interventions or a supportive
    quantitative sudomotor axonal reflex test (QSART)

the development of CRPS. Discontinuing therapy under these circumstances will only make matters worse. Physical therapy should continue, but the approach most likely will be altered. Mobilization of the affected limb is of paramount importance, and often the pain must be aggressively treated to accomplish this, using the regional anesthetic techniques and/or pharmacologic agents discussed later. A gentle approach using heat, massage, vibration, and other mild stimuli helps restore more normal sensory processing. Isometric strengthening should be followed by progressive stress loading, as tolerated. One must be careful when using medication or, in particular, regional anesthesia in conjunction with physical therapy to avoid aggressive range-of-motion exercises and heavy loading of the affected limb. (Chapter 16 contains a full description of physical therapy for patients with CRPS.)

2. Drug treatments

(i) Neuropathic pain medications

Tricyclic antidepressants

Tricyclic antidepressants (TCAs) block the reuptake of norepinephrine and serotonin into the presynaptic terminal from the synaptic cleft. They are effective in treating neuropathic pain syndromes, including postherpetic neuralgia, diabetic neuropathy, and CRPS. The exact mechanism of action of the analgesic effect of these medications is unknown, but it is thought to be multifactorial. Spontaneous pain, shooting pain, and allodynia may all be improved. The effect of TCAs on pain is thought to be separate from that on mood, as the doses required for pain reduction are generally smaller than those required for mood elevation. These agents can, however, facilitate the treatment of pain by improving mood, sleep, and anxiety states. The most commonly prescribed TCAs are amitriptyline, nortriptyline, desipramine, and doxepin. They have somewhat different effects on norepinephrine and serotonin reuptake and therefore somewhat different side-effect profiles (see Chapter 11, Table 1). This should be considered when prescribing these drugs, particularly in the elderly. Refer to Chapter 11 and Appendix VIII for a full description of these drugs.

Anticonvulsants

The anticonvulsants are a heterogeneous group of drugs, some of which have known efficacy for the treatment of neuropathic pain.

Several anticonvulsants have been used successfully for CRPS, including phenytoin, carbamazepine, valproic acid, and gabapentin.

The most popular of these is gabapentin because of its favorable side effect profile. The use of gabapentin for diabetic neuropathy, postherpetic neuralgia, and migraine headaches has been validated in multicenter randomized trials. Although such validation for the use of gabapentin for CRPS has not yet been achieved, recent reports suggest it has considerable efficacy in CRPS patients. Side effects are a significant drawback of the other anticonvulsants, but these may be used if gabapentin does not prove effective. The anticonvulsants are described in Chapter 11.

The mechanism of action of gabapentin is unknown. Because the drug's structure resembles that of the neurotransmitter gamma-aminobutyric acid (GABA), it was originally thought that it acted via GABA receptors. However, it does not in fact interact with these receptors. The drug binds to a calcium channel subunit, but the significance of this action is also uncertain. The most common adverse effects of gabapentin are somnolence, dizziness, ataxia, fatigue, inability to concentrate, gastrointestinal (GI) disturbances, and nystagmus. These side effects can largely be prevented by careful upward titration of dosage to therapeutic levels (see Chapter 11 and Appendix VII).

Local Anesthetics

Mexiletine was developed as an anticonvulsant, but it has been used almost solely until recently as a class Ib antiarrhythmic. It is structurally similar to lidocaine and has been demonstrated to be useful in treating neuropathic pain states. Although few studies exist, it is generally felt that mexiletine may be useful in the treatment of CRPS. At the MGH, a trial of mexiletine is generally preceded by an intravenous (IV) lidocaine trial. If a patient has a good response to a lidocaine infusion, and because of their structural similarity, a trial of oral mexiletine is warranted. Recently, transdermal lidocaine patches have been used successfully in areas of localized neuropathic pain with allodynia and hyperalgesia in postherpetic neuralgia. EMLA (eutectic mixture of local anesthetic) cream is a topical preparation containing both lidocaine and prilocaine. They may both prove to be useful in the treatment of localized areas of hyperesthesia associated with CRPS, but this has not yet been demonstrated.

(ii) Nonsteroidal anti-inflammatory drugs

Nonsteroidal anti-inflammatory drugs (NSAIDs) are not useful as a sole pharmacologic therapy in CRPS because pain relief is generally inadequate, although they may be helpful during the early stages of the disease. However, they may be useful as adjunctive therapy, especially when there is joint and tendon involvement. The decision to use an NSAID is often based on the ability of the patient to tolerate the drug's side effects. GI irritation, sometimes leading to catastrophic GI bleeding, is the most feared NSAID side effect. Other relatively common side effects are renal damage and platelet dysfunction. NSAIDs are therefore contraindicated in patients with a history of peptic ulceration, renal dysfunction, coagulopathy, and known sensitivity to NSAID. They are relatively contraindicated in patients with asthma, cardiac failure, and the elderly. The newer cyclooxygenase (COX)-2 inhibitors are less likely to cause GI irritation and bleeding. A detailed description of the NSAIDs can be found in Chapter 8.

(iii) Opioids

The use of opioids in neuropathic pain states is controversial. Formerly, neuropathic pain was considered to be unresponsive to opioids, although currently opioid responsiveness with a rightward shift of the dose–response curve (indicating efficacy but at higher doses) is accepted. Although there have been no well-controlled trials of opioid therapy in patients with CRPS, it appears that in a significant number of patients the addition of an opioid can improve pain scores markedly. Therefore, if patients have not responded adequately to other treatments, a trial of opioids may be warranted. Opioids should be used only as adjuncts to other treatments, and great care should be taken when prescribing them for patients with a history of substance abuse (see Chapter 30). A full description of opioid drugs can be found in Chapter 9 and in Appendix V.

(iv) Others

Baclofen has been reported to be useful in neurologic diseases involving painful muscle spasm and other neuropathic pain states, thus raising hopes for its utility in the treatment of CRPS. However, further studies are necessary.

Phentolamine, an alpha-adrenergic blocker, is used by IV infusion to test the susceptibility of CRPS to sympathetic blockade. It is reported that approximately 30% of patients with sympathetically mediated pain respond positively to an IV infusion test. In these patients, IV regional blocks that include sympatholytic agents may subsequently prove useful. Oral alpha-blockers have not been found useful in the treatment of neuropathic pain. Side effects, most importantly hypotension and tachycardia, preclude patients from taking any but the smallest doses and severely limit their utility as analgesics.

Clonidine, an alpha-2 agonist, has been shown to have significant analgesic properties. It can be administered systemically or neuraxially, and it has been proven effective for both nociceptive and neuropathic pain. IV regional blockade using 1 μg/kg clonidine can provide marked pain relief in patients with sympathetically mediated pain. Likewise, transdermal clonidine is believed to be useful, particularly when applied to discreet areas of hyperalgesia. Oral clonidine, now rarely used as an antihypertensive, is being evaluated for its role in the treatment of various pain states. Clonidine has both central and peripheral actions and may be a useful adjunct in the treatment of CRPS. Sedation is a significant side effect of clonidine, but patients are unlikely to become somnolent or unrousable. In addition, clonidine may cause hypotension and bradycardia.

Corticosteroids are known to markedly decrease inflammation and have been advocated for use in the early stages of CRPS. Although there are no well-controlled trials, there is recent evidence to suggest a marked inflammatory component to the early stages of CRPS. Thus, if a patient has pain secondary to joint movement and trophic changes, a trial of corticosteroids with a reasonably rapid taper is recommended. Using this approach, one may avoid many of the undesirable side effects of steroids while evaluating and treating the inflammatory component of CRPS early in the disease.

Capsaicin interferes with cutaneous nociceptive C-fiber function by depleting peptides such as substance P and calcitonin gene-related peptide at the nerve terminals. Capsaicin cream should be applied directly to areas of hypersensitivity and, with time, may lead to decreased sensitivity. Unfortunately, it is often difficult to get patients to comply with a trial of capsaicin cream because of the significant pain with the initial applications.

Calcitonin bisphosphonates are sometimes given to patients with CRPS in an effort to bolster their bone density. The additional benefit of decreasing spontaneous pain is sometimes seen. Calcitonin is given by subcutaneous injections days to weeks apart; if there is a positive effect on pain, it is seen early.

3. Regional anesthesia

A number of regional anesthetic modalities have been used in the treatment of CRPS. The primary goal remains alleviation of pain as an adjunct to physical therapy in the process of functional restoration. Regional sympatholysis in patients with sympathetically maintained pain can be both diagnostic and therapeutic (in conjunction with physical therapy).

(i) Sympathetic blockade

Temporary sympatholysis of the upper extremity can be accomplished by a stellate ganglion block or a cervical sympathetic block. A lumbar sympathetic block provides sympathetic blockade in the lower extremities. An increase in temperature of the limb (upper or lower) is always a reassuring sign that the sympathectomy has been achieved (Horner's syndrome by itself is not an indication of limb sympathectomy). The accuracy of these blocks has been greatly increased by fluoroscopic guidance of needle positioning. In addition to providing temporary pain relief, sympathetic blocks can help determine the extent of the sympathetic component of a patient's pain, thereby predicting potential benefit from pharmacologic therapy. However, some degree of somatic blockade is almost certain to occur in conjunction with these blocks, so the test is not entirely clean.

The aim of temporary sympatholysis in CRPS is to achieve sufficient pain relief to allow functional restoration during a course of physical therapy. The endpoint for the combined therapy is either adequate functional restoration, or the point at which the patient is no longer able to increase endurance and workload after sympathetic blockade. A series of blocks may be necessary, in conjunction with the physical therapy sessions.

Sympathetic neurolysis has been advocated for patients with CRPS whose pain has been nearly or completely abolished by temporary sympathetic blockade. It can be accomplished by injecting phenol or absolute alcohol under fluoroscopic guidance. Chemical neurolysis lasts only 3 to 6 months, and patients may then suffer a recurrence, or even worsening, of their original pain. There is also a risk of spread of the neurolytic agent to the sensorimotor fibers in close proximity to the targeted nerves (e.g., phrenic nerve, lumbar plexus). This approach is recommended only for patients who have proved refractory to all other treatments.

More recently, **percutaneous radiofrequency lesioning of the sympathetic trunk** and **endoscopic sympathectomy** have been used in patients with clearly demonstrable sympathetically maintained pain. Long-term evaluation of the efficacy of these treatments has not yet been completed.

(ii) Intravenous regional blockade

Intravenous regional blockade has been attempted with numerous medications with varying reports of success. If a patient has failed other, more conservative therapies, a trial of IV regional medication is warranted. Local anesthetic and clonidine are often used in combination for this purpose. Some have advocated the addition of ketorolac if the patient is in the acute stage of CRPS when there is a significant inflammatory component. In the past, guanethidine, reserpine, bretylium, and other drugs have been used in IV regional blockade. None of these have clearly been shown to be helpful in the treatment of CRPS, and a number are no longer available in the United States. Many patients are unable to tolerate the procedure because of severe pain with limb exsanguination and tourniquet placement.

(iii) Epidural blockade

Lumbar epidural blockade and, less frequently, cervical epidural blockade have been used for extended periods of time to treat cases of CRPS that have been unresponsive to less invasive therapies. Lumbar epidural catheters can be used to provide continuous lumbar plexus blockade for patients who have inadequate pain relief and have been unable to participate in physical therapy. A low concentration of local anesthetic is used, high concentrations tending to produce sensory and motor blockade, which hampers functional restoration. Often, an opioid or clonidine is used in combination with the local anesthetic to augment pain relief. Temporary epidural catheters have been left in place for up to 6 weeks, allowing successful functional restoration. Clearly, there are risks associated with long-term epidural catheters, and sometimes the external infusion system can interfere with the exercise regimen. Implanted epidural infusion systems are more secure and less intrusive, but the risks of the surgical procedure are probably not warranted other than in the most refractory cases.

(iv) Brachial plexus blockade

Continuous brachial plexus blockade for patients with CRPS of the upper extremity has been advocated and can be accomplished with an axillary, infraclavicular, or supraclavicular catheter. The advantage, as with epidural catheters, is that the prolongation of neural blockade enables patients to make relatively rapid progress in physical therapy. Under neural blockade, care should be taken to avoid overextending the passive and active range of motion exercises. As with any catheter treatment, there are risks of dislodgement and infection. A fairly high infusion rate of local anesthetic is needed for successful brachial plexus catheter treatment, which limits the utility of these treatments in outpatients. The treatment is best suited to patients who have been unresponsive to pharmacologic therapy but are likely to have a good and rapid response to physical therapy with adequate sensorimotor blockade.

4. Neuromodulation

(i) Spinal cord stimulation

Spinal cord stimulation has proven useful in patients with refractory CRPS, and in those who have had intolerable side effects from other therapies. Patients must have met government guidelines and specific insurance company stipulations prior to approval of a trial of spinal cord stimulation. Stimulation is conducted at the C5-7 level for the upper extremities, and the T8-10 level for the lower extremities. Approximately 50% of preselected patients with CRPS have a positive response to a trial of stimulation therapy. Approximately 70% of these patients have good to excellent longer-term benefit. A goal of pain relief, rather than full functional restoration, is reasonable in view of the refractory nature of the pain in patients selected for this expensive therapy.

(ii) Peripheral nerve stimulation

Peripheral nerve stimulation has been advocated for use in patients with CRPS II, with symptoms entirely or mainly in the distribution of a single major peripheral nerve, who have been unresponsive to other therapeutic modalities. It is not considered an option for patients with CRPS involving an entire limb or further extension to the trunk or other extremities. Peripheral nerve stimulators present a special problem in that they generally cross several mobile joints and therefore may be dislodged with movement. In select patients, however, early small studies suggest this might be a successful treatment for patients with CRPS II who have been unresponsive to other therapies.

(iii) Psychotherapy

Many patients with CRPS become depressed at some time in the course of their illness. There has been a great deal of discussion regarding whether a premorbid tendency to depression predisposes patients to CRPS, or whether CRPS causes depression or uncovers a preexisting condition, and no consensus has been reached. Early in the illness, only about 10% to 15% of patients with CRPS report being depressed, which is an incidence similar to that of depression in the general population. Furthermore, when psychological tests are conducted at this stage, the results are similar to those in the general population. As CRPS progresses, anxiety and depression play a greater role, as is confirmed by psychological testing. Many patients are already on a TCA for their pain, but the dose may need to be increased. A psychiatrist, psychologist, or social worker familiar with CRPS should be involved in caring for patients at this juncture. Also, a biofeedback program for relaxation and reduction of muscle tension is a useful adjunct to pharmacologic therapy, physical therapy, and psychotherapy.

VI. CONCLUSION

The vast majority of CRPS patients are best managed with a combination of skilled physical therapy with drug or interventional pain therapy. The aim is always to restore functionality as much as possible. A simple drug regimen, or a simple nerve block (usually sympathetic) or series of blocks, is sufficient in all but the most refractory cases. More complicated procedures, including implanted catheters and stimulators, are rarely needed in these patients. With a team approach to the treatment of patients with CRPS, a successful outcome is most likely.

SELECTED READINGS

1. Blumberg H, Janig W. Clinical manifestations of reflex sympathetic dystrophy and sympathetically maintained pain. In: Wall PD, Melzack R, eds. *Textbook of pain,* 3rd ed. Edinburgh: Churchill Livingstone, 1994:685–698.
2. Bossut DF, Perl ER. Effects of nerve injury on sympathetic excitation of A-delta mechanical nociceptors. *J Neurophysiol* 1995;73: 1721–1723.
3. Bruehl S, Harden RN, Galer B, et al. External validation of IASP diagnostic criteria for Complex Regional Pain Syndrome and proposed research diagnostic criteria. *Pain* 1999;81:147–154.
4. Devor M, Wall P, Catalan N. Systemic lidocaine silences ectopic neuroma and DRG discharge without blocking nerve conduction. *Pain* 1992;48:261–268.
5. Eisenach JC, DeKock M, Klimscha W. Alpha-2-adrenergic agonists for regional anesthesia: A clinical review of clonidine (1984–1995). *Anesthesiology* 1996; 85:655–674.
6. Galer BS, Bruehl S, Harden RN. IASP diagnostic criteria for Complex Regional Pain Syndrome: A preliminary empirical validation study. *Clin J Pain* 1998;14:48–54.
7. Harden RN, Bruehl S, Galer BS, et al. Complex regional pain syndrome: Are the IASP diagnostic criteria valid and sufficiently comprehensive? *Pain* 1999; 83:211–219.
8. Janig W, Stanton-Hicks M, eds. *Reflex sympathetic dystrophy: A reappraisal.* Seattle: IASP Press, 1996.
9. Kamibayashi T, Maze M. Clinical uses of alpha 2-adrenergic agonists. *Anesthesiology* 2000;93:1345–1349.
10. Kingery WS. A critical review of controlled trials for peripheral neuropathic pain and complex regional pain syndromes. *Pain* 1997; 73:123–139.
11. Merskey H, Bogduk N, eds. *Classification of chronic pain: Description of chronic pain syndromes and definition of pain terms,* 2nd ed. Seattle: IASP Press, 1994.
12. Mitchell SW, Morehouse GR, Keen WW. *Gunshot wounds and other injuries of nerves.* Philadelphia: JB Lippincott, 1864; and Mitchell SW. *Injuries of nerves and their consequences.* Philadelphia: JB Lippincott,1872. Reprinted in *Clin Orthop* 1982;163:2–7.
13. Stanton-Hicks M, Baron R, Boas R, et al. Consensus report: Complex regional pain syndromes: Guidelines for therapy. *Clin J Pain* 1998;14:155–166.
14. Woolf CJ, Mannion RJ. Neuropathic pain: Aetiology, symptoms, mechanisms, and management. *Lancet* 1999;353:1959–1964.

Back and Neck Pain

Shihab U. Ahmed

Pain wanders through my bones like a lost fire.
—*Theodore Roethke (1908–1963)*

One of the most frequent complaints that brings patients to their doctors is low back pain (LBP), which is estimated to afflict 15% to 20% of U.S. adults and is the most common cause of disability in individuals under the age of 45 years. The direct cost of diagnosis and treatment of LBP in the United States is estimated to be in the billions of dollars, and the indirect cost in terms of loss of work is inestimable. Despite its high prevalence in our community, accurate diagnosis and treatment of LBP remains difficult. Neck pain also occurs frequently, having a point prevalence of nearly 13% and a lifetime prevalence of nearly 50%.

I. DEFINITIONS

The International Association for the Study of Pain (IASP) defines **lumbar spinal pain** as "pain perceived as arising from anywhere within a region bounded superiorly by an imaginary transverse line through the tip of the last thoracic spinous process, inferiorly by an imaginary transverse line through the tip of the first sacral spinous process, and laterally by vertical lines tangential to the lateral borders of the lumbar erectors spinae."

Sacral spinal pain is defined as "pain perceived as arising from anywhere within a region bounded superiorly by an imaginary transverse line through the tip of the first sacral spinous process, inferiorly by an imaginary transverse line through the sacrococcygeal joints, and laterally by imaginary lines passing through the posterior superior and posterior inferior iliac spines." LBP is considered to arise from both the lumbar and sacral locations.

Cervical spinal pain is pain perceived as arising from anywhere within the region bounded superiorly by the superior nuchal line, inferiorly by an imaginary transverse line through the tip of the first thoracic spinous process, and laterally by sagittal planes tangential to the lateral borders of the neck." These definitions are specific to only the location, not to the cause of the pain.

Somatic pain arises from the stimulation of the nerve endings in the skin and musculoskeletal components, such as the bone, ligament, joint or muscle. **Referred pain** is pain perceived as arising or occurring in a region of the body supplied by nerves other than those that innervate the true source of the pain. Referred pain may be perceived in areas relatively distant from the actual source of pain, but when the true source of pain and area of referred pain are adjacent to each other, they seem to be confluent.

Radicular pain is pain that is evoked by stimulation of the sensory dorsal root of a spinal nerve, or its dorsal root ganglion (DRG), and is not synonymous with radiculopathy. **Radiculopathy** is a pathologic condition in which the function of the nerve root is compromised, leading to numbness, motor loss, and pain, depending on which fibers of the nerve root are involved.

It may be difficult to distinguish clinically between radicular pain and somatic pain referred from localized pathology of the spine (e.g., discs, facet joints, ligaments, paraspinus muscles), yet it is important to try to make this distinction. In the case of radiculopathy, pain may arise from the deeper structures (e.g., muscle and bone) innervated by the affected nerve root(s) and not in the predicted dermatomal distribution. Likewise, somatic referred pain often presents with a nondermatomal distribution in the proximal limb. It is helpful to remember that radicular pain in the distal limb (forearm and lower leg) is unlikely to be of somatic origin, whereas in the proximal limb (upper arm and leg), somatic pain frequently mimics radicular pain.

II. ANATOMIC AND PATHOLOGIC BASIS OF BACK AND NECK PAIN

The spine consists of the bony vertebral column and cartilaginous discs, supporting ligaments, muscle, joints, soft tissues, and nervous tissue. The spine not only supports the weight of the head and torso but also supports and cushions the spinal cord, the nerve roots, the sensory and autonomic ganglia, and the peripheral nerves. All the tissues of the spine are innervated and sensitive to pain and other sensations. It is not hard to imagine why the tissue diagnosis of spine pain is so difficult. To understand the pathophysiology of back pain, the goal should be to have a thorough knowledge of the different tissue types in the region, their nerve supply (Figure 1), the biomechanics of the various spinal structures, and the various ways they can be injured.

1. Vertebral bodies

The vertebral bodies, like any other bone in the body, are well innervated with nociceptors, especially in the periosteum. The nerve

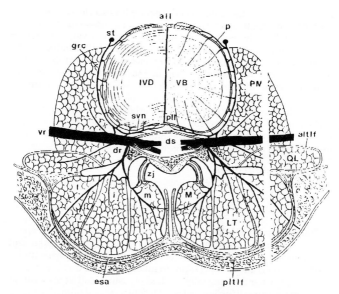

Figure 1. Innervation of the lumbar spine. A cross-sectional view incorporating the level of the vertebral body (VB) and its periosteum (p) on the right, and the intervertebral disc (IVD) on the left. PM, psoas major; QL, quadratus lumborum; IL, iliocostalis lumborum; LT, longissimus thoracis; M, multifidus; altlf, anterior layer of thoracolumbar fascia; pltlf, posterior layer of thoracolumbar fascia; esa, erector spinae aponeurosis; ds, dural sac; zj, zygapophysial joint; pll, posterior longitudinal ligament; all, anterior longitudinal ligament; vr, ventral ramus; dr, dorsal ramus; m, medial branch; i, intermediate branch; l, lateral branch; svn, sinuvertebral nerve; grc, gray ramus communicantes; st, sympathetic trunk.

supply comes from adjacent ligaments and muscles. The major innervation comes from the plexus of the anterior and posterior longitudinal ligaments, which supply the periosteum and the deeper structures. Nociceptive markers such as substance P and calcitonin gene-related peptide (CGRP) have been isolated from bone marrow, periosteum, and the cortex of the bones.

Fracture of the vertebral body is often painful and the cause of the pain may be (a) irritation of the nociceptors caused by distention from the local inflammation or hematoma formation, or (b) chemical stimulation from the inflammatory mediators. Fracture may also cause pain because of structural deformity, which can lead to abnormal stress to nearby structures such as joints, ligaments, and muscles.

Metabolic diseases that affect the vertebral body include osteoporosis, Paget's disease, and osteitis fibrosa. The mechanism of pain in osteoporosis may include microfractures or mechanical irritation of the perivascular sensory nerve within the vertebral spongiosa. The vertebral body can also be affected by primary or secondary tumors. In secondary tumors, multiple vertebral lesions are common, and the tumor usually expands posteriorly. A recently proposed mechanism of vertebral pain is intraosseous hypertension caused by the obstruction and distension of veins, which in turn causes stimulation of the sensory nerves in their adventitia.

The cervical spine in humans consists of seven vertebrae. The first and second vertebrae are modified to provide head movement. Osteoarthrosis of the atlanto-odontoid joint has been found to cause suboccipital pain. Below the C2 level, each vertebra forms an arch with an anterior convexity. One other distinguishing feature of the cervical vertebrae is the uncovertebral joint with its hooklike projections on either side of the superior surface. The uncinate processes are close to the exiting nerves.

2. Intervertebral discs

Intervertebral discs are innervated and a common source of spine pain. Each disc is composed of a central nucleus pulposus surrounded by the peripheral annulus fibrosus and two layers of cartilage, which cover the superior and inferior aspects of the disc.

The nucleus has a semifluid consistency and consists of chondrocytes, collagen fibers, and ground substance. It is avascular and not innervated. The fluid consistency of the nucleus deforms under pressure and transmits pressure in all directions. Thus it works as a shock absorber for vertically applied pressure, and as a semifluid ball bearing during flexion, extension rotation, and lateral bending of the vertebral column.

The annulus fibrosus is composed of concentrically arranged lamellae made of collagen fibers surrounding the nucleus pulposus. The lamellae are thicker in the anterior and lateral portion of the annulus and thinner in the posterior annulus, which is weaker than the rest. The annulus helps to stabilize the interbody joints and acts as a ligament to limit excessive motion. The outer third of the annulus is well innervated. Various studies have documented simple free nerve endings as well as complex sprays, convoluted tangles, and encapsulated nerve endings at the outer annulus. These nerve endings have been found to be immunoreactive to nociceptive neuropeptides such as substance P, CGRP, and vasoactive intestinal polypeptide (VIP). Signals from these nociceptors from the posterolateral segment of the disc travel to the spinal cord via the sinuvertebral nerve.

The anterior disc and part of the lateral disc receive innervation via gray rami communicantes. The vertebral end plate covers the entire nucleus pulposus but does not cover the peripheral annulus fibrosus. The outer annulus inserts by Sharpey's fibers into the smooth outer rims of the vertebral bodies. The vertebral end plate and the inner annulus together surround the nucleus like a capsule made of collagen fibers.

Lumbar discs have long been known to cause LBP. In patients with symptoms, injection of radiocontrast dye into a diseased disc can mimic the patient's pain (provocative discography). On the other hand, it appears that in asymptomatic individuals, provocation by injection into the normal disc does not cause LBP. The lumbar disc may be the source of pain in discitis, torsion injury, or internal disc disruption (IDD). Torsion injury to the disc occurs with forceful rotation of the intervertebral joint. The risk of injury increases if rotation occurs while the spine is flexed, which already causes stress at the annulus.

Degradation of the nuclear matrix and disruption of the annulus characterize the clinical entity of IDD. The proposed diagnostic criteria for IDD include a positive provocation discogram and the presence of a radial tear extending to the outer third of the annulus on postdiscogram computed tomography (CT) (Fig. 2). Based on these criteria, Schwarzer et al. (1995) found the prevalence of IDD among the patients with chronic LBP to be at least 39%.

The cause of IDD remains controversial. One possible mechanism is that the end plate fractures as a result of repetitive motion injury. This theory proposes that the end-plate fracture initiates a progressive degradation process of the nuclear matrix. During the process of degradation, the nucleus loses some of its water content and its ability to sustain pressure. This causes a shift of load to the annulus and makes it susceptible to injury. The degradation process may also spread to the annulus in the form of an annular tear. The nociceptors of the outer annulus are now exposed not only to degradation products and enzymes but also to inflammatory chemicals leading to back pain. Standard imaging studies, including magnetic resonance imaging (MRI), CT, myelography, and discography, may not reveal abnormalities of the annulus. However, injecting radiocontrast dye inside the annulus and taking a postcontrast CT may help identify any annular pathology.

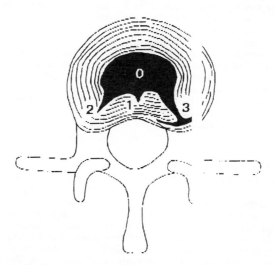

Figure 2. Grades of radial fissures in internal disc disruption.
Grade 0: No disruption is evident in the annulus fibrosus
Grade 1: Disruption extends into the inner third of the annulus fibrosus
Grade 2: Disruption extends as far as the inner two thirds of the annulus
Grade 3: Disruption extends into the outer third of the annulus fibrosus, and may spread circumferentially between the lamellae of collagen.

3. Ligaments

Anterior and posterior longitudinal ligaments

The lumbar sympathetic trunk, gray rami communicantes, and sinuvertebral nerves innervate the anterior and posterior longitudinal ligaments. These ligaments are attached to the annulus fibrosus and may be difficult to separate from disc (annular) pathology as a source of LBP. Kuslich et al. (1991) found that the posterior longitudinal ligament causes central back pain when stimulated.

Spinous ligaments

The spinous ligaments are less likely to cause pain. The **interspinous ligament** is innervated by the medial branch of the posterior primary rami, but clinical studies demonstrate that the ligament is responsible for only a small proportion of LBP. Poor innervation of the **ligamentum flavum** makes it a less likely source of LBP. The **supraspinous ligament** may not be associated with LBP because it is absent at the lower lumbar region.

4. Muscles

Muscles of the back are supplied by the dorsal rami of the spinal nerves. In normal volunteers, injections of hypertonic saline to the back muscles produced LBP and referred pain in the buttocks. The deeper quadratus lumborum and psoas muscles, on the other hand, are supplied by ventral rami of the lumbar plexus and may potentially be a source of pain in the back itself.

Although the exact mechanism is not well understood, LBP from muscles has been attributed to spasm, to sprain and strain, and to trigger points in myofascial pain. Free nerve endings may be stimulated from direct trauma, stretch, pressure, disruption of the fibers, or accumulated metabolites during anaerobic metabolism. Muscle spasm is probably a common cause of nonspecific back and neck pain (pain with no clear cause), and it may also cause worsening of back and neck pain when spasm is triggered by less painful pathology in other structures.

5. Joints

Facet joints

The facet joints (also known as **zygapophysial joints** or **Z joints**) are well innervated by the medial branches from the posterior primary rami. Each joint has a dual innervation, one from the dorsal rami of the same level and one from the level above. The facet joints of the cervical spine, at C2 and below, are located at the lateral edge of the lamina and are richly innervated via the medial branch from the posterior primary rami. The medial branch from the joint above and below innervates each facet joint. The C2-3 facet joints receive innervation from the third occipital nerves and medial branches of the C3 dorsal rami.

In the lumbar region, intra-articular injection of hypertonic saline and contrast medium in volunteers has shown to cause LBP and referred pain. Although facet joints can be affected when disc disease or spondylosis is present, facet joints have also been shown to cause LBP. Among the suggested causes of facet joint pain are trauma, inflammation, synovial impingement, meniscoid entrapment, and chondromalacia. Hyperextension and rotation of the lumbar spine can cause a capsular tear and avulsion, subchondral fracture, or fracture of the articular process or intra-articular hemorrhage. Pain from facet joints tends to be localized to the back with radiation to the buttock and posterior thigh and, occasionally, below the knee joints. Plain radiographs, CT scans, and MRI are usually not useful in the diagnosis of facet joint pain. Diagnosis can be made only by diagnostic blockade with local anesthetic. To avoid a high false-positive response, controlled diagnostic block techniques are recommended. In one study, the estimated prevalence of LBP from facet joint origins among injured workers was found to be 15%.

Sacroiliac joint

The sacroiliac (SI) joint is a synovial joint, and a portion of it contains a synovial lining. Posteriorly, it receives innervation from dorsal rami of L4–5, and S1–2, and there is some controversy about whether it also receives ventral innervation. Sacroiliac joints have been found to cause localized pain over the joint and referred pain to the lower extremity when stressed with contrast medium in healthy volunteers. Various systemic illnesses including ankylosing spondylitis, metabolic derangements, and infectious disease can affect the SI joint and cause pain. Most cases of suspected SI joint pain are considered mechanical in origin, although the exact mechanism remains unclear. The diagnosis of SI joint pain can be made by an injection of local anesthetic intra-articularly. Its prevalence among chronic LBP sufferers is estimated to be 15%.

6. Nerve roots

Nerve roots and DRG, when compressed, can be the source of axial spine pain and extremity pain. It is important to separate radicular pain, which is pain along the distribution of a spinal nerve, from radiculopathy, in which sensory or motor deficits of a spinal nerve distribution are associated with the pain symptoms. Although acute compression of a normal nerve root will cause paresthesia or numbness, it will not generate persistent pain. In contrast, compression of the normal DRG can cause sustained discharge and may provoke radicular pain and radiculopathy.

Chronic compression of the nerve root can cause pain by sensitizing the nerve to both mechanical and chemical irritation. The underlying neural pathology in chronic compression may include focal demyelination, partial axonal damage, or intraneuronal edema. Nuclear material from a disrupted disc can cause chemical irritation with nerve root inflammation (radiculitis), radicular pain, or radiculopathy.

7. Meninges

The dura mater is a well-innervated structure. The nerve supply is more abundant on the ventral aspect and around the nerve root sleeves. Back pain can arise in a patient with a dura mater inflamed by infection or the presence of intrathecal blood. Clinical studies have shown that LBP and referred gluteal pain are associated with stimulation of the dura by both mechanical and chemical irritation. Chemical irritation from the herniated disc material can cause an inflammatory reaction around the dural sleeve and is believed to be the cause of LBP and somatic referred pain. This is distinct from the radicular pain resulting from radiculitis secondary to chemical or mechanical irritation from the herniated disc materials.

III. EVALUATING THE PATIENT WITH BACK AND NECK PAIN

Important principles in the evaluation of back and neck pain are the following:

- Rule out the serious causes of pain (e.g., infection, tumor, trauma).
- The etiology of pain in a significant number of patients with back and neck pain may remain unknown. Nonspecific back or neck pain is a legitimate diagnosis.
- History and physical examination have a limited role in the diagnosis of back and neck pain but are important in ruling out serious pathology.
- It is important to distinguish somatic referred pain from radicular pain and radiculopathy.
- Reassure patients that the vast majority of patients with acute back and neck pain recover within weeks.
- Diagnostic local anesthetic blocks may be the key for making an anatomic diagnosis.
- IDD is the most common cause of axial LBP with or without somatic referred pain.
- Cervical facet joints are by far the most common cause of neck pain.

1. History

General medical history

The first responsibility of the physician presented with a patient with back or neck pain is to seek signs and symptoms that indicate a serious underlying cause for the pain. A careful medical history should include any history of cancer, recent weight loss, immunosuppression, recent back or neck surgery, intravenous drug abuse, anticoagulation, metabolic bone diseases, abdominal aortic aneurysm, and history of trauma. It is also important to ask questions about associated symptoms including bilateral lower extremity pain, numbness, weakness, bowel and bladder incontinence, and perineal numbness, which could suggest a spinal cord or nerve root compression. Worsening pain at night, inability to get relief at rest, and increased pain in the supine position suggest epidural spinal metastasis. It is important to include a social and family history to assess the psychosocial support needed to cope with the chronic pain condition.

Pain history

The pain history should document events surrounding the onset of pain. If a motor vehicle accident is the cause of pain, a thorough history including the use of a seat belt, single or multiple car involvement, and whether impact was from the rear or side of the vehicle can be useful in formulating a differential diagnosis. Cervical facet joint pain has been found to be a common source of pain after acceleration–deceleration (whiplash) injury.

The pain history should also focus on the location of pain, its duration, radiation, character (e.g., deep, superficial, sharp, achy, burning, shooting, pins and needles) and worsening or relieving factors. When more then one site is involved, each pain complaint should be documented separately. Pain history also includes previous interventions for pain symptoms including medications, nerve blocks, surgery, physical therapy, and behavioral therapy. If another pain physician saw the patient, a review of those medical records is quite useful. A brief history of the patient's activities of daily living and limitations resulting from the pain should be documented. This will be helpful in assessing the benefits of future interventions.

2. Physical examination

Comprehensive physical examination

The initial focus of the physical examination should be to determine if there are signs of serious pathology such as fever, spine tenderness, and signs of myelopathy, perineal numbness, loss of anal tone, and pulsatile abdominal mass. If infection or neoplasia is present and there are symptoms of neurologic compromise, an MRI (if available) should be ordered. This will delineate the spread of infection or tumor in the soft tissues. Routine radiographs can help identify bony fractures or destructive bony lesions. A bone scan delineates infection or tumor in bone, although it does not differentiate between the two. In patients with osteoporosis, minor trauma can lead to fracture presenting with significant pain and neurologic deficits.

Examination of the spine

Examination of the spine begins with inspection. The patient's gait, posture, and any obvious deformity of the spine can be examined very easily. The next step should include a closer examination of the entire length of the spine for scars, rash, or swelling. Palpation should begin gently to detect any sensitivity of the skin. Firmer palpation is then used to detect any midline tenderness or mass, paraspinous tenderness, or muscle tightness. Range of motion of the spine should be examined (flexion, extension, and lateral bending). During the range of motion examination, pain with flexion of the spine can be related to disc pathology, whereas pain with extension can indicate facet arthropathy or spinal stenosis. Pain with lateral bending can be a sign of ipsilateral facet disease.

A thorough neurologic examination, including sensory, motor and deep tendon reflexes, helps to rule out associated spinal cord or nerve root pathology. A positive straight leg raising (SLR) test with the patient in a supine or sitting position can point to nerve root irritation. However, nerve root irritation is not always present in patients with LBP or posterior thigh discomfort. In patients with nerve root irritation, a clear bandlike distribution of pain along a dermatomal distribution is typical in the SLR test. Tenderness over the SI joint should raise the suspicion of SI joint etiology. One compression test to detect SI pathology is Patrick's test: the supine patient with flexed leg rests an ankle on the opposite knee, and the examiner presses over the flexed knee to elicit the patient's LBP.

3. Imaging

Radiologic studies for the anatomic diagnosis of neck and back pain have a limited role. A plain film of the spine is indicated when a fracture is suspected, as in the case of trauma, a history of bony metastasis, or the presence of osteoporosis. An urgent MRI is recommended for patients with axial back pain and evidence of neurologic deficit when spinal cord pathology is suspected. If tumor or infection is thought to be the cause of pain, MRI is the imaging study of choice because it delineates the extent of the disease, including epidural spinal compression. Although routine use of MRI for nonspecific axial neck and LBP is controversial, many physicians consider this after initial conservative therapy fails. Provocative intradiscal dye injection (discography) is the most effective way to identify the pathologic disc disease. A postdiscography CT scan is recommended to delineate the anatomic distortion, which may not be seen by routine fluoroscopy.

Further descriptions of history taking, physical examination, and radiologic testing for pain patients can be found in Chapters 4 and 5. Table 1 summarizes the differentiating features of LBP.

IV. CAUSES OF BACK AND NECK PAIN

1. Rare causes

Infection, tumor, aortic aneurysm, sickle cell crisis, retroperitoneal mass, and chronic pancreatitis are among the rare causes of axial spine pain with or without extremity pain. A thorough medical history is critical. Pain often starts suddenly, and it is severe, unrelenting, and not relieved by rest. MRI in most cases is the imaging study of choice, and treatment of the underlying pathology (e.g., surgery, radiation) usually helps to alleviate the pain.

2. No clear cause

In most cases of LBP or neck pain, the anatomic or pathologic diagnosis remains unclear. A thorough history and physical examination is essential to exclude some of the rare but serious causes. LBP and neck pain of unclear etiology is a legitimate diagnosis. In the absence of neurologic symptoms, analgesics such as acetaminophen or nonsteroidal anti-inflammatory drugs (NSAIDs) can be provided.

Patients should be encouraged to continue their usual activity. If no improvement is seen within 3 weeks, physical therapy may be helpful. If axial neck pain or LBP lasts for more then 12 weeks, an attempt should be made to establish an anatomic diagnosis. The etiology of pain can be established in many cases with controlled invasive diagnostic tests with local anesthetics. Schwarzer et al. found that among patients suffering from chronic LBP, 40% have discogenic pain, 15% to 20% have SI joint pain, and 5% to 10% have facet joint pain.

3. Discogenic pain

The patient with LBP or neck pain originating from the vertebral disc often presents with deep, achy, axial midline pain. Pain can be referred to shoulder or scapular regions for cervical discs, and to buttocks and posterior thigh for lumbar discs. Patients with discogenic pain are often young, are otherwise healthy, and may

Table 1. Differentiating features of low back pain

	Trigger point	Sitting intolerance	Sensory or motor deficit	Dermatomal pain pattern	Pain on extension	Pain on flexion	SLR test	Diagnostic test
Discogenic pain	Usually absent	Usually present	Usually absent	Usually absent	May be present	Usually present	Usually absent	Discography
Facet joint pain	May be present	May be present	Usually absent	Usually absent	Usually present	Usually absent	Usually absent	Medial branch block
SI joint pain	Usually absent	May be present	Usually absent	Usually absent	May be present	May be present	Usually absent	Intra-articular anesthetic block
Spinal stenosis	Usually absent	Usually absent	May be present	Usually absent	Usually present	Usually absent	May be present	MRI study
Myofascial pain	Usually present	Usually absent	Usually absent	Usually absent	May be present	May be present	Usually absent	TP injection with anesthetic
Failed back syndrome	May be present	May be present	May be present	May be present	May be present	May be present	May be present	History
Radiculopathy	Usually absent	May be present	Likely to be present	Likely to be present	May be present	May be present	Usually present	EMG

SLR, straight leg raising; TP, trigger point; EMG, electromyography; SI, sacroiliac; MRI, magnetic resonance imaging; EMG, electromyography.

have jobs that require repetitive motion of the affected spine segment (such as package handlers). Onset of symptoms is usually gradual. Pain is experienced while sitting, standing, and bending forward. The referred pain usually remains in the proximal part of the extremity. Results of physical examination are usually nonspecific, with limited range of motion at the affected segment, or pain with movement, particularly on flexion. MRI and CT scans are not usually helpful. The presence of a high-intensity zone on MRI at the posterior aspect of the disc on sagittal plane may indicate the radial fissure of IDD. Provocative discography by injection of radiocontrast dye is utilized to rule out axial disc pathology. Discography is usually done with fluoroscopic guidance, with a second disc as a control. A postdiscography CT scan can provide more detailed information concerning the anatomic abnormality. Treatment for discogenic pain starts with conservative therapy, including physical therapy and oral NSAIDs. Refractory patients may be considered for intradiscal electrothermal therapy (IDET) (see Chapter 13). This is a relatively new technique with some encouraging data suggesting efficacy. Surgical fusion of the spine remains an option, usually as a last resort.

4. Facet joint pain

Axial spine pain originating from the facet joints has a presentation similar to that of discogenic pain. In most cases, the pain starts gradually and is deep, achy, and localized around the midline; there may be some standing and sitting intolerance. Extension and lateral bending of the affected spine are usually painful. Referred pain to the shoulder, buttock, and proximal extremities is common. Most commonly, pain is the result of stress of the facet joint capsule secondary to loss of disc or vertebral height. It can be caused by degenerative change or osteoporosis, and it is also seen after decompression surgery. When pain is secondary to osteoarthritis of the facet joints, it tends to be less severe and is often described as morning stiffness. In rare cases, facet joint pain may originate from fracture or hemarthrosis following trauma.

Physical examination is usually nonspecific, and sensory and motor examination is usually benign. Some patients have paraspinal tenderness and pain on extension and lateral bending. Imaging studies may help identify pathology such as loss of disc or vertebral height, spondylolisthesis, or other degenerative changes. Diagnostic local anesthetic block under fluoroscopic guidance is the most accurate way to isolate the facet joint as the source of axial spine pain (see Chapter 12). Currently, radiofrequency lesioning of the medial branches is considered the most effective long-term therapy for axial spine pain originating from the facet joints.

5. Sacroiliac joint pain

Localized lower back or upper buttock pain is the common presentation of SI joint pain. Pain referred to the posterior thigh and below the knee is rare. In most cases, the cause is unclear. Trauma, infection, and tumor are uncommon causes of SI joint pain. Physical examination may reveal localized tenderness over the joint, and Patrick's test may be positive (see preceding section, "Examination of the Spine"). Degenerative change of the joint on a radiograph is extremely common and nonspecific and not helpful in making a diagnosis. Intra-articular injection of local anesthetic under fluoroscopic guidance with complete pain relief indicates that the SI joint is the probable source of the pain. Treatment for SI joint pain remains controversial. Currently, an intra-articular injection of steroid with local anesthetics is the most common therapy (see Chapter 12).

6. Spinal stenosis

Spinal stenosis includes both central canal narrowing and foraminal narrowing. Symptoms from central canal narrowing tend to be diffuse compared to foraminal narrowing (when the exiting nerve root often produces symptoms in a dermatomal distribution). The clinical presentation of central canal narrowing includes axial spine pain (e.g., LBP) and extremity pain. The degree of axial and extremity pain varies between individuals; pain tends to start at the spine and gradually involve the extremities. The pain tends to be diffuse (nondermatomal) and is usually characterized as achy. It commonly worsens with walking (neurogenic claudication), especially downhill walking, and with extension of the spine. Rest and flexion of the spine usually provide temporary relief. A simple way to distinguish neurogenic from vascular claudication is to exercise patients on a bike. Patients with neurogenic claudication usually have no pain, whereas those with vascular claudication have pain while biking.

Spinal stenosis is more common in older individuals and may be associated with age-related changes of the spine. The pathophysiology includes osteophytes, facet capsular hypertrophy, and diffuse broad-based disc bulge. Foraminal narrowing can be caused by these changes as well as by loss of disc height and by spondylolisthesis. MRI can be useful in delineating the extent and the causes of the narrowing.

In mild to moderate cases, a translaminar epidural steroid injection may be therapeutic. Most patients feel their extremity pain improve sooner then their axial pain. The injection can be repeated for a cumulative benefit. If there is no improvement from epidural steroid injections, a surgical consultation may be sought to evaluate possible decompression surgery. Cervical spinal stenosis symptoms can involve both upper and lower extremities, and an early surgical consultation should be sought.

7. Myofascial pain

Neck pain and low back pain of myofascial origin are fairly common, especially after trauma and repetitive motion injury. Myofascial pain around the neck and low back presents as deep, achy, localized discomfort worsening with activity. Pain is thought to be caused by strain or sprain injury to the muscle. Patients are sometimes able to feel a focal area of tight muscle knot and tenderness on palpation. Patients may complain only of paraspinal muscle discomfort, or the pain may extend to the occiput, scapular, and shoulder areas, or to the buttocks and upper thigh areas. It is important to distinguish somatic referred pain (from disc or facet joint pathology) from pain of muscular origin. Physical examination may reveal a tight muscle band, tender to palpation, and may have a characteristic radiation pattern (trigger point).

Various physiotherapy techniques (e.g., stretching and strengthening exercise, massage, iontophoresis) remain the initial therapy of choice (see Chapter 16). Injection of local anesthetics into the tender points may be very useful, especially if a coordinated physiotherapy program immediately follows the injection. Some physicians add steroid with local anesthetics for this injection. There is a risk of local muscle atrophy with repeated steroid injection. Myofascial pain is described in detail in Chapter 17.

8. Failed back syndrome

The diagnosis of failed back syndrome is given to patients who suffer from chronic pain after spine surgery. The surgery may have been performed only for the purpose of relieving pain, or it may have been done for other reasons including stabilization or decompression to relieve neurologic deficit. Pain may vary significantly, and it may be accompanied by neurologic deficits. The pain is often different in quality and in distribution from the patient's presurgical pain. Epidural scarring is thought to be the primary cause of persistent pain. A thorough history and physical examination are critical to distinguish the nociceptive and neuropathic components of pain. Pain along the distribution of one or more nerve roots may indicate epidural fibrosis. Nociceptive pain from facet or disc disease should be also considered. Up to 40% of postlaminectomy (lumbosacral) patients have LBP originating from facet joints. Scar tissue, early-onset arthritic change, and osteophytes may cause spinal stenosis.

Therapy for failed back syndrome remains controversial. Repeat surgery may not provide the desired pain relief. For patients with neuropathic pain, epidural steroid injection via the foraminal or caudal route can be a useful and relatively benign initial intervention. Other interventional modalities, such as epidural lysis of adhesions via epiduroscopy or by catheter technique (Racz procedure), are not widely practiced because of limited evidence of efficacy. Spinal cord stimulation has been shown to be an effective mode of therapy for neuropathic pain from failed back surgery (see Chapter 13).

9. Whiplash injury

Acceleration–deceleration injury from motor vehicle accidents, commonly known as whiplash injury, frequently causes neck pain. Whiplash is estimated to occur in 1% of the general population, and the pain may become chronic in 10% to 25% of the patients. A controlled study found cervical facet joints to be the most common cause of neck pain after whiplash injury. The authors estimated that in at least 50% (possibly as high as 80%) of high-speed injuries, cervical facet joints are the source of neck pain. The most common cervical segments involved are C5-6 and C2-3. The neck has a large number of muscles, including the neck extensor, flexor, rotator, and lateral flexors. They are well innervated and a common source of neck pain.

The initial office visit should include a history of injury or risk factors for serious pathology. Physical examination has a limited role because of poor reliability and validity of identifying specific causes of pain. It may show limited range of motion, pain with movement, or tenderness over the articular pillars or paraspinous muscles. These signs are nonspecific for making pathoanatomic diagnoses. In the case of trauma, plain films may show fracture or dislocation. MRI and CT are not indicated unless there is a suggestion of impending neurologic compromise. Ronnen et al. (1996) showed that MRI is not useful for diagnosing whiplash-related injury.

Facet joints are the most common cause of neck pain. To formulate an accurate diagnosis of cervical facet joint pain, a control joint block is recommended because of the high rate of false-positive responses from a single diagnostic block. The prevalence of cervical discogenic pain is unknown. Provocative discography may help to identify discogenic pain, although cervical discography has a fairly high level of false-positive responses. A high degree of vigilance and expertise are required when using this technique to avoid infection and injury to vital structures.

V. CONCLUSION

The vast majority of the patients with back and neck pain recover within weeks. The cause of the acute pain remains undetermined in the majority of cases. Neoplasms and infections account for less than 0.7% and 0.01% cases of acute LBP, respectively. History and physical examination should focus on identifying the warning signs of serious underlying pathology. In routine cases, findings include a limited range of motion, pain with activity, and back tenderness; these signs and symptoms are nonspecific and do not help in making a definitive diagnosis. Furthermore, if serious pathology is not suspected, special investigations do not help to make a specific diagnosis. Initial treatment for acute nonspecific back and neck pain should focus on providing reassurance and encouragement, as well as adequate analgesia using simple analgesics and physical treatments, allowing patients to remain active and continue to work.

SELECTED READINGS

1. Barnsley L, Lord S, Wallis B, Bogduk N. False positive rates of cervical zygapophysial-joint blocks. *Clin J Pain* 1993;9:124–130.
2. Bogduk N. Low back pain. In: Bogduk N. *The Clinical anatomy of the lumbar spine and sacrum,* 3rd ed. Edinburgh: Churchill Livingstone, 1999:188–189.
3. Bogduk N. *Acute lumbar radicular pain,* chap 3, p 5. Newcastle, Australia: Cambridge Press, 1999.
4. Bogduk N, Aprill C. On the nature of neck pain, discography and cervical zygapophysial-joint pain *Pain* 1993;54:213–217.
5. Kuslich SD, Ulstrom CL, Michael CJ. The tissue origin of low back pain and sciatica: A report of pain response to tissue stimulation during operation on the lumbar spine using local anesthesia. *Orthop Clin North Am* 1991;22: 181–187.
6. Maigne JY, Aivaliklis A, Pfefer F. Results of sacroiliac joint double block and value of sacroiliac pain provocation tests in 54 patients with low back pain. *Spine* 1996;21:1889–1892.
7. Merskey H, Bogduk N, eds. *Classification of chronic pain,* 2nd ed. Seattle, WA: IASP Press, 1994.

8. Ronnen HR, de Korte PJ, Brink PR, vander Bijl HR. Acute whiplash injury: Is there a role for MR imaging? A prospective study of 100 patients. *Radiology* 1996;201: 93—96.
9. Schwarzer AC, Wang SC, Bogduk N, et al. The false positive rate of uncontrolled diagnostic blocks of the lumbar Z-joints. *Pain* 1994;58:195–200.
10. Schwarzer AC, Aprill CN, Derby R, Fortin J. The prevalence and clinical features of internal disc disruption in patients with chronic low back pain. *Spine* 1995;20:1878–1883.
12. Walsh TR, Weinstein JN, Spratt KF, et al. Lumbar discography in normal subjects. *J Bone Joint Surg* 1990;72A:1081–1088.

Headache

F. Michael Cutrer
and Pramit Bhasin

I have a pain upon my forehead here.
—*Othello Act 3, Scene 3, by William Shakespeare (1564–1616)*

Headache descriptions and treatments can be found in pre-Christian Sumerian and Egyptian writings. Aretaeus of Cappadocia in second-century Turkey wrote of headache sufferers who "hid from the light and wished for death." Headache is still a common affliction; in 1985, a large-scale survey-based study reported the prevalence of headache in the United States to be 78% of women and 68% of men. It is estimated that 40% of adults in North America have experienced a severe debilitating headache at least once in their lives.

Despite its long history and great prevalence in the population, the complaint of recurrent headache is still met with widespread indifference and suspicion among many health care providers. As a result, headache patients must often contend with haphazard and sometimes even inappropriate treatment. This is unnecessary and can even be tragic because not only can headache be the presenting symptom for a serious and even life-threatening abnormality, but also the majority of patients with recurrent headache show a good response to therapy.

I. ANATOMY OF HEAD PAIN

Over 50 years ago, epilepsy surgery performed on the brains of awake patients under local anesthesia indicated that brain tissue itself was relatively insensate to electrical or mechanical stimulation, whereas electrical stimulation of the meninges or meningeal blood vessels produced a severe boring headache. The meninges and meningeal vessels are richly supplied with C fibers (small fibers) and are the key structures involved in the generation of headache. The C fibers from the meninges converge into the trigeminal nerve and project to the trigeminal nucleus caudalis in the lower medulla, where they synapse. From the caudal brainstem, fibers carrying nociceptive signals project to more-rostral trigeminal subnuclei and the thalamus (ventral posterior medial, medial, and intralaminar nuclei). Projections from the thalamus ascend to the cerebral cortex, where painful information is localized and reaches consciousness.

II. PATHOGENIC THEORIES OF HEADACHE

Head pain results from the activation of the pain fibers that innervate intracranial structures regardless of the activating stimulus. In a small number of patients, an identifiable structural or inflammatory source for the headache can be found using neuroimaging or other laboratory investigations. However, the overwhelming majority of patients encountered in clinical practice suffer from primary headache disorders such as migraine or tension headache in which physical examinations and laboratory studies are unrevealing. Research into the pathophysiology of headache has been limited by the subjective nature of the complaints and the paucity of animal models with which to test hypotheses. Theories of migraine pathogenesis fall roughly into two categories, vasogenic and neurogenic. Since the duration of headache frequently exceeds the duration of the initiating stimulus, it is likely that sensitization within the trigeminal and upper cervical pain pathways contributes to the prolongation of headaches. Sensitizing events may occur in both the peripheral and central portions of these pathways.

1. Vasogenic theory

In the late 1930s, investigators observed that cranial vessels appear to be important in the generation of headache. They found that in many patients extracranial vessels became distended and pulsated during a migraine attack, and that vasoconstrictive substances such as ergots could abort the headache, whereas vasodilatory substances such as nitrates tended to provoke the headache. Based on these observations, they theorized that intracranial vasoconstriction is responsible for the aura of migraine, that the headache results from a rebound dilation and distention of cranial vessels. Later, it was postulated that head pain is enhanced by vasoactive polypeptides.

2. Neurogenic theory

The alternative hypothesis holds that migraine is caused by a dysfunction of the brain itself, involving a lowered cerebral thresh-

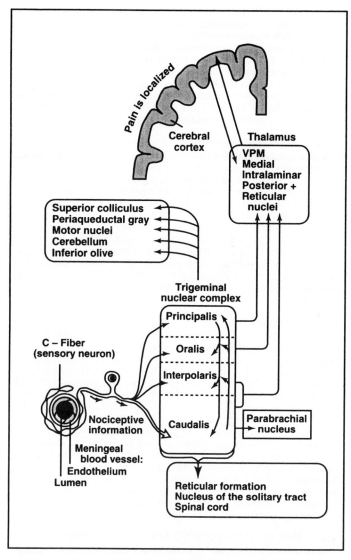

Figure 1. Schematic overview of the mechanism leading to headache pain perception after activation of trigeminovascular nociceptive neurons. VPM, ventral posterior medical.

old to migraine attacks. According to this hypothesis, when precipitating factors exceed this threshold, a migraine attack occurs, and although vascular changes may occur during a migraine attack, they occur as a result rather than the cause of the attack. Proponents of the neurogenic theory point to the broad range of neurologic symptoms associated with a migraine attack that cannot be explained on the basis of vasoconstriction within a single cerebrovascular distribution, as well as the prodromal symptoms such as euphoria, hunger, thirst, or fluid retention that precede the headache, in some individuals by as much as 24 hours.

3. Peripheral sensitization

There is increasing experimental evidence that once activated, C fibers release neuropeptides (e.g., substance P, neurokinin A, calcitonin gene-related peptide) that generate a neurogenic inflammatory response within the meninges. This response consists of increased plasma leakage from meningeal vessels, vasodilation, and activation of mast cells and endothelial cells. Once set into motion, this process may act to lower the threshold of the C fibers to further activation and, as a result, prolong and intensify the headache attack. Drugs known to be effective in ending a migraine attack, such as dihydroergotamine or sumatriptan, have been shown to act at serotonin (5HT) receptor subtypes to block the release of neuropeptides and the development of neurogenic inflammation.

4. Central sensitization

Animal studies indicate that inflammatory or chemical C-fiber activation results in expansion of receptive fields and recruitment of previously non-nociceptive neurons into the transmission of painful information. The changes are clinically reflected as hyperalgesia (lowered pain threshold) and allodynia (the generation of a painful response by normally nonpainful stimuli). Analogous clinical phenomena are seen in headache disorders. For example, minor head movements, bending, or coughing, which normally do not cause pain, are perceived as painful during or in the hours following a migraine attack. Recent studies by Burstein and coworkers have demonstrated that stimulation of meningeal nociceptors causes a lowering of the activation thresholds for convergent, previously nonpainful skin stimulation. Subsequent studies of human subjects during migraine attacks have also demonstrated the development of cutaneous allodynia both within the areas innervated by the trigeminal nerve and in extratrigeminal areas.

III. CLINICAL APPROACH TO ACUTE HEADACHE

When faced with a patient in the emergency department whose primary complaint is that of a severe headache, the first question to ask is whether the headache is symptomatic of a potentially serious underlying abnormality requiring rapid and appropriate treatment. In the vast majority of cases, the headache represents a particularly severe episode in a primary headache disorder. However, the distinction between primary and secondary (symptomatic of another cause) headache must be made as rapidly and accurately as possible. It is crucial to use the history and physical exam to decide whether the patient is at high or low risk, to order diagnostic tests, and to provide therapy accordingly. Laboratory tests and imaging studies ordered without good clinical indication are usually unhelpful and always expensive.

1. Important questions to ask

Is this headache the first of its kind? If the headache is unlike anything experienced previously, the risk increases. If it is similar (even if of greater intensity) to attacks experienced over many months or years, the likelihood that it is a benign process increases. This question becomes increasingly important for patients over 40 years, as the incidence of the first attack of migraine decreases and the incidence of neoplasm and other intracranial pathology increases.

Was this headache of sudden onset? A persistent headache that begins and reaches maximal intensity within a few seconds or minutes is more suggestive of an ominous vascular cause.

Has there been any alteration in mental status during the course of the headache? Generally a family member or friend who has been with the patient must answer this question. Although migraineurs can appear fatigued, especially after prolonged vomiting or analgesic use, obtundation and confusion are more suggestive of meningitis, encephalitis, or subarachnoid hemorrhage.

Has there been recent or coexistent infectious disease? Infection in other locations (e.g., lungs, paranasal or mastoid sinuses) may precede meningitis. Fever is *not* a feature of migraine or a primary headache disorder. Fever may also occur in association with subarachnoid hemorrhage, although usually 3 to 4 days after the actual hemorrhage.

Did the headache begin in the context of vigorous exercise or seemingly trivial head or neck trauma? Although effort-induced migraine or coital migraine certainly exist, the rapid onset of headache with strenuous exercise, especially when minor trauma has occurred, increases the possibility of carotid artery dissection or intracranial hemorrhage.

Does the head pain tend to radiate posteriorly? Pain radiation between the shoulders or lower is not typical of migraine and may indicate meningeal irritation from subarachnoid blood or infection.

Other important points not to be overlooked in a careful history include the following:

Do other family members have similar headache? Migraine has a strong familial tendency.

What medications does the patient take? Certain medications can cause headache. Anticoagulants and oral antibiotics place the patient in a higher risk group for hemorrhage or partially treated central nervous system (CNS) infection.

Does the patient have any other chronic illness or a history of neurologic abnormality? These may confuse the neurologic examination.

Is the headache consistently in the same location or on the same side? Benign headache disorders tend to change sides and locations at least occasionally.

2. Important physical findings

It is crucial to examine each patient carefully, especially when there are atypical elements in the history. A basic neurologic examination should be performed that addresses the following six components:

Mental status: What is the patient's level of consciousness? Is the patient able to maintain normal attention during the examination? Are language and memory normal?

Cranial nerves: Each cranial nerve should be tested separately. Are there asymmetries? Is there papilledema?

Motor: Are motor strength and muscle tone symmetrical and within the normal range? Are there any abnormal involuntary movements?

Sensory: Are there asymmetries of pain, temperature, or proprioceptive sensation?

Coordination: Is there dysmetria or gait ataxia?

Reflexes: Is there asymmetry of reflexes in either the upper or lower extremities?

Three findings on examination should be considered signs of possible serious pathology:

Nuchal rigidity: This can be an indicator of either meningitis or subarachnoid hemorrhage.

Toxicity: Is there a low-grade fever or persistent tachycardia? Does the patient appear more acutely ill than most migraine patients?

Previously unnoticed neurologic abnormality: Subtle findings such as slight pupillary asymmetry, unilateral pronator drift, or an extensor plantar response are significant and should lead to further investigation.

3. When to order laboratory tests or imaging studies

Laboratory tests should be obtained to confirm the presence of abnormalities suspected from the history and physical examination and should be appropriate for the pathology suspected. Laboratory, electroencephalographic, or neuroimaging "fishing trips" are discouraged because they rarely provide useful information, can delay treatment, and can divert attention away from more relevant findings. At the present time computed tomography (CT) is the imaging study most likely to be available in the acute setting. There are three major indications for an urgent CT scan:

- The presence of papilledema
- Any impairment of consciousness or orientation
- The presence of localizing or lateralizing findings on neurologic examination

CT is most useful for identifying recent intracerebral and extracerebral hemorrhages, hydrocephalus, brain abscesses, and other space-occupying lesions.

IV. DIFFERENTIAL DIAGNOSIS OF SECONDARY HEADACHES

Headache can be symptomatic of many underlying abnormalities. The frequency of secondary headaches is smaller than that of primary headache disorders. However, it is vital that these headaches be diagnosed quickly and treated appropriately. The most common causes are listed in Table 1.

Table 1. Secondary headache etiologies

Vascular
  Subarachnoid hemorrhage
  Subdural hematoma
  Cerebellar hemorrhage
  Arteriovenous malformations (AVM)
  Intracerebral arterial occlusion
  Occlusion of cerebral venous sinus (e.g., cavernous sinus
  thrombosis)
  Carotid artery dissection

Infectious
  Meningitis
  Meningoencephalitis
  Brain abscess
  Acute sinusitis
  Upper respiratory or systemic viral infection
  Acquired immunodeficiency disease

Neoplastic

Inflammatory
  Temporal arteritis
  Autoimmune inflammatory process

Hypertensive
  Acute pressor response to an exogenous agent
  Pheochromocytoma
  Malignant hypertension (including hypertensive encephalopathy)
  Preeclampsia or eclampsia

Glaucoma
  Pigmentary glaucoma
  Acute angle-closure glaucoma

Substance abuse headache

Benign intracranial hypertension (pseudotumor cerebri)

V. DIFFERENTIAL DIAGNOSIS OF PRIMARY HEADACHES

In clinical practice, the vast majority of patients investigated because of head pain ultimately prove to have a primary headache disorder (i.e., recurrent headaches for which no underlying structural, infectious, or other systemic abnormality can be found). Migraine and tension-type headaches form the bulk of this population, but cluster headache and other less common syndromes are occasionally seen. To classify and investigate primary headaches, the International Headache Society (IHS) has developed classification and diagnostic criteria for headache and facial pain (Table 2), which are invaluable for clinical research, with the caveat that many patients do not fall neatly into a diagnostic category.

1. Migraine

It is estimated that approximately 16% of women and 6% of men in the United States meet the diagnostic criteria for migraine. Migraine sufferers frequently have family members who also

(*text continues on page 398*)

Table 2.   Diagnostic criteria for common headache types

Headache type	Diagnostic criteria
Migraine without aura	The patient must have had at least five attacks that fulfill each of the following categories: a) Headache attacks lasting 4–72 hours (untreated or treated successfully) b) Headache has at least two of the following: • Unilateral location • Pulsating quality • Moderate or severe intensity (inhibits or prohibits daily activity) • Aggravation by walking stairs or similar routine physical activity c) During headache, at least one of the following: • Nausea and/or vomiting • Photophobia • Phonophobia d) Headaches not correlated to another physical abnormality
Migraine with aura	In addition to fulfilling the criteria of migraine without aura, the patient must have experienced at least two attacks with three of the four following characteristics: a) Attacks associated with reversible aura symptoms indicating focal cerebral cortical and/or brainstem dysfunction b) At least one of the aura symptoms develops gradually over 4 minutes, or two or more symptoms occur in succession c) No aura symptom lasts for more than 1 hour (if more than one aura symptom are present, accepted duration is increased accordingly) d) Headache follows resolution of aura symptoms within 1 hour or less (headache can sometimes begin simultaneously with the aura) e) Neither the headache nor the aura symptoms can be correlated to another physical abnormality

Table 2. *Continued*

Headache type	Diagnostic criteria

Tension-type headache	The patient must have had at least 10 headaches fulfilling each of the following categories:
	a) Headache lasting from 30 minutes to 7 days
	b) Headaches have at least two of the following pain characteristics:
	  • Pressing/tightening (nonpulsatile) quality
	  • Mild or moderate intensity (does not prohibit normal routine)
	  • Bilateral location
	  • No aggravation by routine physical activity
	c) Both of the following
	  • No associated nausea or vomiting
	  • Either photophobia or phonophobia may be present, but not both
	d) Headache not correlated with any other physical abnormality

Cluster headache	The patients must have experienced at least five attacks fulfilling each of the following criteria:
	a) Severe unilateral orbital or supraorbital and/or temporal pain lasting 15 to 180 minutes if treated
	b) Headache is associated with at least one of the following signs on the ipsilateral side:
	  • Conjunctival injection
	  • Lacrimation
	  • Nasal congestion
	  • Rhinorrhea
	  • Forehead and nasal sweating
	  • Miosis
	  • Ptosis
	  • Eyelid edema
	c) Attacks occur with a frequency of at least one attack every other day to eight attacks per day
	d) Headaches not correlated with any other physical abnormality

From the International Headache Society (IHS) Classification and Diagnostic Criteria for Headache and Facial Pain, with permission.

have recurrent headaches. Migraine falls into two categories: **migraine without aura** (previously called common migraine) and **migraine with aura** (previously called classic migraine). Patients with migraine often report prodromal symptoms that begin 24 to 48 hours before a headache attack. These symptoms can include hyperactivity, mild euphoria, lethargy, depression, cravings for certain foods, frequent yawning, and other atypical symptoms. Prodromal symptoms should not be confused with the migraine aura, which occurs within 1 hour of the onset of the headache and consists of specific neurologic symptoms. Typical migraine aura symptoms include the following:

- Homonymous visual disturbance, classically a scintillating scotoma
- Unilateral paresthesias and or numbness, often affecting the distal extremities or the perioral region of the face
- Unilateral weakness
- Aphasia or other language disturbance

The aura symptoms in some patients localize to the brainstem. These include visual symptoms in the temporal and nasal fields of both eyes, dysarthria, vertigo, tinnitus, decreased hearing, double vision, ataxia, bilateral paresthesias, bilateral weakness, and decreased level of consciousness.

Basilar migraine

Patients in whom brainstem symptoms predominate are generally given the diagnosis of basilar migraine. Many of these symptoms are subject to misinterpretation, as they can occur with anxiety and hyperventilation. In many patients, basilar attacks are intermingled with typical attacks. Dizziness is frequently reported as a feature of an otherwise typical attack of migraine with aura.

Migraine with prolonged aura, or complicated migraine

Migraine attacks in which the aura symptoms persist for more than 1 hour, but less than 1 week, and in which neuroimaging studies are normal are diagnosed as complicated migraines.

Familial hemiplegic migraine

Patients who have migraine with aura including hemiparesis, and who have at least one first-degree relative who experiences identical attacks, are given a diagnosis of familial hemiplegic migraine. This form of migraine has been localized to chromosome 19 in several families.

2. Tension-type headache

Tension-type headache is probably the most common primary headache disorder. It has been referred to by many names in the past including muscle contraction headache, essential headache, stress headache, and psychomyogenic headache. The exact pathogenesis of tension-type headache and the importance of muscle contraction to its generation are still poorly understood. Pericranial muscle spasm or tenderness may or may not be present. Tension-type headache occurs in both episodic and chronic forms.

3. Cluster headache

Cluster headaches are much less common than migraine or tension-type headaches. They afflict men five to six times more often than women, and the age of onset is typically 20 to 40 years. The syndrome derives its name from the fact that attacks occur in series lasting for weeks or months (the so-called cluster periods), separated by remissions that usually last for months or years. During cluster periods, headache attacks might be provoked by alcohol, histamine, or nitroglycerine. The pain is very severe, with a throbbing, at times sharp, quality. During a cluster headache, a patient is often agitated and frequently paces, unlike a migraine patient who prefers to avoid movement in a quiet dark room. In some instances, the clustering pattern of the episodic form can change into the chronic form in which there is no remission.

4. Miscellaneous benign headaches

There are several headache syndromes that are unassociated with a structural cause but are distinct from migraine, tension-type, or cluster headaches. The following is a brief listing and description of these syndromes.

Chronic paroxysmal hemicrania is a relatively rare syndrome in which attacks occur that are similar to those of cluster headache. It differs from cluster headache in that attacks occur with greater frequency (>5 per day for more than half the time) and tend to be very brief (5 to 20 minutes), prolonged remissions do not occur, women are affected more frequently than men, and attacks are very responsive to low-dose indomethacin.

Paroxysmal hemicrania is a relatively uncommon syndrome characterized by brief (2 to 45 minutes) and multiple (five or more per day) episodes of unilateral orbital throbbing or stabbing pain of severe intensity. The attacks are associated with ipsilateral autonomic signs (e.g., conjunctival injection, rhinorrhea, tearing, eyelid edema, and ptosis).

Hemicrania continua is a rare headache syndrome in which unilateral orbital or temporal pain is present almost constantly.

Idiopathic stabbing headache, a series of icepick-like jabbing pains, frequently occurs in migraineurs on the side frequently affected by migraine attacks. These attacks often respond to oral indomethacin (25 mg three times per day).

Benign exertional headache can be precipitated by any form of exercise. It is generally bilateral in location and can last from several minutes to 24 hours.

Cold-induced headaches can result from either exposure of the head to low ambient temperatures or passage of a cold liquid or solid material over the palate or posterior pharynx (e.g., "ice cream headache").

Orgasm-induced headache can occur in susceptible individuals with masturbation or sexual intercourse.

Benign cough headache may be diagnosed only after a structural lesion has been excluded with neuroimaging.

VI. REFRACTORY HEADACHES

1. Chronic daily headache

The IHS classifies headaches that are present for at least 15 days per month during at least 6 months per year as chronic. Patients usually describe these headaches as being tension-type in quality, although more severe attacks similar to migraine may be interspersed. Prophylactic therapy in patients taking daily analgesics or ergotamine-containing medications is frequently ineffective. Discontinuation of daily analgesic or ergotamine use often results in improvement.

2. Status migrainosus

Migraine attacks that persist for longer than 72 hours despite treatment are classified as status migrainosus. In-patient treatment is necessary (see section VII, 1, iii).

VII. RATIONAL APPROACH TO PHARMACOLOGIC TREATMENT OF PRIMARY HEADACHES

Pharmacologic treatment of patients with headache can be divided into two broad categories: acute therapy given during an attack to end it, and prophylactic treatment given daily to decrease the frequency and severity of future attacks. The reader is referred to Appendix VIII or to the Physicians Desk Reference (PDR) for more detailed descriptions of the drugs used in the management of headache.

1. Treatment of migraine

(i) Acute therapy for mild or moderate attacks

Acetaminophen. Occasionally, patients have mild attacks that, when caught early, respond to over-the-counter analgesics like acetaminophen (650 to 1,000 mg). Mild to moderate attacks during pregnancy should be treated with acetaminophen in the first instance.

Nonsteroidal anti-inflammatory drugs (NSAIDs) including aspirin (900 to 1,000 mg), ibuprofen (1,000 to 1,200 mg), Naprosyn (500 to 825 mg) and ketoprofen (100 to 200 mg) can be used to treat mild to moderate attacks.

Midrin is a combination medication containing acetaminophen, isometheptene mucate (a mild vasoconstrictor), and dichloralphenazone (a mild sedative). Two tablets should be taken at the onset of headache followed by one each hour until relief occurs or up to a maximum of five capsules within a 12-hour period. Anecdotally, Midrin is less likely than many of the other combination medications to generate a rebound headache syndrome, although daily use of any of these treatments is not recommended.

(ii) Acute therapy for severe attacks

Butalbital is a barbiturate combined with caffeine, acetylsalicylic acid, and/or acetaminophen in several medications (including Fiorinal, Fioricet, Phrenilin, and Esgic). The recommended dosage is two tablets every 4 hours, not to exceed six per day. These medications are best suited for treatment of moderate to severe, infrequent headaches. If used to treat headaches occurring more than twice per month, patients may develop rebound headaches. If prescribing these drugs, physicians should ensure that they are not prescribed in escalating doses.

Oral opioid-containing medications have little place in the treatment of chronic recurrent primary headaches and should be avoided until all other treatment alternatives have been considered. Under certain conditions they are the only viable option, (e.g., pregnancy, severe vascular disease). Physicians should discuss the risks of rebound headache and dependency before prescribing.

Ketorolac is a potent NSAID that is available in injectable form. It can be given intramuscularly (IM) or intravenously (IV) for the treatment of severe migraine attacks with early and prominent vomiting. Although ketorolac is expensive and not clearly superior to cheaper medications, some patients respond well. Because of its potency, the risk of side effects is actually greater than with other NSAIDs, and the manufacturers recommend short-term usage only (see Chapter 8).

Ergotamine-containing medications are available in oral, sublingual, and suppository formulations in the United States. Ergotamines are the classical antimigraine agents and can be effective if patients tolerate the side effects of nausea and peripheral vasoconstriction. They are typically most effective if given early in the migraine attack. A potential problem is overuse, which can result in a chronic daily headache syndrome and in extreme cases the gangrene-like complications of ergotism. If prescribing the suppository, patients should be instructed to cut the suppository in half or into quarters to find the lowest effective dose and thereby reduce ergotamine-induced nausea. Contraindications include coronary artery disease, angina, peripheral vascular disease, Raynaud's phenomenon, uncontrolled hypertension, and severely impaired renal or hepatic function.

Dihydroergotamine (DHE) is a hydrogenated ergot that until recently was the mainstay of nonopioid treatment of acute severe headache attacks. It has fewer potent peripheral arterial vasoconstrictive effects and can be effective even when given well into the attack. It is associated with less nausea than ergotamine, but an antiemetic given prior to treatment is usually required. DHE is available in injectable and intranasal formulations. To give DHE in the acute setting, early in the attack, administer 1 to 2 mg IM or subcutaneously (SC), repeated up to a further 3 mg in 24 hours. Well into a severe attack, administer prochlorperazine 5 mg IV, or metoclopramide 10 mg IV, followed in 5 to 10 minutes by DHE 0.75 to 1 mg IV over 2 to 3 minutes. If the attack has not subsided after 30 minutes, an additional 0.5 mg of DHE may be given IV.

Sumatriptan (Imitrex) and the "triptans." Sumatriptan is the prototype of the new triptan class of drugs that selectively bind to $5HT_{1B/D/F}$ receptors. It exerts both direct vasoconstrictor and antineurogenic inflammatory effects on dural vessels. Sumatriptan treatment is also associated with improvement in the nausea, vomiting, photophobia, and phonophobia that accompany many migraine attacks. It has been shown to be effective when given up to 4 hours after the onset of a headache attack. Sumatriptan is available in injectable (6 mg SC) oral (25 and 50 mg) and intranasal (20 mg) as well as oral formulations.

Newer $5HT_{1B/D/F}$ receptor agonists that have recently become available include **naratriptan (Amerge), zolmitriptan (Zomig),** and **rizatriptan (Maxalt)**. The overall efficacy and side-effect profiles of these new agents do not vary greatly from those of sumatriptan. However, there are differences in half-life, relative affinity for the $h5HT_{1D}$ and $h5HT_{1B}$ receptor subtypes, and blood–brain barrier penetrance. Naratriptan (2.5-mg tablets) has been reported to have an overall lower incidence of side effects than sumatriptan, but the onset appears to be somewhat slower. Duration may be longer, however. The side-effect profiles of both **zolmitriptan** (2.5- and 5-mg tablets) and **rizatriptan** (5- and 10-mg tablets and rapidly dispersible wafers) are similar to sumatriptan, but trials suggest that the onset of action may be slightly faster than oral sumatriptan. Three more triptans, **eletriptan**, **frovatriptan**, and **almotriptan**, await approval from the U.S. Food and Drug Administration (FDA). These drugs are now widely available and have become the de facto drugs of choice in the outpatient treatment of moderate to severe migraine attacks in patients without risk factors for coronary disease or prolonged neurologic symptoms.

Neuroleptics, including chlorpromazine, prochlorperazine, and droperidol, have been used as an alternative to meperidine or vasoactive medications in the emergency department for the treatment of severe migraine attacks. Droperidol given by repeated IV injection is frequently effective in the treatment of status migrainosus. The protocol for patients with intractable migraine attacks is as follows: Give 2.5 mg IV and repeat twice at 30-minute intervals if the headache persists (total dose, 7.5 mg). To avoid akathisia, pretreat with benztropine (Cogentin), 1 mg PO (orally), followed by 1 mg PO twice daily. The risks of hypotension, sedation, and akathisia limit the use of neuroleptics.

Opioids. Meperidine is the opioid most frequently chosen by emergency department physicians for the treatment of severe migraine headache. It is commonly given in combination with an antiemetic. The choice of meperidine, or in fact any opioid, is questionable for this indication, and there is no evidence in the literature to support this practice. In fact, in one double-blind comparison study, meperidine was found to be inferior to chlorpromazine for aborting a migraine attack. Its main beneficial effect may be that of induction of sleep with resultant resolution of the attack. The use of parenteral opioids should be limited to patients with infrequent attacks, or patients in whom other treatments are contraindicated. The use of meperidine is generally discouraged because of the toxicity of its metabolite normeperidine, and because of the preference of addicts for this particular opioid (see Chapter 9). Suitable alternatives would be morphine or hydromorphone.

(iii) Treatment of status migrainosus

If efforts to end a migraine attack in the emergency department are unsuccessful and the patient requires hospitalization, IV treatment with DHE is the treatment of choice if there are no contraindications. The following protocol is recommended:

1. Metoclopramide 10 mg IV plus DHE 0.5 mg IV is given over 2 to 3 minutes.
2. If the headache stops but nausea develops, no DHE is given for 8 hours, then 0.3 or 0.4 mg DHE plus 10 mg metoclopramide is given every 8 hours for 3 days.
3. If the head pain persists and no nausea develops, 0.5 mg DHE is repeated in 1 hour. If headache is relieved but nausea develops, DHE 0.75 mg IV every 8 hours for 3 days plus metoclo-

pramide 10 mg is given. If headache is relieved and no nausea develops, DHE 1.0 mg every 8 hours plus metoclopramide 10 mg for 3 days is given.
4. If headache stops and no nausea develops, DHE 0.5 mg plus metoclopramide 10 mg IV is given every 8 hours for 3 days.

The DHE should be given undiluted through an IV Hep-Lock. Metoclopramide may be discontinued after six DHE doses.

Diarrhea is a common side effect of the DHE protocol and can be controlled with oral diphenoxylate (Lomotil). Contraindications to IV DHE include Prinzmetal's angina, pregnancy, coronary artery disease or uncontrolled hypertension, peripheral vascular disease, and severe renal or hepatic disease.

When patients are hospitalized and given IV DHE, special attention should be given to the amount of analgesic medications they were taking prior to admission. Status migrainosus is frequently associated with overuse of abortive medications, and patients should be watched carefully for evidence of barbiturate or opiate withdrawal. If no prophylactic regimen is in place in a patient with episodes status migrainosus, then initiation of prophylactic therapy is appropriate.

(iv) Prophylactic therapy

Acute drug treatment of headache is largely to relieve symptoms and has no benefit beyond the single attack. In the many patients who have infrequent attacks, an effective abortive agent is sufficient. However, the frequent use of abortive agents rapidly becomes a part of the problem. Once a patient has slid into the insidious cycle of analgesic rebound, prophylactic therapy may be futile and the headaches just keep on getting worse.

If attacks occur more than once or twice per month and are sufficiently severe to prohibit normal activities, or the patient's dread of the attacks is intrusive, then prophylactic therapy should be considered (Table 3). The regimen should be individualized to the patient. Concurrent medical problems may contraindicate certain prophylactic medications, or occasionally the prophylactic medicine can be used to treat migraine as well as a preexistent illness. Prophylactic medications are empiric treatments, and to date, their mechanism of action is unknown. Most of these medications were originally used for other indications and their antimigraine effects were found coincidentally. It is likely that in many cases their effect in migraine is unrelated to the action for which they were originally prescribed. Most prophylactic agents are associated with increased appetite and patients should be warned about potential weight gain.

Prophylactic medications fall into a two-tiered hierarchy. First-line agents are those that are likely to be effective without intolerable side effects. Second-line agents may be effective when the first-line agents have failed, but they carry the risk of more frequent or potentially serious side effects.

First-Line Agents

Adrenoceptor blockers. Beta-blockers shown to be effective migraine prophylactic agents in clinical trials include propranolol, nadolol, atenolol, timolol, and metoprolol. The antimigraine

Table 3.   Prophylactic medications useful in migraine

Drug	How supplied (mg)	Daily oral dose (mg)
Beta-blockers	10, 20, 40, 80	40–240
Propranolol (Inderal)	20, 40, 80, 120, 160	20–80
Nadolol (Corgard)	25, 50, 100	50–150
Atenolol (Tenormin)	5, 10, 20	20–60
Timolol (Blocadren)	50, 100	50–300
Metoprolol (Lopressor)		
NSAIDs		
Naproxen sodium (Aleve, Anaprox)	220, 275, 550	480–1,100
Naprosyn (Naprosyn)	250, 500	750–1,000
Ketoprofen (Orudis)	25, 50, 75	150–300
Aspirin	375	1,000–1,300
Antidepressants		
Amitriptyline (Elavil)	10, 25, 50, 75, 100, 150	10–120
Calcium channel blockers		
Flunarizine	Not available in U.S.	
Verapamil (Calan)	40, 80, 120	120–480
Anticonvulsants		
Divalproex sodium (Depakote)	125, 250, 500	250–1,500
Gabapentin (Neurontin)	100, 300, 400, 600	600–3,600
Serotonin antagonist		
Methysergide (Sansert)	2	4–8
Monoamine oxidase inhibitor		
Phenelzine (Nardil)	15	30–60

activity of these medications does not depend on CNS penetration, cardioselectivity, or 5HT binding. The only common pharmacologic property that separates the beta-blockers effective in migraine prophylaxis from those that are ineffective is the lack of partial sympathomimetic activity. Because of differences in pharmacologic properties among the various agents, failure of one agent is not an indicator of failure of others. Side effects occur in 10% to 15% of patients and include hypotension, fatigue, dizziness, gastrointestinal (GI) disturbance (diarrhea, constipation), depression, insomnia, and memory disturbance. Contraindications include asthma, congestive heart failure, chronic obstruction pulmonary disease, peripheral vascular disease, cardiac conduction defects, and brittle diabetes.

NSAIDs. Although NSAIDs inhibit platelet function as part of their spectrum of activities (see Chapter 8), it has been difficult to correlate prophylactic efficacy with inhibition of platelet function. NSAIDs that have been shown to exhibit prophylactic effects in controlled clinical trials include aspirin, naproxen/naproxen sodium, tolfenamic acid, ketoprofen, mefenamic acid, and fenoprofen.

There have been no trials comparing different NSAIDs for migraine prophylaxis. The only agent shown to be effective in controlled studies for treatment of menstruation-associated migraine is naproxen sodium. This, coupled with its proven efficacy in double-blind studies, makes it the first choice among the NSAIDs for migraine prophylaxis.

Antidepressants. The only antidepressant with significant evidence of efficacy in migraine prophylaxis is the tricyclic antidepressant amitriptyline, which inhibits reuptake of both norepinephrine and 5HT. However, reuptake inhibition does not appear to correlate with efficacy in migraine. Clinical trials also indicate that the antimigraine activity of amitriptyline is unrelated to its antidepressant activity. In fact, the doses generally useful in the treatment of migraine are well below those required to treat depression. The tricyclic antidepressants are described in detail in Chapter 11.

Calcium channel blockers prevent the transmembrane influx of calcium ions through slow voltage-dependent channels. They were first introduced for use in the treatment of migraine on the basis of their presumed blockade of the vasospastic phase in a migraine attack, although vasospasm is now considered an unlikely cause of migraine. Of the available blockers, only verapamil has sufficient evidence of efficacy to warrant its use in migraine.

Anticonvulsants are the most recent addition to the migraine prophylactic armamentarium. Valproic acid, an anticonvulsant known to inhibit gamma-aminobutyric acid (GABA) aminotransferase, reduces headache frequency and severity. It should be reserved for use as a second-line agent because of its association with birth abnormalities (neural tube defects) in the offspring of women taking it during the first trimester of pregnancy, and with polycystic ovarian syndrome. Gabapentin, a GABA analog, has recently shown efficacy in migraine prophylaxis, and is generally well tolerated, although it may be associated with dizziness and sedation. Although gabapentin has a very favorable side-effect profile, the general experience is that it is less efficacious in the treatment of recurrent headaches than valproic acid. However, until information from head-to-head trials is available, any definitive statement as to relative effectiveness is premature. The anticonvulsants are fully described in Chapter 10.

Second-Line Agents

Methysergide, an ergot derivative, was one of the first drugs used for migraine prophylaxis. It was thought to have an effect via inhibition of $5HT_2$ receptors. However, recent evidence indicates that potent selective $5HT_2$ antagonists are weak or ineffective in migraine. Double-blind clinical trials have shown methysergide to be effective in reducing the frequency, severity, and duration of migraine attacks. Unfortunately, it is associated with the serious complication of retroperitoneal, pericardial, or pleural fibrosis. Because of the risk of this potentially fatal side effect, methysergide should be reserved for severe cases that are refractory to other prophylactic regimens. Since the fibrotic complications are reversible early in the process, methysergide should be discontinued for 6 to 8 weeks every 6 months. The early symptoms of retroperitoneal fibrosis include decreased urine output and leg or back pain.

Phenelzine is a monoamine oxidase inhibitor that has been shown to be effective in patients with severe migraine. The potential for the generation of a hypertensive crisis after dietary intake of tyramine-containing foods should limit its use to patients with severe migraine who have been refractory to other treatments and who are committed to strict dietary monitoring.

2. Treatment of tension-type headache

(i) Acute treatment

The majority of tension-type headaches are of mild to moderate severity, and many patients use nonprescription medications quite effectively. NSAIDs are the mainstay of treatment (see Chapter 8). Those commonly used are listed in Table 4. Acetaminophen in both 650- and 1,000-mg doses has been reported to be superior to placebo in the treatment of headache.

Muscle relaxants are sometimes used to treat tension-type headache. Such agents include diazepam, baclofen, dantrolene sodium, and cyclobenzaprine hydrochloride. There are no clinical trials of these medications in the treatment of acute tension-type headaches; therefore, their use is largely empiric. The one exception is

Table 4.   NSAIDs commonly used in tension-type headache

Medication	Initial dose (mg)	Repeat dose (mg)
Aspirin (325 mg)	650–975	975
Ibuprofen	600–800	600
Ketoprofen	50–75	50
Naprosyn	500–750	500
Naproxen sodium	550	275
Ketorolac (oral)	20	10
Indomethacin (suppository)	50	—

tizanidine, which has recently been shown to be effective in chronic tension-type headache. In our experience, doses of 4 to 16 mg may be effective.

(ii) Prophylactic treatment

Tricyclic antidepressants are generally considered the first-line agents for prophylaxis. Amitriptyline is the drug of choice. Other medications that are sometimes selected for prophylaxis include NSAIDs, atypical antidepressants, and valproate, although evidence supporting their use in this situation is scanty.

Amitriptyline has been shown to affect headache improvement in double-blind placebo-controlled studies. Dosage ranges from 10 to 100 mg per day or higher if tolerated. In some patients, its use is somewhat limited by its anticholinergic side effects (i.e., sedation, dry mouth, tachycardia, constipation, or urinary retention). To minimize sedation, the drug can be given in a single dose 1 to 2 hours before bedtime. It should be started at a low dose (10 mg per day) and slowly increased over several weeks (10-mg increments at intervals of 1 to 2 weeks).

3. Treatment of cluster headache

(i) Acute treatment

Oxygen inhalation is a safe and effective treatment for individual attacks of cluster headache in many patients. The patient most likely to respond to oxygen treatment is one with episodic-type cluster headaches who is under the age of 50 years.

Oxygen is delivered at a rate of 8 liters per minute for 15 minutes via a loose-fitting facemask. Nasal biprongs are less effective because of greater air entrainment and lower oxygen concentration delivered. Patients who respond to oxygen do so usually within 10 minutes. The mechanism of effect of oxygen is unknown.

Ergotamine has been used since the 1940s to treat cluster headache attacks. The sublingual and inhalational routes appear to be superior to oral tablets. Ergotamines are effective and well tolerated in many patients with cluster headaches. DHE may also be of use in the acute treatment of cluster headaches.

Sumatriptan has been found to be effective in reducing both the pain and conjunctival injection of cluster headache within 15 minutes. It is well tolerated in patients with cluster headache. However, sumatriptan is contraindicated in patients with coronary artery disease, which is quite common among middle-aged men who make up the majority of cluster headache sufferers.

(ii) Prophylactic treatment

In general, prophylactic treatment for cluster headache is given only during the cluster period. Once a remission is established, in most cases within 3 to 6 weeks, the prophylactic agents is tapered and withdrawn.

Verapamil is frequently used in cluster headache, and in many patients it has a good effect with few side effects. The recommended dose is 240 to 480 mg/day.

Ergotamine tartrate is the traditional agent used in the prophylactic treatment of cluster headache. In doses of 2 to 4 mg/day in either oral or suppository form, ergotamine is an effective, well-tolerated medication for many of these patients.

Methysergide prophylaxis is efficacious in about 70% of patients with episodic cluster headache. The development of retroperitoneal, pleural, or pericardial fibrosis, which limits its use in migraine, is not as likely to occur in these patients because the length of use is considerably shorter. In patients with cluster headache, methysergide should be discontinued for 4 to 6 weeks after 2 to 3 months of treatment.

Lithium carbonate has been shown in over 20 open clinical trials to be effective in the treatment of chronic cluster headache. Because of its rather narrow therapeutic window, it is important to monitor serum lithium levels during periods of treatment. The serum level should be obtained 12 hours after the last dose and should not exceed 1.0 mmol/L (therapeutic range is usually from 0.3 to 0.8 mmol/L). Certain medications can interact with lithium to increase the serum level, including the NSAIDs and the thiazide diuretics. Average daily doses range from 600 to 900 mg but should be titrated according to serum concentrations.

Steroids are widely used in the treatment of both the episodic and chronic forms of cluster headache, even though documentation of their effect is largely limited to open trials.

4. Indomethacin-sensitive headaches

There are several headache syndromes that frequently respond to prophylactic treatment with indomethacin. Indomethacin, a potent NSAID, is not effective in migraine and has significant GI side effects. The syndromes for which indomethacin can be effective include chronic paroxysmal hemicrania, hemicrania continua, benign cough headache, effort and coital migraine, and idiopathic jabbing headaches. It is not known why these headaches respond to indomethacin when others do not. Clinical features that indomethacin-sensitive headaches share include a tendency to be provoked by certain movements or activities, relatively brief duration, and severe intensity.

To treat these syndromes, an initial dose of 25 mg twice a day is increased over several days until the attacks cease (sometimes requiring up to 150 mg to 250 mg per day). After relief is stable for several days, the dose should be titrated downward to the lowest effective maintenance dose (usually 25 to 100 mg daily). There is great variation between individuals in the maintenance dose required.

Indomethacin can have potentially serious GI side effects when given over long periods of time. These include dyspepsia, peptic ulcer, and GI bleeding. Other potential side effects include dizziness, nausea, and purpura.

VIII. NONPHARMACOLOGIC TREATMENT OF HEADACHE

Nonpharmacologic treatments include very old treatments such as application of pressure, heat, or cold directly to the head, as well as electrical stimulation, dental treatment, acupuncture, hypnosis, relaxation training, biofeedback, and cognitive therapy. All of these techniques have proponents, but the inherent difficulties in designing and carrying out blinded, unbiased studies make it almost impossible to make strong statements regarding their efficacy. At this point, it is impossible to predict whether an individual patient will benefit.

IX. HINTS FOR SUCCESSFUL HEADACHE MANAGEMENT

Less is More

In prescribing prophylactic therapy, start with a small dose and titrate upward using small increments at 1- to 2-week intervals. This will allow you to determine the lowest effective dose.

Don't Abandon Ship

If a prophylactic medication does not work at a modest dose, titrate upward slowly and systematically. Listen to the patient, and let side effects be your guide.

Pregnancy and Prophylaxis Potentially Precipitate Problems

Women who intend to become pregnant should be withdrawn from prophylactic treatment because the effects of many of these drugs on the fetus (especially in the first trimester) are not known. In many cases, pregnancy induces a remission in migraine attacks.

All Headaches are not Created Equal

Just because a patient has intermittent severe migraine attacks does not mean that every headache is a migraine requiring aggressive abortive therapy. Many migraineurs have frequent simple tension-type headaches intermixed, and the frequent use of ergotamines, analgesics, or barbiturate-containing medications can result in an iatrogenic rebound syndrome.

Prophylaxis is not a Life Sentence

Once a patient has been headache free for several months, begin discussions about tapering down the medications.

SELECTED READINGS

1. Burstein R, Cutrer FM, Yarnitsky D. The development of cutaneous allodynia during a migraine attack. *Brain* 2000;123: 1703–1709.
2. Burstein R, Yamamura H, Malick A, Strassman AM. Chemical stimulation of the intracranial dura induces enhanced responses to facial stimulation in brain stem trigeminal neurons. *J Neurophysiol* 1998;79:964–982.
3. Edmeads J. Emergency management of headache. *Headache* 1988;28:675–679.
4. Forsyth PA, Posner JB. Headaches in patients with brain tumors: A study in 111 patients. *Ann Neurol* 1992;32:289.
5. Gabai IJ, Spierings EL. Prophylactic treatment of cluster headache with verapamil. *Headache* 1989;29:167–168.
6. Mathew NT, Stubits E, Nigam MP. Transformation of episodic migraine into daily headache. *Headache* 1982;22:66–68.
7. Medina JL, Diamond S. Cluster headache variant: Spectrum of a new headache syndrome. *Arch Neurol* 1981;38:705–709.
8. Olesen J, ed. IHS classification and diagnostic criteria for headache disorders, cranial neuralgias and facial pain. *Cephalalgia* 1988;8(suppl 7):9–92.
9. Olesen J, Teelft-Hansen P, Welch KMA, eds. *The headaches.* New York: Raven Press, 1993.
10. Quality Standards Subcommittee of the American Academy of Neurology. Practice Parameter: The utility of neuroimaging in the

evaluation of headache in patients with normal neurologic examinations (summary statement). *Neurology* 1994;44:1353–1354.

11. Raskin HN. *Headache.* New York: Churchill Livingstone, 1988.

12. Raskin HN. Treatment of status migrainosus: The American experience. *Headache* 1990;30(suppl 2):550–553.

13. Sjaastad O, Spierings ELH. "Hemicrania continua": Another headache absolutely responsive to indomethacin. *Cephalalgia* 1984;4:65–70.

14. Taylor H, ed. *The Nuprin report.* New York: Louis Harris & Associates, 1985.

15. Thomas JE. Rooke ED, Kvale WF. The neurologist's experience with pheochromocytoma. *JAMA* 1966;197:754–758.

16. Welch KM. Drug therapy in migraine. *N Engl J Med* 1994;329: 1476–1483.

29

Facial Pain

Martin A. Acquadro
and Avine M. Lydon

Pain is the most urgent of symptoms.
—Henry K. Beecher, first chairman of anesthesia at MGH (1904–1976)

Many medical, dental, and other health specialists are involved in the identification of facial pain, often exposing the patient to a variety of referrals and interventions. Although facial pain is commonly the result of a complex process, it is often approached from the bias of one particular specialty, when a multidiscipline or multidimensional approach would provide a more comprehensive treatment. The many specialists involved in the treatment of facial pain, the rich synaptic connections with the limbic and autonomic systems, the social function of the face, and the highly visible and expressive nature of the face, all together make facial pain unique.

I. NEUROANATOMY AND NEUROPHYSIOLOGY

In the head and neck, afferent inputs converge on the trigeminal brainstem sensory nuclear complex within the pons (analogous to, but cephalad to, the dorsal horn of the cervical spinal cord) and on other cranial nerve nuclei. Multiple areas of convergence and interconnections are present between cranial nerves, cervical nerves, and autonomic nerves within the brainstem, comprising the trigeminal sensory nucleus and extending to the level of C5. Lateral thalamic projections assist in location discrimination, while medial thalamic projections mediate emotional and perceptual responses to pain. Ascending pathways project from the trigeminal sensory nucleus to the thalamus, reticular formation, and hypothalamus.

Depending on the specific sensory, autonomic, or neurochemical input, nociception can be suppressed or facilitated by modulating inputs from above and below the level of the trigeminal nucleus, altering the patient's perception of pain. Clinical features such as referral patterns, autonomic signs, interference with sleep/wake patterns, and the effect of emotional stimulation can be better understood in the context of this rich area of neural interchange. Peripherally, many facial structures are innervated by branches of multiple nerves producing pathways for referred pain. For example, the periauricular area receives sensory innervation from cranial nerves V, VII, IX, and X and from cervical roots C2 and C3, with referral patterns to the neck, eye, and face. Anatomically encapsulated areas such as the middle ear, the eye, dental pulp, and the closed calvaria are susceptible to compression, potentially expressed as facial pain.

II. PSYCHOLOGICAL ASPECTS

The face and the treatment of facial pain are the most visible examples of the biophysical psychosocial model of pain. The face is a window through which we view the world and, in turn, are viewed. Facial pain is therefore a highly visible form of pain, etched on the most expressive area of the body for all to see. This visibility is emphasized by the term for trigeminal neuralgia, *tic douloureux*. The lack of privacy encountered by sufferers of facial pain compounds the increased rates of anxiety and depression found in many chronic pain states. In addition, facial pain sufferers may be perceived as angry, sad, or socially negative as a result of the effects of pain on their facial expression.

Psychological factors present before the onset of pain (primary) and as a result of the pain (secondary) are important in the patient's perception of pain. Modification of the psychological factors can modulate the pain experience. Treatment of anxiety, depression, and sleep disruption should always be undertaken in conjunction with treatment of the primary pain source.

III. TEMPOROMANDIBULAR JOINT DYSFUNCTION, TEMPOROMANDIBULAR MUSCLE DYSFUNCTION, AND MYOFASCIAL DYSFUNCTION

1. Diagnostic features

It is useful to distinguish between true temporomandibular joint (TMJ) abnormalities, temporomandibular muscle dysfunction (TMD: dysfunction and pain of the muscles of mastication), and myofascial dysfunction originating in muscles other than those involved directly with mastication. Myofascial dysfunction with pain is a primary muscle disorder featuring pain and inflammation. When it involves the face, the source of pain may be the head and facial muscles, or muscles of mastication.

Because of their neuroanatomy, muscles of the shoulders and neck can have referral patterns to the face, sinuses, or head. Just as there are involuntary mechanical and muscle compensations in the lower back, hips, and knees associated with lower back and extremity musculoskeletal pathology, so there are instigating, contributing, and perpetuating factors of myofascial pain of the head, neck, and orofacial areas from outside these areas.

2. Clinical characteristics

Temporomandibular joint dysfunction

True pathologic derangement of the TMJ as the principle cause for pain is not common. TMJ damage can be the result of direct trauma, wear and tear from chronic pathologic occlusal forces, extreme limits of TMJ motion, acute dislocation, cancer or some other tissue-destructive process, surgical intervention, or arthritis.

Just as magnetic resonance imaging (MRI) abnormalities of the lumbar spine can be found in patients who are asymptomatic, so demonstrable TMJ pathology can be found in asymptomatic individuals. Many subjects have an "abnormal" TMJ that "clicks" or has a deviation or displacement during opening and closing of the mandible, but few have accompanying pain. True TMJ dysfunction with pain deserves assessment by an oral surgeon.

Temporomandibular muscle dysfunction

It is useful to separate TMD from other myofascial pain, as treatment focuses additionally on jaw and occlusal activities. TMD is defined by tenderness in one or more masticatory muscle. Additional clinical features include a reduced mandibular range (<35 mm) between incisors and a clicking or popping of the joint. The pain is commonly described as a dull ache exacerbated by chewing, fluctuating in intensity daily, and associated with remissions lasting months.

A range of terms exists, with a variety of classifications. These include myofascial dysfunction, masticatory myositis, masticatory myalgia, tendomyositis, and fibromyalgia. TMD is characterized by dull aching pain exacerbated by mandibular use, muscle tenderness in at least two masticatory muscle groups, and often a decreased mandibular range of motion. The absence of clinical features referable to the TMJ and the presence of muscle tenderness distinguish this from primary TMJ disorders, although secondary TMJ changes can occur. Tendomyositis involves inflammation and pain at the tendon insertion points at the zygomatic and coronoid arch area following spasm of the temporalis and masseter muscles, often precipitated by prolonged mouth opening during dental treatments.

Myofascial dysfunction

Dysfunction of the muscles of the shoulders, neck, head, and face is relatively common in the general population, and it can aggravate headaches, sinus area pain, and orofacial pain. Fibromyalgia, a type of myofascial dysfunction distinguished as a systemic disease, is characterized by muscle pain and tenderness exacerbated by stress, anxiety, and weather changes; it is accompanied by a variety of generalized symptoms such as fatigue, morning stiffness, irritable bowel syndrome, and migraine. The patient with fibromyalgia may initially present with facial pain and tenderness in the muscles of mastication; it is important to question patients for systemic features and not simply focus on the local complaint. Trauma is a possible trigger of myofascial dysfunction, and a history of trauma should be sought. Direct trauma and whiplash injuries to muscles cause tears, bleeding, and edema, and muscle recruitment results in extension of pain into the neck and shoulders.

3. Epidemiology

Myofascial pain syndromes occur predominantly in women. Masticatory myalgia and myositis occur in younger women (late teens to 40 years), whereas the peak age of presentation of fibromyalgia is older (45 to 55 years). The prevalence of TMD ranges from 6% to 12% of the North American population. Patients complaining of

TMD pain are likely to be female (9:1), with an average age of 40 (±16) years. Pain produced by direct trauma to facial muscles is notable for its greater frequency in men (3:1).

4. Diagnostic evaluation, imaging studies, and laboratory tests

There are no imaging techniques or laboratory markers that are useful in the diagnosis or management of myofascial pain syndromes. Radiographs frequently show abnormalities of the TMJ disc position in asymptomatic joints and thus are unhelpful. No specific laboratory tests indicate TMJ or TMD pain. An erythrocyte sedimentation rate (ESR) should be obtained if there is suspicion of temporal arteritis, and concerns about other rheumatologic or immunologic diagnoses dictate additional studies and referral to the appropriate specialist.

Diagnostic evaluation includes a careful and thorough history and physical, focusing on global musculoskeletal pain, myofascial pain of the shoulders, neck, and head, and myofascial pain of TMD and TMJ. Evaluation should include a review of a history of headaches, surgeries, trauma, and psychosocial events and stressors. A review of vocational and avocational activities along with posture, repetitive movements, habits, and sleep patterns should be included. A history of bruxism (clenching and grinding of teeth), awakening in the morning with sore jaw muscles, clicking or grating noises when opening the mouth, and recent or extensive dental work should be elicited. Eating habits, medications, exercise routines, and activities that help or worsen myofascial discomfort should be ascertained.

The physical exam should focus on range of motion of the shoulders, arms, neck, and mandible. An exam of the oral cavity for any lesions that may cause a reflex avoidance pattern, pain on extreme opening of the mandible, and abnormal bite should be checked. Teeth sensitivity, painful muscles, and painful points of insertion should be examined.

5. Treatment

Physical therapy

Treatment modalities include physical therapy consultation and treatment, and an active exercise program, with guidance from a physical therapist.

Pharmacologic therapy

Pharmacologic therapy includes judicious use of nonsteroidal anti-inflammatory drugs (NSAIDs), and very selective use of triclyclic antidepressants (TCAs), analgesics, muscle relaxants, anxiolytics, and, rarely, narcotics. NSAIDs may be used for both their analgesic and their anti-inflammatory properties. There is marked interpatient variability in response to different agents, necessitating trials until the optimal response is obtained. Because of the ceiling effect of NSAIDs, increasing doses beyond the recommended maximum is not useful. NSAIDs are of no proven value in the long-term management of TMJ pain, although large doses may provide short-term relief. Patients who are unable to tolerate NSAIDs may use tramadol hydrochloride, a weak and nonaddicting μ agonist, in a dose of 50 to 100 mg every 6 hours as needed.

Centrally acting muscle relaxants include cyclobenzaprine (Flexeril) and carisoprodol (Soma). These agents decrease excess electromyographic (EMG) activity and muscle spasm. The tertiary amine amitriptyline and the secondary amines desipramine and nortriptyline, in low doses, may improve sleep and act as indirect analgesics by augmenting midbrain serotonin levels. Benzodiazepines such as diazepam decrease muscle spasm, improve sleep, and are anxiolytic. A dose of 5 mg twice daily is useful in initial therapy. Prolonged use of benzodiazepines should be avoided because of their addiction potential.

In patients requiring prolonged treatment of anxiety symptoms, buspirone (BuSpar) 5 mg three times daily is effective with little addiction potential, but it has no muscle relaxant effects. Opioids are useful in decreasing pain in refractory cases but are associated with risks of tolerance, addiction, and dependence.

Trigger point injections and physical therapy

Pressure on active trigger points causes acute pain and produces muscle spasm when the muscle is used, decreasing the range of motion. Trigger points can be localized by pressure and then inactivated by the topical application of vapocoolant spray (dichlorodifluoromethane), allowing stretching exercises to restore muscle mobility. Refractory trigger points can be disrupted physically by dry needling. The injection of local anesthetic (0.5 mL of 0.5% procaine or 1% lidocaine per trigger point), or selected trigger point injections of a mixture of equal volumes of lidocaine 1% and bupivacaine 0.5% can be performed with subsequent physical therapy. This provides more prolonged analgesia, allowing the patient a pain-free period to commence physical therapy, with subsequent use of vapocoolants and stretching exercises at home. Corticosteroids, such as triamcinolone acetonide (Kenalog) in a final concentration of 0.1% can be added to the mixture. Steroid injections should not be repeated any sooner than 6 weeks, as a *peau d'orange* cosmetic defect may occur.

Psychological therapy

Psychological intervention including biofeedback, relaxation techniques, and cognitive behavioral therapy addressing aversive behaviors when they exist should be considered.

TMH and TMD splint therapy

Advocates of splint therapy suggest that bite occlusion mechanically unloads the TMJ and limits masticatory muscle activity and symptoms of TMD and TMJ. Many anecdotal examples of benefit exist, but clinical studies have not provided evidence to support this traditional practice.

TMJ surgery and dental treatment

Surgery of the joint, including arthroscopy and surgical implants, is associated with high morbidity and a lack of efficacy, unless proper and careful patient selection is utilized by an experienced oromaxillofacial surgeon. Missing teeth and dental malocclusions have an inconsistent relationship to TMJ and TMD pain. Oral appliances such as bite blocks to prevent tooth grinding are not always helpful or predictive in the treatment of TMJ and TMD pain. Dental and occlusal evaluation by an experienced dental specialist is required.

Suggested TMD home treatment regimen

Temporary rest of the TMJ is sometimes helpful. A liquid and soft diet is instituted, and gum chewing is stopped. Wide, uncontrolled opening of the jaw is discouraged. Yawning, coughing, laughing, and the eating of large sandwiches is minimized. A hand or fist placed under the chin helps to hold the jaw in place.

Heat therapy can be useful: a heating pad, warm face cloth, or warm water bottle placed to the sides of the jaw and TMJ area has a soothing and relaxing effect on the muscles. Gentle midline opening and closing exercises of the mandible help to retrain and relax muscles. Use of a vapocoolant spray may also be helpful in reducing movement-induced pain so that exercises designed to improve joint mobility can be tolerated.

Judicious use of NSAIDs may also help. Consider acetaminophen in patients with NSAID sensitivity, or cyclooxygenase-2 (COX-2) inhibitors in patients with a serious risk of bleeding or other relevant history. The use of additional medication should be directed by the physician.

IV. DENTAL DISEASE AND DYSFUNCTION

1. Diagnostic features

Because of the rich innervation of the mouth, pain resulting from tooth or periodontal disease can present with numerous features including local pain, headache, or eye symptoms (photophobia, lacrimation, conjunctival injection). A differential diagnosis should include trigeminal neuralgia, sinusitis and other sinus disease, central nervous system (CNS) pathology, cluster, migraine, and muscle contraction tension-type headaches, and myofascial pain of the shoulders, neck, head, and masticatory muscles with referral.

2. Epidemiology

Dental disease is common in men, women, and children of all ages.

3. Diagnostic evaluation, imaging studies, and laboratory tests

During the history and physical examination, dental pathology must be adequately assessed. If dental disease is obvious, then the appropriate referral should be made. However, if dental disease, oral mucosal disease, and pathologic occlusal forces have been ruled out, other pathology must be considered. Problems such as sinusitis; undiagnosed sinus diseases such as cysts, Wegener's granulomatosis, mucocele, or latent fungal or bacterial infections; undiagnosed and uncategorized headache; chronic allergies; and CNS pathology can mimic dental pain. Computed tomography (CT) or MRI may be indicated.

4. Treatment

Patients should be referred to a dentist, otolaryngologist, or neurologist for further management to rule out organic and treatable pathology. If treatable conditions have been ruled out, however, and there are no obvious sources except a prior history of disease and pain, peripheral or central neuroplastic changes or deafferentation should be considered. Treatment should be directed toward a comprehensive and neuropathic approach, with due consideration of the biophysical psychosocial model of pain treatment. In addition, a late-declaring dental or other problem may appear and be treatable.

V. PARANASAL SINUS AREA PAIN AND HEADACHE

1. Diagnostic features

Acute sinusitis presents with bilateral or unilateral throbbing or sharp facial pain. In the acute setting, diagnosis is usually straightforward. Frequently, pain is exacerbated by leaning forward. A sense of pressure is described by 74% of patients. Medial orbital pain with radiation to the temple is a feature of ethmoid sinusitis. Frontal sinusitis features forehead pain and headache; maxillary sinusitis is suggested by pain over the maxilla, or it may be referred to the occiput, forehead, or orbit.

Chronic sinus area pain presents more of a diagnostic dilemma. Pain that is perceived as emanating from the sinuses can have other causes, including referred pain from dental, dural, and musculoskeletal areas. The differential diagnosis includes myofascial pain, vascular and other types of headache, neuralgias, allergies, and dental disease. Other diagnostic features of sinusitis include purulent discharge from the nasal passages or nasopharynx, intermittent fever, smell or taste disorder, tenderness on tapping the maxillary teeth, and tenderness over the maxillary, frontal, or ethmoidal sinuses. A history of recurrent injury in the form of upper respiratory tract infections and allergies may be elicited. A combination of history, anterior endoscopic examination, and CT findings is required to accurately diagnose sinusitis, particularly prior to embarking on surgical treatments.

2. Epidemiology

There are no distinctive epidemiologic features.

3. Imaging studies and laboratory tests

Endoscopic examination is useful in demonstrating inflamed turbinates, sinus ostia edema, and purulent nasopharyngeal discharge. CT imaging reveals opacification of the sinuses and occluded ostiomeatal complexes. Additional abnormalities may be demonstrated on imaging, including chronic maxillary atelectasis, mucocele, ossifying fibroma of the maxilla, and fungal involvement. Of note, even the common cold can cause mucosal thickening of the sinuses sufficient to be seen on MRI. Elevations in ESR and C-reactive protein are independently predictive of sinusitis but are nonspecific. Recent clinical research from Johns Hopkins has raised the possibility of an underdiagnosed genetic predisposition for subclinical cystic fibrosis in some patients with symptoms of chronic sinusitis. A chromosome gene analysis of a buccal smear to look for the defect found in cystic fibrosis, followed by a sweat chloride test if indicated, may provide a diagnosis.

4. Treatment

Otolaryngologic consultation should be obtained. Endoscopic surgery should be considered when a 6-month trial of medical therapy has failed, or immediately in the case of a significant abnormality on imaging. With careful patient selection, endoscopic sinus surgery can achieve relief of pain in 56% of patients, and substantial improvement in a further 29%. Difficulties arise in patients with chronic sinus area pain that mimics sinusitis but may not be true sinusitis. When imaging repeatedly demonstrates normal sinuses, and there is a lack of any objective evidence for sinusitis, a multidisciplinary, multidimensional approach, including the specialties of neurology, psychiatry, and behavioral medicine, is required. These patients are unlikely to benefit from surgical intervention.

VI. TRIGEMINAL NEURALGIA

1. Diagnostic features

Trigeminal neuralgia is characterized by sudden, stabbing, severe unilateral facial pain in one of the three divisions (most frequently the second) of the trigeminal nerve. Onset is frequently triggered by mechanical stimulation such as talking, chewing, touch, or cold (e.g., cold wind). Attacks can last from several seconds to minutes. Periods of attacks can last weeks or months, followed by periods of remission of months or years. Carbamazepine responsiveness is considered a diagnostic feature.

2. Epidemiology

Incidence increases with age, peaking at 75 years, and thus more commonly presenting in women.

3. Diagnostic evaluation, imaging studies, and laboratory tests

MRI is an important diagnostic test for excluding intracranial masses and multiple sclerosis (MS), particularly in younger patients. MS should be considered in women younger than 30 years. An MRI can show demyelinating lesions of the white matter associated with MS. Symptoms such as diplopia, weakness, and clumsiness are suggestive of MS.

4. Treatment

Carbamazepine is the drug of first choice in treatment, with a beneficial response in more than 75% of patients. Its mechanism is depression of excitatory transmission in the brainstem trigeminal nucleus. Carbamazepine should be started at a dose of 200 mg daily and increased in increments of 200 mg until pain relief or side effects occur. The usual therapeutic dose range is 600 to 1,200 mg per day. Phenytoin is a less effective alternative but can be a useful adjunct to carbamazepine. Baclofen potentiates the action of carbamazepine at the trigeminal nucleus and can be a useful adjunct. It can be started at a dose of 30 mg daily, increasing to 50 to 60 mg daily. Gabapentin is a safe and well-tolerated adjunct to carbamazepine, titrated to effect from a starting dose of 300 mg at night to a usual range of 900 to 3,000 mg daily. Other agents used less frequently include tocainide, clonazepam, and sodium valproate.

Surgical approaches to the treatment of trigeminal neuralgia include microvascular decompression and radiofrequency electrocoagulation. Microvascular decompression relieves pulsatile compression of the trigeminal nerve at the cerebellopontine angle, achieving immediate pain relief in 79% and long-term relief in 73% of patients. Radiofrequency electrocoagulation is performed either by a percutaneous or open partial cranial rhizotomy, achieving immediate pain relief in more than 90% of patients. Unfortunately, this treatment is associated with pain recurrence in 80% of patients, occurring anytime from weeks to years after treatment. The key to a high success rate is ensuring that the patient fits a very rigorous definition for trigeminal neuralgia.

VII. BURNING MOUTH SYNDROME

1. Diagnostic features

Glossodynia is characterized by burning pain of the mucous membranes of the tongue (most commonly), mouth, hard palate, or lips. The onset of pain is gradual with no precipitating event, and it is usually bilateral. Associated symptoms are altered taste and dry mouth. Physical examination of the mouth is normal and excludes causes such as infection and trauma. Although nutritional and menopausal factors, abnormal glucose tolerance, and chronic mechanical irritation have all been suggested as causes, there is inadequate evidence to pinpoint these factors as the origin of burning mouth syndrome. Recent evidence suggests that peripheral nerve injury of the chorda tympani produces pain as a result of loss of inhibition of the trigeminal nerve.

2. Epidemiology

The prevalence rate is 1.5% to 2.5% in the general population. Patients are more likely to be female (3 : 1) and older than 50 years.

3. Diagnostic evaluation, imaging studies, and laboratory tests

There are no useful radiographic or laboratory examinations. As always, a careful history and physical examination are required to rule out other treatable causes.

4. Treatment

Fifty percent of patients experience spontaneous resolution within a variable length of time, up to several years after onset. Tricyclic antidepressants such as amitriptyline, nortriptyline, and desipramine (titrated in 10-mg increments to a range of 30 to 75 mg) and the serotonin reuptake inhibitor sertraline may be effective. In a study of 30 patients, clonazepam given at a dose of 0.5 to 1.5 mg daily lessened pain in 70% of patients; clonazepam was also found to be effective when applied topically to the mouth. A number of drugs including angiotensin-converting enzyme inhibitors and antihypertensives have been associated with burning mouth syndrome that is reversible with discontinuation of the drug. As pharmacologic therapy is unsuccessful in many patients, psychological support is important.

VIII. DEAFFERENTATION PAIN

1. Diagnostic features

Teeth and dental nerves are commonly amputated. Phantom tooth pain is similar to other phantom pain syndromes, producing pain in previously extracted teeth. Pain is constant with sharp exacerbations and is associated with local allodynia. Notably, sleep is undisturbed. The onset of pain can usually be related to a procedure such as dental extraction or sinus surgery.

2. Epidemiology

Phantom tooth pain prevalence rates of 3% closely match those of phantom pain following limb amputation (5%). Given the relative frequency of dental procedures when compared to limb amputation, phantom tooth pain is a common cause of facial pain. There is equal distribution between sexes, and although all ages are affected, occurrence in children is rare.

3. Diagnostic evaluation, imaging studies, and laboratory tests

Radiographs frequently demonstrate dental intervention but do not assist in diagnosis or management. History and physical exam are important as they pertain to extent of dental work and other trauma or surgeries in the area. History of prior severe dental pain of an extracted tooth or teeth, as well as prior sinusitis pain and traumatic pain, may suggest possible peripheral or central neuroplasticity.

4. Treatment

Pain therapies are targeted at both the central and peripheral components of deafferentation pain. The centrally acting drug of choice is gabapentin, starting at a dose of 300 mg at bedtime and increasing to a dose range of 900 to 3,000 mg daily. Some patients may be too sensitive, needing to start at 100 mg each evening and slowly titrate to higher doses. Other membrane-stabilizing agents such as carbamazepine and phenytoin are usually ineffective in phantom tooth pain, and efficacy of these agents suggests a diagnosis of trigeminal neuralgia. Clonazepam 1 to 3 mg daily and baclofen 30 to 60 mg daily are useful adjunctive agents. Amitriptyline and other TCAs, 10 to 75 mg daily, are effective, particularly when combined with a phenothiazine, such as perphenazine, in severe cases. A fixed daily dose of a narcotic agent such as oxycodone has been used successfully but is associated with a risk of dependence and addiction.

Peripherally acting agents include topically applied drugs and nerve blocks. Ketamine, capsaicin, and clonidine have been applied topically with mixed results. Nerve blocks with local anesthetic agents and low-dose steroids are effective but may require a number of trials to determine optimal injection sites for an individual patient. Surgical procedures are ineffective in treatment of phantom tooth pain and may actually increase pain severity.

IX. ACUTE AND POSTHERPETIC NEURALGIA

1. Diagnostic features

Acute herpetic neuralgia (AHN) arises as a result of herpes zoster infection (shingles) stimulating an acute inflammatory process of the dorsal root ganglion and peripheral nerves. Pain and cutaneous vesicles are located along the distribution of the affected peripheral nerve or nerves. Areas commonly affected are thoracic dermatomes (50%), ophthalmic division of the fifth cranial nerve (10% to 20%), and cervical dermatomes (10% to 20%). Shingles is almost always unilateral and may be recurrent (1% to 8%), usually in the same site.

Pain is described as burning, itching, well localized to the dermatome, with lancinating episodes, and it is associated with hyperesthesia and hyperalgesia. Intense lancinating pain and paresthesia usually diminish in the second or third week as the skin lesions begin to heal. In contrast, the pain of postherpetic neuralgia (PHN) is diffuse, dull, and aching, with a superficial dysesthetic sensation evoked by clothes or light touch. Pain persisting for longer than 1 month after complete healing of the acute herpes zoster lesions is considered PHN.

PHN is believed to result from deafferentation and hypersensitivity in the dorsal horn of the spinal cord. There is evidence that first-order neuron C-fiber death occurs both in the periphery and centrally in the substantia gelatinosa (lamina II) of the spinal cord. This may be followed by ingrowth of first-order neuron A-beta fibers from laminae III and IV into lamina II, which may explain the dysesthesia with normally non-noxious stimuli.

2. Epidemiology

PHN, ophthalmic involvement, and nervous system complications such as stroke, cranial neuropathy, and myelitis are associated with increasing age and an immunocompromised state.

3. Diagnostic evaluation, imaging studies, and laboratory tests

Diagnosis is clinical and based on the presence or history of vesicles, although complications such as stroke should be completely evaluated with CT or MRI.

4. Treatment

Early effective treatment of acute herpes zoster shortens the acute episode, decreases acute pain, and decreases the incidence of PHN. Antiviral therapy with acyclovir intravenous (IV) 5 mg/kg every 8 hours for 5 days, begun within 72 hours of the shingles eruption, is effective, and is particularly useful in immunocompromised individuals. The timely use of antiviral therapy has been shown to be effective in reducing both AHN and PHN. Amitriptyline, NSAIDs, doxepin, trazodone, and fluoxetine are useful for controlling the pain of AHN; if pain remains uncontrolled, narcotic agents can be added. Subcutaneous local anesthetic and steroid injections reduce acute and chronic symptoms but should be used with care in the immunocompromised patient.

TCAs are the mainstay of treatment in PHN. The efficacy of amitriptyline and desipramine has been confirmed in controlled clinical trials. Topical agents, such as a 5% lidocaine patch or salicylate prepared as 700 mg aspirin dissolved in 15 to 30 mL of chloroform or diethyl ether, can produce substantial pain relief with minimal systemic absorption. Anxiolytics and anticonvulsants have been used with less success. Narcotics should be reserved for patients who are unresponsive to other agents. Capsaicin is often poorly tolerated because of cutaneous sensitivity. A transcutaneous electrical nerve stimulator is associated with minimal morbidity and sometimes produces significant benefit; it is under utilized and should always be considered for patients with PHN.

X. PERIOCULAR PAIN

1. Diagnostic features

Ophthalmic pain results from stimulation of pain fibers related either directly or indirectly to the orbit. Cranial nerves involved may include the trigeminal, facial, vagus, and glossopharyngeal. The trigeminal sensory complex communicates actively with these cranial nerves, as well as the limbic and autonomic systems, and dips down to the level of C6. As a result, pain may be poorly localized, or it may be referred from other anatomic structures and areas with shared innervation peripherally and centrally. Pain can be classified as ocular, orbital, or referred.

Ocular pain

Corneal irritation or damage is associated with local pain, photophobia, and lacrimation, together with the sensation of a foreign body. Anterior scleritis presents with severe ocular pain, whereas posterior scleritis is characterized by less well defined orbital pain; either may be associated with a systemic collagen vascular disease. A triad of red eye, increased intraocular pressure, and a mid-dilated pupil is pathognomonic for acute angle glaucoma. Severe ocular pain is associated with headache, and it may radiate to the sinuses and teeth and be associated with systemic features such as nausea and vomiting. Atherosclerotic disease of the carotid may present with ocular ischemic pain. Uncorrected refractive error produces pain from excess ciliary body tone, pain that radiates to the head and brow. Photo-oculodynia is an uncommon pain syndrome of unknown cause in which ocular pain is precipitated by light.

Orbital pain

Orbital cellulitis presents acutely with pain exacerbated by palpation and movement. Orbital pseudotumor is an inflammatory process of unknown cause that presents with pain, chemosis, diplopia, and red eye. Trochleitis is characterized by orbital pain with movement, together with exquisite superonasal point tenderness. Retro-ocular pain and diminished vision are features of optic neuritis, which may occur alone or as a symptom of a demyelinating disease.

Referred pain

The proximity and convergence of afferent pain fibers produce referred pain. Direct and indirect noxious stimulation of the trigeminal nerve and its divisions produce primary and secondary trigeminal neuralgia. Occasionally, pain from the area of the greater occipital nerve radiates from the occiput to the eye and face (secondary trigeminal neuralgia), because of convergence and communication between the greater occipital nerve, C2, and C3, and the trigeminal sensory complex. Trigeminal neuralgia associated with a red eye, lacrimation, rhinorrhea, and Horner's syndrome is known as Raeder's syndrome. Cervical spondylitis may produce secondary trigeminal neuralgia presenting as orbital pain caused by the cervical branches in the spinal tract of the trigeminal nerve converging with the ophthalmic and maxillary divisions of the trigeminal nerve. Migrainous headache, sinusitis, otitis, mastoiditis, and dental pain can all be referred to the eye. Temporal arteritis presents with visual loss and ipsilateral facial pain and is diagnosed on temporal artery biopsy.

2. Epidemiology

Carotid occlusive disease, glaucoma, and temporal arteritis are more common in the elderly, whereas optic neuritis occurs predominantly in young adults, and MS with optic neuritis is seen in young to middle age adults.

3. Diagnostic evaluation, imaging studies, and laboratory tests

MRI is indicated to detect MS as a cause of optic neuritis. Raeder's syndrome requires imaging to rule out a parasellar mass or carotid dissection as causes. Doppler flow studies are useful in detecting carotid stenosis as a cause of orbital ischemia. An ESR greater than 100 mm/hour, and increased C-reactive protein and fibrinogen levels are strongly associated with temporal arteritis.

4. Treatment

If temporal arteritis, optic neuritis, or orbital pseudotumor is suspected, high-dose corticosteroids should be started immediately (e.g., methylprednisolone 1g IV or prednisone 60 mg orally), and the patient should be referred to an ophthalmologist or a rheumatologist, depending on the suspected diagnosis. All patients with suspected eye pathology should be seen by an ophthalmologist. Keratitis and orbital cellulitis are treated aggressively with topical and systemic antibiotics, and with surgical drainage of collections and sinusitis as required. Acute-angle glaucoma requires urgent ophthalmologic referral and topical pupillary constriction, with or without laser iridotomy.

XI. PERIAURICULAR PAIN

1. Diagnostic features

Otitis media presents with either dull aching or sudden exquisite pain, with or without aural discharge, an inflamed tympanic membrane, and systemic evidence of infection (malaise and pyrexia). Otitis externa can be exquisitely painful, and it is generally an acute process. Mastoiditis and otitis pain may be referred to the eye, pharynx, and neck as a result of involvement of cranial nerve VII (supplying branches to both the eye and the ear), convergence with the trigeminal sensory complex, and the shared innervation of C2 and C3 and the petrous bone (Gradenigo's syndrome). A common cause of otalgia that is frequently overlooked is referred myofascial pain from muscles of the neck, pharynx, and mastication.

2. Epidemiology

Otitis media presents more frequently in childhood and should always be considered in the immunocompromised patient. Mastoiditis and infected cholesteatoma are found more frequently in children and young to middle-aged adults.

3. Diagnostic evaluation, imaging studies, and laboratory tests

Elevated white cell count is supportive but nonspecific evidence of otitis media. CT and MRI are invaluable for mastoiditis and cholesteatoma. History and physical examination should direct an appropriate otolaryngologic referral.

4. Treatment

In general, urgent consultation with an otolaryngologist is required. Evidence of petrosal involvement requires broad-spectrum IV antibiotics. Referrals to a pain specialist are often from an otolaryngologist who has successfully treated the immediate pain problem, but the patient still suffers from chronic pain, together with frequent myofascial pain of the neck, head, and orofacial muscles. Treatment is multidimensional and comprehensive, covering possible neuropathic and nociceptive pain. Attention is directed to the common myofascial pains.

XII. HEAD AND NECK CANCER

1. Diagnostic features

Head and neck cancers present with a wide variety of symptoms. Frequently, a multidimensional approach is required during diagnosis, treatment, and recovery. Nociceptive and neuropathic pain may occur at any time during the course of disease and treatment, and coordination between surgical, dental, psychiatric, physical therapy, and oncologic consultations are frequently required.

Characteristic effects of the various manifestations of malignant disease and its treatment are as follows:

- Local tumor growth and invasion results in local tissue destruction, secondary infection, nerve compression with mononeuropathy and plexopathy, secondary myofascial pain from distorted mouth opening and function, diplopia, and ptosis.
- Surgical resection and reconstruction results in acute postoperative pain, nerve damage and resection, inadequate vascularization of myocutaneous flaps, and sacrifice of the accessory nerve.
- Chemotherapy with vincristine and cisplatinum results in nerve damage and neuritis.
- Radiotherapy results in mucositis of the gastrointestinal tract, osteoradionecrosis, cheilosis (tissue breakdown at the corners of the mouth), loss of salivary glands, secondary infection (fungal and bacterial), and loss of range of motion of the neck, facial and masticatory muscles (including limited mouth opening and remodeling of the TMJ, with secondary severe myofascial pain and dysfunction).
- Nutritional deficiencies (secondary to pain, loss of appetite, poor caloric intake, and mismatch between metabolic demands

and intake) result in poor fit of dental prostheses (with or without pain) and in pyridoxine, B_{12}, and other specific vitamin and mineral deficiencies.

- Secondary infection results in tissue breakdown and pain.
- Psychosocial factors contribute to the overall pain response inducing fear, anxiety, lack of self esteem; there are also cosmetic concerns, and fears of tumor recurrence lead to patients' misinterpreting symptoms as tumor recurrence rather than the expected secondary complications of therapies.

2. Epidemiology

Head and neck cancer occurs predominantly in older adults, although lymphoma, adenocarcinoma of the sinuses, and squamous cell carcinoma do occur in younger adults. Smoking and chewing of tobacco; alcohol; chronic irritation and injury of the intraoral mucosa secondary to habits, damaged dentition, and poorly fitting fixed and removable prostheses; and sun exposure and fair skin are strongly associated with the development of head and neck cancers.

3. Diagnostic evaluation, imaging studies, and laboratory tests

Radiologic imaging techniques of CT and MRI, endoscopy, biopsy, and surveillance are invaluable in the management of head and neck cancer.

4. Treatment

Pain due to head and neck cancers should be treated following the same principles as those outlined in Chapter 32. With particular reference to head and neck cancer, physical therapy can improve range of motion of the neck, mouth, and TMJ. Myofascial pain of the shoulders, neck, and head, and headache are frequent secondary occurrences and may also respond to physical therapy. Nutritional consultation may be helpful, as may dental consultation to aid with oral function and cosmesis.

XIII. CONCLUSION

Facial pain has a vast number of complex causes, and its successful treatment requires contributions from many different specialties. This pain is one of the most distressing of all painful syndromes and warrants aggressive and appropriate treatment in a multidisciplinary setting. This chapter outlines some of the causes, diagnostic features, and treatments of facial pain.

SELECTED READINGS

1. Acquadro MA. Headache and sinusitis. *Curr Opin Otolaryngol Head Neck Surg* 1998;6:2–5.
2. Barker FG 2nd, Jannetta PJ, Bissonette DJ, et al. The long term outcome of microvascular decompression for trigeminal neuralgia. *N Engl J Med* 1996;334:1077–1083.
3. Bohr TW. Fibromyalgia syndrome and myofascial pain syndrome: do they exist? *Neurol Clin* 1995;13:365–384.
4. Graff-Radford SB. Facial pain. *Curr Opin Neurol* 2000;13:291–296.

5. Hu JW, Tsaj CM, Bakke M, et al. Deep craniofacial pain: Involvement of the trigeminal subnucleus caudalis and its modulation. In: Jensen TS, Turner JA, Wiesenfeld-Hallin Z, eds. *Proceedings of the Eighth World Congress*. Seattle: IASP Press, 1997;497–506.
6. Huang W, Tothe MJ, Grant-Kels JM. The burning mouth syndrome. *J Am Acad Dermatol* 1996;34:91–98.
7. Marbach JJ. Medically unexplained chronic orofacial pain: Temporomandibular pain and dysfunction syndrome, orofacial phantom pain, burning mouth syndrome and trigeminal neuralgia. *Med Clin North Am* 1999;83:691–710.
8. Marbach JJ. Orofacial phantom pain: theory and phenomenology. *J Am Dental Assoc* 1996;127:221–229.
9. Marbach JJ, Lennon MC, Link BG, et al. Losing face: Sources of stigma as perceived by chronic facial pain patients. *J Behav Med* 1990;13:583–604.
10. Merrill RL. Orofacial pain mechanics and their clinical application. *Dent Clin North Am* 1997;41:167–187.
11. Truelove E, Sommers E, LeResche L, et al. Clinical diagnostic criteria for TMD. *J Am Dent Assoc* 1992;123:47–5

Opioid Therapy in Chronic Nonmalignant Pain

Scott M. Fishman and Jianren Mao

> Thou only givest these gifts to man, and thou hast the keys of Paradise,
> O just, subtle and mighty opium!
> —*Thomas De Quincey (1785–1859)*

Chronic nonmalignant pain (CNMP) refers to a broad spectrum of chronic pain states associated with a variety of disease processes. CNMP can be categorized as follows:

- Chronic nociceptive pain (e.g., arthritic pain)
- Neuropathic pain [e.g., complex regional pain syndrome (CRPS), postherpetic neuralgia]
- Pain with mixed nociceptive and neuropathic components (e.g., low back pain with radiculopathy)
- Pain with an unknown etiology, termed idiopathic pain (e.g., fibromyalgia)

Opioids are still the gold standard of the currently available analgesics, yet their use in CNMP is controversial. The decision to initiate opioid therapy in patients with CNMP should be patient specific and based on the rationale for treatment, observable treatment endpoints, and the potential for side effects and addiction. Each of these considerations is discussed in this chapter. The general pharmacology and dosing schedules for opioid therapy as well as issues of opioid addiction, abuse, and adherence are discussed in Chapters 9 and 35. In general, long-acting opioids are preferred. Short-acting opioids are avoided so that patients can learn to utilize other means of controlling their pain when they experience breakthrough pain.

Whether or not long-term opioid treatment is beneficial for patients with CNMP is debated, with a scarcity of convincing scientific data to persuasively argue for either side. Since the endpoint of analgesic therapy is often difficult to quantitatively monitor, managing chronic opioid therapy can be a formidable undertaking, fraught with the challenges of measuring the positive and negative impact of treatment on quality of life. Patients who use opioids for CNMP range from those using consistent amounts of opioid with little variation to those whose needs are seemingly never satisfied and whose dosages frequently escalate. Resistance to chronic opioid therapy is often founded on social, medical, and legal stigmata. Concerns in this patient population include questions of efficacy, adverse side effects, toxicity, addiction and abuse potential, tolerance and physical dependence, fear of regulatory scrutiny, possible neuropsychiatric deterioration, reinforcement of pain behavior, and even possible immunosuppression.

I. RATIONALE

Opioid therapy can be an integrated part of a multidisciplinary approach for CNMP management, which includes any possible combination of interventions with many other analgesic drug groups, interventional procedures, and other modalities of psychological and physical rehabilitation. Much of the debate concerning the role of opioid therapy in CNMP management has been centered on the issue of whether opioid therapy should be used as a first-line treatment. Should pain physicians withhold opioid therapy until other treatment options are exhausted? Although there is a lack of consensus on this important issue, opioid therapy tends to be used as a second-line treatment for CNMP for the following reasons:

1. CNMP may respond to nonopioid pharmacologic interventions such as nonsteroidal anti-inflammatory drugs (NSAIDs) for arthritic pain and anticonvulsants or tricyclic antidepressants for postherpetic neuralgia.
2. At times, interventional analgesia can be more effective than chronic drug management; for example, sympathetic nerve blockade may provide better therapeutic outcomes than opioids in certain types of CNMP (e.g., CRPS types I and II, postherpetic neuralgia).
3. Considering the significant side effects and liability profiles of opioid treatment (see later), the assessment of risks versus benefits often suggests that some patients with CNMP are not good candidates for opioid therapy.

Opioid therapy should not, however, be withheld in patients with CNMP whose pain is not relieved by other interventions. Although the effectiveness of opioid therapy in certain types of CNMP remains controversial (in Chapter 35, see the section "Opioid Responsiveness"), there is no evidence suggesting that opioid therapy is contraindicated in these circumstances. Preclinical studies have shown a right shift of the opioid dose–response curve in neuropathic pain, suggesting that higher opioid doses may be required for patients primarily suffering from neuropathic pain. Thus, a limiting factor for opioid therapy in neuropathic pain treatment may be related to the development of significant side effects associated with the high doses of opioids needed. It is possible that methadone may be an optimal choice as an opioid for neuropathic pain because of its N-methyl-D-aspartate (NMDA) blocking effects.

In summary, opioid therapy may be initiated in patients with CNMP when a thorough evaluation of the risk-to-benefit ratio supports this intervention. This requires a clear sense of purpose;

clear, observable endpoints of treatment; and an exhaustive trial of other potentially effective therapies that have less risk. In addition, combination analgesia (e.g., an opioid in combination with an NSAID) can have opioid-sparing effects by taking advantage of nonopioid analgesic actions that have synergistic effects with the opioids, increasing analgesia at lower doses of each, and helping reduce the side effects of each.

II. TREATMENT ENDPOINTS

There are two critical issues related to treatment endpoints in opioid therapy for CNMP:

1. What should be considered a positive outcome after a trial of opioids?
2. When should opioid therapy be discontinued (or tapered) if the treatment is either effective or ineffective?

Clinical studies in this area are limited.

Markers of benefit in patients treated with opioids for CNMP include subjective pain reduction and objective evidence of improvement in functional status and quality of life. However, psychological and social factors, as well as the status of coexistent disease, may influence pain perception, suffering, and entitlement, crucially altering the overall assessment. Unfortunately, not all these issues will improve concomitantly and proportionately following the initiation of opioid therapy.

For example, it is well recognized that psychological factors may influence pain perception. Conceivably, the reduction of pain from an opioid trial may not be as robust in a patient who has not adequately resolved other psychological amplifiers of pain perception. Also, pain reduction and improvement of functional status resulting from effective opioid analgesia may not be simultaneous. Thus, other than requiring objective evidence of efficacy, determining treatment endpoints during an opioid trial usually requires some flexibility in considering the many possible variations in functional gain and improvement in quality of life. Pain reduction is always subjective and, as such, can only serve as a single aspect of adequate chronic opioid therapy.

Consider the patient who has daily pain rated 6 on a pain severity scale of 1 to 10, with significant disability associated with the pain. Although opioid therapy may reduce subjective pain scores by only one point (from 6 to 5), the treatment is clearly successful if there is evidence of increased function such as return to work and improved ability to participate in physical rehabilitation. On the other hand, an opioid trial characterized by subjective reports of marked pain relief but no observable functional gains, and possibly even signs of functional loss such as sedation, loss of job, dysfunctional interpersonal relationships, or diminished physical activity, suggests that the improvement in subjective analgesia has not improved the quality of life and may have worsened it overall.

When function worsens, it is imperative to assess the possible contribution of opioid side effects, including addiction. Signs of dysfunction always warrant consideration of, but do not confirm, possible addiction (see later). It is only with careful assessment of objective treatment endpoints that side effects can be recognized and managed, allowing chronic opioid therapy to be safe, with minimal adverse effects.

Another critical issue is when to discontinue opioid therapy if the treatment is deemed unsatisfactory. Determination of treatment failure requires consideration of many possible contributing factors, including the following:

- Inadequate dose
- Inappropriate dosing schedule
- Improper drug delivery route
- Opioid-insensitive pain relating to the nature of the pain generator (e.g., neuropathic pain)
- Involvement of unresolved contributors to pain, such as physical, psychological and social disability
- The development of significant side effects limiting the dose escalation

Some patients appear resistant to one opioid and sensitive to another; a possible solution, therefore, is to try a different one.

How long effective opioid therapy should be continued remains a question with little science to guide decision making and no clear consensus among practitioners. Pharmacologic tolerance to opioids can develop during treatment (see later) and may necessitate an increase in dose to maintain the same therapeutic effect. Although some clinical studies have suggested a plateau of opioid dose requirement following an initial escalation, it is possible that progressive dose escalation may be required during prolonged opioid treatment. This implies that periodic opioid dose escalation would be expected even in patients experiencing effective pain relief. Clearly, decisions regarding the duration of effective opioid therapy should be made on the basis of each patient's need, with full consideration of treatment efficacy relative to adverse effects as well as to the progression or regression of underlying pathology. Once opioid therapy is started, it may not be possible to know how much pain would be present without it, unless opioids are discontinued (by slow taper.)

III. SIDE EFFECTS

The most common side effects of opioids are constipation, nausea, vomiting, sedation, pruritus, and respiratory depression. Any adverse effects from opioids may significantly limit therapy and some can present with life-threatening consequences. Unfortunately, there are few ways to predict which patients will experience which side effects, and which particular opioids will produce them. It is sensible to expect side effects and to take preventive action. As not all opioid-related side effects can be prevented, patients should be followed closely with a high level of suspicion. Effective management includes anticipation of adverse effects and preventive measures (such as laxatives for constipation), choosing the best medication with careful administration, and clear communication with the patient, family, or nurse to ensure prompt recognition of and response to adverse effects.

1. Constipation

Constipation is the most common side effect of opioids. Whereas tolerance develops to most other side effects, it does not develop to constipation, which can be expected throughout the duration of opioid administration. Preventive therapy with cathartics and adequate fluid intake is the mainstay of therapy and should be offered at the time opioids are started and continued throughout opioid treatment. Stool softeners and bulking agents such as bran or psyllium derivatives alone will be inadequate because opioid-related constipation results from decreased gut motility. Thus, active stimulating laxatives are effective and passive ones are not.

Severe constipation may respond to oral administration of an opioid antagonist such as naloxone. This maneuver exploits the extensive metabolism of naloxone after oral administration that limits its systemic bioavailability. Unfortunately, there is uncertainty about the dosing regimen. It is suggested that an initial oral naloxone dose should not exceed 5 mg. Start with 1.2 mg to 2.4 mg orally (four to six small ampules) every 4 hours until the first bowel movement, or for five doses. If ineffective, another series with a higher dose (3 to 5 mg per dose) may be tried.

Oral naloxone usually works only when the constipation is related solely to opioids. When concurrently used nonopioid drugs contribute to this side effect, the constipation is not reversed by naloxone (e.g., the anticholinergic side effect of tricyclic antidepressants).

Because constipation can be mitigated by direct effects of opioid antagonists on the bowel, opioids that are delivered without direct bowel contact may induce less constipation. Some evidence shows that certain opioid products that are absorbed without contact to the gastrointestinal (GI) tract, such as transdermal fentanyl, may induce less constipation than equivalent oral morphine. In one study of cancer patients, the incidence of constipation was reduced by up to two thirds by switching from oral morphine to transdermal fentanyl.

Drugs that cause diarrhea are usually well balanced with constipating opioids. Misoprostol (Cytotec), a drug that is marketed to protect the gastric mucosa from NSAID toxicity, is commonly associated with diarrhea but is a compelling addition to combination therapy with opioids and NSAIDs.

2. Nausea and vomiting

Although nausea and vomiting is a common early side effect of opioids, severe protracted nausea and vomiting caused solely by opioids is rare. Addition of antiemetics, or reduction of the opioid dose to the minimum that produces acceptable analgesia, is usually effective. A change in the route of administration may also alleviate symptoms. Fortunately, nausea and vomiting often becomes less significant within several days of administering opioids, at which time antiemetic therapy can be discontinued.

Although it remains unclear why one opioid should produce nausea and vomiting in an individual patient while another does not, the change to a different opioid often reduces or eliminates emetic side effects. A history of severe nausea with previous opioid treatment may prompt pretreatment with an antiemetic or avoidance of the previous offending opioid. There is rarely a need to discontinue or avoid opioid treatment, since the nausea and vomiting is usually responsive to dose reduction and/or antiemetic treatment.

Opioid-induced nausea and vomiting is thought to result from activation within the medullary chemoreceptor trigger zone (CTZ), a brainstem area responsible for afferent input to the emetic center. This anatomic area is rich in specific receptors responsive to various neurotransmitters. Effective antiemetic agents include the antihistamines (e.g., hydroxyzine), serotonin antagonists (e.g., ondansetron), dopamine antagonists (e.g., droperidol, haloperidol, and metoclopramide), and anticholinergics (e.g., scopolamine). It is not clear which of these drug classes is most effective for opioid-induced nausea and vomiting, so the choice is usually made on a try-it-and-see basis.

Opioid-related nausea may be related to orthostasis or ambulation, perhaps suggesting vestibular involvement. There are many other causes of nausea and vomiting that can occur concomitantly but which are unrelated to opioids. These include chemotherapy (particularly cisplatin), radiation therapy, metastases (particularly to brain and GI tract), increased intracranial pressure, peptic ulcer disease, esophagitis, gastritis, electrolyte and acid–base imbalance, uremia, liver disease, infection, pregnancy, and fear or anxiety. Since predicting the most effective antiemetic is not always possible, an agent may be chosen for its secondary benefits such as its promotility, sedative, antipruritic, anxiolytic, or antipsychotic properties.

3. Sedation

Opioid-related sedation is very common, and it can indicate either excess drug or even delirium. Opioid-induced sedation is usually temporary, resolving over time as the patient accommodates to a new opioid drug or a new dose. In those with significant sedation, the opioid dosage should be reduced to the minimal level required for adequate analgesia.

In some cases, where sedation occurs late in treatment, medication may be accumulating and, if so, it will be necessary to either increase the dose interval or change to a different agent. Also, in such cases, consider other causes of sedation such as other sedating drugs and encephalopathy. For unremitting sedation that limits therapeutic options, stimulants such as dextroamphetamine or caffeine can reduce sedation.

4. Pruritus

Pruritus is uncommon in association with oral opioid use, somewhat more common in patients treated with intravenous (IV) or intramuscular opioids, and frequent in patients treated with intrathecal and epidural opioids. Such effects often vary with the specific agent and dosage. Parenteral opioid-induced pruritus is usually mild, although it may rarely be moderate to severe. Fortunately, tolerance usually occurs quickly. Opioid-related pruritus is often localized to the face and less often to the perineum, but it can become generalized. The mechanism is not well understood. Suggested hypotheses include mu receptor stimulation, histamine release, local excitation of dorsal horn neurons, and central migration of spinal opioids to the brainstem.

Opioid-induced pruritus may respond to a change in opioid agent. Mini-doses of naloxone are effective for opioid-related pruritus and should not interfere with analgesia (5 μg/kg IV every 10 minutes;

repeat as needed, and hold if analgesia decreases). Antihistamines may also be effective. Since nonsedating antihistamines are less effective than sedating antihistamines, the antipruritic efficacy of antihistamine therapy may be related in part to sedation.

5. Respiratory depression

Depressed respiration is one of the most feared opioid side effects. Tolerance to opioid-induced respiratory depression usually develops early in the course of chronic therapy, so with long-term therapy, respiratory depression is rarely a problem. However, depression of respiratory drive may occur more rapidly when oral or intravenous opioids are combined with epidural or intrathecal opioids. Likewise, combining opioids with other sedating drugs can worsen the respiratory depressant effect of the opioid.

Significant acute respiratory depression can be managed with the opiate receptor antagonist naloxone. The dosage of naloxone for treating respiratory depression is 0.04 mg IV (one 0.4-mg ampule diluted in 10 mL) repeated every few minutes until a response is seen. Although naloxone may provide a brisk response, its duration of action is short, often requiring frequent dosing or continuous IV administration. Particular care must be given to the rapid administration of naloxone in a patient who has had prolonged opioid exposure, as this can precipitate an aggressive and possibly dangerous withdrawal. In special cases, particularly in a patient predisposed to pulmonary edema (congestive heart failure, adult respiratory distress syndrome), reversal of opioid actions can promote pulmonary edema.

IV. OPIOID TOLERANCE, PHYSICAL DEPENDENCE, AND ADDICTION

Pharmacologic tolerance and physical dependence are pharmacologic properties of a drug and are not synonymous with addiction. Both can develop following opioid treatment. Sustained analgesia at stable doses is also seen, especially in patients treated with opioids for CNMP. It is not clear why tolerance and physical dependence develop in some individuals and not others, although these phenomena tend to be associated more with the rapidly accelerating and large doses used to treat cancer pain than with those used to treat CNMP. (See Chapter 35, the section "Opioids and Addiction," for a full account of distinguishing between physical dependence, tolerance, and addiction.)

1. Tolerance

Tolerance occurs when a fixed dose of opioid produces decreasing analgesia so that a dose increase is required to maintain a stable effect. Just as tolerance develops to analgesic effects, so it may also occur to opioid side effects. Either changing the opioid or increasing the dose can usually compensate decreased analgesic efficacy in a tolerant patient. A patient who has become tolerant to one opioid drug may respond with adequate analgesia to another. Mechanisms underlying this clinical observation are not completely understood; it may relate to the differential opioid receptor profiles of different opioid agonists. Equianalgesic dosages are not applicable in the opioid-tolerant patient. When starting a new opioid agent in a tolerant patient, begin with half the equianalgesic dose and titrate to effective analgesia.

Recent studies have demonstrated the involvement of the NMDA receptor in mechanisms of opioid tolerance. It may be beneficial to combine an NMDA receptor antagonist with an opioid to attenuate tolerance. Such agents include dextromethorphan and ketamine. Appropriate ratios for such combinations for tolerance reduction are yet to be determined. In addition, methadone may be useful in opioid tolerance presumably because of its agonist effects on opioid receptors and its antagonism at NMDA receptors.

2. Physical dependence and withdrawal

Physical dependence applies to many drugs that are and are not addictive (e.g., morphine, clonidine.) Physical dependence relates to the expression of a withdrawal syndrome upon sudden drug cessation. It may reflect a biochemical adaptation from chronic exposure to a drug. Thus, duration of opioid treatment is probably a significant factor contributing to the development of opioid-related physical dependence. Cellular and intracellular mechanisms of opioid-related physical dependence have been proposed, including a rebound increase in cyclic adenosine monophosphate (cAMP), increased release of endogenous NMDA receptor agonists (namely, glutamate and aspartate), and changes in the NMDA receptor property following repeated opioid exposure. Fear of opioid dependence may lead to undertreatment.

Opioid withdrawal is rarely life-threatening and usually occurs with a systematic progression of symptoms. The least severe withdrawal symptoms typically appear earlier than the most severe. Withdrawal begins with increased irritability, restlessness, anxiety, insomnia, yawning, sweating, rhinorrhea, and lacrimation, and it progresses to dilated pupils, gooseflesh, tremor, chills, anorexia, muscle cramps, nausea, vomiting, abdominal pain, agitation, fever, tachycardia, and other features of heightened sympathetic activity. Laboratory data may reveal leukocytosis, ketosis, metabolic acidosis and respiratory alkalosis, and electrolyte imbalance.

The withdrawal syndrome may be seen with discontinuation or antagonism of any opioid. However, sudden discontinuation of shorter-acting opioids such as morphine or hydromorphone is more likely to produce withdrawal symptoms than discontinuation of agents with longer plasma half-lives, such as methadone or transdermally administered fentanyl. Slow, systematic tapering of opioids at a rate of 10% to 15% every 48 to 72 hours can usually prevent withdrawal. Usually a 2- to 3-week period is necessary for completion of the taper. Once the tapering is accomplished, withdrawal may be reversed by reintroducing the opioid at dosages of 25% to 40% of the previous daily dose.

Slow weaning of bedtime doses may help avoid the sleep disturbances that are often associated with opioid cessation. Signs of sympathetic hyperactivity may be treated with sympatholytics. Effective sympatholytics include clonidine (0.2 to 0.4 mg/day) and beta-blockers although these agents can produce hypotension. Clonidine may produce sedation and its anti-withdrawal effects may be antagonized by tricyclic antidepressants.

When abrupt discontinuation of a chronic opioid is necessary, clonidine detoxification can effectively blunt objective findings of sympathetic hyperactivity. It remains controversial whether clonidine or other sympatholytics increase or mask subjective symptoms of withdrawal such as anxiety, insomnia, and restlessness. Such treatment is often begun at dosages of 10 to 20 µg/kg/day in three divided doses, with subsequent adjustments to reduce signs of withdrawal while limiting hypotension. Clonidine may be maintained for between 4 days for short-acting opioids and 14 days for long-acting opioids. Tapering of clonidine can then occur over 4 to 6 days.

3. Opioid addiction and pseudoaddiction

This topic is discussed in greater detail in Chapter 35. Opioid addiction is a disorder characterized by compulsive use of opioids resulting in physical, psychological, and/or social dysfunction to the user and continued use despite that dysfunction. Opioid addiction should be distinguished from pseudoaddiction, a phenomenon that results from undertreatment. Whereas addiction is marked by dysfunction with the use of the drug that stimulates the disease, pseudoaddiction resolves when increasing the drug that the patient seeks, resulting in improved function.

V. CONCLUSION

To date, there is no consensus on whether, when, and how opioid therapy should be administered in CNMP patients. Rational and individualized opioid treatment regimens should be formulated according to the general guidelines presented here. Safe opioid therapy requires a program for ongoing close monitoring of functional gains and possible side effects.

SELECTED READINGS

1. American Pain Society. Principles of analgesic use in the treatment of acute pain and chronic cancer pain, 2nd ed. *Clin Pharm* 1990;9:601–611.
2. Carr DB. Pain. In: Firestone LL, Lebowitz P, Cook C, eds. *Clinical anesthesia procedures of the Massachusetts General Hospital,* 3rd ed. Boston: Little Brown, 1988:571–585.
3. Foley KM. Controversies in cancer pain. Medical perspectives. *Cancer* 1989;63: 2257–2265.
4. Fishman SM, Yang J, Reisfield G, et al. Adherence monitoring and drug surveillance with chronic opioid therapy. *J Pain Symptom Manage* 2000;20:293–307.
5. Fishman SM, Bandman T, Edwards A, Borsook D. The opioid contract in the management of patients on chronic opioid therapies. *J Pain Symptom Manage* 1999;18:27–37.
6. Mao J. NMDA and opioid receptors: Their interactions in antinociception, tolerance and neuroplasticity. *Brain Res Rev* 1999; 30:289–304.
7. Mao J, Price DD, Mayer DJ. Mechanisms of hyperalgesia and opioid tolerance: A current view of their possible interactions. *Pain* 1995;62:259–274.
8. National Institutes of Health Consensus Development Conference: The integrated approach to the management of pain. *J Pain Symptom Manage* 1987;2:35–41.
9. Portenoy RK. Chronic opioid therapy in nonmalignant pain. *J Pain Symptom Manage* 1990;5:S46–S62.
10. Wall PD, Melzack R, eds. *Textbook of pain,* 3rd ed. New York: Churchill Livingstone, 1998.

Pain in Acquired Immunodeficiency Syndrome

Steven P. Cohen

Oh, write of me, not "Died in bitter pain,"
But "Emigrated to another star!"
—*Helen Hunt Jackson (1830–1885)*

  I. Etiology of pain in patients with AIDS
 II. Pain syndromes in patients with AIDS
   1. Gastrointestinal pain
   2. Thoracic pain
   3. Rheumatologic manifestations of AIDS
   4. Neurologic pain manifestations of AIDS
   5. Herpes zoster
III. Treatment options
   1. Opioid management for the HIV-positive patient
   2. Nonopioid pain adjuvants
   3. Nerve blocks and regional anesthesia
   4. Nonpharmacologic interventions

Pain is a common reason for the hospitalization of patients with acquired immunodeficiency syndrome (AIDS). The prevalence of pain in patients with AIDS has been reported to be between 40% and 60% in hospitalized patients, somewhat higher (around 70%) in ambulatory patients, and 97% in terminally ill patients. The incubation period of the human immunodeficiency virus (HIV) ranges from a few years to more than 10 years since the advent of new antiviral therapy and prophylactic treatment for opportunistic infections (OIs). As the life expectancy of these patients continues to increase, issues related to quality of life, including adequate pain control, take on increasing importance. It is therefore incumbent on physicians responsible for treating patients with AIDS to be familiar with the myriad of pain syndromes with which they present, and to provide adequate treatment.

This chapter reviews the etiology of pain manifestations in HIV-positive patients in different organ systems and discusses appropriate treatment strategies. Pain treatment is based on the underlying cause, when possible. Symptomatic measures, however, should not be delayed while the workup for the underlying cause is in progress or if the underlying cause cannot be treated effectively. Specific problems of pharmacologic and nonpharmacologic symptomatic pain relief in HIV-positive patients are also discussed. Figure 1 outlines a possible approach to the treatment of pain in these patients.

I. ETIOLOGY OF PAIN IN PATIENTS WITH AIDS

Pain in patients with AIDS may be caused by the direct effects of the human immunodeficiency virus on the nervous system, by OIs, by tumors related to immunosuppression, or by the various therapies for HIV and its associated disorders. Several studies

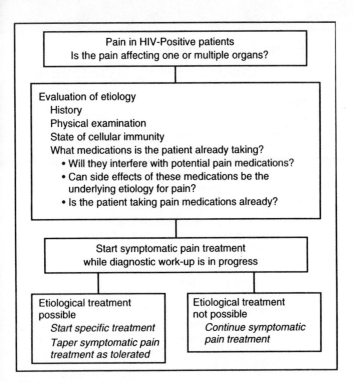

Figure 1.   An approach to the treatment of pain in patients with AIDS.

have examined the incidence of various types of pain syndromes in HIV-positive patients. Although the exact prevalence varies according to patient population, study methodology, and the extent of disease progression, the most common pain diagnoses are headaches, abdominal pain, peripheral neuropathies, and rheumatologic manifestations such as myalgias and arthralgias. When pain was classified by mechanism, Hewitt et al. found that 45% of pain syndromes were somatic, 15% were visceral, 19% were neuropathic, and 4% were unknown. Seventeen percent of pain complaints were headaches and could not be classified into these categories. Figure 2 represents a breakdown by location of the different pain syndromes in patients with HIV infection.

II. PAIN SYNDROMES IN PATIENTS WITH AIDS

1. Gastrointestinal pain

Pain in HIV disease can arise anywhere in the gastrointestinal (GI) tract, including the oral cavity, esophagus, anus and rectum, hepatobiliary system, and pancreas.

(i) *Oral cavity*

Between 20% and 50% of HIV-infected patients develop oral lesions during the course of their illness. These lesions often provide

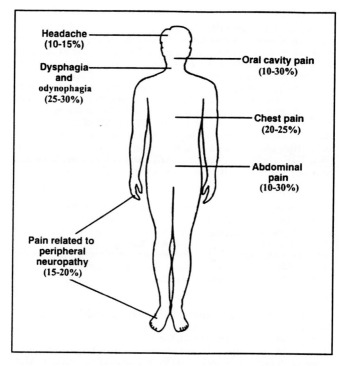

Figure 2. Pain symptoms, according to location, in AIDS patients.

the first clue to infection with the virus and may herald disease progression and immunologic decline. Oropharyngeal candidiasis occurs in up to one third of HIV-positive individuals and over 90% of patients with AIDS. Because of its high incidence, *Candida* infections are the most common cause of pain in the oral cavity, even though most patients are asymptomatic. At least four different types of presentations have been described: hyperplastic, erythematous, angular cheilitis, and pseudomembranous or "thrush," the most common kind.

Treatment is important, as pain and dysphagia may impair oral intake and contribute to wasting and overall deterioration. For mild cases, therapy includes topical antifungal agents, with systemic agents being reserved for more extensive disease.

Oral ulcers are common in individuals infected with HIV and may result from a variety of organisms, including viruses, fungi, and the bacteria implicated in necrotizing ulcerating infections (gingivitis, periodontitis, and stomatitis). Some of the antivirals used in the treatment of HIV infection such as zalcitabine (ddC) can also precipitate stomatitis. When oral ulcers are unresponsive to conventional therapy, the use of steroids and thalidomide may prove beneficial. In many cases, topical anesthetics and systemic analgesics are necessary for pain management.

(ii) *Esophagitis*

Approximately one third of patients with AIDS develop dysphagia and odynophagia. Candidal esophagitis is the most common cause of esophageal pathology, with the treatment of choice being systemic antifungal agents. The absence of oral involvement does not exclude a diagnosis of esophageal candidiasis.

Ulcerating and nonulcerating lesions of the esophagus can be caused by a wide variety of different pathogens including fungi, bacteria, and viruses. Cytomegalovirus (CMV) is the most commonly implicated, being present in 10% to 40% of all biopsies of esophageal ulcers. This pathogen can manifest as a single ulcer, as multiple ulcers, or as a diffuse esophagitis. Medications used to treat HIV, such as zidovudine (AZT) and zalcitabine, have also been implicated as being a cause of esophageal lesions.

(iii) *Abdominal pain*

Abdominal pain is a frequent complaint in patients with HIV, with an incidence of greater than 25% in some studies. The wide array of possible causes can pose a diagnostic dilemma for the clinician. Some are specific to the immunocompromised state of patients with AIDS, such as infections, neoplasms, and the side effects of drug treatments. Others are more common, such as peptic ulcer disease and gastroenteritis.

(iv) *Hepatobiliary disease*

Among the pathogens that affect the hepatobiliary tree in HIV infection, the most common is the *Mycobacterium avium-intracellulare* complex (MAC), found in the liver of 20% to 50% of patients at autopsy. Other organisms affecting the liver include *M. tuberculosis* and sexually transmitted organisms. AIDS cholangiopathy is a syndrome characterized by sclerosing cholangitis with or without papillary stenosis. Patients typically present with abdominal pain, fever, nausea, and vomiting. When a pathogen can be isolated, the most commonly found are CMV and *Cryptosporidium.* Sphincterotomies performed endoscopically have produced excellent results in the relief of pain.

Cholecystitis may occur coincidentally in AIDS patients with gallstones. More common, though, is acalculous cholecystitis resulting from OIs. The most common causes of AIDS cholangiopathy are CMV and *Cryptosporidium,* with MAC and Kaposi's sarcoma (KS) being less frequently implicated.

(v) *Pancreatitis*

In HIV-infected patients, pancreatitis is most commonly associated with medications. OI agents such as CMV, *Toxoplasma,* and mycobacteria; neoplasms; and perhaps even the HIV virus itself can also cause pancreatitis.

(vi) *Neoplasms*

Kaposi's sarcoma and non-Hodgkin's lymphoma (NHL) are the two neoplasms that most commonly affect patients with AIDS. These tumors can occur anywhere in the GI tract, from the oral cavity to the liver, pancreas, and bowel. Among patients with skin or nodal KS, 40% also have GI involvement, giving rise to a wide range of GI symptoms including appendicitis, obstruction, perforation, and bleeding. In addition, the radiation used to treat KS can cause painful, ulcerating sores.

In the oral cavity, pain from NHL is usually from aggressively growing masses that can result in the destruction of bone and soft tissue. In the lower GI tract, lymphoma can cause abdominal pain, bowel obstruction, perforation, and bleeding. Treatment is with radiation therapy and systemic cancer chemotherapy.

(viii) Anorectal pain

In one study of 340 homosexual and bisexual men with AIDS, 34% were found to have anorectal disease. These patients can present with painful perirectal abscesses, fissures, fistulas, and hemorrhoids. Infectious causes of proctitis include herpes simplex virus (HSV), CMV, and other sexually transmitted organisms. A slight increase in anorectal carcinoma has also been noted in HIV-positive homosexual men. Therapy is directed at the underlying cause and includes surgery, antibiotics and stool softeners.

2. Thoracic pain

(i) *Pulmonary*

Because of its prevalence, pneumonia is the most common cause of chest pain in patients with AIDS. Although *Pneumocystis carinii* (PCP) is the most frequent pathogen found, patients with AIDS are susceptible to infection by a wide range of other organisms as well. Lung malignancy can also cause chest pain, with the two most important ones being KS and NHL. The presentation of pulmonary KS can be similar to that of OIs and includes cough, fever, pleuritic chest pain, dyspnea, and infiltrates on chest radiograph. Further adding to the difficulty in diagnosing malignancy is the fact that up to 50% of patients with pulmonary malignancy have superimposed infection.

Nonsteroidal anti-inflammatory drugs (NSAIDs) may be helpful in treating the pain associated with pulmonary disease. Opioids should be used with caution as they may further compromise an already tenuous respiratory status.

(ii) *Cardiac*

Pericarditis, myocarditis, and, in the intravenous (IV) drug–abusing population, endocarditis all occur with increased frequency in HIV-infected patients. Chest pain is a more salient feature in pericarditis than in myocarditis and endocarditis, although it may be conspicuously absent in chronic disease. Its prevalence in HIV-positive patients ranges from as low as 3% to as high as 26.9%. Patients with heart disease may be sensitive to the hemodynamic effects of opioids and poor candidates for treatment with tricyclic antidepressants. In the absence of renal disease or coagulation defects, NSAIDs can be a useful adjuvant.

3. Rheumatologic manifestations of AIDS

It has been widely documented that musculoskeletal complaints occur with increased frequency in patients with HIV infection. In one series involving 101 patients in various stages of HIV disease, musculoskeletal involvement was noted in 72% of cases. Reiter's syndrome was the first rheumatic disease reported in patients with

HIV infection, and it is frequently claimed to be the most prevalent. The most common presentation of Reiter's syndrome is oligoarthritis, preferentially affecting the large, weight-bearing joints in the lower extremities.

Septic arthritis and psoriatic arthritis arthropathy may also occur with greater frequency in patients with AIDS and should be treated the same way as in the non-HIV-infected population. An HIV-associated arthritis has also been described. The onset of this oligoarthritis tends to be gradual, ranging from 1 to 6 weeks, with the duration averaging about a month. The joints of the lower extremities are most frequently affected, although any joint in the body can be involved.

Therapy for rheumatologic arthropathies generally begins with the traditional NSAIDs, although in severe cases they alone may be insufficient. Second-line agents that have proven useful include gold, sulfasalazine, phenylbutazone, and certain antimalarial drugs. In refractory cases, the use of steroids, either systemically or via intra-articular injection, may be necessary.

An association between HIV infection and inflammatory muscle disease (myalgias and myopathies) was first recognized in 1983, with the most common disorder being polymyositis. Patients with polymyositis generally present with progressive muscle weakness, the lower extremities being more frequently affected than the arms. Myalgias and muscle cramps are also prominent complaints. Drugs used to treat HIV disease, particularly AZT, have been known to cause a toxic myopathy indistinguishable from that of polymyositis. This scenario classically develops after 6 to 12 months of treatment with doses exceeding 500 mg/day, and there is usually improvement after the drug is discontinued. Most patients with myalgias respond well to NSAIDs, although an aggressive physical therapy program may be needed if weakness exists. In severe cases, moderate doses of steroids for 4 to 6 weeks may be indicated.

4. Neurologic pain manifestation

Neurologic complications are common in HIV-infected patients: at least 10% present with neurologic symptoms. Perhaps because of its affinity for the central nervous system (CNS) and the ease with which the virus is able to cross the blood–brain barrier, involvement of the nervous system has been found in 30% to 63% of patients over the course of the illness.

(i) *Headache*

Patients with HIV infection frequently report headache, with an incidence varying from 17% to over 50% in patients with documented neurologic involvement. Because the cause varies according to the stage of disease and the medications being taken, knowledge of these factors can provide important clues to diagnosis. In otherwise healthy HIV carriers with normal CD4 counts, no prior opportunistic infections, and an absence of other neurologic manifestations, headaches are unlikely to be the result of serious neurologic disease. Common causes of headaches in healthy HIV carriers include tension headaches, migraines, and sinusitis.

Headaches in HIV-infected patients can also result from medication therapy. Antiretroviral therapies as well as drugs used to treat OIs have both been documented to cause headaches.

Although it is often difficult to ascertain the precise incidence of drug-induced headaches, results from one study revealed a 16% prevalence of AZT-induced headaches.

(ii) *Nonfocal brain disorders*

HIV encephalopathy, also known as AIDS dementia complex (ADC), refers to a constellation of cognitive, behavioral, and motor symptoms that is thought to be caused by HIV-1. Headaches are not unusual in ADC and are usually attributed to aseptic meningitis. Another fairly common nonfocal CNS infection is CMV encephalitis, with early autopsy studies showing evidence of CMV infection in about 25% of brains. Although many of these patients are asymptomatic, some suffer a fulminant course with significant morbidity and mortality. In addition to headaches, symptoms of CMV CNS infection include confusion, delirium, seizures, and ataxia.

The most likely cause of meningitis in HIV patients is infection with the fungus *Cryptococcus,* estimated to affect between 5% and 15% percent of patients. The clinical symptoms of this entity vary widely, from none at all to the more classic picture of headache, nausea, vomiting, malaise, confusion, and signs of meningeal irritation such as neck stiffness and photophobia.

Probably the second most common cause of meningitis in the HIV-infected population is aseptic meningitis, believed to be caused by the virus itself. Both acute and chronic forms have been reported. Aseptic meningitis commonly occurs during the transition from asymptomatic to symptomatic disease, as the CD4 count is falling. Whether HIV meningoencephalitis is a distinct entity is still being debated. Nevertheless, symptoms of this controversial illness are usually self-limited and include headache, photophobia, and occasionally nausea. Pain treatment is symptomatic and includes NSAIDs, tricyclic antidepressants (TCAs), and calcium channel blockers.

(iii) *Focal brain disorders*

Cerebral toxoplasmosis is the most common focal brain lesion in AIDS, occurring in 5% to 10% of HIV-positive patients. Another frequent cause of focal CNS disease is progressive multifocal leukoencephalopathy (PML), with an incidence of 4% to 5%. Although there is no specific and reliable treatment for PML, there are numerous reports of spontaneous remission after the institution of highly active antiretroviral therapy. Primary CNS lymphoma is the third major focal brain disorder encountered in patients with AIDS, accounting for between 2% and 7% of CNS complications in HIV disease. Other malignancies such as Kaposi's and other sarcomas also occur with increased frequency in patients with AIDS.

Symptoms of focal brain lesions generally relate to mass effect and include headaches, cognitive changes, seizures, and focal neurologic deficits. Cranial involvement and impingement on pain-sensitive neurovascular structures can cause constant headaches. Therapies include specific treatment directed at the organism responsible, radiation, and chemotherapy. Steroid therapy may be beneficial, reducing cerebral edema and mass effects. Adequate pain therapy can often be achieved using mild analgesics such as NSAIDs and tramadol, although stronger opioid therapy may occasionally be required for severe pain.

(iv) *Central pain*

The International Association for the Study of Pain (IASP) defines central pain as pain that is caused by a lesion or dysfunction in the CNS. Central pain may occur almost immediately following injury, or it may take years to develop. When delayed, the onset frequently coincides with changes in subjective sensory abnormalities. Characteristics of this phenomenon include continuous, spontaneous pain that is sometimes described as burning, shooting, or aching. It is often accompanied by allodynia, hyperesthesia, and hyperalgesia, and it may be exacerbated by cold temperatures. Some common causes of central pain in patients with AIDS include HIV myelopathy, infarcts, cerebral abscesses, neurosyphilis, and malignancies.

Unfortunately, there is no truly effective means of eradicating central pain. However, combination therapy with TCAs, antiseizure and antiarrhythmic agents, opioids, N-methyl-D-aspartate (NMDA) antagonists such as dextromethorphan, and alpha-2 agonists can often provide substantial relief.

(v) *Peripheral neuropathies*

Peripheral neuropathies have been reported to affect up to 35% of patients with AIDS, with the incidence increasing in advanced stages of the disease. The clinical spectrum of HIV-associated neuropathies is broad, with sensory neuropathies being most commonly encountered. Because of their insidious onset and the progressive nature of HIV disease, peripheral neuropathies often go unreported in this population.

Distal symmetrical polyneuropathy is the most common neuropathy complicating HIV disease, with symptoms usually starting in the toes (and later the fingers), and extending proximally. The most common type of distal polyneuropathy is that caused by the retrovirus itself; it is often referred to as HIV-related distal sensory polyneuropathy (HIVR-DSPN). The goal of treatment for this disorder is symptomatic relief with medications for neuropathic pain such as TCAs and anticonvulsants. For allodynia, the local application of lidocaine cream can be helpful. Although isolated reports exist touting its benefits, traditional treatment with antiretroviral therapy has not been shown to be effective.

Perhaps the second most common neuropathy is caused by medications used to treat HIV-infected patients. Although some patients with neurotoxic distal sensory polyneuropathy complain of a deep or aching pain in their distal extremities as opposed to the typical burning or shooting pain of HIVR-DSPN, in most cases the two are clinically indistinguishable. Affected patients typically present with complaints of burning, tingling, or numbness beginning in the distal parts of the extremities. Occasionally, superimposed shooting pains and allodynia are noted. If a neurotoxic neuropathy is suspected, the offending agent should be stopped immediately. In most cases, the effects are reversible, although improvement may take weeks or even months.

Deficiencies of vitamin B_{12} may produce DSPN characterized by pain, numbness, and paresthesias. In one study, 16% of HIV-infected patients were noted to have either low serum levels of B_{12} or impaired absorption, although other studies have failed to duplicate these results. The treatment of B_{12} neuropathy is replenishment of the vitamin.

Progressive polyradiculopathy (sacral ascending polyradiculopathy) typically occurs late in the course of HIV disease, when CD4 counts are low and OIs are present. This progressive neuropathy is one of the most devastating and dramatic neurologic complications of AIDS. Yet its response to early therapy is good, and this, as well as its fulminant course if left untreated, demand prompt recognition and timely treatment. Progressive polyradiculopathy classically strikes abruptly, with the initial abnormalities being present in the lumbosacral nerve roots. This typically manifests as pain and paresthesias in the buttocks and legs, with back pain being another symptom that is often encountered early. Over the next several weeks, this may be followed by rapid progression to paraparesis, ascending sensory loss, bowel and bladder dysfunction, and areflexia. If left untreated, these abnormalities can extend to the trunk and arms. The large majority of cases of progressive polyradiculopathy appear to be caused by CMV infection, which can sometimes be detected in the cerebrospinal fluid. However, because of the rapidly progressive course, treatment should be started immediately on the basis of clinical evidence. The mainstay of therapy is with antiviral agents.

Patients with focal mononeuropathies present with asymmetrical multifocal motor and sensory symptoms in the distribution of cutaneous nerves, mixed nerves, and nerve roots. In many patients, coexisting cranial neuropathies are present. In HIV-positive patients who are otherwise healthy, the disorder tends to be self-limited, with symptoms being restricted to one or two peripheral nerves. Some patients who develop symptoms early in their illness may even experience spontaneous remission. In patients with more widespread disease, the neuropathy may involve three or more nerves. In these individuals, CMV can often be isolated from nerve biopsies. Though the mainstay of treatment for CMV focal neuropathy is specific antiviral therapy, symptomatic treatment with neuropathic medications may also prove beneficial. In some patients, therapy with IV immunoglobulins, plasmapheresis, and in some cases corticosteroids may be indicated.

5. Herpes Zoster

Several studies have shown the incidence of acute herpes zoster (AHZ) to be higher in the HIV-positive population (from 5% to 10%) than in the general population. Outbreaks of the disease generally correlate with a declining state of immunity and are unusual in healthy persons under 50 years. Therefore, young patients with AHZ should be evaluated for causes of immunodeficiency.

Patients with herpes zoster normally present with pain and/or dysesthesias that typically precede a rash by 3 to 4 days. Infrequently, pain occurs without the development of visible lesions. Unlike non-HIV-infected patients with shingles, HIV-infected patients with shingles exhibit a high prevalence of atypical lesions and frequent recurrences.

In immunocompromised patients, varicella zoster virus (VZV) infections can be life-threatening, and prompt treatment is essential. As in the non-HIV-infected patient, the treatment of choice is anti-herpes-virus agents. Administration of the live attenuated viral vaccine is contraindicated in HIV-infected individuals.

Since the severity of pain during the acute phase of herpes zoster infection is predictive of the development of chronic pain, adequate pain management early in the disease is of paramount importance. Symptomatic pain therapy in acute attacks of AHZ includes treatment with NSAIDs, anticonvulsants such as gabapentin and topiramate (Topamax), and antidepressants. In addition to relieving pain, TCAs have been shown in randomized controlled studies to be effective in reducing the incidence of postherpetic neuralgia (PHN).

Nerve blocks that have been reported to be effective in shingles include intercostal nerve blocks for thoracic involvement, epidural analgesia, and subcutaneous infiltration with and without steroids. Although blocking sympathetic ganglia early in the course of the disease has been reported by some authors to be an effective treatment, a recent critical review of the literature found scant evidence for this view. In those patients refractory to conventional therapy, the use of narcotics may be indicated.

PHN is defined as pain in the affected dermatomes that persists longer than 3 months after crusting of the herpes lesions. Perhaps because of the association with a decline in immune status, AIDS patients with AHZ may be at a slightly higher risk for development of PHN, with an incidence between 10% and 15%. Two other factors that appear to influence the development of PHN include the severity of pain and the duration of lesions. The pain of PHN is often described as burning, aching, or tearing, with superimposed shooting sensations. The scars themselves and the areas around them are often hypoesthetic, but paradoxically, patients may present with allodynia, hyperesthesia, or hyperpathia. As with chicken pox, a severe form of pruritus may ensue.

The only pharmacologic therapies shown to be effective in randomized clinical trials in patients with PHN are TCAs, gabapentin, topical agents, and opioids. Empirical therapies with other anticonvulsants have yielded mixed results. Recently, topical local anesthetics such as the lidocaine patch, with or without capsaicin, have been demonstrated to be of benefit in the treatment of PHN-associated allodynia. Good results have also been obtained with opioids. In spite of isolated reports to the contrary, in most cases local anesthetic blocks have limited value in the treatment of PHN. Transcutaneous electrical nerve stimulation (TENS) is associated with almost no adverse side effects and may be beneficial in some situations. Finally, in patients who continue to have refractory pain, surgical therapies such as spinal cord stimulation and neuroablative procedures may be considered.

III. TREATMENT OPTIONS

These pain treatments are more fully described in Chapters 8-11.

1. Opioid management of the HIV-positive patient

In the United States, approximately 25% of HIV-infected patients have a history of IV drug abuse. Yet for many of these patients, the diseases they have and the pain they are faced with necessitates treatment with opioids. When treating these patients, the fundamental principle of pain management is the same as that for other patients: pain complaints should be taken seriously and treated aggressively. In one study, IV drug addicts were not found to complain more of pain or require larger doses of opioid analgesics than non–drug abusers.

For patients with chronic pain, long-acting opioids provide a steady state of analgesia and are associated with less euphoria than short-acting narcotics. Consequently, they also tend to have a lower abuse potential when used therapeutically. The fentanyl patch has perhaps the lowest potential for abuse, although innovative addicts have found methods to abuse even this.

When patients in methadone maintenance programs or those taking long-acting opioids for chronic conditions present with acute nociceptive pain, long-acting medications can be continued and patient-controlled analgesia can be added to provide additional analgesia for the acute phase and as a means of measuring opioid requirements. Mixed agonist–antagonists should be avoided in these patients as they may trigger withdrawal. In patients with inadequately treated pain, pseudoaddiction can be misinterpreted as drug-seeking behavior (see Chapter 30). Finally, only when the patient's pain is under control should an attempt be made to treat addiction in motivated patients wishing to change their lifestyle.

2. Nonopioid pain adjuvants

The NSAIDs and acetaminophen provide safe and effective analgesia in many cases of mild to moderate pain. Advantages of these medications are their relative safety, their availability, and their low potential for abuse. Even in conditions that require stronger therapy, the opioid-sparing properties of these medications make them a good addition to any multimodal pain regimen. However, in view of the multiple organ system dysfunction patients with AIDS may suffer, clinicians must be aware of the toxic effects of these drugs. Acetaminophen carries a dose-dependent risk of hepatotoxicity and less commonly causes renal tubular necrosis. It may also decrease the clearance of AZT. In some situations, the newer specific cyclooxygenase-2 (COX-2) inhibitors, which have a more favorable side effect profile than traditional NSAIDs, may be preferable.

In light of the high prevalence of neuropathic pain and depression in HIV-infected patients, it is not surprising that TCAs often play a prominent role in pain therapy. In addition to their use in the treatment of neurogenic pain and some causes of headache, the side effects of decreased peristalsis and sedation may be helpful in patients with refractory diarrhea and insomnia.

The anticonvulsants carbamazepine and phenytoin have long been successful in neuropathic pain conditions, but both can interact with other drugs commonly used by patients with AIDS, such as isoniazid and TCAs. Newer agents, such as gabapentin and lamotrigine, and the antiarrhythmic mexiletine may be preferred in some patients.

Topical creams such as capsaicin for arthralgias, and lidocaine for PHN are not absorbed systemically and are thus associated with minimal side effects. However, both are expensive and it may not be feasible to apply them to large areas of skin several times each day.

3. Nerve blocks and regional anesthesia

Nerve blocks and regional anesthesia often prove to be useful adjuncts in AIDS patients in whom analgesics have failed to alleviate pain or who cannot tolerate them because of side effects. However, there are some special considerations that need to be addressed before proceeding with nerve blocks. Patients with HIV have a greater incidence of potentially progressive neurologic problems than the general population. Although it is not an absolute contraindication, for many pain specialists the existence of progressive neurologic disease mitigates against the use of spinal and epidural agents in patients who might otherwise be suitable candidates for neuraxial blockade.

Another concern is infection. One study found a higher infection rate in patients with AIDS who had had epidural catheters inserted for chronic pain than in the general population. But two other studies failed to reproduce the findings of an increased complication rate during epidural treatment in HIV-infected patients for labor analgesia and postdural puncture headaches (epidural blood patches). Certainly, the risks and benefits of steroid injections must be carefully balanced in these patients, especially those in the later stages of disease who are already markedly immunosuppressed.

Finally, patients with AIDS often present with thrombocytopenia and other coagulopathies, because of both their disease and their treatments. Coagulopathy is a contraindication to regional anesthesia. Other contraindications are systemic or local infection at the site of needle puncture, and leukopenia.

4. Nonpharmacologic interventions

Because of the nature of the immunodeficiency virus and its modes of transmission, a large percentage of HIV-positive patients are faced with the daunting paradox of being young and having an incurable disease. Consequently, many are emotionally unprepared for dealing with a fatal illness. Both psychological and social factors play a major role in the pain experience, necessitating a multidisciplinary approach to the AIDS patient with pain.

Unlike the plethora of medications these patients are often compelled to take, most noninterventional pain treatments are devoid of side effects. These treatments include self-hypnosis, biofeedback and other relaxation techniques, acupuncture, and group therapy. Physical therapy and other functional restoration programs can help reduce musculoskeletal pain and maintain strength and mobility. Finally, a good therapist who focuses on the cognitive and behavioral aspects of pain and illness can be indispensable in this population.

SELECTED READINGS

1. Dolin R, Masur H, Saag MS, eds. AIDS therapy. Philadelphia: Churchill Livingstone, 1999.
2. Holloway RG, Kieburtz KD. Headache and the human immunodeficiency virus type 1 infection. *Headache* 1995;35:245–255.
3. Merigan TC Jr, Bartlett JG, Bolognesi D, eds. *Textbook of AIDS medicine,* 2nd ed. Baltimore: Williams & Wilkins, 1999.
4. Patton LL, van der Horst C. Oral infections and other manifestations of HIV disease. *Infect Dis Clin North Am* 1999;13:879–900.

5. Simpson DM, Olney RK. Peripheral neuropathies associated with human immunodeficiency virus infection. *Neurol Clin* 1992;10: 685–711.
6. Wormser GP, ed. *AIDS and other manifestations of HIV infection*, 3rd ed. Philadelphia: Lippincott-Raven, 1998.
7. Hewitt DJ, McDonald M, Portenoy R, et al. Pain syndromes and etiologies in ambulatory AIDS patients. *PAIN* 1997;70:117–123.

Pain Due to Cancer

Pain in Adults with Cancer

Jeffrey A. Norton and Annabel D. Edwards

We must all die. But that I can save him from days of torture, that is what I feel as my great and ever new privilege. Pain is a more terrible lord of man than even death.
—*Albert Schweitzer (1875–1965)*

The American Cancer Society estimates that in the year 2000, 1.2 million new cases of invasive cancer will be diagnosed in the United States alone. Of all the symptoms that a person experiences while living with cancer, pain is the most feared. At least one third of cancer patients have pain at the time of their diagnosis. Up to two thirds of patients with advanced cancer rate their pain level as moderate to severe. A large portion (about 90%) of all cancer patients with pain can be treated effectively with the multidisciplinary modes of treatment currently and readily available.

I. DEFINING CANCER PAIN

The term *cancer pain* does not have a specific definition. In fact, cancer patients as a group have some of the most diverse types of pain. Their pain can stem from any of the following:

- Tumor invasion or compression of other tissues by tumor
- Surgery and biopsies
- Radiation damage to tissues
- Neuropathies caused by chemotherapy or other treatments
- Ischemia
- Inflammation
- Blocked or damaged organ structures (visceral pain)
- Decreased mobility and arthropathies (musculoskeletal pain)
- Pathologic fractures

Some pain occurs in direct temporal relationship to an event such as surgery. Other types of pain start days or months after an initiating event and get worse with time, as may happen with peripheral neuropathy induced by chemotherapy. It is common for many types of pain to coexist in patients with cancer. In addition, some pains are constant, whereas others are incidental to specific movements, and still others are intermittent and resulting from physiologic factors. Timing issues related to pain occurrence influence the therapeutic approach used.

Common words used to describe pain, such as *chronic pain,* often do not lead to an understanding of the basic mechanism of the pain. It is important to avoid using such phrases casually, as they can inhibit effective evaluation and treatment. The success of pharmacologic pain therapy lies primarily in the proper match between a specific pain mechanism and the pharmacologic effect of the chosen medication. The success of nonpharmacologic adjuvant pain therapies, such as relaxation or self-hypnosis, depends on the patient's abilities and beliefs, practice (or use over time), the modality chosen, and sometimes the pain mechanism.

Another aspect of pain is related to the patient's sense of wellness. Psychic pain, or suffering, can play a major role in a patient's overall quality of life. Ignoring this type of "pain" is as harmful as ignoring somatic pain. Physical pain and psychic pain are so closely entwined that it makes no sense to treat one without the other. The abolition of physical pain means little when a patient is unable to derive pleasure from life.

II. BARRIERS TO APPROPRIATE CANCER PAIN MANAGEMENT

Unfortunately, many barriers still exist to the effective treatment of cancer pain, despite the fact that most cancer pain can be treated relatively easily with basic pain management techniques. These barriers are multifactorial and include the following:

- Lack of knowledge about the various mechanisms behind cancer pain syndromes
- Lack of knowledge about the variety of medications used to treat the various mechanisms of pain
- Failure to properly assess the patient in pain
- Fears (of the patient, the patient's family, and healthcare providers) about addiction and the use of controlled substances
- Fear of complications or side effects of opioid analgesics
- Lack of respect for or knowledge of nonpharmacologic therapies
- Fear that use of opioids may hasten death near the end of life

Patients may, in fact, create significant barriers to their own care, which is why a careful assessment of their attitudes and worries is necessary. Cancer patients have stated in a number of surveys that they see pain as inevitable and that they should be able to tolerate it. They worry that physicians will be distracted from treating the cancer if they mention the pain, or that they will be seen as complainers. Often, denial is a factor because many patients see worsening pain as a sign of worsening disease, so they do not want to think about it or admit to it. Some patients cannot afford the medications prescribed and instead of asking if there is an alternative that is less expensive, they simply do not fill their prescriptions. There are also patients who just do not want to take multiple pills.

Problems in the healthcare system can also impact on pain management efforts. Insurance coverage may make specific forms of therapy unattainable. The availability of medications may be restricted by insurance or pharmacy willingness to carry various products. Instruction about pain and its management is not common in medical schools and is barely mentioned in the majority of textbooks. In addition, practitioners who *do* provide pain management are often poorly reimbursed for their time.

Some problems that foster poor pain management may well be addressed over the next year or two as the new Joint Commission for the Accreditation of Hospital Organizations (JCAHO) regulations relating to pain management are put into place and graded. These regulations will impact all types of healthcare facilities examined by the JCAHO (for website, see Appendix III).

III. PAIN ASSESSMENT

Proper assessment of the nature of a patient's pain or pains and the probable cause or causes is essential for effective treatment. Each pain needs to be evaluated separately, as the mechanisms may differ and require different treatments. Because new pain can develop and old pain can worsen or improve (e.g., with disease progression, new health problems, treatment of the disease), the pain situation should be reassessed regularly.

Pain is a combination of sensory and emotional reactions to intense stimuli. It is inherently a subjective experience. Thus a large part of a pain assessment comes from the information the patient provides. The diagnosis of cancer brings with it many emotional responses that may strongly overlay the patient's report. Perhaps this plays a role in the tendency of providers to underestimate pain. Understanding how the cancer patient thinks of himself or herself and the disease can be important.

1. Pain descriptions

The two major pieces of information that the patient provides include the level of pain and the description of the pain (i.e., what it feels like). Pain level is measured on a scale, most commonly from 0 to 10 (where 0 is no pain and 10 is the worst pain imaginable). Scales can be verbal or written; they may use colors, numbers, lines, or faces; or they may rely on behavioral cues. The key is to find a scale that works for the individual patient and to use that scale consistently. Levels of pain cannot be compared between patients. The scale can only measure changes (e.g., evaluate the effect of interventions) in an individual patient.

A general goal is to try to get a patient below a 5/10 level of pain, but this is purely empirical. Some patients are content with a 5/10 level, whereas others are miserable. The ultimate goal is to achieve a reasonable level of comfort while minimizing side effects; patients and providers need to decide together when this goal has been reached.

Patients' descriptions of pain help determine the mechanisms of pain. When pain is primarily from a recent injury (nociceptive), words like sharp and throbbing are often used and the patient can often point directly to a place that hurts. Pain that derives from damaged nerves may elicit descriptors like shooting, burning, electrical, painful numbness, or pins and needles. This type of pain tends to be more diffuse or to travel from one place to another. These verbal indicators are not precise but they are helpful. Clinical knowledge and experience inform treatment decisions as well.

2. Specific elements of the history and physical examination

All the usual features of the history and physical examination are relevant (Chapter 4). The following aspects of the history and physical are of particular importance in cancer patients.

Review of medications

Ask about herbal or home remedies (which are very popular and widely advertised to cancer patients) so that adverse interactions can be avoided and the treatment plan can be simplified. A careful determination of all pain medications that have been prescribed, whether in the past or recently, is also warranted, so that the patient is clear about which medications to take.

Treatment history

About 20% of cancer patients have pain secondary to treatment, so the history of treatments is crucial. Pain caused by treatments may confuse the clinical picture for the practitioner and make a patient less willing to continue with the therapeutic plan.

Pain secondary to radiation includes plexopathy, myelopathy, mucositis, and bone necrosis. Mechanisms include fibrosis, tissue ischemia, necrosis, and inflammation.

Pain secondary to chemotherapy may be caused by peripheral neuropathy, mucositis, bone necrosis, or herpes zoster. Vincristine, cisplatin, and paclitaxel (Taxol) commonly cause neuropathies. Methotrexate, 5-flurouracil deoxyribonucleoside, and many other drugs can cause mucositis, which usually starts 1 to 2 weeks into therapy. Mechanisms include inflammation and nerve damage.

Pain secondary to procedures or surgery includes acute pain, phantom pain, stump pain, postdural puncture headache, and nerve injury pain (particularly after nephrectomy and thoracotomy). Mechanisms are usually nociceptive or neuropathic.

History of concomitant disease

Concomitant diseases can be responsible for a cancer patient's pain. For example, shingles: often affects cancer patients because of their immunocompromised state. Pain occurs during acute shingles and can become chronic (postherpetic neuralgia). This very debilitating and distressing pain state is extremely difficult to treat. Early and aggressive treatment of the shingles and associated acute pain is important (see Chapter 25, IV, 1, iii).

Pain history

Some pain syndromes are more likely to occur with specific cancers. For example, bone metastases occur commonly with neoplasms of the lung, bronchus, prostate, breast, rectum, and colon. Frequent sites of disease include the long bones, spine, pelvis, femur, and skull. The pain is usually well-localized somatic pain that is often aggravated by movement (incidental pain). The clinician should be aware of the possibility of completed or impending pathologic fracture, as well as the presence of potentially life-threatening hypercalcemia that can accompany widespread bony metastases.

Compression of the spinal cord by epidural or spinal metastases is a medical emergency. If treatment for cord compression is initiated when the patient is ambulatory, neurologic function is usually maintained. On the other hand, only 50% of patients who have paraparesis before treatment regain ambulatory function. Patients who are frankly paraplegic rarely if ever regain motor strength. The following points about the syndrome of spinal cord compression are important:

- Approximately 5% to 10 % of cancer patients develop vertebral body metastases.
- In up to 8% of patients, vertebral metastasis and back pain are the presenting symptoms of cancer.
- Dull, aching, midline back pain presents first in 90% of patients with epidural metastases.
- Symptoms may progress to sharp radicular pains, and neurologic deficits can appear approximately 6 to 7 weeks after initial symptoms.
- Changes in bowel or bladder function, as well as sensory changes, may herald spinal cord compression.
- Treatment includes immediate high-dose steroids, emergent radiation therapy, and occasionally surgical decompression or stabilization.
- Patients exhibiting classic warning symptoms of impending or actual cord compression should be sent to the emergency room immediately.

Table 1 presents a summary of the characteristics of this and other pain syndromes.

Psychological assessment

The diagnosis of cancer, regardless of type or prognosis, often brings with it a series of automatic assumptions and expectations, mostly negative. It is important to clarify these concerns and to help patients obtain help if necessary (e.g., support groups, counseling, family discussion).

Neurologic examination

A neurologic examination often reveals early or previously missed cancer or cancer treatment effects. Small changes in sensation or strength may be a clue to new or extended tumor involvement. One survey demonstrated that over 60% of the cancer patients sent to a pain management center had previously undetected lesions that were picked up in the assessment process.

3. Helpful diagnostic studies

(i) Radiologic

Imaging studies are helpful in filling out the details of the evaluation of a patient with cancer pain. These studies should be acquired and evaluated early in the course of treatment. They provide a baseline for measuring disease progression or regression, and they also provide essential information to the various specialists who become involved in the patient's care. Examples include the following:

Conventional radiology, or plain films are excellent for diagnosis of fracture or other bony abnormalities. Some soft-tissue tumors and visceral pathology can be seen on plain films.

Table 1. Characteristics of pain syndromes in patients with cancer

Area of involvement	Typical cancers involved	Common pain description	Potential pain issues: descriptions and management considerations
Long bones Shoulder Pelvis Hip	Br, C, R, L, B, P L, B, Br C, R, P C, R, P	Sharp, achy, throbbing, pressure	Increased pain with use, localized, may fracture, consider plain film, and ±bone scan
Cervical vertebrae	Br, MM	Sharp	Can radiate to posterior skull. Can cause sensory/motor loss in upper extremity
Chest wall	Br, L, B	Sharp, throbbing, achy, pressure	Localized, may progress to ribs, intercostal nerves, vertebrae, brachial plexus
Abdomen	C, R, P, Pa, Ov, Ut	Crampy	If retroperitoneal, bending or curling may reduce pain. May radiate to groin, shoulder, back
Abdominal carcinomatosis	P, C, R	Crampy, dull, colicky, ache	May see diarrhea, constipation, ascites, nausea, obstruction
Ribs, intercostal nerves	L, B, Br	Burning, shooting, electric shock	Can increase with deep breath or movement, radiate along nerve root, cause sensory loss
Brachial plexus	Br, L, B	Burning, shooting, electrical	Can radiate down arm, cause numbness, hyperalgesia, allodynia. May progress into epidural space
Lumbar plexus	C, R, P	Burning, shooting, electrical, ache, pressure	Can radiate into anterior or posterior thigh and groin. May cause numbness, edema, weakness, paresthesias
Sacral plexus	P, C, R, Gu, Gyn	Burning, shooting, dull, aching	Mainly felt low back midline. May see bowel and bladder dysfunction, impotence, perianal sensory loss

Syndrome	Tumor	Quality	Description
Spinal cord	Br, L, P, B, K, C, R, MM, ST, Bn, GI	Aching, dull, bandlike, tight	Pain in back worse when lying down, coughing, weight bearing. Can be emergency if indicates impending cord compression
Postmastectomy pain syndrome	Br	Burning, tight	Can start 1–3 months after surgery. Worse with motion
Post-thoracotomy pain syndrome	L, B	Ache, burn, constant, electrical	Can have numbness and scar tenderness. Worse with movement. May represent new tumor growth
Painful peripheral neuropathy	(Postchemo) Br, P, L, B, C, R	Tingling, burning	Mild stimuli can be painful. May see loss of reflexes and hand/foot distribution. Pain may resolve as neuropathy resolves
Pain associated with steroid use	Br, P, L, B, C, R	Aching, tenderness, throbbing	Mostly transient, in muscles and joints, may be related to taper. May cause aseptic throbbing, necrosis of femur/humerus. Worse with motion, may require surgery
Upper extremity radiation fibrosis	Br, L, B	Burning	Can start 6 mo to 20 yr after radiation. May feel numbness, tingling, and neurologic deficits. Pain may also mean tumor recurrence
Lower extremity radiation fibrosis	C, R, P	Burning, pulling	Can start 1–30 years after radiation. May feel numbness, tingling, and neurologic deficits. Bone necrosis may occur
Radiation myelopathy		Aching	Can start 5–30 months after radiation treatment. Not reversible. Must rule out impending cord compression

Bn, bone; Br, Breast; B, bronchus; C, colon; Gyn, gynecologic; Gu, genitourinary; GI, gastrointestinal; K, kidney; L, lung; MM, multiple myeloma; Ov, ovarian; P, prostate; R, rectal; ST, soft tissue; Ut, uterus.
Source: *Adapted from McCaffery and Pasero, with permission.*

Computed tomography is excellent for bony abnormalities and metastatic lesions.

Magnetic resonance imaging is excellent for soft-tissue abnormalities, and very useful for analysis of spinal pathology and bony metastatic disease.

Bone scan, using radioactive compound to detect areas of increased bone growth or turnover, is extremely useful for detection of bony metastases.

(ii) Neurophysiologic

See Chapter 7 for a description of these studies.

Electromyography is used to examine muscle activity to detect an abnormality that may demonstrate nerve pathology.

Nerve conduction studies are useful for the detection of neuropathy or other disease of the nervous system. They can help clarify, for example, whether tumor is involved in the plexus.

Quantitative sensory testing includes a variety of noninvasive studies that explore the functioning of sensory nerve pathways. The results can often expose abnormal functioning in specific components of the pain pathway thus, helping to clarify possible mechanisms of pain.

IV. CANCER PAIN MANAGEMENT

1. Primary treatment of malignancy

Primary treatment of malignancies with surgical resection, radiation therapy, or systemic chemotherapy is often a successful treatment for cancer-related pain. However, analgesic medication or other pain treatment added during the primary treatment helps to improve a patient's experience with the cancer treatment, and can be tapered when it is no longer needed. Pain treatment also helps patients to remain compliant with treatment protocols that are difficult. Early intervention helps prevent long-term pain problems such as postherpetic neuralgia and phantom limb pain.

2. Pharmacotherapy

To raise awareness of functional pain management treatment protocols for cancer pain, the World Health Organization (WHO) developed a stepwise treatment algorithm, which was widely disseminated around the world (Fig. 1). This WHO analgesic ladder is composed of three basic steps that can be outlined as follows:

Step 1: Start with nonopioid analgesics for mild pain.

Step 2: Begin using opioids such as hydrocodone or codeine for mild to moderate pain, with or without nonopioid analgesics.

Step 3: Use the more potent opioids such as morphine or hydromorphone (Dilaudid) for moderate to severe pain, with or without nonopioid analgesics.

Other adjuvant medications (see later) can be added at any step of the ladder. This logical guide to cancer pain treatment has proved extremely helpful throughout the world. It has provided a simple algorithm to direct cancer pain therapy using widely available and inexpensive medications.

However, in the United States and other advanced countries, there is now debate about whether the stepladder should be modi-

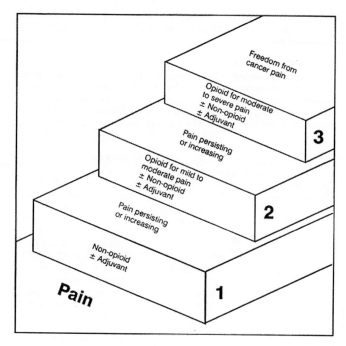

Figure 1. WHO analgesic ladder.

fied. For example, it has been suggested that the concept of "mild" opioids in the second step should be abandoned because these are really "strong" opioids in formulations that have dose limitations because of the addition of acetaminophen or aspirin. Would it actually be preferable to give opioids and nonopioids separately, especially since the advent of more potent and safer nonopioid analgesics? Also, because the safety and tolerability of long-acting opioids is well established, should the use of "mild" opioids in the second step be abandoned in favor of long-acting opioids?

Also, the stepladder concept has been extended by some to include two possible higher-level step interventions. Step 4 would be the use of devices as epidural catheters, implanted opioid pumps, and spinal cord stimulators. A fifth step might include cryotherapy, radio-frequency lesioning, and neurosurgical treatment techniques.

Some practitioners worry that the ladder concept may be misconstrued, resulting in the treatment of all patients with the same protocol despite differences in pain levels and mechanisms of pain. For example, some patients may present with severe pain and need to be treated at a higher step of the ladder rather than the first step. However, it should be clear that the WHO analgesic ladder is meant to act as a guide not a predetermined treatment plan.

The various classes of medications commonly used to treat cancer pain and related symptoms are summarized in Table 2 and discussed next.

(i) Nonopioid analgesics

This group comprises the nonsteroidal anti-inflammatory agents (NSAIDs), acetaminophen, and tramadol. (Tramadol is difficult to classify because it does have mu opioid receptor activity, but this is not its sole analgesic activity, and the drug does not behave like the standard opioids.) Unlike the opioids, these medications do not

Table 2.   Drugs commonly used in the management of cancer pain

Chemical class	Drug	Recommended adult dose
Long-acting opioids	OxyContin	Starting dose 10 mg PO BID, with upward titration as needed
	MS Contin/ Oramorph	Starting dose 15 mg PO BID, with upward titration as needed
	Transdermal fentanyl	Starting dose 25 μg per hour, changed every 72 hours
	Methadone	Starting dose 5 to 10 mg PO every 8 to 12 hours
Short-acting opioids	Oxycodone	5 to 10 mg every 3 to 4 hours prn
	Morphine	10 to 30 mg every 3 to 4 hours prn
	Dilaudid	1 to 3 mg every 4 hours prn
	Hydrocodone	5 to 10 mg every 4 hours prn
Laxatives	Senna	1 to 2 tablets up to BID
	Lactulose	15 to 30 mL up to TID prn
	Oral naloxone	0.8 to 4 mg PO every 4 hours until four doses or bowel movement
Psychostimulants	Dextro-amphetamine	5 to 10 mg every morning, occasionally repeated at 2 P.M.
	Methylphenidate	10 mg titrated up to maximum of 40 mg before midday
Nonsteroidal anti-inflammatory drugs		
Nonspecific	Ibuprofen	400 to 800 mg every 8 hours

Table 2. *Continued*

Chemical class	Drug	Recommended adult dose
	Naproxen	250 to 500 mg every 8 to 12 hours
	Ketorolac	15 mg IV or IM every 6 hours
	Choline magnesium Salicylate	500 to 750 mg every 8 to 12 hours
Selective COX-2 inhibitors	Celecoxib	100 to 200 mg once or twice a day
	Rofecoxib	12.5 to 25 mg once a day
Adjuvant medications		
Tricyclic antidepressants	Amtriptyline, nortriptyline, doxepin	10 to 50 mg nightly
	Desipramine	10 to 50 mg every morning
Anticonvulsants	Gabapentin	300 to 3,600 mg per day in three divided doses
Other analgesics	Tramadol	50 to 100 mg up to every 6 hours as needed

PO, orally; BID, twice daily; TID, three times a day.

cause physiologic dependence, but they all have ceiling effects (in contrast to the opioids). As they are synergistic with opioids, the two types of drugs can be used together in lower doses than either one alone, which may reduce the potential toxicity of each. They are widely prescribed and often provide real benefit.

It is common for liver or kidney function to be impaired in cancer patients, so caution must be used when prescribing these medications (see Chapter 8). This caution extends to the use of combination therapies such as Percocet, Percodan, Vicodin, and Vicoprofen, which contain NSAIDs or acetaminophen. Accidental overdoses of acetaminophen associated with the use of these combination therapies have occurred because of a lack of awareness of their constituents. As widely used as these medications are, they can cause harm.

There are two classes of NSAIDs on the market at this time, the nonselective COX inhibitors (e.g., aspirin, ibuprofen, naproxen sodium), and the cyclooxygenase-2 (COX-2) selective inhibitors (e.g., celecoxib and rofecoxib). The nonselective group causes a higher incidence of side effects related to gastric distress and platelet dysfunction. The COX-2 selective group causes a lower incidence of these problems, but it is not free of them. These newer agents have been available in United States only in the last few years, and they are still being assessed in cancer patients. It will be a few more years before we can evaluate their role, determine their risk, and decide if they should be emphasized in place of traditional therapies such as choline magnesium salicylate (Trilisate).

Ketorolac is the only NSAID that can be given parenterally for analgesia in the United States. This medication is rarely used for chronic pain, but it is useful for the short-term management of acute pain and is as efficacious as morphine for mild to moderate pain. It should be used for only 3 to 5 days. Gastric distress and bleeding are the major potential problems with its use.

Acetaminophen is a useful analgesic and antipyretic, but it should be avoided in patients with impaired liver function because it is potentially hepatotoxic.

Tramadol is useful for mild to moderate pain, especially for patients who do not wish to take opioids. It is occasionally useful for severe pain in combination with other nonopioid analgesics and/or adjuncts in patients who cannot tolerate opioids. It is known to lower seizure thresholds, so it must be used with caution in patients with seizure disorders or brain pathology. Tramadol competes for protein-binding sites and may potentiate the effects of Coumadin.

(ii) Opioids

Opioids are the mainstay of cancer pain treatment and their use can markedly improve the quality of life of these patients. Fears of addiction are unwarranted in cancer patients, and they (and their family and caregivers) should be reassured of this so that fear of addiction does not prevent appropriate opioid use. Another related fear is that death will be hastened at the end of life by using opioids. In fact, the contrary is true, and it has been demonstrated that the lives of terminally ill patients can be prolonged and the quality of their final days improved by opioid analgesia. Caregivers should not hesitate to use appropriate doses of opioids at the end of life, guided by the patient's level of pain and distress.

a) *Choice of opioid*

The WHO has designated morphine the standard for the treatment of cancer-related pain on the basis of its efficacy, its ready availability throughout the world, widespread familiarity with its use, and its low cost. However, multiple opioids exist, both naturally occurring and synthetic, and each has advantages and disadvantages in the clinical care of cancer pain patients. Factors affecting the choice of an opioid agent may include drug potency, half-life, toxicity, and available routes of administration.

b) *Short-acting versus long-acting*

Another consideration in drug choice relates to the pattern and timing of the patient's pain. For example, if a patient's pain is primarily related to specific and infrequent activities, the use of an intermittent short-acting opioid preparation is preferred. Examples include MSIR (morphine sulfate, immediate release), oxycodone, and Dilaudid. If, on the other hand, a patient's pain is constant throughout the day, then long-acting opioid preparations should be emphasized, reserving short-acting opioid medications for intermittent exacerbations of the pain (often referred to as breakthrough pain). Examples of long-acting opioids include MS Contin, OxyContin, and methadone. See Chapter 9 for a full description of these drugs.

Methadone is an excellent analgesic; it is very inexpensive, it has additional benefits in the dorsal horn, and it is completely legal to use for pain provided that the words *For Pain* appear on the prescription. It does, however, tend to accumulate (because of its affinity for protein-binding sites and its slow rate of metabolism), and it may require a downward dose adjustment 5 to 10 days after initiating its use or after a dose increase.

Breakthrough pain is defined as a transitory exacerbation of pain superimposed on a background of otherwise stable pain treated with analgesic. Reported by 50% to 66% of cancer patients, it can be related to movement (e.g., bony metastases), general activity, time of day, other physiologic changes, or possibly disease progression. Whenever possible, moments in which breakthrough pain are likely to occur should be anticipated and treated 30 to 45 minutes ahead of time (e.g., as before taking a shower each morning or changing a dressing).

c) *Route of administration*

Oral administration of opioids is always preferred and usually easily accomplished early in the treatment of cancer-related pain. However, as disease progresses or enters the terminal phase, it may become necessary to use other routes of administration. Patients with face and neck pathology may not be able to swallow, and those with gastrointestinal tract pathology may not be able to reliably absorb oral preparations.

Fentanyl in the form of the Duragesic patch provides a 3-day sustained-release opioid therapy that can be useful for patients with stable pain who have trouble using oral medications or who are active and find regular oral dosing inconvenient. As with any long-acting preparation, breakthrough medication should be provided in addition. There may be problems with this treatment choice in cancer patients. First, doses are not readily titrated (up or down) because of the absorption characteristics of both the patch and the subcutaneous depot (see Chapter 9). Changes (up and down) may take up to 18 hours to be complete. Some patients are sensitive to the adhesives in the patch and develop skin irritations. Some cancer patients become cachectic, losing their subcutaneous body fat, which may alter the absorption rate of the fentanyl. There may be less constipation because the oral route is avoided.

Parenteral opioids can be delivered intramuscularly (IM), intravenously (IV), or subcutaneously (SC). The IM route is irritating, painful, and not needed. SC infusions of opiates are satisfactory if the IV route is not available, although serum levels are not as stable and depend on local perfusion and absorption. The use of the SC route limits the volume of medication that can be delivered (volumes over 10 mL/hr tend to cause local irritation and poor absorption), thereby limiting drug choice (e.g., methadone cannot be concentrated to more than 10 mg/mL; Dilaudid and morphine are available in highly concentrated forms). Many cancer patients have some form of intravenous access in place, and it can be utilized for pain medications.

Patients who are alert and wish to have control over their own analgesia often benefit from using a patient-controlled analgesia (PCA) device. This provides flexibility and can be used for continuous infusion, intermittent injection, or a combination of the two. The patient can carry the device around with in a fanny pack, a small backpack, or a pocket. The most commonly used PCA opioids are morphine and Dilaudid. Other opioids such as fentanyl, methadone, and, rarely, meperidine (Demerol) can be used.

More invasive opioid delivery systems include epidural and intrathecal catheter systems. These treatments often benefit cancer patients who require relatively large doses of systemic opioid, especially when side effects are intolerable, because neuraxial doses are much smaller. Approximately one-tenth the IV dose is needed for epidural delivery and one-hundredth for intrathecal delivery. The addition of a local anesthetic agent such as bupivacaine can provide supplementary analgesia and reduce the amount of opioid needed. Catheters can be used with an external injection port for intermittent injections, with an external infusion pump (PCA is also an option), or with a totally implanted delivery system. Unfortunately, catheter placement is contraindicated in patients with infection or coagulopathy. A backup plan should always be in place because most catheter problems, if they arise, cannot be fixed at home, requiring a trip to the hospital and a delay before treatment can be reinstated.

d) *Side effects*

The opioids have a number of well-recognized and often troublesome side effects including respiratory depression, nausea, slowing of bowel movements, sedation, euphoria, dysphoria, and pruritus. By slowly increasing opioid doses in cancer patients as pain levels increase, most side effects can be avoided, including respiratory depression, which is rarely a problem.

Two side effects of opioids, however, remain potentially significant for cancer patients despite dosing changes: constipation and sedation. Constipation can usually be avoided by placing the patient on a bowel regime consisting of stimulating laxatives [e.g., senna concentrate (Senokot), two tablets, twice daily]. Bulk-forming laxatives do not reverse the problem of slowing of bowel movements and may actually make matters worse.

However effective opioids are in controlling cancer pain, some patients are reluctant to use them because they would rather have pain than feel drowsy and confused. For these patients, feeling alert and interactive (especially with family members) is so important that they reject pain medication. The addition of a stimulant (e.g., dextroamphetamine, methylphenidate) can help relieve these symptoms without compromising analgesia. Alternatively, nonopioid and adjunctive treatments can be maximized to allow for lower opioid doses.

e) *Tolerance*

Some degree of tolerance to opioids is common in cancer patients because these drugs are often used over long periods of time (tolerance is not addiction—see Chapter 9). As tolerance increases, dosage escalations are necessary to achieve the same level of comfort. Very high opioid doses may be reached in an attempt to meet the analgesic requirement, and sometimes these high doses result in toxicity, in particular, myoclonus. It may be beneficial in such cases to try to reduce tolerance and, at the same time, the opioid dosage. This can be attempted in a number of ways:

Opioid rotation: Switching from one opioid to another may be helpful because of partial cross-tolerance between opioids. Switching to methadone may be the best choice because of methadone's additional *N*-methyl-D-aspartate (NMDA) receptor antagonism (see Chapter 9). It is often possible to reduce the equivalent dose of the new opioid to half or one quarter, or, in the case of methadone, even to one tenth. This is our most common response to tolerance.

Resting period off opioids: In the case of mild to moderate cancer pain, it is sometimes possible to discontinue opioid medication altogether for a while, substituting nonopioid analgesics and/or adjuvants. A 1- to 2-week rest from opioids may allow the opioid receptors to reset, thereby reducing or eliminating tolerance.

NMDA antagonists: Tolerance is known to be dependent on NMDA receptor activity. Some clinical studies have shown that the co-administration of NMDA antagonists may reduce opioid tolerance. The NMDA antagonist most often used for this purpose is dextromethorphan, which is now available as an over-the-counter medication.

(iii) Adjuvant analgesics

Whereas the nonopioid analgesics and the opioids just described are used for their primary analgesic effects, there are other drugs that have useful secondary analgesic effects. These are referred to as the adjuvant analgesics and they come from such drug classes as antidepressants, anticonvulsants, antispasmodics, local anesthetics, and corticosteroids. A full description of these drugs can be found in Chapters 10 and 11. In cancer pain patients, these drugs can be used particularly to treat a neuropathic pain component (e.g., gabapentin), to treat pain-associated depression or insomnia (e.g., tricyclic antidepressants), or to shrink a tumor mass that may be causing pain (steroids).

NOTE: Cancer patients are often on complex treatment protocols requiring that they take a number of medications. When possible, the treatment regimen should be kept simple or simplified. Try to choose medications that give more than one benefit at a time. For example, nortriptyline, a tricyclic antidepressant, has been shown to be beneficial in the treatment of neuropathic pain and it has the secondary benefit of augmenting sleep. In the upper dosage range, it can also treat depression.

(iv) Bisphosphonates and calcitonin

Severe bone pain frequently accompanies bone metastases. Although this pain does respond somewhat to opioids and NSAIDs, it is often useful to think in terms of treating the causative pathology. External beam radiation can be extremely helpful, as can systemic radioisotopes (see Chapter 20). Bone pain caused by osteoclast-induced bone resorption by tumor (typically breast metastases) may also be responsive to agents that inhibit bone resorption, such as the bisphosphonates (e.g., pamidronate) and calcitonin. These agents are also used to treat hypercalcemia of malignancy. Although these agents appear to be beneficial in some patients, other patients show no response. Study findings are mixed, and additional studies are warranted to define criteria that may predict clinical efficacy.

3. Anesthetic techniques

Research in pain management has shown that peripheral and central sensitization are involved in most types of clinical pain syndromes. In addition, certain forms of chronic cancer pain may be mediated by the sympathetic nervous system. Both somatic and sympathetic nerves can be blocked in the treatment of cancer pain. It is important when referring to nerve blockade to note whether it is an anesthetic (reversible) or a neurolytic/neuro-destructive (more permanent) block. (For a full description of diagnostic and therapeutic procedures used in pain management see Chapters 12 and 13.)

Perhaps the most rewarding block for cancer patients is the celiac plexus block for the treatment of pain associated with pancreatic cancer and other intra-abdominal malignancies. This is usually a two-stage procedure. After needle placement, a local anesthetic is injected. If the pain is significantly abated, a lytic agent such as alcohol or phenol is injected. The local anesthetic usually wears off after a few hours. The lytic part of the block may not become effective for a couple of days. This block has a pain-relieving efficacy rate of greater than 80% and can be repeated if necessary. Most patients with pancreatic pain get several months of pain relief from this procedure.

4. Neurosurgical techniques

With the advent of implantable devices for neuraxial analgesics, neurosurgical procedures for the management of pain are rarely used. These procedures are indicated in a few select patients and can be complicated by neurologic dysfunction. Examples of these procedures (see also Chapter 14) include the following:

- Peripheral neurectomy
- Anterolateral cordotomy, usually for contralateral somatic pain below the C5 dermatomal level
- Dorsal rhizotomy
- Hypophysectomy, best used for widespread hormonally mediated metastatic cancer (i.e., breast or prostate)

V. CONCLUSION

Cancer pain is almost always multifactorial and variable, making ongoing assessment critical to good care. Careful and regular assessment also helps to ensure the best quality of life for cancer patients. From the initial diagnosis of disease to the final stages of life, pain management techniques can relieve pain in the vast majority of cancer patients. It is often helpful to refer patients to a multidisciplinary pain treatment center when they present with a complex pain picture, preferably before the pain and associated symptoms are out of control.

SELECTED READINGS

1. Ahmedzai S. Pain control in patients with cancer. *Eur J Cancer* 1997;33:555–562.
2. Cutson TM. Management of cancer pain. *Prim Care* 1998;25: 407–420.
3. Du Pen SL, Kharasch ED, Williams A, et al. Chronic epidural bupivacaine-opioid infusion in intractable cancer pain. *Pain* 1992; 49:293–300.
4. Fitzgibbon DR, Galer BS. The efficacy of opioids in cancer pain syndromes. *Pain* 1994;58:429–431.

5. Grond S, Radbruch L, Meuser T, et al. Assessment and treatment of neuropathic cancer pain following WHO guidelines. *Pain* 1999;79:15–20.
6. Levy M. Pharmacologic treatment of cancer pain. *N Engl J Med* 1996;335:1124–1130.
7. Mercadante S. Opioid rotation for cancer pain: rationale and clinical aspects. *Cancer* 1999; 86:1856–1866.
8. Patt RB, ed. *Cancer pain.* Philadelphia: JB Lippincott, 1993.
9. Payne R. Mechanisms and management of bone pain. *Cancer* 1997;80(8 suppl):1608–1613.
10. Portenoy R, et al. Breakthrough pain: Characteristics and impact in patients with cancer pain. *Pain* 1999; 81:129–134.
11. Portenoy R, Portenoy RK, Hagen NA. Breakthrough pain: Definition, prevalence and characteristics. *Pain* 1990;41:273–281.
12. World Health Organization Expert Committee. *Cancer pain relief and palliative care.* Geneva: World Health Organization, 1990.

Control of Pain in Children with Chronic and Terminal Disease

Alyssa A. LeBel and Christine N. Sang

Infants do not cry without some legitimate cause.
—*Omnibonus Fenarius*

I. Presentation of chronic and terminal pain in children
   1. Children with cancer
   2. Children with other chronic and terminal illnesses
II. Developmental issues and the pain system
   1. Maturity of the nervous system
   2. Cognitive development
III. Assessment of pain
   1. General principles
   2. Self-report
   3. Pain behavior and physiologic variables
IV. Pain management
   1. Pharmacologic treatment
   2. Regional anesthesia and analgesia
   3. Other techniques
V. Conclusion

Pain is the overwhelming concern in children with terminal disease. These patients have complex presentations of acute and chronic somatic, visceral and neuropathic pain associated with severe illnesses: cancer, acquired immunodeficiency syndrome (AIDS), cystic fibrosis, congenital heart disease, neuromuscular disease, and neurodegenerative disorders. Treatment and procedure-related pain is prominent and includes such problems as mucositis, pleurisy, pathologic fracture, phantom limb pain, chemotherapy-associated neuropathy, prolonged postdural puncture headache, abdominal pain from intractable vomiting, and radiation dermatitis. As well, the child's sensory experience is accompanied by emotional and behavioral responses modified by parental fears and beliefs, social context, and past experiences.

I. PRESENTATION OF CHRONIC AND TERMINAL PAIN IN CHILDREN

1. Children with cancer

A prospective study assessing the prevalence and etiology of pain in children and young adults with cancer treated by the pediatric branch of the National Cancer Institute over a 6-month period demonstrated that pain was present in 54% of hospitalized patients and 25% of outpatients. The individual frequencies of the various causes of pain differed markedly from those reported in a similar adult series. Tumor-related pain accounted for 34% of the pain experienced by hospitalized children and only 18% of the pain experienced by outpatients. Treatment-related pain was commonly reported in both inpatient and outpatient children. Even in patients with active malignancy, tumor-associated pain accounted for only 46% of the pain experienced, and therapy-related pain accounted for 39%; pain from both causes was reported by 14% of the patients.

Several obvious differences between adult and pediatric malignancies contribute to these reported differences:

1. The spectrum of malignancies seen in children is different from that in adults. The most common malignancies seen in children (acute lymphoblastic leukemia, primary brain tumors, rhabdomyosarcoma, neuroblastoma, and other soft-tissue and bone sarcomas) are rarely seen in adults, whereas carcinoma, the most common adult malignancy, rarely occurs in children.
2. Most pediatric malignancies become widely metastatic and are rapidly fatal once they become refractory to standard therapy. An adult, on the other hand, may survive for many years with advanced disease.
3. Most pediatric cancers are initially managed with aggressive multimodal treatment regimens that combine surgery, radiation therapy, and chemotherapy. These treatments are highly effective in inducing tumor remission, but they also result in considerable morbidity.
4. When conventional therapy is no longer effective, many children continue to receive anticancer treatment (often investigational treatment) until shortly before their death. This approach is designed to test new treatment strategies; however, it inevitably leads to an increase in treatment-related morbidity and pain for children.

2. Children with other chronic and terminal illnesses

In other chronic and terminal illnesses in children, such as AIDS, cystic fibrosis, and congenital heart disease, pediatric patients may have the more "adult" experience of prolonged disability with superimposed acute exacerbations and intervention-related distress.

II. DEVELOPMENTAL ISSUES AND THE PAIN SYSTEM

1. Maturity of the nervous system

Until recently, many clinicians assumed that "neurologic immaturity" prevents very young children from experiencing pain. Current research disputes this contention. Pain transmission pathways develop during fetal life. Nerve tracts in the spinal cord and brainstem begin to myelinate around the gestational age of 22 weeks and are completely myelinated by 28 to 30 months after birth. More specifically, myelination is complete up to the thalamus by 30 weeks' gestation, and the thalamocortical pain connections to the cortex are myelinated by 37 weeks' gestation. Thus, pathways that conduct noxious information from nociceptor to cortex are present in the newborn infant.

The majority of neurotransmitters and neuromodulators are present in the fetus. Calcitonin gene-related peptide (CGRP) and substance P are present at 8 to 10 weeks' gestation, and others such as enkephalin and vasoactive intestinal peptide (VIP) appear 2 to 4 weeks later. Catecholamines are present in late gestation, and, in the human fetus, serotonin has been found at 6 postnatal weeks. Neurotransmitters that enhance the perception of pain are produced earlier in the fetus than are endogenous opioids.

It appears, therefore, that pain processing in the mature fetus and newborn is adequately developed so that the infant may exhibit behavioral and physiologic responses to noxious stimuli and may even have enhanced nociception. The misconception that neonates and infants do not feel pain, combined with a fear of using opioids in very young children, has resulted in gross undertreatment of pain in this population. Recent research has emphasized the importance of providing adequate pain control in newborns and young infants. It is now clear that the undertreatment of pain can have both short- and long-term adverse psychological and pathologic effects on these young patients.

2. Cognitive development

Piagetian theory is often used to describe the developmental levels of understanding pain in school-age children; these levels are listed in Table 1. Speculations about younger children have been extrapolated from that framework. However, recent findings have shown that younger children have a more sophisticated understanding of pain than was previously reported. Children of 18 months of age can express and localize pain. Although younger children may recover more frequently from surgery and report less pain after surgery, they typically have more pain from needle procedures than older children. Young children's limited cognitive development may preclude an understanding of the context of the needle pain, the realization that the pain will be over quickly, and the use of effective cognitive coping strategies.

Coping strategies are influenced by cognitive development. Children as young as 18 months indicate, through structured play sessions, the awareness of ways to eliminate their pain, generally by seeking hugs and kisses and asking for medicine. Children who are 3 to 4 years of age spontaneously use distraction and also report that play makes them feel better. Although they may use this tech-

Table 1. Development sequence of children's understanding of pain

Age	Expression of pain
6–18 mo	Fear of painful situations; use of simple words associated with pain; development of localization of pain
18–24 mo	"Hurt" used to describe pain
24–36 mo	Describes pain and external cause of pain
36–60 mo	Defines intensity of pain; use of descriptive adjectives and emotional terms
5–7 yr	Clear differentiation of levels of pain intensity
7–10 yr	Explanation of why pain hurts
>11 yr	Explanation of the value of pain

Source: Adapted from McGrath PJ, Craig KD. Developmental and psychological factors of children's pain. *Pediatr Clin North Am* 1989;36:823–836.

nique spontaneously, children cannot deliberately distract them-selves or use self-initiated cognitive strategies to decrease pain before the age of about 5 years. Cognitive and behavioral strate-gies, such as relaxation, are generally beyond their capabilities.

Communicating pain is also influenced by cognitive development (see the following section).

III. ASSESSMENT OF PAIN

1. General principles

The assessment of pain in children should be systematic, and it requires reevaluation throughout the course of the illness. Because infants cannot communicate verbally, behavioral and physiologic responses can be used to assess pain in the very young, including facial expression, tachycardia, and stress-related hormones. How-ever, these signs may not be specific to pain. The child's cognitive development and ability to understand pain influence the choice of suitable measurement tools.

In children, pain measurement must take the following into ac-count (taken from McGrath and Craig 1989):

- The child's report of pain is the best indicator of pain.
- Pain that appears to be unexplained by known causes may indicate disease progression or other factors and should be investigated.
- The denial of pain when there is evidence of tissue damage should be investigated.
- Neonates and infants feel pain.
- Developmental factors should be considered before selecting the appropriate measures of pain intensity (this is more diffi-cult younger than 2½ years).

2. Self-report

Children as young as 18 months can indicate their pain and give a location, but it is not possible to obtain a self-report of intensity of pain before about 3 years of age. Children who are 3 years of age can give a gross indication, such as "no pain," "a little pain," and "a lot of pain." Similarly, many children at this age can use concrete measures such as "poker chips" of "pieces of hurt" to convey the in-tensity of their pain. The use of more abstract self-report instru-ments, such as the "smiling faces scale" (see Fig. 1 of Chapter 6), are generally not valid for use in children under 5 years of age.

Simple self-report measures are recommended for children older than 6 years of age. Among the most useful scales for measuring intensity of pain are visual analog scales, either vertical or hori-zontal, and simple numeric scales. For example, "If 0 means no hurt or pain and 10 means the biggest pain you ever have, what is your pain now?" The use of adjectival categorical scales such as "mild," "moderate," "severe," and "excruciating" are not recom-mended for children younger than 13 years of age.

3. Pain behavior and physiologic variables

Behavioral observations should not be used in lieu of self-report. However, behavioral observations are invaluable when self-report is not available—for example, in children younger than 2 years of age or in children without verbal ability as a result of disability or disease. In the presence of noxious stimuli, behavioral pain indicators may arouse suspicion and prompt investigations even in the absence of a verbal report of pain. Behavioral indicators of pain are listed in Table 2.

Neonates and infants feel pain, and neonates are no less sensitive to noxious stimulation than are older children and adults. Therefore, assessment of pain, although more complex than in older children, should be considered essential in the care of neonates and infants. In infants, reliance on facial expression, crying, posture, and physiologic variables such as heart rate, respiratory rate, blood pressure, and palmar sweating are important as potential indicators of pain, and scoring systems, such as the CRIES scale described by Krechel and Bildner (1995) are useful. There are currently no physiologic measures that reliably indicate pain, and pain treatment should never be withheld because of a lack of physiologic evidence alone.

IV. PAIN MANAGEMENT

The administration of analgesics to children with cancer and terminal illness follows the general principles of the WHO analgesic ladder, a stepwise approach to prescribing analgesics depending on the intensity of pain (see Chapter 32).

1. Pharmacologic treatment

Table 3 lists the pediatric dosages for common pain medications.

(i) *Acetaminophen and the nonsteroidal anti-inflammatory drugs*

Acetaminophen has been shown to be safe even for newborns, in whom the immature hepatic metabolism system is protective, with decreased production of toxic metabolites. In children who are unable to take acetaminophen by mouth, the rectal route is the next option. However, in the child with cancer, bacterial seeding is a concern.

Aspirin, salicylates (such as choline magnesium trisalicylate), and several nonsteroidal anti-inflammatory drugs (NSAIDs), including ibuprofen (Motrin) and naproxen (Naprosyn), are used, particularly for children with pain of inflammatory origin. Early experience with the use of the selective cyclooxygenase-2 (COX-2) inhibitors, such as rofecoxib (Vioxx) and celecoxib (Celebrex), is

Table 2.   Behavioral indicators of pain

Crying
Fussing, irritability
Withdrawal from social interaction
Sleep disturbance
Facial grimacing
Guarding
Not easily consoled
Reduction in eating
Reduction in play
Reduction in attention span

Adapted from McGrath PJ. An assessment of children's pain: A review of behavioral, physiological, and direct scaling techniques. *Pain* 1987;31:147–176.

Table 3. Analgesic medications in children

Drug	Dose	Route	Frequency
Acetaminophen	10–15 mg/kg	PO (PR)	q4h
Amitriptyline	0.2–3 mg/kg	PO	every night
Aspirin	10–15 mg/kg	PO	q4h
0.1% Bupivacaine	2–7 mL/hr	Epidural	continuous
Choline magnesium salicylate	10–15 mg/kg	PO	q4h
Codeine	0.5–1 mg/kg	PO	q4h
Fentanyl	0.5–2 µg/kg	IV	q1–2h
2 µg Fentanyl/ 0.1% bupivacaine mix	2–7 mL/hr	Epidural	continuous
Gabapentin	5–45 mg/kg/day	PO	3 divided doses
Ibuprofen	4–10 mg/kg	PO	q6–8h
Morphine	0.01–0.05 mg/kg/hr	IV, SQ	continuous
	0.08–0.1 mg/kg	IV	q2h
	0.1–0.15 mg/kg	IV, IM	q3–4h
	0.2–0.4 mg/kg	PO	q4h
Morphine sustained release	0.3–0.6 mg/kg	PO, PR	q12h
Meperidine	0.8–1.3 mg/kg	IV	q2h
	0.8–1 mg/kg	IV, SQ	q3–4h
Methadone	0.1 mg/kg	IV, PO	q4h × 2, then q6–12h
Naproxen	5–7 mg/kg	PO	q8–12h
Naloxone	0.5–1 µg/kg	IV	q10–15min

Source: Adapted from Berde CB, Ablin A, Glazer J, et al. Report of the Sub-committee on Disease Related Pain in Childhood Cancer. *Pediatrics* 1990; 86:818–825.
PO, orally; PR, rectally; IV, intravenously; IM, intramuscularly; SQ, subcutaneously; q, every.

promising. The use of these medications, however, is limited in the child with thrombocytopenia, coagulopathy, or gastritis.

(ii) *Opioids*

Although there is a history of avoidance of opioids in the treatment of newborns and infants, our current understanding dictates that there are few contraindications to opioid treatment in the very young. Physiologic factors, such as the immaturity of the nervous system, liver, and kidneys, force us to alter the method of providing opioid analgesia but do not preclude the use of these important and effective analgesics.

As in adults, opioid analgesics are the drugs of choice for moderate to severe pain. For infants 3 to 6 months of age, clearance and analgesic effects of morphine, fentanyl, sufentanil, and methadone resemble those for young adults. Six-month-old infants show no more respiratory depression from fentanyl than do adults. All opioids, including morphine, appear to have a wide margin of safety and excellent efficacy for most children older than 6 months with cancer pain and resistant chronic pain.

Premature and term infants show reductions in clearance of most opioids. The sensitivity of newborns to morphine is the result, in part, of kinetic factors, including a smaller volume of distribution, diminished clearance, and, possibly, increased entry through the blood–brain barrier. An increased sensitivity on a pharmacodynamic basis, associated with immaturity of ventilatory responses to hypoxemia and hypercarbia, may also be present.

For nonintubated infants younger than 3 to 6 months, opioids must be used with caution and only with close observation. The dose should be approximately one third to one fourth of that used for children. In contrast to respiratory effects, the cardiovascular depressant effects of opioids in newborns are mild and may actually be beneficial in some situations.

For children with cancer, the oral route is most effective. However, the use of this route may be limited by nausea, mucositis, and difficulty with swallowing pills or elixirs. The principles of opioid therapy (see Chapter 9) apply equally to adults and children. Long-acting preparations are used as the basis of chronic opioid therapy, and short-acting opioids are reserved for breakthrough pain. However, in small children (<20 kg), the use of long-acting preparations is limited by the lack of availability of low-dose preparations. Tramadol (Ultram), a weak opioid agonist (chiefly at the mu receptor) with additional norepinephrine and serotonin reuptake inhibition, is an option for oral analgesia with somewhat fewer side effects than pure opioid agonists. However, the concomitant use of standard opioids, or use in opioid-dependent patients, should be avoided because of unpredictable interactions.

When parenteral administration is required, the intravenous or subcutaneous route can be used. Intramuscular injections should not be used because they are painful and frightening, and children may accept pain in preference to asking for a "shot." In cases of severe pain in a patient whose dose requirement is unknown, 0.05 to 0.1 mg/kg of morphine can be given; the patient is reassessed every 15 minutes, and additional increments of 0.05 mg/kg are administered until relief is obtained. Intermittent bolus injections of morphine can then be provided around the clock. Continuous infusions of morphine may begin at a starting dose of 0.01 to 0.05 mg/kg per hour for children older than 6 months of age. Occasionally, an alternative opioid may be indicated, in which case equianalgesic doses can be substituted for morphine (see Appendix VIII). Patient-controlled analgesia (PCA) is effective for children and adolescents aged 5 years and older (see Chapter 22). However, some children and adolescents may not have the cognitive, emotional, or physical resources to use PCA.

The pharmacologic approach to the management of side effects is similar to that in adults. However, children may have difficulty communicating subjective symptoms that reflect difficulties with pruritus, nausea, and dysphoria. Therefore, if an infant or child becomes restless or irritable with an increased opioid dose, treatment of side effects is suggested empirically, as is a change to an alternative opioid. For acute respiratory depression, as dictated by professional judgment, children may receive naloxone titrated to the desired effect. The initial dose of naloxone in a child is 0.5 to 1.0 μg/kg.

(iii) *Adjuvant medications*

Adjuvant medications such as tricyclic antidepressants and stimulants are beneficial as co-analgesics in children with cancer pain, with dosages extrapolated from the adult dosage by weight (see Chapter 32 and Appendix VIII). In general, the starting dose is low, approximately 0.2 mg/kg of amitriptyline (Elavil), with an increase to approximately 1 to 3 mg/kg per day. A baseline electrocardiogram may be useful in patients who have received other cardiotoxic medications. Neuropathic pain may respond to anticonvulsant or sodium channel blocking agents such as gabapentin (Neurontin), up to 45 mg/kg/day, titrating from every hour of sleep (5 mg/kg) to three times daily, and mexiletine, 2 to 3 mg/kg, two to three times a day. The starting dose for stimulants, such as dexamphetamine and methylphenidate, is 0.05 mg/kg. Corticosteroids are helpful because of their anti-inflammatory, antiemetic, and mood-altering effects.

2. Regional anesthesia and analgesia

Regional blockade techniques have been developed for children of all ages, including newborns, and are generally performed with sedation or light general anesthesia because of patients' fear of needles. Regional, caudal epidural, and lumbar epidural blockade provide excellent analgesia with wide margins of safety. Hemodynamic and respiratory effects of epidural or subarachnoid blockade in infants are mild. The distribution and clearance of bupivacaine and lidocaine following regional blockade in children older than 6 months resemble those in adults. Bupivacaine clearance is mildly delayed in newborns. Epidural and subarachnoid infusions of opioid and local anesthetics have been effectively used in infants and children who have refractory cancer pain, deafferentation pain, and complex regional pain syndrome, type I (CRPS-I). It is important to administer local anesthetic slowly in children, with constant assessment for clinical signs of intravascular effect.

Infants and children may also receive viscous lidocaine for mucosal analgesia. A single mucous dose of lidocaine should not exceed 4 mg/kg; a repeated oral administration of up to 2 mg/kg is generally safe. Infants and young children should receive dilute lidocaine sprays, such as 1% in neonates and 2% in children (compared to the 4% to 10% used in adults). A transdermal 5% lidocaine patch (Lidoderm) applied to dermal areas of localized peripheral neuropathic pain (one to three patches per 12 hours) is currently being studied in children.

3. Other techniques

Children are excellent subjects for hypnosis, relaxation, and biofeedback training, all of which are especially useful for recurrent pain such as headache and for brief painful medical procedures.

Some of these techniques are described in Chapter 22. Children over the age of 7 years generally benefit from such programs, but some behavioral treatment strategies have applied to children as young as 3 to 4 years.

CONCLUSION

Thankfully, chronic pain and serious illness are rare in the pediatric population of the Western world. However, when they occur, their effects are devastating, not only to the children but also to their families and caregivers. Pain treatment in this population is challenging for many reasons, including caregivers' insecurity over pediatric dosing, difficulties in assessing pain, and resistance to opioid use because of misguided fears. It is, however, critically important to give the benefit of adequate analgesia to these vulnerable patients, even though this may require the involvement of experts in developing safe and effective treatment regimens.

SELECTED READINGS

1. Anand KJS, Hickey PR. Pain and its effects in the human neonate and fetus. *N Engl J Med* 1987;317:1321–1329.
2. Berde CB. The treatment of pain in children. In: MR Bond, Charldon JE, Woolf CJ, eds. *Proceedings of the Seventh World Congress on Pain.* New York: Elsevier, 1991:435–440.
3. Berde CB, Ablin A, Glazer J, et al. Report of the Subcommittee on Disease Related Pain in Childhood Cancer. *Pediatrics* 1990; 86:818–825.
4. Beyer JE, Wells N. Assessment of cancer pain in children. In: Patt RB, ed. *Cancer Pain.* Philadelphia: Lippincott, 1993:57–84.
5. Burrows FA, Berde CB. Optimal pain relief in infants and children. *Br Med J* 307:815–816, 1993.
6. Eliott K, Foley KM. Neurologic pain syndromes in patients with cancer. *Neurol Clin* 1989;7:333–360.
7. Ferrell BR. The experience of pediatric cancer pain. Part 1: Impact of pain on the family. *J Pediatr Nurs* 1994;9:368–379.
8. Krechel SW, Bildner J. CRIES: A new neonatal postoperative pain measurement score. Initial testing of validity and reliability. *Paediatr Anaesth* 1995;5:53–61.
9. Leahy S, Hockenberry-Eaton M, Sigler-Price K. Clinical management of pain in children with cancer: Selected approaches and innovative strategies. *Cancer Pract* 1994;2:37–45.
10. McCarthy PJ, Beyer J, Cleeland C, et al. Report of the Subcommittee on Assessment and Methodologic Issues in the Management of Pain in Childhood Cancer. *Pediatrics* 1990;36:814–817.
11. McGrath PJ, Craig KD. Developmental and psychological factors in children's pain. *Pediatr Clin North Am* 1989;36:823–836.
12. Yaster M, Krane EJ, Kaplan RF, et al. *Pediatric pain management and sedation handbook.* St. Louis: Mosby–Year Book, 1997.
13. Zeltzer LK, Altman A, Cohen D, et al. Report of the Subcommittee on the Management of Pain Associated with Procedures in Children with Cancer. *Pediatrics* 1990;86:826–831.

Palliative Medicine

Andrew T. Putnam and J. Andrew Billings

You are outside life, you are above life, you are afflicted with ills the ordinary person does not know, you transcend the normal level and that is what people hold against you, you poison their quietude, you corrode their stability. You feel repeated and fugitive pain, insoluble pain, pain outside thought, pain which is neither the body, nor the mind, but which partakes of both. And I share your ills, I am asking: who should dare to restrict the means that bring us relief?
—*Antonin Artaud*

I. WHAT IS PALLIATIVE CARE?

Palliative care is comprehensive interdisciplinary care that focuses on quality of life for patients with a life-threatening or terminal disease and for their families. Care is comprehensive because it addresses all the sources of suffering, including not only pain and other disagreeable physical symptoms but also emotional, sociocultural, and spiritual distress. A core palliative care team typically consists of a physician, nurse, social worker, and chaplain, who meet regularly to provide coordinated, interdisciplinary care and promote a patient-derived concept of quality of life. Teams may also include a bereavement counselor, a volunteer coordinator, volunteers, a nutritionist, a physical therapist, and so on. The goals of care grow out of an exploration of the patient's notions of living well until death comes—an individualized and changing view of a "good death"—and from a commitment to address all forms of suffering. Palliative medicine is the branch of medicine encompassing the physician's knowledge, attitudes, and skills requisite for practicing on such a palliative care team.

Palliative care should not be confused with the dismissal or abandonment conveyed when physicians say to a dying person, erroneously and perhaps cruelly, "Nothing more can be done." It is not "comfort measures only" but rather an aggressive, active, hopeful team approach to making the best of limited time. Palliative care is based on the hospice philosophy of care, but it is not subject

Supported in part by grants from the Robert Wood Johnson Foundation and the National Cancer Institute.

to regulations that limit hospice care in the United States to persons with a prognosis of 6 months or less who have decided to forego all "aggressive," expensive, and life-prolonging interventions. Indeed, palliative care has a role in the earliest phases of management of a life-threatening or terminal illness. It coexists comfortably with curative or life-prolonging measures, and it aggressively pursues comfort and support through all appropriate means in even the final days of life.

II. WHAT IS A GOOD DEATH?

Although all medical decisions should reflect patient values and goals, nowhere in medicine are individualized notions of good care—and of a good death—more important to recognize than in palliative medicine. Patient wishes for comfort, enjoying family, or being at home may be equally or more important than such common medical goals as prolonging life or trying to cure an illness. Weighing benefits and burdens often leads to a decision to discard a variety of "aggressive" interventions—diagnostic or therapeutic maneuvers that would seem appropriate at most times of life but not when one is dying. Simple measures (e.g., sublingual medication for a patient unable to swallow rather than an intravenous line) are often favored because they are easier to carry out at home, and they do not entail regular nursing attention or much discomfort or expense.

Areas typically addressed in a palliative care plan of care include the following:

Pain and symptom control: Dying patients often experience a bewildering array of disagreeable physical symptoms that interfere with their ability to function and enjoy remaining life. These symptoms include not only pain but also nausea, vomiting, anorexia, dyspnea, weakness, fatigue, and bowel and bladder problems. The fear of unrelieved pain and suffering can be enormously disturbing and make patients wish they were already dead. While studies of what patients and family members want most when they are terminally ill tend to identify primarily nonphysical matters, excellent pain and symptom control are essential substrates that allow good psychosocial and spiritual coping and a good death. Attention to all physical symptoms and meticulous treatment of even minor distress can contribute greatly to the patient's overall well-being.

Sense of control: Control of different aspects of life is very important to many individuals. From the time a terminal illness intrudes into one's existence, more and more of that control is lost. People may feel diminished when they sense they are being treated as merely patients, subject to the orders of doctors and nurses and requiring family for assistance with everyday tasks. An individualized care plan reflecting sensitivity to concerns about control helps patients feel more fully themselves rather than passive victims. For example, using a patient-controlled analgesia (PCA) device rather than relying on nurses or family to bring medications may bolster a patient's sense of active involvement in the care process.

Patient-centered decisionmaking: By current bioethical standards, competent adults can choose which medical treatment to accept. They have the right to refuse any proposed life-sustaining treatment. More important, to identify a plan of care that meets their personal values and goals, patients have the right to be helped to understand all reasonable diagnostic and treatment options and the likely consequences of carrying out such procedures.

Patients need professional help in making choices—shared decision making. If the patient is incapable of making decisions or prefers to delegate them, then a designated proxy or, by default, the closest family member, needs to consider carefully what the patient would want. For an incompetent patient, a process called substituted judgment is requested, asking the proxy to determine what the patient would choose if he or she were able to make a decision. The proxy might be asked, "Has the patient ever said anything about similar diagnostic or treatment options in the past? Would she want to live this way? How did she react to other people's decisions in such situations or their deaths?" Answers to these sorts of questions provide clues to how substituted judgment can be carried out. Importantly, substituted judgment does not require the proxy or family to decide what they think is right or what they want; it asks them simply to express the patient's values so that these values can be applied to decisions made by the healthcare team. Only when no such information about patient preferences is available is the proxy or family asked to help make a decision on behalf of the patient, based on what they think is right. Finally, when no proxy is available, decisions in the best interest of the patient are left to the medical team, sometimes assisted by a patient representative, an ethics consultant, or, occasionally, a court-appointed guardian.

Avoid inappropriate prolongation of dying when life is no longer enjoyable or meaningful: Patients and families fear painful, depersonalized, costly, prolonged dying. Many fear a medical system that uses technology to keep a patient alive but does not know when to stop. Patients and families should be reassured that wishes not to have the dying process prolonged will be honored. At the same time, they should never feel abandoned or that the intensity of support and attention to their comfort will be lessened because they have rejected any management options.

Great importance may be placed on protecting the patient from a bad death. Would it make more sense to let the patient die from a potentially reversible infection or metabolic disorder rather than to rescue him briefly from death but leave him to face great pain and suffering? Is an effective treatment, perhaps involving prolonged hospitalization or invasive procedures, less desirable than a simple, easily handled approach that can be carried out in the home? Neither excess reliance on medical technology nor crude and inflexible dismissal of the most elaborate technical approaches is appropriate.

Identify meaning and purpose in life and find hope for the remaining time: Paradoxically, facing death involves seeking meaning and purpose in life. Patients who recognize their terminal condition regularly ask spiritual questions: "Why me? Did I live a good life? What happens after I die? Will I be remembered?" Exploring these questions, perhaps in the context of religious beliefs, is part of making sense of mortality and facing death. The answers to these questions are also the basis of hopes for the future—not necessarily hopes to live forever, but to live longer or to make the best of whatever time is left. Patients often hope to fulfill key duties or wishes in their remaining time. Putting one's affairs in order or surviving long enough to see a new grandchild or to attend a family wedding may be attainable goals. Reconciliation with loved ones may be important. Patients can be helped by asking about unfinished business: "If you died tonight, what would be left undone?" or "What do you still hope to accomplish?"

Assistance in preparation for death: Dying persons may want assistance with such practical issues as writing a will or making funeral arrangements. Many patients are hesitant to ask about their future or to share their worries about the dying process, although they harbor deep fears (e.g., of a crescendo of intractable pain, or of suffocation). Although clinicians cannot foresee the future, they can reassure patients about providing comfort and nonabandonment, and they often can reassure patients about unnecessary fears (e.g., "You really do not need to worry about suffocation with this kind of cancer.") They can ask, "What are your concerns now? Have you had thoughts about what the future holds? Are you thinking about death? What are your worst fears?"

Psychosocial and spiritual care of the family: Because the patient's medical condition usually takes center stage, professional caregivers may overlook the suffering of family and friends. While the patient is dying, the people standing around the bed may already be grieving, each struggling with his or her own loss. They also benefit from caring and support. Would a chaplain or priest be welcome at the bedside? Would a social worker be able to assist the family in coping better with their grief? How will they manage the financial burden of the illness or the needs of assisting the patient at home? Unhappy memories of a relative's difficult death or the perception that an expected role was not fulfilled can cause suffering long after the patient dies. Family support should extend through the period of intense bereavement.

III. ALTERNATIVES TO AN ACUTE-CARE HOSPITAL

Patients and their families commonly wish to be home for most or all of the course of a terminal illness. In the United States, hospice programs specialize in offering appropriate end-of-life care in the home. Such programs have been shown to provide improved outcomes at lower cost for dying persons in the final 6 months of life. Unfortunately, government-mandated admission requirements, including a likely prognosis of 6 months or less and a rejection of costly, "aggressive" measures, have hindered appropriate referral of patients to hospice. Most patients use such services only in the last few weeks of life. Palliative care programs—well-established features of care throughout the United Kingdom, Australia, and Canada, and currently developing in many academic centers in the United States—are more flexible in serving patients and families earlier in the course of the illness and are willing to entertain all forms of diagnostic and therapeutic interventions that might benefit the patient.

Home care: At home, the patient often finds comfort, privacy, and security. The close involvement of family and friends and the convenience of being home are also appreciated. Most patients express the wish to be cared for and often even to die at home. Home hospice generally provides medications, durable medical equipment, occasional nursing visits, home health aide visits, and 24-hour on-call assistance, while offering support from volunteers, chaplains, social workers and bereavement coordinators. For the majority of the day, families are usually the direct caregivers in the home. When properly arranged, home hospice can be a rewarding experience and a powerful source of satisfaction for the family, leaving them with the feeling that they did everything they could for their loved one.

Institutional care: When the patient's medical condition and comfort requires more attention or skilled care than is available in the home from trained health service providers and the informal assistance of family and friends, institutional sites of care are required. Inpatient hospices and palliative care units provide such an option, typically located in acute-care hospitals, chronic care hospitals, or nursing homes. These units ideally provide not only a homelike atmosphere (with ready access to family, friends, and pets) but also consistent professional assistance. By unburdening the family of difficult patient-care responsibilities that are often physically and psychologically burdensome, these units allow the family to support a loved one in a more comfortable, appropriate manner.

Discharge planning from an acute-care facility is a process, not a single event. Patients and their families, assisted by various health professionals, need to be educated about providing care and the common problems they might encounter. Arrangements for professional help and durable medical equipment need to be completed. Medication management is often tricky, but regimens can frequently be simplified. How can anxiety be lessened and crises averted by educating the patient and family about common problems they might face? How will they obtain assistance when new concerns arise? If the patient is going to die at home, whom does the family call at the time of death?

IV. PAIN MANAGEMENT AT THE END OF LIFE

Pain is frequently a problem at the end of life. Important principles in pain management in this situation include the following:

Opioids are the mainstay of cancer pain treatment. Many terminally ill patients with pain can be successfully managed with opioids alone, without resort to other analgesics or to interventional treatments. Some patients benefit from adjunctive therapies such as NSAIDs, neuropathic pain medications, and various psychotropic medications. A small number with unremitting, poorly controlled pain may benefit from an interventional procedure. The celiac plexus block is simple to perform and helpful for patients with intra-abdominal malignancies, particularly pancreatic cancer. Simplicity is the key in terminally patients, because many home caregivers are nonprofessionals who are easily overwhelmed by fancy treatments. Treatment choices are described in Chapter 32.

Many patients prefer the oral route. The oral route for pain relief generally allows the greatest freedom and comfort for the patient and greatest ease for home management. Long-acting forms are convenient. In general, avoid (a) painful intramuscular injections; (b) intravenous injections that require skilled personnel, regular monitoring, and continuous access; and (c) epidural or intrathecal pumps that often intimidate families and home health nurses, that may fail at home, and that are unacceptable at some post–acute-care facilities.

If a patient loses the ability to swallow pills and liquids, concentrated opioid elixirs can be taken sublingually. Analgesia from sublingual administration of morphine or oxycodone is roughly equivalent to that from oral administration of the same dosage.

Use simple alternatives to the oral route when patients cannot swallow.

1. *Transdermal* administration of medications is commonly used for pain control at the end of life when patients cannot swallow reliably, or earlier in the course of an illness when the oral route is not feasible. The fentanyl patch may provide basal pain control, while the sublingual or rectal route is reserved for as-needed medication. The smallest patch (25 µg/hr) is roughly equivalent to 90 mg of oral morphine over 24 hours. Clinicians should avoid the temptation to start the patch when the patient's opioid requirements are significantly lower than this daily dosage of morphine. Transdermal preparations of other medications, including opioids, are popular in some hospice practices, although little evidence supports their efficacy.

2. The *rectal* route may be useful. A few opioids are available commercially as suppositories, but a pharmacist can often prepare suppositories of a desired medication and dosage. Analgesic levels from rectal administration are generally comparable to that achieved with the same dosage given orally. Limited experience with long-acting opioids suggest that they can be used by the rectal route.

3. *Subcutaneous infusion* should be considered in place of intravenous or intramuscular medication for patients being managed at home, in a subacute care facility, or when intravenous access is problematic. Both intermittent and continuous infusions can be used, generally delivered through an intravenous infusion needle or a specially designed needle placed in the subcutaneous tissue. These needles are easily inserted, and accidental removal poses no hazard of bleeding. Absorption appears roughly equivalent to that achieved with an intravenous infusion, if somewhat delayed. Considerable experience has now accumulated in combining opioids with other agents in subcutaneous infusions. Subcutaneous administration of fluids (hypodermoclysis) can also be considered.

Minimization of tolerance. Many terminal patients take opioids for long periods of time. Tolerance and the need for high dosages may lead to inconvenient regimens with many pills or patches. Toxicity, including sedation or other side effects, particularly myoclonus, is not infrequent. Opioid rotation—switching from one drug to another—may allow for use of lower dosages or occasionally leads to better pain control, either from improved analgesia or from reduced toxicity. Methadone is often chosen when a component of neuropathic pain is suspected. The opioid equivalency found in equianalgesic tables (Appendix VIII) is not appropriate once a patient has developed opioid tolerance because there is incomplete cross-tolerance between the opioids. A dose that is one half to one quarter of the equivalent dose is normally used when a different opioid is started, (one tenth in the case of methadone), with slow upward titration, if necessary, to achieve the desired effect. The principle of opioid rotation and alternative ways to control tolerance are described in Chapter 32 (IV, 2, (ii)).

Appropriate use of opioid infusions. Continuous intravenous opioid infusions are regularly used in inpatient settings to ensure good analgesia, relieve breathlessness, and/or provide sedation in the last few days of life. Common indications include (a) inability to take oral medication (vomiting, dysphagia) or uncertain oral absorption, and (b) a need for fine-tuning or rapid titration of analgesics, including for breakthrough or incidental pain, dyspnea, or even agitation. For patients with severe distress, analgesic effects may need to be monitored every 5 to 15 minutes.

When prescribing continuous opioid infusion for a dying patient, write orders for a generous dose range so that the patient's fluctuating symptoms can be quickly relieved. In addition to the constant infusion, there should be orders for boluses "as necessary" (e.g., morphine sulfate 1 to 8 mg every 15 minutes) to be used whenever the patient complains of severe pain. Providing relief immediately with a bolus injection is preferable to waiting for the effects of an increase in infusion rate. Boluses can be via a PCA pump or by injection, remembering that very ill patients may not have the capacity to control PCA.

Inappropriate fears of hastening death. All health professionals are concerned about causing a patient's death. Unfortunately, some clinicians avoid opioids or prescribe them at ineffective dosages to avoid any hint of hastening death. In reality, opioids prescribed and titrated appropriately for physical distress rarely produce life-threatening toxicity, except perhaps constipation. Dosages required to alleviate severe pain or dyspnea generally are not associated with serious sedation.

In unusual situations, clinicians are faced with a difficult choice in prescribing the right dose of an opioid. Higher opioid dosages that produce good symptom control may cause serious sedation (generally when nonsedating analgesics and psychostimulants have been ineffective), whereas lower opioid dosages allow greater alertness but do not control symptoms well. Patient goals and values should play an important role in deciding the appropriate therapy.

In situations where sedation or, more rarely, respiratory depression is a desirable goal and may conceivably hasten death, clinicians should be familiar with the **principle or rule of double effect,** which makes a distinction between intended effects and foreseeable but unintended effects. This principle, widely accepted by bioethicists and medicolegal experts, indicates that when comfort is the primary goal of medical management, a treatment for achieving comfort is justifiable even if that treatment has the potential for causing serious, predictable, but unintended side effects. The principle of double effect justifies the use of opioids or the upward titration of opioids even if the doses necessary for the patient to be comfortable cause unintended but foreseeable harm to the patient. The importance of keeping a patient comfortable at the end of life is arguably the most important responsibility of the clinician and justifies the risks of medications necessary for that comfort.

In very unusual circumstances, physical or emotional suffering near the end of life is so severe and refractory to usual medications that *"sedation for intractable suffering in the dying patient"* (often called by the misleading term, *terminal sedation*) is necessary. In these situations, continuous infusions of barbiturates (e.g., pentobarbital) or anesthetics (e.g., propofol) may be used alone or added to opioid regimens. Opioid dosages should be continued to ensure adequate pain relief.

V. NON–PAIN-SYMPTOM CONTROL

To convey the complexity and richness of non–pain-symptom control, Table 1 lists a few of the major interventions that are regularly employed by palliative medicine practitioners. Details of evaluation and treatment are included in some of the texts in the Selected Reading list at the end of this chapter. In all cases, consideration of the underlying etiology, diagnostic testing, and potential specific treatments is appropriate, but purely symptomatic approaches make sense for many patients nearing death.

Table 1.   Non–pain-symptom control

Agitation: Haloperidol can help organize the patient's thoughts and reduce agitation, and it generally produces less somnolence than other antipsychotics. Chlorpromazine is favored when sedation is desirable.

Anorexia: Common treatments include megestrol and glucocorticosteroids. Gastroparesis is a common complication of cancer, and can be treated with metoclopramide. Dronabinol is occasionally useful. Patients and families often require intensive counseling that improve nutrition, including total parenteral nutrition, will neither improve well-being nor prolong life, and thus the patient should eat for pleasure.

Anxiety: Benzodiazepines are usually the anxiolytics of choice, but they can lead to confusion, paradoxical agitation, and excess somnolence, especially in the elderly. Hydroxyzine or diphenhydramine can be effective. In more severe or unresponsive anxiety, haloperidol or chlorpromazine is indicated, or a newer "atypical" neuroleptic.

Ascites: Diuretic treatment can be useful early, but monitoring of hydration and mineral balance may be burdensome. Paracentesis provides symptomatic relief but ascites usually recurs quickly. The procedure should be performed as infrequently as tolerated, since repeated paracentesis can deplete serum proteins, thus aggravating the ascites, and also may lead to infection. Indwelling peritoneal catheters are useful for selected patients requiring regular paracenteses.

Asthenia: Treat the underlying cause if possible (e.g., metabolic disturbances, anemia). Patients may be counseled on reducing unnecessary exertion and saving strength for key activities. Otherwise, corticosteroids and psychostimulants may provide some short-term relief.

Cachexia: Treatments focus on anorexia, if present, as described above, but no treatments for progressive wasting due to cancer have proven to increase length of life.

Table 1. Continued

Constipation: Laxatives, such as senna and magnesium salts, are the mainstay of treatment, especially for a patient on opioids. For difficult opioid-induced constipation, oral naloxone is helpful.

Cough: Remove airborne irritants. Nebulized saline may be effective as a mucolytic agent. Opioids are the mainstays of treatment, and anticholinergic agents may assist in reducing respiratory secretions.

Dehydration: This common late-stage consequence of cancer is generally not uncomfortable as long as good mouth care is maintained. Hydrating a patient often causes more distress in the form of excessive edema and increased GI or respiratory secretions.

Depression: This syndrome is common in the course of a terminal illness but is often dismissed inappropriately as a normal response to dying. Conventional SSRI and tricyclic antidepressants are often effective but require considerable time to achieve therapeutic benefit. For most dying persons, a psychostimulant, such as methylphenidate or dextroamphetamine, can alleviate depression within a few days.

Diarrhea: Loperimide or diphenoxylate are the most common symptomatic treatments for patients not receiving opioids.

Dyspepsia: Antacids, H_2-receptor antagonists, proton pump inhibitors, and gastrokinetic agents are the most common treatments. The choice depends on the likely cause and the severity of the discomfort.

Dysphagia: Appropriate treatments for candidiasis or mucositis may be helpful. In patients with head and neck cancers, alternate feeding routes are often appropriate. In some patients dietary manipulation may be sufficient, especially near the end of life.

Dyspnea: This unpleasant subjective feeling of difficulty breathing, not to be confused with tachypnea, is usually associated with anxiety. An open window or a cool breeze from a fan often helps. Opioids are the treatment of choice; treat dyspnea like pain. Benzodiazepines help the symptom by treating the anxiety. Corticosteroids can act as bronchodilators or can alleviate dyspnea due to cancer in the lungs. Studies of nebulized morphine have not indicated convincing benefit. When massive hemoptysis or other catastrophic events lead to severe breathlessness or a sense of suffocation, vigorous use of opioids and benzodiazepines is recommended to ensure prompt, deep sedation.

Hepatic failure/encephalopathy: In a dying patient, dietary protein restriction and oral lactulose are the mainstays of treatment. Oral neomycin may also be helpful and can replace some lactulose when diarrhea from this laxative is troubling.

Hiccups: Common bar remedies, such as quickly swallowing a tablespoon of sugar, are worth trying. Protracted, unresponsive hiccups can often be relieved with chlorpromazine. Gastric irritation is a common cause, and may respond to antacid regimens. Many other agents have been reported as useful, including baclofen and nifedipine.

Insomnia: When this symptom cannot be attributed to physical discomfort, anxiety, depression, drug side effects, or one of the many other causes of a sleep disorder, patients should be counseled on good sleep hygiene and offered a short-acting benzodiazepine.

continued

Table 1.   *Continued*

Malignant small-bowel obstruction: Most patients will not require nasogastric suction and intravenous fluids. Ongoing oral liquids, perhaps supplemented with small amounts of parenteral fluids, and time often lead to resolution. Regardless, prescribe opioids for pain, antispasmodics for cramps, and antiemetics for nausea and vomiting. For symptomatic treatment, octreotide can reduce the amount of GI secretions. A venting gastrostomy may be considered for patient comfort.

Nausea and vomiting: Consider the common causes of the nausea and treat with an appropriate medication. Common causes are gastric stasis (use metoclopramide), chemoreceptor trigger zone (CTZ) stimulation (treated with phenothiazines, haloperidol, or 5-HT$_3$ receptor antagonists), intestinal irritation or vestibular stimulation communicated to the emesis center (use antihistamines, antimuscarinic agents, or treatments for CTZ stimulation), cortical causes (modified by benzodiazepines), or cerebral edema (reduced by corticosteroids and mannitol).

Pressure ulcers: The best treatments are preventive: relieve pressure, avoid friction, and keep the skin dry and clean. Active treatment should be appropriate to the stage of the ulcer. When terminal patients are not bothered by decubiti, difficult and often painful treatment may be forgone.

Pruritus: When the cause cannot be reversed or specific treatments are not available (e.g., cholestyramine for cholestasis), corticosteroids or antihistamines (H$_1$ and possibly H$_2$ blockers) often provide relief.

Putrid wounds: Powdered metronidazole sprinkled over the wound will often control the growth of the anaerobes causing the smell.

Somnolence: Methylphenidate or amphetamines can reduce medication-induced sedation or somnolence due to other causes.

Stomatitis: Preventative treatment is the mainstay. Keep the mouth clean and moist. Topical anesthetics for pain and appropriate treatments for candidiasis or other infections are important.

Xerostomia: Vaseline to the lips and artificial saliva to the mouth provide effective symptom control.

VI. COMMUNICATION WITH PATIENTS AND FAMILIES

Taking care of a patient with a terminal disease can be stressful for us as clinicians. We naturally feel distress when someone is suffering greatly from an incurable disease. Patients whom we particularly like or who are similar to ourselves or to our loved ones can make us particularly uncomfortable, reminding us of our mortality and that of persons close to us. Some clinicians believe that they or the medical system have failed dying patients, and so they feel ashamed or guilty. Others believe that since we cannot cure the illness, there is "nothing more to do." Consequently, clinicians often unconsciously avoid spending time with dying patients or do not talk with them about emotionally charged matters. Yet many terminally ill persons wish to share their concerns about dying and find few people who will really listen. They turn to their physicians for help with their fears and concerns.

Talking with a dying patient is similar to talking with any patient. Confusional states are very common, particularly near the end of life, so the mental status should be assessed carefully. Rather than knowing what to say, communication primarily requires basic listening skills.

Introduce yourself. Patients meet many clinicians in the hospital. They cannot always read nametags or remember names. The clinician should always introduce herself and explain her role in the patient's care.

Sit down for a discussion of any length. Studies show that patients feel the seated clinician has given them more attention and has been present for a longer time. Try to sit at roughly the same eye level as the patient.

Body language conveys interest in what is being said. For example, lean towards the speaker, make good eye contact, and nod to show you are listening.

Physical contact can be positive if the clinician and patient feel comfortable with it. A light touch on the arm or shoulder for emphasis or to comfort the patient or family member can help form an important connection.

Avoid jargon. Use words and expressions that the patient knows. Explain complicated matters in clear, simple language. The clinician is responsible for being sure that the patient understands the substance of the conversation.

Open-ended questions allow patients to tell their stories and to feel that they are being heard. More directed and closed-ended questions are useful for clarification after the patient has laid out a broad response to open-ended questions. Clinicians tend to cut off the patient early and concentrate on topics they consider important, thus missing what the patient wants to convey.

Avoid interruptions and tolerate silence. Asking another question before the patient has finished answering a previous one can give the impression that you are not interested in the answer. Let the patient tell his or her story at his or her own pace. Avoid the normal tendency to fill up silences with your own words or new questions. Tolerating silence can be especially difficult for busy clinicians who generally prefer quick, fact-oriented history-taking. But silence encourages the patient to lead a conversation, and can also convey tolerance of difficult feelings.

Listen for and respond to the affect. Patients quickly learn from their medical interviewers whether feelings are supposed to be part of an interview. History-taking should not be just about "the facts." Acknowledge affect ("So that really upset you" or "I can see how troubling that must have been") and encourage its expression ("How did that make you feel?").

Facilitate conversation and support the patient. Statements of encouragement ("Yes, good, go on" or "Say more") or nonverbal encouragement through head-nodding also help patients feel attended to and encourage them to deepen the conversation.

Encourage the patient to talk with clinicians, family, and friends. Many dying persons do not talk unless encouraged, feeling that others do not wish to listen. Families often have a hard time talking about death and may need gentle encouragement.

Giving permission to both family and patient to discuss the dying process can be among the most important interventions a clinician makes.

VII. THREE KEY QUESTIONS FOR PATIENTS FACING A TERMINAL ILLNESS

1. *If you become temporarily or even permanently unable to make decisions for yourself—perhaps from a stroke or because of medications—whom would you like to make decisions on your behalf?* Does this person know you want him or her to take responsibility? Does he or she accept the role? Have you created a formal healthcare proxy document?

Have you discussed the preferences you would have if various situations arose and if decisions need to be made about using cardiopulmonary resuscitation or artificial ventilation or similar life-sustaining procedures? I strongly advise you to review advanced care planning documents with your proxy and family, and to consider writing out a living will or similar document.

2. *How much information about your illness would you like to have?* Do you want the frank truth or do you prefer to be shielded from distressing information? Would you like to be told everything first or would you prefer that we talk with someone else of your choosing who would decide what to share with you?

3. *Strong pain medicines can sometimes make people sleepy or confused. In general, we can control pain without causing serious mental clouding. However, in some circumstances, pain treatment can interfere with alertness. Given the choice, would you rather have some pain and a clear mind, or would you rather have no pain even if that required enough medicine to make you sleepy or confused?*

VIII. FAMILY MEETINGS

Meetings between family members and health professionals, either with or without the patient, provide an important means for sharing key information, assessing family coping, and providing family support. The communication strategies described earlier are also important when talking with families. Table 2 lists guidelines for breaking bad news.

Begin a meeting by making sure that everyone knows everyone else present. State the general purpose of the meeting such as "to help determine how Mr. Smith would wish to be taken care of now." Next, find out what the family knows by asking them their understanding of the patient's current medical condition and how they think he is doing. Some of the health professionals may then give their own views on how the patient is doing. Consider inviting a nurse or physical therapist who has had close contact with the patient. Clear up any important misconceptions. Ask the family to express their concerns. Listen for questions that have not been fully expressed, and speak about worries that are not being said out loud. If possible, do not ask that any important decisions be made immediately after bad news is delivered.

At the end of the meeting, quickly review the discussion. If some decisions will have to be made soon, make that explicit. Also, plan how to be in contact again. A family spokesperson is helpful for disseminating information in larger families.

Table 2. Guidelines for breaking bad news

1. Choose an appropriate setting: quiet, private, comfortable, no interruptions.
2. Consider involving family or other health professionals, but beware that the family's information needs may differ dramatically from those of the patient.
3. Ask yourself what the patient absolutely needs to know now. Very little new, distressing information can be absorbed in a single meeting. What would be better shared over time as the patient becomes capable of or interested in absorbing more information?
4. Begin by asking what the patient and family already know. Consider reviewing the facts as they have developed up to the present.
5. Ask what they wish to know, including who should be hearing it.
6. Fire a warning shot: "I'm afraid I have some bad news."
7. Keep it very simple and clear. Often a few sentences are quite adequate. Avoid jargon.
8. Encourage questioning. Let the patient's understanding, concerns, and questions guide further discussion.
9. Listen carefully. What sense are they making of the news?
10. Maintain honesty. Avoid both false reassurance and excessive bluntness.
11. Repeat key points.
12. Support the patient and family. Reassure them of your continuing attention to their well-being.
13. To minimize helplessness, try to explain the next steps or offer a realistic plan for making the best of things in this changed situation.
14. Arrange for prompt follow-up that addresses information-sharing and support.

IX. EUTHANASIA AND PHYSICIAN-ASSISTED SUICIDE

"Doctor, I do not want to live anymore. Can you help me?" Physicians usually dread hearing those words, and they often manage to cut off patients from expressing such common sentiments near the end of life. Society and physicians are divided about whether a physician may, in certain circumstances, be the agent of a patient's death. Regardless of how one feels about helping a patient take his own life, clinicians should foster discussions about hastening death and even ask patients directly if they are entertaining such thoughts.

Once the topic is broached, further inquiry is productive. What are the factors that make life intolerable? What sort of relief for physical and emotional suffering might make life bearable or even worthwhile? Is the patient troubled by current treatable pain or symptoms, or perhaps frightened by the possibility of future, accelerating symptoms? Can we treat a depression or a delirium? Is dependency on others intolerable? Are there worries about burdening the family with physical or emotional demands of personal care or its financial implications? Sit with the patient and try to explore the fear and sadness that led to this call for help. How can we maximize the quality of the life that is left to the patient? What does the patient value that may lead to a wish to live? In many instances, psychiatric consultation can be helpful.

Once the clinician explores and responds to these issues, few patients persistently request for death to be hastened. Data from Oregon and the Netherlands, where physician-assisted suicide is legalized, suggest that difficulty tolerating dependency and lack of control is the major reason that patients seek to hasten death. A very small portion (around 0.1% of dying patients) request and are offered assisted suicide and about half of them actually commit suicide.

X. CONCLUSION

In the context of caring for terminally ill patients, pain physicians are called upon to offer expert advice about pain management, possibly but rarely involving interventional therapy. The guidance of the palliative care team is indispensable for formulating reasonable treatment plans that fit the patients' needs as well as those of families and other caregivers, often within the constraints of caring for patients at home, with or without the aid of hospice.

SELECTED READINGS

1. Abrahm JL. *A physician's guide to pain and symptom management in cancer patients.* Baltimore: Johns Hopkins University Press, 2000.
2. Berger A, Portenoy RK, Weissman DE. *Principles and practice of supportive oncology.* Philadelphia: Lippincott-Raven, 1997.
3. Block SD for the ACP-ASIM End-of-Life Care Consensus Panel. Assessing and managing depression in the terminally ill patient. *Ann Intern Med* 2000;132:209–218.
4. Block SD, Billings JA. Patient requests to hasten death: Evaluation and management in terminal care. *Arch Intern Med* 1994; 154:2039–2047.
5. Cassell ES. The nature of suffering and the goals of medicine. *N Engl J Med* 1982;306:639–645.
6. Cassem EH. The person confronting death. In: Nicholi AM Jr. *The new Harvard guide to psychiatry.* Cambridge, MA: Harvard University Press, Belknap Press, 1998:728–758.
7. Doyle D, Hanks GWC, MacDonald N, eds. *Oxford textbook of palliative medicine,* 2nd ed. New York: Oxford University Press, 1998.
8. Farr WC. The use of corticosteroids for symptom management in terminally ill patients. *Am J Hospice Care* 1990;7:41–46.
9. MacDonald N, Boisvert M, Dudgeon D, Hagen N, eds. *Palliative medicine: A case-based manual.* Oxford: Oxford University Press, 1997.
10. Waller A, Caroline NL. *Handbook of palliative care in cancer.* Boston: Butterworth-Heinemann, 2000.
11. Wanzer SH, Federman DD, Adelstein SJ, et al. The physician's responsibility toward hopelessly ill patients: A second look. *N Engl J Med* 1989;320:844–849.
12. Woodruff R. *Palliative medicine: Symptomatic and supportive care for patients with advanced cancer and AIDS,* 3rd ed. Melbourne: Oxford University Press, 1999.

Special Situations

Chronic Opioid Therapy, Drug Abuse, and Addiction

Barth L. Wilsey and Scott M. Fishman

He jests at scars that never felt a wound.
—*Romeo and Juliet, act 2, scene 2, by William Shakespeare (1564–1616)*

Using opioids for chronic nonmalignant pain (CNMP) remains controversial in the midst of growing awareness of the necessity to help patients manage pain. Much of the controversy surrounding the prescribing of these medications is related to addiction. State boards of medical examiners have proposed that the mere exposure of patients to opioids induces psychological dependence. Within the last decade, a national survey of members of these boards revealed a prevalent belief that physicians who prescribe opioids to patients with CNMP for over 6 months should undergo investigation. Probably no factor impedes the appropriate prescribing of controlled substances as much as the periodic disciplining of practitioners mandated by these misconceptions. Attempts by regulatory bodies to prevent addiction produce significant barriers to effective pain management, and clinicians who treat pain are often fearful of their efforts to deliver adequate analgesia.

Beyond regulatory scrutiny, treating pain has its own intrinsic difficulties stemming from pain's subjective nature and the lack of conclusive objective markers. For instance, a history of substance abuse or the manifestation of prescription drug abuse are two areas that require special attention, for they pose special dilemmas for even the most experienced physician. Working together with patients on these and other issues that involve potential problems can be an arduous task. Questions arise daily and specific answers remain elusive. This chapter will explore the rational use of opioids in relation to addiction and monitoring of adherence. We hope to help the clinician develop an approach to opioid use that allows substantial suspicion of potentially adverse effects while suspending judgment and maintaining compassion in the service of effective analgesic intervention.

I. OPIOID USE IN THE ATMOSPHERE
OF REGULATORY OVERSIGHT

States regulate the prescription of controlled substances, and all physicians prescribing these drugs should be familiar with the regulations in their states. The California triplicate prescription law, established in 1939 for controlled substances, is the longest continuously running multiple-copy prescription program in the United States. The rationale for multiple-copy or serialized prescriptions is to provide a means of tracking these medications, thereby reducing their illicit use. Unfortunately, this law has not led to a reduction in illicit drug trafficking. One possible reason for this is that the vast majority of drug abusers [i.e., those meeting the criteria of the Diagnostic and Statistical Manual of Mental Disorders (DSM-III) for the diagnosis of abuse of schedule II drugs] obtain the drugs from sources other than their physician. Regulatory scrutiny seeks to prevent the misuse associated with addiction, but it risks producing suffering by its secondary disincentive for adequate pain management. Probably the most difficult question is what degree and type of regulation actually controls addiction and illicit drug use, and what merely stands in the way of adequate pain treatment.

Concerns over forgery, theft, excessive dosages, regulatory investigation, and addiction are cited as reasons why pharmacists are asked to uphold the "letter of the law" and are often reluctant to fill prescriptions for strong opioids. Prohibiting preferred drug regimens, restricting allotment to a 30-day maximum supply, and allowing only a 3-day emergency supply limits access to medications. It is not surprising that regulations and their ramifications have discouraged the prescribing of schedule II drugs. Recently, there have been proposals that would seek the enactment of electronic data transfer (EDT) of pharmacy information to centralized processing points so that unscrupulous physicians and patients with multiple prescribers can be identified. Individual state governments are also considering modifying their approaches to drug abuse by adopting the revised Uniform Controlled Substances Act and/or establishing state pain initiatives. Taken together, these programs may someday alleviate the need for regulations requiring restriction of pain prescriptions to a specific number of dosage units and/or using multiple-copy prescriptions for controlled substances.

To avoid misinterpretation by regulatory agencies, physicians contemplating long-term opioid therapy for patients with chronic pain may be well advised to follow clear and consistent procedures to limit diversion of medications and drug abuse. At the very least, it is advisable to perform a thorough initial history and physical examination, to maintain a written treatment plan, and to consult as needed with knowledgeable colleagues. Minimum assessment should include substance abuse, social, and psychiatric histories. This is significant because a history of substance abuse or a lifestyle in which drug use is accepted or pervasive might indicate the need for additional measures before and after initiating opioid therapy.

On the physical exam, note the patient's affect and mood, evidence of loss of interest in personal grooming, needle marks, and any signs of intoxication or withdrawal. If any of these signs are detected, proceed with a laboratory evaluation. This examination should include a gamma glutamyl transpeptidase level for evidence of hepatocellular damage, a red cell volume for evaluation of megaloblastic anemia associated with alcoholism, and, in the case of positive signs of intravenous drug use, hepatitis B and C antigen titers and a human immunodeficiency virus (HIV-1) ribonucleic acid level. Because opioids never cure the underlying disorder that causes pain, consultation with a specialist in the area of the patient's pain problem may be necessary when initiating opioid therapy. Although all these steps go a long way toward minimizing the risk of regulatory action for the patient and the clinician, the practitioner must also maintain skills for recognizing and responding to possible prescription drug abuse.

II. PRESCRIPTION DRUG ABUSE

Careful assessment for possible prescription drug abuse is essential to limit a physician's liability with regard to regulatory scrutiny. Many practitioners rely on their impression of the patient's "drug-seeking behavior" to provide them with a rationale to refuse prescribing opioids. But there is controversy about the meaning of "drug-seeking behavior," as the term is often used pejoratively and signs of these behaviors can easily be based on false impressions and lead to false conclusions. Repeated prescription loss, multiple prescribers, and requests for early refills may simply be manifestations of inadequate analgesia by a patient who is attempting self-medication to alleviate pain.

Pseudoaddiction, a related phenomenon first described in patients with cancer, also results in "drug-seeking behavior" when the patient suffers and cannot endure his or her pain any longer. Unlike addiction, this behavior resolves once adequate opioid therapy is prescribed.

The psychiatric and addiction literature has, until recently, been a source of confusion regarding addiction in the patient with chronic pain. To diagnose addictive disease, the DSM-IV Diagnostic Criteria for Substance Dependence required evidence of certain drug-seeking behaviors whereby "important social, occupational, or recreational activities were given up or reduced because of substance use." But classic evidence of compulsive opioid use may be missing in pain patients because opioid medication is being prescribed and thus readily available. In addition, pain patients usually do not have to compromise their lifestyle or run the risk of endangering their lives to obtain the prescribed opioid. Likewise, an illicit lifestyle (i.e., involvement in criminal activity, drug diversion) is generally not seen in patients with chronic pain. The form of addiction seen in the pain patient is different from the type seen in the street addict. The subtle signs of prescription drug abuse (Table 1) are deciphered from multiple observations and encounters.

If there is evidence of emotional distress accompanying prescription drug abuse, visits to a mental health provider should be encouraged to evaluate psychosocial issues. In cases of comorbid addiction and chronic pain requiring opioid therapy, it may be prudent to coordinate care with both a pain and an addiction specialist.

Table 1. Signs of prescription drug abuse

Self-escalation of dosage
Repeated prescription loss with classic excuses
    "The pills fell into the toilet bowl."
    "I left the prescription in the changing room."
    "The airline lost my luggage."
    "The dog ate it."
    "The vial was stolen from my medicine cabinet."
    "The pills were ruined in the laundry."
Multiple prescribers
Frequent telephone calls to the office
Multiple drug intolerances described as "allergies"
Focusing mainly on opioid issues during visits
Visiting office without an appointment

III. DISTINGUISHING BETWEEN PHYSICAL DEPENDENCE, TOLERANCE, AND ADDICTION

Recently it has become possible to decipher the chemical "trigger zones" in which individual drugs of abuse initiate their habit-forming actions. Addiction and physical dependence are believed to be subserved by distinct anatomic areas within the central nervous system. Dissimilar drugs such as heroin, cocaine, nicotine, alcohol, phencyclidine, and cannabis all activate a common reward circuitry in the brain. The area of the rat brain responsible for opioid reward, the ventral tegmental dopaminergic area (mesolimbic pathway) is anatomically distant from the locus coeruleus, a noradrenergic area in the periventricular gray matter thought to have a major role in maintaining physical dependence. Several lines of evidence support the involvement of noradrenergic neurons in the development of withdrawal phenomena. Norepinephrine levels change in the brain following opioid dependence. Furthermore, administration of an alpha-2-agonist, such as clonidine, or a beta-antagonist, such as propranolol, reduces the severity of opioid withdrawal. The disparate anatomic and biochemical bases of addiction and withdrawal complement their differentiation in the clinical setting.

Despite the substantial differences between addiction and the pharmacological states of physical dependence and tolerance, these concepts and labels are frequently misunderstood and used inappropriately. Physical dependence is characterized as a physiologic state in which abrupt cessation of a drug results in a strong counterreaction called withdrawal. Such reactions are common to many drugs such as alcohol, benzodiazepines, and caffeine. Physical dependence also occurs with drugs that have almost no abuse potential such as clonidine.

Opioid withdrawal can result from abrupt cessation of administration of an opioid antagonist. The withdrawal syndrome for opioids is often characterized as a "flulike" condition, with runny nose, chills, yawning, sweating, aching muscles, abdominal cramps, nausea, and diarrhea. It is self-limited, usually lasting 3 to 7 days. To avoid the syndrome, medications can be tapered by 10% to 15% every 48 to 72 hours. Usually, a 2- to 3-week period is necessary for completion of the taper. Occasionally, it is also necessary to add clonidine 0.2 to 0.4 mg per day to ward off particularly bothersome symptoms of withdrawal in selected patients.

The Committee on Pain of the American Society of Addiction Medicine defined *tolerance* as a form of neuroadaptation to the effects of chronically administered opioids (or other medications). Tolerance occurs when exposure to the opioid results in a higher dose requirement to sustain the same level of effect. Although this is a common feature of chronic opioid therapy in animal models, in clinical circumstances it is not commonly a barrier to effective opioid analgesia. Dose escalation can alternatively indicate other problems such as disease progression. Fortunately, tolerance to the nonanalgesic effects of opioids (e.g., sedation, cognitive impairment, decreased motor reflexes) appears to occur more reliably.

Addiction in the context of pain treatment with opioids was defined by this same Committee on Pain of the American Society of Addiction Medicine as being characterized by a persistent pattern of dysfunctional opioid use. This could involve adverse consequences, loss of control over the use of opioids, and/or preoccupation with obtaining opioids despite the presence of adequate analgesia. Addiction implies a psychiatric or behavioral state in which the subject pursues a self-indulgent drug effect despite its damaging impact. Although the term *addiction* may include the signs and symptoms of physical dependence and tolerance, physical dependence and/or tolerance are not synonymous with addiction. In the patient with chronic pain who is chronically taking opioids, physical dependence and tolerance can be anticipated; however, the maladaptive behavior changes associated with addiction do not necessarily follow.

Most authorities seem to agree that the presence of problem behaviors in the patient with chronic pain is tantamount to addiction. The occurrence of dysfunction appears to be a critical component of addiction. It is of major importance to recognize the distinction between the dysfunction that marks addiction and the improved function that marks effective pain management. Thus, addiction and effective pain treatment have diametrically opposite endpoints and are distinguishable.

Addiction to opioid analgesics is estimated to occur in between 3% and 16% of patients with chronic pain. The exact number is difficult to calculate because of unclear terminology and ongoing changes in the nomenclature. Doctor shopping, multiple prescribers, prescription loss, visiting without an appointment, frequent telephone calls to the clinic, self-reported multiple drug intolerances or "allergies," and frequent dose escalations are the common manifestations of addiction in patients with pain. However, there is rarely a single behavior or event that confirms the diagnosis of addiction. Making this diagnosis requires careful consideration of diverse information and firm conclusions cannot always be supported. The diagnosis of addiction can range from crystal clear to murky and elusive. Often, the decision to alter or discontinue opioid therapy is based on partial suspicion of dysfunction and addiction but may be more securely based on the collateral finding of insufficient gains in function from the therapeutic trial of opioids.

IV. DIFFERENTIATING ADDICTION FROM EFFICACY IN OPIOID THERAPY

Restoration of function should be one of the primary treatment goals for the patient with chronic pain (Table 2). Unlike the patient whose level of function is impaired by substance use, the chronic pain patient's level of function may improve with adequate, judicious use of medications, including opioids. Analgesic trials for chronic pain should use function as an objective outcome, and lack of functional gain or malfunction should indicate treatment failure. As in the case of treatment failure in any therapeutic trial, the possibility of toxicity being responsible for the failure must be considered. An increase in function means that the patient's activities of daily living increase or improve in quality as a result of therapy. Specific improvements (e.g., increasing participation in recreation, time spent shopping, socializing with friends and relatives, performing yard work, or doing household chores) should be sought. Return to work is another outcome that might be sought in specific cases.

Improvements in functionality should be made part of the patient's treatment plan and reviewed on each visit after initiating therapy with opioids. Often, it is necessary to gather collateral information from family members or others. Using improvement as the main outcome goal of prescribing opioids allows pain to be de-emphasized and provides a behavior-oriented program to induce desirable outcomes. On the other hand, acknowledging that a patient is not becoming more functional may forgo sanctioned dose escalations and eventually lead to tapering the patient from these medications.

V. HISTORY OF SUBSTANCE ABUSE

Until relatively recently, a history of substance abuse has been considered a virtual contraindication to opioid therapy for CNMP. A recent retrospective review shed light on this issue by reviewing the records of 20 patients with a history of substance abuse treated with chronic opioid therapy for CNMP. Almost half the group developed prescription drug abuse. Individuals who developed abusive behavior (see Table 1) were more likely to have a prior history of opioid abuse or a recent history of polysubstance abuse, whereas patients with either isolated alcohol abuse or a remote history of polysubstance abuse were more likely to manage their medications appropriately. Thus, isolated alcohol abuse and past polysubstance abuse do not appear to be absolute contraindications to opioid therapy for CNMP.

Prescription drug abuse has also been evaluated prospectively by comparing patients with a history of substance abuse to those

Table 2. Desirable functional outcomes

Participating in recreation
Shopping
Socializing with friends and relatives
Performing yardwork
Doing household chores
Returning to work

without. Of all the patients studied, 34% met one criterion, and 27% met three or more of the abuse criteria listed in Table 1. On psychological testing, no differences were identified between those who developed drug abuse and those who did not. Most interestingly, the incidence of previous drug or alcohol abuse did not differ between the abusers and the nonabusers.

Together, these studies point to the feasibility of using chronic opioid therapy in certain patients with a remote history of drug abuse. This seems especially true in the case of patients with a remote history of alcohol abuse. Concurrent monitoring by an addiction specialist or psychiatrist is advisable.

VI. LONG-ACTING VERSUS SHORT-ACTING OPIOIDS

Whether long-acting opioids offer less risk of inducing addiction has not been well studied. However, a preponderance of diverted street opioids are found to be short-acting, and it is logical that with their fast onset and high peak serum levels they are better suited than long-acting opioids for inducing psychoactive nonanalgesic effects. Theoretically, at least, this euphoric effect of short-acting opioid preparations (e.g., oxycodone, hydrocodone, codeine) might foster addiction. The use of long-acting opioids (e.g., sustained release preparations of morphine and oxycodone, transdermal fentanyl, and soon-to-be-available sustained-release preparations of hydromorphone) have been championed because of their gradual onset and the reduced chance that a euphoric effect may be produced. To reduce the incidence of prescription opioid abuse, it can be argued that all patients who are receiving opioids for CNMP should be utilizing long-acting opioids. Whether or not the use of long-acting opioids actually reduces the incidence of prescription drug abuse is not definitely known and awaits validation with clinical trials.

For ongoing intractable pain, short-acting opioids require frequent administration; this undermines attempts to improve functionality by minimizing attention to analgesic dosing. Long-acting opioids maintain steady opioid serum levels (and a steady level of analgesia) with fewer doses, and the need for fewer analgesic interventions helps to remove the focus on pain. Although long-acting opioids may be preferable for CNMP in general, there are a few exceptions. For opioid-naive patients or those with significant pulmonary disease or sleep apnea, short-acting opioids may be the most appropriate agents, at least initially. In addition, since opioid-induced disorientation and confusion is common in patients with underlying cognitive deficits, persons suspected of having these conditions should be started, and possibly maintained, on a short-acting preparation.

Patients who reject long-acting opioids and find acceptable analgesia only with frequent daily dosing of short-acting opioids are not necessarily difficult or addicted. However, this behavior suggests abuse and should prompt close observation and the use of methods to monitor adherence discussed next.

VII. MONITORING ADHERENCE TO AN OPIOID REGIMEN

A wide variety of prescription opioids are available on the street. The markup from pharmacy cost can be considerable (e.g., from $0.25 to $75 per pill). Given the high value placed on diverted drugs, a degree of suspicion for diversion should always be maintained, particularly if there is evidence of abuse. If suspicions appear to be correct, closer control of opioid prescribing is indicated and clearly defined parameters must be maintained. This may include obtaining random urine samples to determine if the patient is taking the prescribed drug or, alternatively, to establish the taking of illicit substances. Recurrent excuses about lost or stolen prescriptions should increase the index of suspicion; this may suggest drug diversion if random urine testing reveals a lack of evidence of medication intake. Requests for specific drugs with a high street value or requests for "name brands" only (e.g., Dilaudid, Percocet) may also indicate a problem, although occasionally the preference my be a conditioned response to a particular drug and due to a placebo effect (see Chapter 3). A high level of suspicion should be balanced by efforts to avoid erroneous assumptions. Valuable information may be gathered from family members, friends, or pharmacists, and if appropriate, prescription requests may be validated by documentation such as police reports of theft or airline tickets for unexpected travel.

Conventional methods of measuring compliance such as tablet counts, diaries, and patient interviews usually overestimate adherence to prescription regimens. Because of the possibility of deception, laboratory testing plays a larger role in the assessment of compliance in the patient suspected of prescription drug abuse. Although opioid levels can be detected in multiple body compartments (serum, urine, hair, and saliva), urine screening is the most commonly used method for routine drug surveillance. The advantages of testing urine include the relative ease of sampling, simpler testing method, lower cost, and longer duration of a positive result compared to that in serum. Unfortunately, routine urine assays provide only qualitative results (i.e., a representative from a specific drug class—such as opioid, benzodiazepine—was or was not present). The routine urine assays is simply a screening method, which needs to be followed by a second confirmatory test. The preliminary test result must be validated when the consequences of a false-positive result are critical, such as in the case of ongoing litigation. The second confirmatory testing is aimed at providing drug identification (e.g., morphine, Dilaudid, codeine) rather than simply identifying that a class of substances is present.

Screening methods for opioids include urine immunoassays and thin layer chromatography. Technically more complex confirmatory tests include high-pressure liquid chromatography and gas chromatography–mass spectrometry.

Results from urine analysis of opioids must be interpreted with knowledge of each laboratory's specific procedures because toxicology laboratories have differing handling practices for screening and confirmatory tests. It is imperative to become knowledgeable about local laboratory policies (e.g., whether they automatically proceed with the confirmatory test or if this must be determined by the physician ordering the test). In addition, a negative screen can rule out only those opioids that are detectable by that particular assay. For example, some assays detect oxycodone and oxymorphone only at very high concentrations. Consequently, patients taking normal dosages of oxycodone may test negative by urine opioid screen and might therefore be suspected of diversion of medication. Other opioids (including buprenorphine, butorphanol, and pentazocine) are not detected by common opioid assays. Urine screening may also produce false-positive results; for example, recent ingestion of poppy seeds can return a positive screen for morphine.

Following ingestion, opioids may be detected in urine for approximately 10 days. However, this is only an estimate that depends on many factors. For example, dehydration and impaired renal function may slow drug clearance, thereby prolonging the duration of a positive urine result. Consumption of large amounts of fluid can accelerate clearance, a tactic sometimes employed by individuals wishing to foil drug screen detection.

VIII. OPIOID AGREEMENTS

Agreements or contracts are often employed in the chronic administration of opioids and are intended to improve adherence to a treatment regimen. The Massachusetts General Hospital Pain Center opioid agreement is presented in Figure 1. In addition to enhancement of adherence or compliance, contracts provide education and informed consent. The "opioid contract" often includes clear descriptions of what constitutes medication use and abuse, terms for random drug screening, consequences of contract violations, and measures for opioid discontinuation should this be required.

The efficacy of opioid contracting is not known. Studies reviewing use of contracts for patients in methadone programs suggest a positive benefit. Mandatory structured contingency contracting systems involving weekly urine toxicology screens have been scrutinized in this population. When the participants continued to use illicit drugs, the initial contingency was to lower their methadone dose. Tapering (detoxification) and discharge followed subsequent violations. Illicit opioid use decreased significantly for subjects utilizing such stringent contracts.

Anecdotal reports have described the implementation of similar formal treatment agreements for patients with pain. Key features included acknowledgement that previous treatment strategies had failed, listing of side effects and the risks of opioid therapy (including the potential for addiction), and the contingencies of treatment including the importance of pain relief coupled to enhanced function via the active participation in other therapies. A survey comparing opioid contracts from major academic centers disclosed substantial consistency among many contracts across the country. The major impetus of contracting was to improve care through distribution of information, facilitating a mutually agreed-upon course, and enhancing compliance with medications. Thus, although there is limited scientific evidence to support successful contracting in the pain population, the practice seems to be widespread.

A model for tracking prescription drug abuse with a log for monitoring contract violations has been championed. In these models, known as "three strikes and you're out," patients are given a maximum of three minor events (e.g., early refills, multiple prescribers, self-escalation of dosage) before they are tapered and discharged from care. Other prescribers are more stringent, tapering and discharging after one or two instances of prescription drug abuse.

MGH Pain Center Agreement on the Use of Chronic Opioids

Dr. _____ has explained to me the risks and benefits of opioid therapy for pain control.

I _____, understand that I must comply with the following rules of the MGH Pain Clinic in receiving opioids.

1. I will use the opioid pain medications only as directed.

2. I will NOT incease my opioid usage, nor abruptly stop my opioid usage, without a pain clinic doctor's permission.

3. I will NOT receive opioid pain medications outside of the MGH Pain Center.

4. I will receive opioids ONLY at scheduled pain clinic visits. I will NOT receive opioid pain medications from the clinic by mail, or over the phone.

5. I will call the pain center if I think I need to schedule a more urgent appointment, or having side-effects or problems from the opioids.

6. I may be asked to submit to drug testing during opioid therapy. If my drug testing results are unsatisfactory, I understand that my doctor may elect to decrease or discontinue my opioid therapy.

7. I will NOT use illegal drugs with my opioid pain medications, sell my pain medications, allow others to use my medications, alter my medication prescriptions, use my medications in unintended ways, or allow my medications to become damaged.

8. I will file a local police report if my opioids are lost or stolen before they are replaced at the pain center (Opioids are controlled substances, US Drug Enforcement Administration).

9. I will notify my doctor if I am considering pregnancy, or become pregnant.

10. I understand that opioids can impair motor skills. Caution is urged when driving and operating heavy equipment.

11. If it is felt that I am not complying with the opioid agreement, my doctor may elect to decrease my opioids, or have addiction services assist in my care.

I understand that my doctor may also choose to discontinue my opioid therapy if he/she believes that my pain is not improving on opioids, my use of opioids is escalating, or I am experiencing unacceptable side-effects.

_____   _____
patient signature   date

_____   _____
physician signature   date

Figure 1.   The Massachusetts General Hospital Pain Center opioid agreement.

Certainly, unlawful activities such as forging prescriptions, selling drugs, or resumption of alcohol or illicit drug intake are considered grounds for such a lower threshold for tapering and discharge.

IX. OPIOID RESPONSIVENESS

There is disagreement about the overall beneficial effect of opioids on the treatment of patients with chronic pain. Many open-label trials have been performed in which opioids have been shown to be effective. Several clinical trials have demonstrated the efficacy of opioids in chronic pain.

However, there are also reports of improvement in pain level when patients are detoxified from opioids. In the latter studies, neither psychological profiles nor a history of substance abuse differentiated the groups that improved after opioid withdrawal. Most patients were said to have experienced an improved sense of well-being with abstinence.

These conflicting outcomes are explicable by assuming that there is a spectrum of patients with chronic pain. Patients who are successfully treated with opioids often experience analgesia without noticeable side effects or functional deterioration. The studies in which patients improved after withdrawal of opioids may have had a selected population referred to them for that purpose—patients who abused their medications, prompting their physicians to refer them for detoxification. It is possible that these patients became dysfunctional while receiving opioids, and only improved after withdrawing from these medications. This supports the practice of using function as a primary determinant of long-term treatment of CNMP with opioids in order to simultaneously gauge analgesic efficacy and addictive side effects.

X. CONCLUSION

Regulations and social stigma that seek to prevent addiction have had a "chilling effect" on opioid prescribing. There are many tools and strategies that can make chronic opioid therapy less risky for clinicians and more efficacious for patients. At the heart of rational chronic opioid therapy is the recognition that function is an important outcome measure, and lack of functional improvement (or dysfunction) is a sign of treatment failure and possible addiction.

SELECTED READINGS

1. Chabal C, Erjavec M, Jacobson L, et al. Prescription opiate abuse in patients with chronic pain: Clinical criteria, incidence, and predictors. *Clin J Pain* 1997;13:150–155.
2. Dunbar S, Katz N. Chronic opioid therapy for nonmalignant pain in patients with a history of substance abuse: Report of 20 cases. *J Pain Symptom Manage* 1996;11:163–171.
3. Fishman SM, Wilsey B, Yang J, et al. Adherence monitoring and drug surveillance in chronic opioid therapy. *J Pain Symptom Manage* 2000;20:293–307.
4. Fishman SM, Bandman TB, Edwards A, Borsook D. The opioid contract in the management of chronic pain. *J Pain Symptom Manage* 1999;18:27–37.
5. Joranson DE, Ryan KM, Gilson AM, Dahl JL. Trends in medical use and abuse of opioid analgesics. *JAMA* 2000;283:1710–1714.
6. Portenoy R. Opioid therapy for chronic nonmalignant pain: A review of the critical issues. *J Pain Symptom Manage* 1996;11:203–217.
7. Wilsey B, Fishman SM. Issues of addiction in opioid therapy. *Prog Anesthesiol* 2000;14:71–83.

Pain and Affective Disorders

Daniel M. Rockers
and Scott M. Fishman

Happiness is not being pained in body or troubled in mind.
—*Thomas Jefferson (1743–1826)*

The majority of patients in chronic pain have comorbid psychiatric conditions, ranging from mild (anxiety, adjustment, depression) to severe (delusional, psychotic). The chronology of these conditions often makes it difficult to determine whether the pain caused the psychiatric diagnosis, the psychiatric condition caused the pain, or they occur simultaneously. Depression and anxiety are known to enhance perceptions of pain and may be a predominating component of some pain syndromes. Some psychiatric conditions may even manifest as pain or pain-like symptoms. For example, it has been suggested that complex regional pain syndrome is a conversion-like disorder (Ochoa, and Verdugo 1995).

Many psychiatric conditions are caused by or are accompanied by neurochemical abnormalities. These abnormalities may significantly affect the pain medications prescribed and may affect the pain condition in a significant manner. For example, serotonin is considered an important factor in pain as well as mood states. The dramatic overlap of the drugs used to treat both pain and psychiatric disorders suggests that common mechanisms may be at work in each. Because of this, comprehensive pain management requires an understanding of basic principles of psychiatric diagnoses and how they might affect or be affected by pain.

I. MOOD DISORDERS

Mood disorders are often split into two general categories: unipolar and bipolar disorders. Unipolar disorders include major depression and dysthymia (a less severe variant of depression). Bipolar disorders include bipolar I (combination of manic and depressive episodes), bipolar II (combination of depressive and hypomanic episodes), and cyclothymia (a less severe variant of bipolar disorder).

1. Major depression

Depression is the psychological issue most frequently associated with chronic pain. Major depression is found in 8% to 50% of patients with chronic pain, and dysthymia may be seen in greater than 75% of patients with chronic pain. At particular risk for major depression are women, those of lower socioeconomic status, those separated or divorced, those with a family history of depression, those with negative stressful events, those not having a confidant, and those living in urban areas.

For a clinical diagnosis of depression, the following are required: (a) at least 2 weeks of either depressed mood or anhedonia (loss of interest) in nearly all activities, and (b) four of the following additional symptoms: changes in appetite or weight, sleep difficulties, changes in psychomotor activity, decreased energy, feelings of worthlessness or guilt, difficulty thinking, and recurrent thoughts of death or suicide. In addition, these symptoms must significantly impair an individual's social, occupational, or other functioning.

It is important to distinguish between depression and other naturally occurring mood states, such as bereavement or normal states of sadness. The use of rapid assessment instruments such as the Beck Depression Inventory or the Hamilton Rating Scale for Depression (HAM-D) augments and documents interview impressions but does not replace them. Use collateral information as well; patients themselves may be poor historians or not recognize when these feelings began to emerge—remember that some of the symptoms include an inability to think, concentrate, or make decisions and may impact the ability to recall. Keep in mind that depression may manifest in a number of various symptom constellations; for example, children may experience depression more in terms of somatic complaints, social withdrawal, or irritability.

Concerns

Suicide risk is greatest for those depressed patients with psychotic functioning, a history of past attempts, family history of completed suicides, or concurrent substance abuse. The astute practitioner is aware when a depressed patient exhibits a loss of impulse control or when cognitive faculties are compromised to the point of poor judgment. When patients are judged to be a significant suicide risk, take standard precautions such as having them sign a written contract to not harm themselves, identify appropriate social support, and help elucidate reasons to continue living. For patients who cannot be left alone, secure family or a friend's assistance, or consider hospitalization. For those in imminent danger of harm to themselves or others, most state laws mandate that any treating clinician, including a pain specialist, must take action to ensure safety as well as formal psychiatric evaluation.

Course and treatment

Symptoms may develop over days or weeks; there may be a prodromal phase characterized by slight anxiety or light depressive symptoms. Duration is variable. An untreated depression typically lasts 6 months or longer, regardless of age at onset. Although the majority of patients experience remission, a significant minority (20% to 30%) continue to have symptoms over a period of 1 to 2 years. In addition, two out of three experience a recurrence.

There are many contemporary models of depression, including cognitive, learned helplessness, reinforcement, biogenic amine, neurophysiologic, and final common pathway. Cognitive or psychological models suggest cognitive and behavioral treatments, whereas biologic models tend to suggest pharmacologic treatments. Beck's characterization of a cognitive triad of depression is that the self is seen in a negative light, the current situation is viewed negatively, and the future is viewed negatively. These cognitions are very common in a chronic tormenting condition such as pain. Seligman's learned helplessness model is that one's responses to the environment are ineffective—that they will not bring relief.

Many patients with chronic pain experience depressive hopelessness about their pain condition, and it is easy to experience negative thoughts or feelings of helplessness when faced with ceaseless pain. The pain seems to (and frequently does) control life. The experience is one of a tormenting, unremitting taskmaster. Psychosocial treatment of unipolar depression consists of behavioral therapy, cognitive-behavioral therapy, or interpersonal therapy. These treatments, discussed in Chapter 15, can result in significant reduction in depressive symptoms and maintain their effect after treatment is terminated. The goal in these treatments is to restructure negative beliefs and enable the patient to experience some sense of self-efficacy in life. Acceptance of the pain condition is often difficult, but it allows movement out of the current depressive state.

Pharmacologic treatment of depression is typically accomplished through antidepressant drugs (see Chapter 11) such as tricyclic antidepressants (TCAs), selective serotonin reuptake inhibitors (SSRIs) (which have recently gained in favor because of their safety and reported efficacy), and a third class called atypical antidepressants. There are documented analgesic effects of TCAs that are independent of the antidepressant effects. To date, the SSRIs have not consistently demonstrated such effects.

2. Dysthymia

When an individual experiences less severe depressive symptoms that persist for a long time (2 years), they may be diagnosed with dysthymia. Many of the symptoms are the same as for depression, but individuals typically experience fewer vegetative symptoms (i.e., sleep difficulties, weight change, psychomotor agitation, or psychomotor retardation). Dysthymia is a risk factor for major depression—75% of those diagnosed with dysthymia go on to develop major depression within 5 years. Women are two to three times more likely to develop dysthymia than men. Lifetime prevalence is approximately 6%.

3. Bipolar disorder

Diagnosis

Bipolar disorder is characterized by a cyclic mood fluctuation between mania and depression. These fluctuations may be predominately manic, with depressive episodes (bipolar I) or depressive episodes may predominate, with hypomanic episodes also occurring (bipolar II). Risk factors for bipolar I include higher socioeconomic status, being separated or divorced, and having a family history of bipolar I. The first episode in men is likely to be manic, whereas the first episode in women is likely to be depressive.

A manic episode is a discrete period in which a number of somatic and cognitive responses are accelerated. Patients in a manic phase experience an elevated, expansive, or irritable mood. They may have an expanded or grandiose sense of themselves or have flights of ideas or racing thoughts. Vegetative or behavioral symptoms include a decreased need for sleep, talkativeness, an increase in goal-directed activity, and excessive involvement in pleasurable activities such as unrestrained buying sprees or sexual indiscretions. Judgment is often impaired. At its extreme, the mania degenerates into psychotic behavior. A depressive episode meets criteria for major depression, as described earlier. The same caveats for depression diagnosis apply to bipolar disorders, and collateral information is a very important aspect, as patients may be poor historians when manic or depressed.

Concerns

Suicide attempts are made by 25% of those with bipolar disorder and 10% to 15% complete suicide—it is a genuine and important concern. There may be abuse or violent behavior when an individual is in a manic episode, as well. Safety may be a paramount concern in fulminant cases. Many drugs common to pain management, such as corticosteroids or antidepressants, can induce mania and must be used with caution.

Course and treatment

Mean age of onset for a manic phase is 20, although some patients begin younger and some have begun as late as 50. Sleep deprivation or abrupt changes in sleep/wake cycles can initiate manic or depressive episodes. The course is chronic; 90% of those with one manic episode go on to have future episodes. The frequency and intensity of episodes tend to decrease as an individual ages. It is important to recognize that manic episodes and depressive episodes can "color" perceptions of pain, so a patient's pain may look like a different animal when the bipolar condition is treated.

A leading conceptualization of bipolar disorder is that it is a disorder of biologic regulation that is activated or maintained by stressful or negative life events. Thus, treatment should be both pharmacologic and psychosocial. As a dysregulation of biology, the primary treatment is pharmacologic. Lithium is the classic agent for treating bipolar disorder, although recently many other agents such as anticonvulsants have gained popularity. Maximize pharmacologic treatments by using medications that target both the pain and the bipolar condition, if possible. For example, membrane stabilizers used for neuropathic pain are often mood stabilizers as well (see Chapter 11).

Psychosocial treatments include psychoeducation, individual psychotherapy, and family therapy. Psychosocial treatments are especially important because bipolar disorder can have devastating effects on an individual's life as well as on family. For example, it is not unusual for an individual to acquire thousands of dollars of debt during a manic phase. Individual psychotherapy helps patients understand their condition better, decrease relapses, and remain adherent to pharmacologic therapies.

Chronic pain patients with comorbid bipolar disorder need appropriate education about both bipolar disorder and chronic pain.

The challenge is to maintain the course through speeding highs and dark immobilizing lows. This includes maintenance of medication for both disorders and the clear overarching knowledge that the current phase will eventually change.

II. ANXIETY DISORDERS

In the spectrum of comorbid pain and affective disorders, anxiety ranks high. For some, the anxiety is a manifestation of the response to the pain, and for others it is a separate entity that can amplify and distort pain and pain perception. There are many disorders with the common characteristic of anxiety. This section includes generalized anxiety disorder (GAD), panic disorders, and post-traumatic stress disorder (PTSD).

1. Generalized anxiety disorder

GAD is considered the "basic" anxiety disorder. It is characterized by excessive anxiety and worry lasting for at least 6 months, often about routine things. The amount of worry and anxiety is out of proportion to the likelihood of the negative consequences occurring, and the individual has much difficulty controlling the worry. Diagnosis requires at least three of the following: restlessness, easy fatigability, difficulty concentrating, irritability, muscle tension, sleep disturbance.

Current models of GAD advocate that there exists a biologic and psychological vulnerability. That, combined with the feeling that situations are outside one's control, leads to neurobiologic changes and excessive self-evaluation. This further fuels the feelings of external control, and the cycle intensifies.

Lifetime prevalence estimates are around 5%. Be aware that some cultures tend to display anxiety in more cognitive symptoms, while others have more somatic symptoms. It is uncommon for GAD to begin after age 20. The course is chronic but tends to worsen in times of stress.

Treatment

Studies of psychological treatments have shown that active treatments are superior to nondirective treatments. The most common successful therapies involve some variant of relaxation therapy combined with cognitive therapy. The task is to bring the stress under the individual's control, which is often done through cognitive restructuring and exposure through graded practice. Several studies have shown cognitive–behavioral therapy superior to benzodiazepine treatment.

Although clinicians typically perceive GAD as a "worry" or an otherwise cognitive disorder, many of the symptom manifestations are somatic. As noted, there may be associated muscle tension, trembling, twitching, muscle aches, soreness, nausea, diarrhea, sweating, headaches, or irritable bowel symptoms. It is possible for an individual to present in the pain clinic with undiagnosed GAD.

2. Panic disorders

Panic attacks are periods of intense fear or discomfort that develop rapidly and reaches a peak within 10 minutes. They are commonly characterized by a number of discrete cognitive or somatic symptoms, such as the following: palpitations, sweating, trembling or shaking, shortness of breath or sensations of smothering, feelings of choking, chest pain, nausea, dizziness, derealization (the surrounding environment seems unreal), depersonalization (the individual feels unreal, but the environment seems real), fear of losing control or "going crazy," fear of dying, paresthesias (numbness or tingling), chills, or sweats.

Panic disorder and its variants (e.g., with agoraphobia, without agoraphobia) are the actual diagnoses that involve panic attacks. To meet criteria for panic disorder, the symptoms should not be attributable to the use of substances such as stimulants or caffeine. For diagnosis, there must be at least one panic attack (at least four of the preceding symptoms, manifesting and peaking within 10 minutes) followed by at least 1 month of persistent concern of having another attack. Patients with this diagnosis usually have other intermittent feelings of anxiety, and they may have a sense of being demoralized. This is because (a) the attacks are often crippling, (b) they may appear to arise of their own accord, and (c) the individual begins to feel little self-efficacy and is unable to get things done.

(i) Course and treatment

Patients usually first experience panic disorder in their teens or early twenties. There may be prodromal symptoms of mild anxiety, or the attack may simply erupt. There is often no way for a patient to predict when the next attack will occur, which leads to anticipatory anxiety. A current leading model of anxiety disorders suggests that an individual has a biologic predisposition, and when placed in a stressful situation involving loss of control, anxiety and panic occur. Lifetime prevalence figures indicate that panic disorder with or without agoraphobia occurs in about 3.5% of the population.

Between 50% and 65% of individuals with panic disorder also have a diagnosis of major depression. Some individuals may treat their anticipatory anxiety, panic, or depression with other substances such as alcohol, thereby developing a comorbid substance abuse disorder. The physician should be careful not to unwittingly treat panic symptoms with analgesics.

Treatment involves educating the patient about the nature of anxiety and panic, coping skills acquisition, and in vivo exposure. Patients are often taught relaxation and diaphragmatic breathing techniques to help combat physiologic symptoms. The course fluctuates and some symptoms may persist even after treatment. The main goals are to decrease subjective anxiety while improving objective function and the ability to travel.

It is not uncommon to see diagnosable panic disorder in the pain patient. Chronic pain often shares with panic disorder a component of apparent uncontrollability. Many patients begin to experience panic or extreme anxiety about impending pain. As the pain begins to emerge, they fear it as an entity in itself; the pain is often experienced as a tormenting aspect with its own volition. Patients with pain should also understand that stimulants may exacerbate both pain and anxiety and so should be utilized with caution.

3. Post-traumatic stress disorder

When subjected to extreme traumatic stressors, individuals may develop PTSD, a characteristic disorder that involves ongoing residual anxiety. Diagnostic criteria require that the traumatic stressor be extreme, and the individual's response involves intense fear, helplessness, or horror. Examples of extreme traumas include involvement in hostage situations, terrorist attacks, torture, war combat, physical or sexual abuse, and automobile accidents. The residual anxiety manifests in re-experiencing events related to the stressor, avoidance of reminders of events, and persistent increased autonomic system arousal. The hyperarousal may show up in sleep disturbance, irritability, hypervigilance, or an exaggerated startle response. Avoidance is accomplished by avoiding thoughts of, or feelings about, the event. It may also show up as amnesia for a part of the event. Diagnosed individuals may also have a restricted range of affect and feel detached from others.

Associated with PTSD is an increase in somatic complaints such as pain, or increased autonomic nervous system arousal. On the pain service, it is not unusual to have war veterans and assault or abuse victims as patients. Lifetime prevalence of PTSD is estimated at 8% of the adult population. About half of those diagnosed with PTSD experience complete recovery in 3 months.

Treatment

Accepted and empirically supported treatment for PTSD is exposure therapy plus anxiety management techniques. Exposure therapy usually consists of imagery as well as exposure-type treatments (*in vivo*), whereas anxiety management techniques include relaxation, breathing retraining, trauma education, guided self-dialogue, cognitive restructuring, and anger management. Pharmacologic therapies may involve treatments with antidepressants as well as other psychiatric drugs.

III. CONCLUSION

As there is an affective component to all pain, there is a common comorbidity of affective disorders and chronic pain. In addition, a chronic stressor such as pain taxes the affective regions of the psyche, which can manifest as an affective disorder. Conversely, an affective disorder can present as a pain disorder. Regardless of primacy, attempts to identify and treat affective disorders should occur simultaneously with identification and treatment of somatic pain disorders.

SELECTED READINGS

1. American Psychiatric Association. *Diagnostic and statistical manual of mental disorders,* 4th ed, text revision. Washington, DC: American Psychiatric Association, 2000.
2. Maxmen JS, Ward NG. *Essential psychopathology and its treatment,* 2nd ed. New York: WW Norton, 1995.
3. Nathan PE, Gorman JM. *A guide to treatments that work.* New York: Oxford University Press, 1998.
4. Ochoa JL, Verdugo RJ. Reflex sympathetic dystrophy. A common clinical avenue for somatoform expression. *Neural Clin* 1995; 13:351–363.

Emergencies in the Pain Clinic

Asteghik Hacobian and Milan Stojanovic

Though an arrow is always approaching its target it never quite gets there, and Saint Sebastian died of fright.
—*Tom Stoppard (1937–)*

I. Procedure-related emergencies
    1. Vasovagal syncope
    2. Systemic local anesthetic toxicity
    3. Complications of epidural and intrathecal procedures
    4. Hypotension
    5. Hypertension
    6. Pneumothorax
II. Medication-related emergencies
    1. Anaphylaxis
    2. Opioid overdose
    3. Opioid withdrawal
    4. Steroid overdose and adrenal insufficiency
III. Conclusion

The use of fluoroscopic guidance and contrast injection markedly decreases the complication rate of pain procedures. However, complications do occur and can have disastrous consequences if the clinic is not prepared to deal with these emergencies. This chapter reviews some of the emergency problems encountered in the pain clinic. Every pain management clinic specializing in interventional pain management procedures should be equipped with emergency equipment, including an airway cart, oxygen tanks, resuscitation equipment, and emergency medication, and all providers in the pain clinic should be familiar with their use and their location. Personnel trained in resuscitation should always be present in the clinic when patients are undergoing or recovering from procedures. Finally, a safety officer should be identified and given the responsibility for a regular check and documenting of the emergency equipment.

I. PROCEDURE-RELATED EMERGENCIES

1. Vasovagal syncope

Syncope is one of the most common reactions that occur in a pain clinic. Patients commonly fear needles and procedures. The best prevention is reassurance. If there is any suspicion that the patient may be very anxious, insertion of an intravenous (IV) line, with the consent of the patient, is recommended. Sometimes, an anxiolytic agent prior to the procedure is helpful, although anxiolytic agents may provide pain relief and diminish the diagnostic value of blocks. Unfortunately, vasovagal syncope can occur even during minor procedures.

Vasovagal syncope is always associated with brachycardia. During any kind of procedure, standard monitors, including non-invasive blood pressure cuff, pulse oximetry, and, in most cases, three-lead electrocardiography (ECG), should be used and patient baseline values documented.

To avoid possible patient injury from a fall due to loss of consciousness, avoid performing procedures in the standing and sitting position.

Symptoms and Signs

Pre-syncopal symptoms and signs include nausea, epigastric distress, perspiration, lightheadedness, confusion, tachycardia, and pupillary dilatation. Syncopal signs include loss of consciousness, generalized muscle weakness, loss of postural tone, pallor or cyanosis, and brief tonicoclonic seizure-like activity. Hypotension can also occur.

Treatment

In the event of any complaint from the patient, including feeling faint, nauseated, or sweating, do the following:

1. Place the patient in the Trendelenburg position.
2. Administer oxygen, evaluate and protect the airway, and support ventilation, depending on the severity of the case.
3. Monitor oxygenation, ventilation, and vital signs.
4. Establish IV access (if not present), and administer atropine 0.4 to 1 mg IV for a heart rate of less than 45 beats per minute or for a rapidly decreasing heart rate.
5. Apply standard monitors and evaluate an ECG tracing for other possible causes of bradycardia (e.g., junctional rhythm).
6. Continue to monitor, and keep patient supine.
7. Make sure all the vital signs are stable and the patient is stable before being discharged home.

2. Systemic local anesthetic toxicity

Systemic local anesthetic toxicity can manifest as minor symptoms such as tinnitus, a metallic taste in the mouth, numbness of the lips, lightheadedness, or visual disturbance, or it may progress to loss of consciousness, seizure activity, and decrease in myocardial contractility.

Toxicity, which depends on the dose of local anesthetic being absorbed into the systemic circulation, may result from an accidental intra-arterial injection, an overlarge bolus, a high infusion rate, or too-frequent boluses. Toxicity can present either with central nervous system (CNS) manifestations or with cardiovascular symptoms, or with both. Cardiotoxic effects of local anesthetic include a depression of myocardial contractility and refractory arrhythmias. The CNS symptoms can progress to loss of consciousness, generalized seizure activity, or even coma.

Treatment

1. The airway should be protected.
2. Oxygen should be administered by mask or bag with the first sign of toxicity; in mild cases, this may be the only treatment needed.

3. Airway, breathing, and circulation should be assessed and standard monitoring should be applied.
4. If seizure activity interferes with ventilation, or if it is prolonged, give midazolam 1 to 2 mg IV or diazepam 5 to 10 mg IV.
5. If the patient's airway is compromised, give thiopental 50 to 200 mg and intubate the trachea; succinylcholine 1.5 mg/kg IV may be given to facilitate intubation; muscle relaxation abolishes muscle activity but the neuronal seizure activity continues.

Treatment of cardiovascular toxicity

1. Airway, breathing, and circulation should be supported according to the acute cardiac life support (ACLS) protocol; oxygen should be administered and emergency assistance should be called.
2. Ventricular tachycardia should subside over time as a result of drug distribution; adequate circulatory support, including lidocaine 100 mg IV, should be provided in the meantime.
3. Bupivacaine-induced ventricular arrhythmia may be more responsive to bretylium 5 to 10 mg/kg IV every 15 to 20 minutes, to a maximum of 30 mg/kg, followed by lidocaine; prolonged cardiopulmonary resuscitation (CPR) or cardiopulmonary bypass may be required until the cardiotoxic effects subside.

3. Complications of epidural and intrathecal procedures

(i) Epidural hematoma

Epidural hematomas are extremely rare if coagulation parameters are normal. However, in a patient with rapid onset of neurologic deficit and severe back pain, the diagnosis it should be entertained. Sometimes the only symptom is severe pain in the back. The treatment includes immediate magnetic resonance imaging (MRI), steroids, and emergent surgical consult for decompression and laminectomy to evacuate hematoma.

(ii) Epidural abscess

Epidural abscess is a rare complication but it should be considered a possibility in a patient with severe back pain, local back tenderness, fever, and leukocytosis with or without neurologic deficit after an epidural or intrathecal injection or catheter placement. An immediate MRI, preferably with gadolinium enhancement, emergency surgical consult for possible decompression laminectomy, and IV antibiotics will be needed.

(iii) High spinal anesthetics

With fluoroscopy and contrast dye, the incidence of this complication is rare. However, it may still occur as a result of an unintentional subarachnoid injection of local anesthetic during an epidural, a celiac plexus block, a lumbar sympathetic block, a stellate ganglion block, or an occipital nerve block.

Symptoms and signs

These may include nausea, vomiting, hypotension, bradycardia, dyspnea, and high sensory level, and they can progress to apnea and unresponsiveness.

Treatment
1. Establish an adequate airway, administer oxygen, assess sensory and motor level.
2. Support ventilation if muscles of respiration are affected; if the airway cannot be protected, endotracheal intubation may be necessary.
3. Support blood pressure and heart rate until the local anesthetic wears off.

(iv) Accidental overdose via neuraxial pump

Intrathecal or epidural pumps implanted on the anterior abdominal wall are a common mode of continuous delivery of opioids into the intrathecal or epidural space. Some of these pumps have two ports, the catheter access port and the drug reservoir port. In case of accidental overdose of morphine (the most common opioid used for intrathecal pump delivery), the patient may experience respiratory depression with or without CNS depression.

In the event of possible morphine overdose, do the following:

1. Establish airway access, breathing, and circulation.
2. Intubation may be necessary.
3. Give naloxone 0.04 to 2 mg IV.
4. Withdraw 30 to 40 mL of CSF through the catheter access port to decrease the concentration of morphine in the CSF.
5. Stop the pump infusion.
6. Monitor the patient's vital signs.
7. Repeat the dosage of naloxone every 2 to 3 minutes. Since the half-life of naloxone is considerably shorter than that of intrathecal or epidural morphine, repeated administration or continuous infusion may be necessary.

In severe cases, intrathecal naloxone may be indicated.

4. Hypotension

Acute systemic causes of hypotension include vasovagal syncope, allergic reaction, myocardial ischemia, adrenal insufficiency, and pulmonary embolism. Patients with a preexisting condition such as hypothyroidism, cardiac dysrhythmias, left ventricular dysfunction, or sepsis are predisposed to hypotension. Iatrogenic causes include the following:

- Intrathecal or subdural injection of local anesthetic
- High neuraxial block
- Celiac plexus block (neurolytic or with local anesthetic) without adequate pre-block hydration
- Lumbar sympathetic block
- Tension pneumothorax
- Rapid release of tourniquet during Bier block, causing release of drugs such as labetalol, guanethidine, and bretylium
- IV phentolamine

Symptoms and signs include pallor, lightheadedness, vomiting, tachycardia, tachypnea, pupillary dilation, confusion, and decreased muscle tone.

Treatment
1. Give supplemental oxygen.
2. Put the patient in the Trendelenburg position or elevate lower extremities.

3. Immediately establish IV access (if not already present).
4. Give IV fluid (boluses of lactated Ringer's solution) if not contraindicated.
5. Monitor the patient's vital signs, ECG tracing, oxygen saturation, and verbal communication.
6. Administer if necessary; administer ephedrine 10 mg every 5 to 10 minutes, or phenylephrine in a bolus of 50 to 100 μg IV, or start a phenylephrine infusion of 100 μg/min and maintain at 40 to 60 μg/min.
7. Depending on the cause, the patient may need to be transferred to an inpatient cardiology unit.

5. Hypertension

Hypertension could be the result of acute pain or an exacerbation of chronic pain. Anxiety, preexisting disease, and essential hypertension are other common causes. Rebound hypertension after a sudden discontinuation of alpha-blockers (e.g., clonidine) or beta-blockers (e.g., propranolol) can cause hypertension, and both these drugs are occasionally used as pain treatments. Drug interactions can cause hypertension (e.g., monoamine oxidase inhibitor interactions with meperidine, tricyclic analgesics, and ephedrine). Accidental vascular injection of vasopressors (e.g., epinephrine in local anesthetic solutions) or absorption of vasopressors from topical solutions (e.g., cocaine) can also induce hypertension. Other causes include hypoxia and hypercarbia.

Treatment

1. Give supplemental oxygen.
2. Ensure adequate ventilation.
3. Treat underlying cause.
4. Cancel planned procedures for diastolic blood pressure greater than 110
5. Treat with nifedipine 10 mg sublingual or labetolol 2.5–5 mg IV every 5 to 10 minutes
6. Depending on the severity, the patient may need to be transferred to an inpatient facility or be followed up with primary care physician

6. Pneumothorax

This may occur as a complication of intercostal nerve block, stellate ganglion block, celiac plexus block, intrascalene nerve block, supraclavicular nerve block, and trigger point injections in the chest and anterior abdominal wall. The incidence of pneumothorax with intercostal nerve blocks is actually rare in experienced hands. Pneumothorax has been reported with transforaminal selective thoracic epidural blocks. However, again in experienced hands, the incidence is very rare.

Symptoms and signs

A small pneumothorax usually causes no symptoms, although chest pain and dyspnea may occur. Depending on the severity of the pneumothorax, signs on physical examination include tachypnea, asymmetrical expansion of the chest on the affected side, deviation of the trachea away from the pneumothorax, hyper-resonance to percussion, and diminished breath sounds on the affected side.

Despite these very specific diagnostic features, pneumothorax is actually very difficult to diagnose with a stethoscope, and a chest radiograph (taken in the upright position and at the end of maximal expiration) is often needed to confirm the diagnosis. Tension pneumothorax manifests as decreased breath sounds, wheezing, hypotension, and circulatory collapse.

Treatment

1. If the situation is life-threatening and cardiovascular collapse is imminent, a large-bore 14-gauge catheter should be inserted in the midclavicular line in the second intercostal space just above the rib. To prevent air from entering the intrapleural space, a syringe should be placed over the catheter before insertion, followed by insertion of a chest tube with placement of waterseal and suction.
2. Airway breathing and circulation should be supported and standard monitoring used. Oxygen should be administered.
3. A small pneumothorax occupying less than 25% of the hemithorax in asymptomatic individuals can be treated on an outpatient basis without removing the area. Serial chest radiographs to exclude nonexpansion should be obtained. The pneumothorax should spontaneously resolve in 7 to 10 days.

II. MEDICATION-RELATED EMERGENCIES

1. Anaphylaxis

Signs and symptoms

Anaphylaxis presents with cardiovascular manifestations including hypotension, tachycardia, and dysrhythmias; pulmonary manifestations including bronchospasm, dyspnea, pulmonary edema, laryngeal edema, hypoxemia, and cough; and dermatologic manifestations including urticaria, facial edema, and pruritus. In its mildest form, there may simply be urticaria; in its worse form, there is complete cardiovascular collapse usually with severe bronchospasm.

Treatment

1. Stop the administration of the drug.
2. Administer oxygen.
3. Assess the airway and ventilation.
4. Intubate the patient if necessary.
5. Administer epinephrine, the absolute treatment of choice, 50 to 100 µg IV; for persistent bronchospasm, give 0.5 µg/min IV, then titrate against the patient's response.
6. Administer IV fluids.
7. H_1 blocker (Benadryl 50 to 100 mg IV), H_2 blocker (cimetidine 50 to 300 mg IV) may be used.
8. Steroids, hydrocortisone 5 mg/kg IV or dexamethasone 1 to 5 mg/kg IV may be used.

In the event of circulatory collapse

1. Perform endotracheal intubation.
2. Administer epinephrine 1 to 5 mg IV, or via endotracheal tube if no IV access; titrate to response.
3. For cardiac arrest, follow ACLS protocol.

2. Opioid overdose

Symptoms and signs

Symptoms and signs include miosis, sedation, hypoventilation, apnea, and coma.

Treatment

First establish an airway, support ventilation and give supplemental oxygen. Give naloxone 0.04 to 0.4 mg IV. If the patient has been on chronic opioid therapy, it is wise to administer no more than 0.04 mg every 2 minutes, which will help avoid inducing a withdrawal syndrome. Because naloxone has a half-life of 1 hour, monitoring and repeated injections might be needed. Close monitoring and a naloxone infusion (0.5 to 1.2 mg/hr) might be required, depending on the half-life and mode of administration of the opioid being reversed. Because vomiting is associated with naloxone administration, it is safer to keep the patient in the lateral decubitus position to prevent aspiration (endotracheal intubation should also be considered).

When treating a patient on chronic opioid therapy, in whom opioid overdose is causing sedation but not significant hypoventilation, observation for a few hours is the best therapeutic approach.

3. Opioid withdrawal

Opioid withdrawal rarely causes life-threatening symptoms. The exception is the patient on chronic opioids who receives naloxone.

Signs and symptoms

- Hypertension, nausea, vomiting
- Aspiration pneumonia (a possible complication)
- Fever, chills, runny nose, yawning, sweating, irritability, diarrhea, abdominal cramping, and muscle aches

Treatment

Resumption of opioid treatment, in general, is the best way to stop the withdrawal syndrome. Generally, 25% to 40% of the previous dose aborts most of the symptoms. In severe cases, clonidine 0.2 to 0.4 mg/day can be added. For symptomatic treatment of nausea, use prochlorperazine, metoclopramide, or droperidol. For treatment of muscle aches, use nonsteroidal anti-inflammatory drugs and for (see Appendix VIII for prescribing information). It may be helpful to admit the patient to an addiction service unit and taper the drug with monitoring.

For a full description of opioid tolerance and withdrawal, see Chapter 30 (IV).

4. Steroid overdose and adrenal insufficiency

When used inappropriately and excessively in a cyclical weekly fashion, epidural triamcinolone (150 to 300 mg) has been shown to suppress adrenal production of cortisol and the pituitary synthesis of endogenous corticotropin.

Symptoms and signs

Adrenal insufficiency presents as weakness, fatigue, hypotension, weight loss, and anorexia. In its ultimate form—adrenal crisis— nausea, vomiting, and abdominal pain may become persistent.

Lethargy may deepen to somnolence. Hypovolemic shock may be precipitated, with a poor hemodynamic performance, although the latter is usually not evident when exogenous hormone is available because mineralocorticoid activity of the adrenal medulla is still maintained.

Treatment

Patients who have been treated with repeat epidural steroid injections within the last month may benefit from supplemental stress-dose steroids before major surgery, or if other stressors develop (e.g., infection, hypoglycemia in diabetes). Some authorities, however, do not give supplementary steroids unless their patients have been on high-dose systemic steroids. Most surgeons at Massachusetts General Hospital do not give prophylactic steroids to patients who have received epidural steroid injections.

Should acute adrenal insufficiency occur, immediate treatment is necessary. First-line therapy is fluid and electrolyte resuscitation and steroid replacement.

III. CONCLUSION

Many of the unwanted sequelae of pain procedures are life-threatening and require immediate and expert intervention. It is important to be prepared for these events in terms of personnel training, equipment available, equipment maintenance, and protocol development. Bad events are rare, but vigilance and preparedness are necessary to avoid adverse outcomes.

SELECTED READINGS

1. Barash PG, Cullen BF, Stoelting RK, eds. *Clinical anesthesia.* Philadelphia: Lippincott, 1989.
2. Cousins M, Bridenbaugh P, eds. *Neural blockade in clinical anesthesia and management of pain,* 2nd ed. Philadelphia: Lippincott, 1988.
3. Isselbacher K, Braunwald E, Wilson JD, eds. *Harrison's principles of internal medicine,* 13th ed. New York: McGraw-Hill, 1994.
4. Kay J, Findling JW, Ralf H. Epidural triamcinolone suppresses the pituitary-adrenal axis in human subjects. *Anesth Anal* 1994;79: 501–505.
5. Levy JH. Allergic reactions during anesthesia. *J Clin Anesth* 1988;1:39–46.
6. Moore DC. *Regional block: A handbook for use in the clinical practice of medicine and surgery,* 4th ed. Springfield, IL: Thomas, 1965.
7. Orkin FK, Cooperman LH, eds. *Complications in anesthesiology.* Philadelphia: Lippincott, 1988.
8. Wyngaarden JB, Smith LH Jr, Bennett JC, eds. *Cecil's textbook of medicine.* Philadelphia: WB Saunders, 1992.

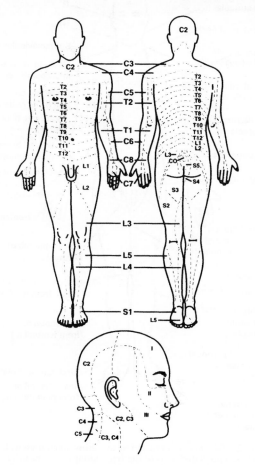

Figure 1. Sensory dermatomes. I, II, and III are the 3 divisions of the trigeminal nerve (cranial nerve V).

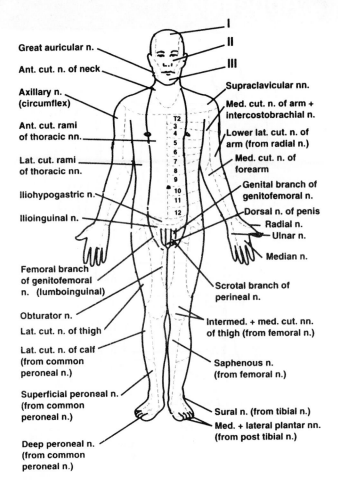

Figure 2.   Sensory innervation of the skin—partial view. I, II, and III are the 3 divisions of the trigeminal nerve (cranial nerve V).

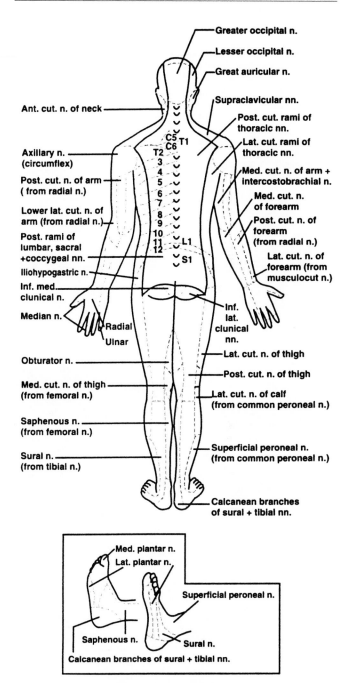

Figure 3. Sensory innervation of the skin—posterior view.

IASP Classification of Chronic Pain Syndromes

The following outline is adapted from the International Association of Pain (IASP) Classification of Chronic Pain Syndromes.

I. Relatively generalized syndromes
 1. Peripheral neuropathy
 2. Stump pain
 3. Phantom pain
 4. Complex regional pain syndrome I (reflex sympathetic dystrophy)
 5. Complex regional pain syndrome II (causalgia)
 6. Central pain (including thalamic and pseudothalamic pain)
 7. Syndrome of syringomyelia (when affecting the head or limb)
 8. Polymyalgia rheumatica
 9. Fibrositis or diffuse myofascial pain syndrome
 10. Rheumatoid arthritis
 11. Osteoarthritis
 12. Calcium pyrophosphate deposition disease
 13. Gout
 14. Hemophilic arthropathy
 15. Burns
 16. Pain of psychological origin
   a. Muscle tension
   b. Delusional or hallucinatory
   c. Hysterical or hypochondriacal
 17. Factitious illness and malingering

II. Neuralgias of the head and face
 1. Trigeminal neuralgia (tic douloureux)
 2. Secondary neuralgia (trigeminal) from CNS lesions
 3. Secondary trigeminal neuralgia from facial trauma
 4. Acute herpes zoster (trigeminal)
 5. Postherpetic neuralgia (trigeminal)
 6. Geniculate neuralgia (cranial nerve VII): Ramsay Hunt syndrome
 7. Glossopharyngeal neuralgia (cranial nerve IX)
 8. Neuralgia of the superior laryngeal nerve (vagus nerve neuralgia)
 9. Occipital neuralgia

III. Craniofacial pain of musculoskeletal origin
 1. Acute tension headache
 2. Tension headache: chronic form (scalp muscle contraction headache)
 3. Temporomandibular pain and dysfunction syndrome
 4. Osteoarthritis of the temporomandibular joint
 5. Rheumatoid arthritis of the temporomandibular joint

IV. Lesions of the ear, nose, and oral cavity
   1. Maxillary sinusitis
   2. Odontalgia: toothache 1: due to dentinoenamel defects
   3. Odontalgia: toothache 2: pulpitis
   4. Odontalgia: toothache 3: periapical periodontitis and abscess
   5. Odontalgia: toothache 4: tooth pain not associated with lesions (atypical odontalgia)
   6. Glossodynia and sore mouth (also known as burning tongue or oral dysesthesia)
   7. Cracked tooth syndrome
   8. Dry socket

V. Primary headache syndromes
   1. Classic migraine
   2. Common migraine
   3. Migraine variants
   4. Carotidynia
   5. Mixed headache
   6. Cluster headache
   7. Chronic paroxysmal hemicrania (chronic stage)
   8. Chronic cluster headache
   9. Cluster-tic syndrome
   10. Posttraumatic headache

VI. Pain of psychological origin in the head and face
   1. Delusional or hallucinatory pain
   2. Hysterical or hypochondriacal

VII. Suboccipital and cervical musculoskeletal disorders
   1. Myofascial syndrome: cervical sprain or cervical hyperextension injury (whiplash)
   2. Myofascial syndrome: sternocleidomastoid muscle
   3. Myofascial syndrome: trapezius muscle
   4. Stylohyoid process syndrome (Eagle's syndrome)

VIII. Visceral pain in the neck
   1. Carcinoma of thyroid
   2. Carcinoma of larynx
   3. Tuberculosis of larynx

IX. Pain of neurologic origin of neck, shoulder, and upper extremity
   1. Prolapsed disc
   2. Osteophyte: cervical spondylosis
   3. Intraspinal tumor
   4. Fracture or collapse of cervical vertebrae
   5. Epidural abscess
   6. Vertebral tumor
   7. Herpes zoster: acute
   8. Postherpetic neuralgia
   9. Syphilis: tabes dorsalis and hypertrophic pachymeningitis
   10. Meningitis and arachnoiditis
   11. Traumatic avulsion of nerve roots
   12. Superior pulmonary sulcus syndrome (Pancoast's tumor)
   13. Thoracic outlet syndrome
   14. Cervical rib or malformed first rib

15. Pain of skeletal metastatic disease of the arm or shoulder girdle

X. Lesions of the brachial plexus
1. Tumors of the brachial plexus
2. Chemical irritation of the brachial plexus
3. Traumatic avulsion of the brachial plexus
4. Postradiation
5. Painful arms and moving fingers

XI. Pain in the shoulder, arm, and hand
1. Bicipital tendinitis
2. Subacromial bursitis (subdeltoid bursitis, supraspinatus tendinitis)
3. Rotator cuff tear: partial or complete
4. Lateral epicondylitis (tennis elbow)
5. Medial epicondylitis (golfer's elbow)
6. De Quervain's tenosynovitis
7. Osteoarthritis of the hands
8. Carpal tunnel syndrome
9. Pain of psychological origin in the shoulder and arm
   a. Tension
   b. Delusional or hallucinatory
   c. Hysterical or hypochondriacal

XII. Vascular disease of the limbs
1. Raynaud's disease
2. Raynaud's phenomenon
3. Frostbite and cold injury
4. Erythema pernio (chilblain)
5. Acrocyanosis
6. Livedo reticularis

XIII. Collagen disease of the limbs
1. Scleroderma
2. Ergotism

XIV. Vasodilating functional disease of the limbs
1. Erythromelalgia
2. Thromboangiitis obliterans
3. Chronic venous insufficiency

XV. Arterial insufficiency in the limbs
1. Intermittent claudication
2. Rest pain

XVI. Pain in the limbs of psychological origin
1. Tension
2. Delusional
3. Conversion

XVII. Chest pain
1. Acute herpes zoster
2. Postherpetic neuralgia
3. Postinfectious and segmental peripheral neuralgia
4. Angina pectoris
5. Myocardial infarction
6. Pericarditis
7. Aneurysm of the aorta
8. Disease of the diaphragm
   a. Infection: chest or pulmonary source
   b. Neoplasm: chest or pulmonary source
   c. Musculoskeletal

        d.   Infection: gastrointestinal source
        e.   Neoplasm: gastrointestinal source
        f.   Cholelithiasis
    9.   Fracture or collapse of thoracic vertebrae
  10.   Slipping rib syndrome
  11.   Postmastectomy pain: acute and subacute
  12.   Postmastectomy pain: chronic nonmalignant
  13.   Last postmastectomy pain or regional carcinoma
  14.   Post-thoracotomy pain syndrome

XVIII. Chest pain of psychological origin
    1.   Muscle tension
    2.   Delusional
    3.   Conversion

XIX. Chest pain: referred from abdominal or gastrointestinal tract
    1.   Subphrenic abscess
    2.   Herniated abdominal organs
    3.   Esophageal motility disorders
    4.   Esophagitis
    5.   Reflux esophagitis with peptic ulceration
    6.   Carcinoma of esophagus
    7.   Gastric ulcer with chest pain
    8.   Duodenal ulcer with chest pain
    9.   Thoracic visceral disease with pain
        a.   Referred to abdomen
        b.   Pericarditis
        c.   Diaphragmatic hernia

XX. Abdominal pain of neurologic origin
    1.   Acute herpes zoster
    2.   Postherpetic neuralgia
    3.   Segmental or intercostal neuralgia
    4.   Twelfth rib syndrome
    5.   Abdominal cutaneous nerve entrapment syndrome

XXI. Abdominal pain of visceral origin
    1.   Cardiac failure
    2.   Gallbladder disease
    3.   Postcholecystectomy syndrome
    4.   Chronic gastric ulcer
    5.   Chronic duodenal ulcer
    6.   Carcinoma of the stomach
    7.   Carcinoma of the pancreas
    8.   Chronic mesenteric ischemia
    9.   Crohn's disease
  10.   Chronic constipation
  11.   Irritable bowel syndrome
  12.   Diverticular disease of the colon
  13.   Carcinoma of the colon

XXII. Abdominal pain syndromes of generalized diseases
    1.   Familial Mediterranean fever
    2.   Abdominal migraine
    3.   Intermittent acute porphyria
    4.   Hereditary coproporphyria
    5.   Variegate porphyria

XXIII. Abdominal pain of psychological origin
    1.   Muscle tension

2. Delusional or hallucinatory
3. Conversion
XXIV. Diseases of the uterus, ovaries, and adnexa
    1. Mittelschmerz
    2. Secondary dysmenorrhea
        a. With endometriosis
        b. With adenomyosis or fibrosis
        c. With congenital obstruction
        d. With acquired obstruction
        e. Psychological causes
    3. Primary dysmenorrhea
    4. Endometriosis
    5. Posterior parametritis
    6. Tuberculous salpingitis
    7. Retroversion of the uterus
    8. Ovarian pain
    9. Chronic pelvic pain without obvious pathology
XXV. Pain in the rectum, perineum, and external genitalia
    1. Neuralgia of iliohypogastric, ilioinguinal, or genitofemoral nerves
    2. Tumor infiltration of the sacrum and sacral nerves
    3. Rectal, perineal, and genital pain of psychological origin
XXVI. Backache and pain of neurologic origin in the trunk and back
    1. Prolapsed intervertebral disc
    2. Acute herpes zoster
    3. Postherpetic neuralgia
    4. Intraspinal tumor
    5. Fracture of lumbar vertebrae
    6. Collapse of lumbar vertebrae
    7. Epidural abscess
    8. Vertebral tumor
        a. Nerve involvement: thorax
        b. Musculoskeletal involvement: thorax
        c. Nerve involvement: abdomen
        d. Musculoskeletal involvement: abdomen
        e. Nerve involvement: low back
        f. Musculoskeletal metastasis: low back
    9. Retroperitoneal tumor
  10. Syphilis
  11. Meningitis and arachnoiditis
  12. Meningeal carcinomatosis
  13. Tumor infiltration of the lumbosacral plexus
XXVII. Back pain of musculoskeletal origin
    1. Osteophyte
    2. Lumbar spondylolysis
    3. Spinal stenosis
    4. Sacralization or lumbarization (transitional vertebra)
    5. Abnormal articular facets (facet tropism)
    6. Acute low back strain
    7. Recurrent low back strain
    8. Trauma: acute
    9. Chronic mechanical low back pain

Source: With permission from the *International Association for the Study of Pain (IASP)*.

Useful Addresses and Web Sites

AMERICAN ACADEMY OF HEAD, NECK AND FACIAL PAIN

Focus on the diagnosis and treatment of TMJ.
Executive Secretary: Cordelia Mason
520 West Pipeline Road
Hurst, TX 76053
Phone: 800-322-8651
Fax: 817-282-1501
E-mail: central@aahnfp.org
www.aahnfp.org

AMERICAN ACADEMY OF OROFACIAL PAIN

Organization of health care professionals dedicated to alleviating pain and suffering through the promotion of excellence in education, research and patient care in the field of orofacial pain and associated disorders.
19 Mantua Road
Mount Royal, NJ 08061
Phone: 856-423-3629
Fax: 856-423-3420
E-mail: aaopco@talley.com
www.aaop.org

AMERICAN ACADEMY OF PAIN MANAGEMENT

Information and Referral, National Pain Data Bank.
Richard S. Weimer, Ph.D., Executive Director
13947 Mono Way #A
Sonora, CA 95370
Phone: 209-533-9744
Fax: 209-533-9750
E-mail: aapm@aapainmanage.org
www.aapainmanage.org

AMERICAN ACADEMY OF PAIN MEDICINE

Organization for physicians practicing the specialty of pain medicine in the United States.
Jeffrey W. Engle, C.M.P., Account Executive
4700 West Lake Avenue
Glenview, IL 60025-1485
Phone: 847-375-4731
Fax: 847-375-4777
E-mail: aapm@amctec.com
www.painmed.org

AMERICAN ALLIANCE OF CANCER PAIN INITIATIVES

Dedicated to promoting cancer pain relief nationwide by supporting the efforts of state cancer pain initiatives.
1300 University Avenue, Room 4720
Madison, WI 53706
Phone: 608-265-4013

Fax: 608-265-4014
E-mail: aacpi@aacpi.org
www.aacpi.org

AMERICAN CHRONIC PAIN ASSOCIATION

ACPA is a support and informational system for people with chronic pain. Has over 800 peer support group chapters worldwide; written materials available.
P.O. Box 850
Rocklin, CA 95677
Phone: 916-632-0922
Fax: 916-632-3208
acpa@pacbell.net
www.theacpa.org

AMERICAN COLLEGE OF OSTEOPATHIC PAIN MANAGEMENT & SCLEROTHERAPY

Organization that provides training and education for physicians interested in practicing prolotherapy/sclerotherapy.
5002 East Woodmill Drive
Wilmington, DE 19808
Phone: 302-996-0300

AMERICAN COUNCIL FOR HEADACHE EDUCATION

Publishes quarterly newsletter; other printed material available; books and videos for sale; 50 support groups nationwide; will provide list of physicians who specialize in headache.
19 Mantua Road
Mount Royal, NJ 08061
Phone: 856-423-0258 or 800-255-ACHE (255-2243)
Fax: 856-423-0082
achehq@talley.com
www.achenet.org

AMERICAN PAIN FOUNDATION

Information, resource and patient advocacy organization serving people with pain.
111 South Calvert Street, Suite 2700
Baltimore, MD 21202
www.painfoundation.org

AMERICAN PAIN SOCIETY

Multidisciplinary organization of basic and clinical scientists, practicing clinicians, policy analysts and others to advance pain related research, education, treatment, and professional practice.
4700 West Lake Avenue
Glenville, IL 60025-1485
Phone: 847-375-4715
Fax: 877-734-8758
E-mail: info@ampainsoc.org
www.ampainsoc.org

AMERICAN SOCIETY OF ADDICTION MEDICINE

The nation's medical specialty society dedicated to educating physicians and improving the treatment of individuals suffering

from alcoholism and other addictions. The goals of the Society are to improve access to care, as well as to increase its quality and effectiveness for patients and their families.
4601 North Park Avenue, Arcade Suite 101
Chevy Chase, MD 20815
Phone: 301-656-3920
Fax: 301-656-3815
www.asam.org

AMERICAN SOCIETY OF LAW, MEDICINE & ETHICS

Educational information at the nexus of law, medicine and ethics, access to research projects on pain under treatment.
765 Commonwealth Avenue
Boston, MA 02215
Phone: 617-262-4990
Fax: 617-437-7596
E-mail: info@aslme.org
www.aslme.org

AMERICAN SOCIETY OF PAIN MANAGEMENT NURSES

Organization of professional nurses dedicated to promoting and providing optimal care of patient with pain through education, standards, advocacy, and research.
7794 Grow Drive
Pensacola, FL 32514
Phone: 888-34-ASPMN
Fax: 850-484-8762
Email: aspmn@puetzamc.com
www.aspmn.org

AMERICAN SOCIETY OF REGIONAL ANESTHESIA

Information, schedules of upcoming meetings, information about fellowships in pain management, consensus statement on Neuraxial Anesthesia and Anticoagulation.
Michael Mulroy, M.D., Current President
PO Box 11086
Richmond, VA 23230-1086
Phone: 804-282-0010
Fax: 804-282-0090
E-mail: asra@societyhq.com
www.asra.com

ARTHRITIS FOUNDATION

Has written material; support groups; will provide list of arthritis specialists in patient's area.
1330 West Peachtree
Atlanta, GA 30309
Phone: 404-872-7100 or 800-283-7800
help@arthritis.org
www.arthritis.org

CANCER CARE, INC.

Has written material; Phone support groups and counseling; will locate other community services in patient area.

275 7th Avenue
New York, NY 10001
Phone: 212-221-3300 or 800-813-4673
www.cancercareinc.org

CANCER PAIN EDUCATION RESOURCE (CAPER)

A resource for use by various educators regarding cancer pain. A twenty-eight member interdisciplinary team designed The Cancer Pain Education Resource (CAPER) world wide web site.
E-mail: cemmp@es.nemc.org
www.caper.tufts.edu

CANDLELIGHTERS CHILDHOOD CANCER FOUNDATION

Candlelighters Childhood Cancer Foundation was founded in 1970 by concerned parents of children with cancer. Provides information, support, and advocacy.
National Office
3910 Warner Street
Kensington, MD 20895
Phone: 800-366-2223 or 301-962-3520
Fax: 301-962-3521
E-mail: info@candlelighters.org
www.candlelighters.org

CFIDS ASSOCIATION OF AMERICA

Advocacy, Information, Support Group Index, Research on Chronic Fatigue Syndrome.
PO Box 220398
Charlotte, NC 28222-0398
Info Line: 800-442-3437
Resource Line: 704-365-2343
Fax: 704-365-9755
E-mail: info@cfids.org
www.cfids.org

COMMISSION ON THE ACCREDITATION OF REHABILITATION FACILITIES (CARF)

Accredits comprehensive inpatient and outpatient pain management programs. A list of accredited programs can be obtained by contacting CARF.
4891 East Grant Road
Tucson, AZ 85712
Phone: 520-325-1044
E-mail: webmaster@carf.org

INTERNATIONAL ASSOCIATION FOR THE STUDY OF PAIN

International, multidisciplinary, non-profit professional association dedicated to furthering research on pain and improving the care of patients in pain.
IASP Secretariat
909 NE 43rd Street, Suite 306
Seattle, WA 98105-6020
Phone: 206-547-6409
Fax: 206-547-1703

E-mail: IASP@locke.hs.washington.edu
www.halcyon.com/iasp

INTERSTITIAL CYSTITIS ASSOCIATION

Has written material; 100 support groups nationwide; will do physician referrals.
51 Monroe St., Suite 1402
Rockville, MD 20850
Phone: 301-610-5300 or 800-HELP-ICA
Fax: 301-610-5308
E-mail: icamail@ichelp.org
www.iche1p.com

JAMA MIGRAINE INFORMATION CENTER, THE JOURNAL OF THE AMERICAN MEDICAL ASSOCIATION

www.ama-assn.org/special/migraine/newsline/newsline.htm

JOINT COMMISSION ON ACCREDITATION OF HEALTHCARE ORGANIZATIONS

An independent, not-for-profit organization, the Joint Commission is the nation's predominant standards setting and accrediting body in health care.
One Renaissance Boulevard
Oakbrook Terrace, IL 60181
Phone: 630-792-5000
Fax: 630-792-5005
www.JCAHO.org

LAST ACTS WEB SITE

An online community dedicated to improving end-of-life care.
www.lastacts.org

LAST ACTS E-MAIL DISCUSSION GROUP

Health care professionals, educators, authors, clergy, and consumers discuss strategies on the national, state and local level to improve care at the end of life. To join the discussion, send an e-mail to join-lastacts-discussion@lists.lyris.net

MAYDAY PAIN RESOURCE CENTER

Inspired and supported by a philanthropic volunteer movement, and dedicated to the prevention, treatment and cure of cancer and other life threatening diseases through innovative research and patient care. City of Hope Pain/Palliative Care Resource Center has nursing research and education materials.
City of Hope National Medical Center
1500 E. Duarte Road
Duarte, CA 91010
http://mayday.coh.org
www.cityofhope.org/medinfo/mayday.htm

MEDICAL MATRIX GUIDE TO INTERNET CLINICAL MEDICINE RESOURCES

Clinical medicine resources database.
www.medmatrix.org/index.asp

NATIONAL CHRONIC PAIN OUTREACH ASSOCIATION

Has initial information packet; books, cassette, videos for sale; currently updating national support group list; will do physician referrals.
7979 Old Georgetown Road, Suite 100
Bethesda, MD 20814-2429
Phone: 301-652-4948
Fax: 301-907-0745
http://neurosurgery.mgh.harvard.edu/ncpainoa.htm

NATIONAL FOUNDATION FOR THE TREATMENT OF PAIN

Not-for-profit organization dedicated to providing support for patients who are suffering from intractable pain, their families, and friends, resource for medical professionals and attorneys.
1330 Skyline Drive, #21
Monterey, CA 93940
Phone: 831-655-8812
Fax: 831-655-2823
www.paincare.org

NATIONAL HEADACHE FOUNDATION

Has written material; about 25 support groups nationwide; will mail list of physicians in patient area.
428 W. St. James Place, 2nd Floor
Chicago, IL 60614-2750
Phone: 888-NHF-5552
E-mail: info@headaches.org
www.headaches.org

NATIONAL NETWORK OF LIBRARIES OF MEDICINE

Provides U.S. health professional with equal access to biomedical information, improve public access. Program is coordinated by National Library of Medicine.
8600 Rockville Pike, Bldg. 38, Room B1-E03
Bethesda, MD 20813
Phone: 301-496-4777
Fax: 301-480-1467
www.nnlm.nlm.nih.gov/

NATIONAL MULTIPLE SCLEROSIS SOCIETY

Has written material; support groups and physician referrals through local chapters.
733 3rd Avenue
New York, NY 10017-3288
Phone: 800-344-4867
E-mail: info@nmss.org
www.nmss.org

NATIONAL VULVODYNIA ASSOCIATION

Organization created to improve the lives of individuals affected by vulvodynia.
PO Box 4491 Silver Springs, MD 20914-4491
Phone: 301-299-0775
Fax: 301-299-3999
E-mail: mate@nva.org
www.nva.org

NEUROPATHY ASSOCIATION

Organization established by people with neuropathy and their families or friends to help those who suffer from disorders that affect the peripheral nerves

60 E. 42nd Street, Suite 942
New York, NY 10165
Phone: 212-692-0662
E-mail: info@neuropathy.org
www.neuropathy.org

ONCOLINK

OncoLink is the first multimedia oncology information resource placed on the Internet. OncoLink's mission is consistent with that of the University of Pennsylvania Medical Center, and the University of Pennsylvania Cancer Center, which has sanctioned its use and development. OncoLink is accessible worldwide to anyone with Internet access, and there is no charge for its use.

E-mail: editors@oncolink.upenn.edu
www.oncolink.com

PAIN ONLINE JOURNAL

The official publication of the International Association for the Study of Pain, publishing original research on the nature, mechanisms and treatment of pain.

www.elsevier.nl/homepage/sah/pain/

PAINLINK

PainLink is a virtual community of health professionals working in institutions that are committed to alleviating pain. Membership benefits for healthcare institutions include technical assistance, teaching cases, access to pain resources and member discussions.

www.edc.org/PainLink/

PEDIATRIC PAIN: SCIENCE HELPING CHILDREN

Research, pediatric pain management information, self-help for children in pain and their parents, Pediatric Pain Letter.

Pediatric Pain Research Lab, Psychology Department
IWK Grace Health Centre, Dalhousie University
Halifax, Nova Scotia, Canada
http://is.dal.ca/~pedpain/pedpain.html

REFLEX SYMPATHETIC DYSTROPHY SYNDROME ASSOCIATION

Has written material; about 100 support groups nationwide; will send list of physician in patient area.

PO Box 821
Haddonfield, NJ 08033
Phone: 856-795-8845
www.rsds.org

SICKLE CELL DISEASE ASSOCIATION OF AMERICA, INC.

Has written materials; will provide list of physicians in patient area, chat room.

200 Corporate Pointe, Suite 495
Culver City, CA 90230-8727

Phone: 310-216-6363 or 800-421-8453
Fax: 310-215-3722
E-mail: scdaa@sicklecelldisease.org
www.sicklecelldisease.org

SOCIETY FOR NEUROSCIENCE
World's largest organization of scientists and physicians dedicated to understanding the brain, spinal cord, and peripheral nervous system.
11 Dupont Circle, NW, Suite 500
Washington, DC 20036
Phone: 202-462-6688
E-mail: info@sfn.org
www.sfn.org

TMJ ASSOCIATION, LTD
Has written material; 29 support affiliates; hotline will refer to other patients; no physician referrals.
PO Box 26770
Milwaukee, WI 53226-0770
Phone: 414-259-3223
Fax: 414-259-8112
E-mail: info@tmj.org
www.tmjassociation.com

TRIGEMINAL NEURALGIA ASSOCIATION
Has written materials; 23 support groups nationwide; phone contact network of patients: limited specialist referral.
PO Box 340
Barnegat Light, NJ 08006
Phone: 609-361-6250
Fax: 609-361-0982
E-mail: tna@csionline.net
www.tna-support.org

THE VULVAR PAIN FOUNDATION
Information, research seminars, personal support and resource network.
PO Drawer 177
Graham, NC 27253
Phone 336-226-0704
Fax: 336-226-8518
www.vulvarpainfoundation.org

VZV RESEARCH FOUNDATION
Has written material on zoster / shingles pain; no support groups; no physician referrals.
40 E. 72nd Street, 4B
New York, NY 10021
Phone: 212-472-3181 or 800-472-8478
Fax: 212-861-7033
Vzv@vzvFoundation.org
www.Vzvfoundation.org

Standards of Treatment: The American Pain Society's Quality Assurance Standards for Relief of Acute and Cancer Pain

In the majority of patients with acute pain and chronic cancer pain, comfort can be achieved with the attentive use of analgesic medications. Historically, though, the outcomes of analgesic treatment have often not been satisfactory, largely because clinical care units have had no systems in place to ensure that the occurrence of pain is recognized and that when pain persists, there is rapid feedback to modify treatment. These suggested standards are offered as one approach to developing such a system. Individual facilities may wish to modify these standards to suit their particular needs.

The guidelines are intended for hospitals and chronic care facilities in which only conventional analgesic methods are used (e.g., intermittent parenteral or oral analgesics) as well as for those using the most modern technology for pain management. In either case, a dedicated pain management team would enhance the quality of pain control if its personnel acquire special training in pain relief. Newer, more aggressive methods of pain control, such as patient-controlled analgesia, epidural opiate administration, and regional anesthetic techniques, may provide better pain relief than intermittent parenteral analgesics in many patients, but they carry their own risks. Should institutions choose to use these methods, they must be delivered by an organized team with frequent follow-up and titration and adequate briefing of the primary caregivers. Such teams should be organized under one of the recognized medical departments of the facility. Specific standards for such methods, monitored by that department, might well augment the general guidelines articulated here.

I. RECOGNIZE AND TREAT PAIN PROMPTLY

Chart and Display Pain and Relief (Process)

A measure of pain intensity and a measure of pain relief are recorded on the bedside vital signs chart or a similar record that facilitates regular review by members of the healthcare team and is incorporated in the patient's permanent record.

1. The intensity of pain or discomfort is assessed and documented on admission, after any known pain-producing procedure, with each new report of pain, and at regular intervals that depend on the severity of pain. Each clinical unit will select a simple, valid measure of intensity. For children, age-appropriate pain-intensity measures will be used.
2. The degree of pain relief is determined after each pain management intervention, once sufficient time has elapsed for the

treatment to reach peak effect (e.g., 1 hour for parenteral analgesics and 2 hours oral analgesics). Each clinical unit will select a simple, valid measure of intensity.

Define Pain and Relief Levels to Trigger Review (Process)

Each clinical unit will identify values for pain intensity rating and pain relief rating that will elicit a review of the current pain therapy, documentation of the proposed modifications in treatment, and subsequent review of its efficacy. This process of treatment review and follow-up should include participation by physicians and nurses involved in the patient's care. As the general quality of treatment improves, the clinical unit will upgrade this standard to encourage a continuous process of improvement.

Survey Patient Satisfaction (Outcome)

At regular intervals to be defined by the clinical unit and the quality assurance committee, each clinical unit will assess a randomly selected sample of patients who have had surgery in the past 72 hours, have another acute pain condition, or have a diagnosis of cancer. Patients will be asked whether they have had pain during the current admission. Those patients who have experienced pain will then be asked about the following:

1. Current intensity of their pain
2. Intensity of the worst pain they experienced in the past 24 hours (or other interval selected by the clinical unit)
3. Degree of relief obtained from pain management interventions
4. Satisfaction with the staff's responsiveness to their reports of pain
5. Satisfaction with relief provided

II. MAKE INFORMATION ABOUT ANALGESIC READILY AVAILABLE (PROCESS)

Information about analgesics and other methods of pain management, including charts of relative potencies of analgesics, is situated on the unit in a way that facilitates writing and interpreting orders. Nurses and physicians can demonstrate the use of this material. Appropriate training to treat their patients' pain is available to health professionals and is included in continuing education activities.

III. PROMISE PATIENTS ATTENTIVE ANALGESIC CARE (PROCESS)

Patients are informed on admission, verbally and in written form, that effective pain relief is an important part of treatment, that their communication of unrelieved pain is essential, and that health professionals will respond quickly to their reports of pain.

IV. DEFINE EXPLICIT POLICIES FOR USE OF ADVANCED ANALGESIC TECHNOLOGIES (PROCESS)

Advanced pain control techniques, including intraspinal opioids, systemic or intraspinal patient-controlled anesthesia or continuous opioid infusion, local anesthetic infusion, and inhalational analgesia, are governed by policy and standard procedures that define the acceptable level of monitoring patients and define appropriate roles and limits of practice for all groups of healthcare providers involved. Such policy includes definitions of physician accountability, nurse responsibility to the patient and the physician, and the role of pharmacy.

V. MONITOR ADHERENCE TO STANDARDS (PROCESS)

1. An interdisciplinary committee, including representation from physicians, nurses, and other appropriate disciplines (e.g., pharmacy), monitors compliance with the preceding standards, considers issues relevant to improving pain treatment, and makes recommendations to improve outcomes and their monitoring. Where a comprehensive pain management team exists, its activities are monitored through the parent department's quality assurance body. In a nursing home or very small hospital where an interdisciplinary pain management committee is not feasible, one or several individuals may fulfill this role.
2. At least the chairperson of the committee has had experience working with issues related to effective pain management.
3. The committee meets at least every 3 months to review the process and outcomes related to pain management.
4. The committee interacts with clinical units to establish procedures for improving pain management where necessary and reviews the results of these changes within 3 months of their implementation.
5. The committee provides regular reports to the administration and to the medical, nursing, and pharmacy staffs.

Appendix V

Massachusetts General Hospital Pain Center Guidelines on Prescribing Controlled Substances for Patients with Nonmalignant Chronic Disease

1. Controlled substance prescriptions are not sent by mail.
2. Prescriptions are not written as "brand name medically necessary" or "no substitution" unless it is absolutely necessary.
3. When chronic opioid therapy is initiated, the primary referring physician must concur with this decision and continue to monitor the patient as well. If, as the patient is observed, there is no demonstrable benefit to the patient's function or quality of life, then the opioid should be tapered. Before starting to taper the drug, the Pain Center physician should discuss the plan in advance with the primary referring physician if one can be identified and if the patient has been seen by that physician during the past year. The concurrence of the primary referring physician with the decision to start or taper opioids must be documented in the chart.
4. Where there is no primary physician, the Pain Center provides the patient with the opportunity to secure such a physician. We do not become the primary source of general medical care for any patient.
5. Discovery that the patient has obtained concurrent prescriptions for controlled substances from multiple doctors results in termination of the Pain Center's relationship with the patient.
6. The second instance of a lost or otherwise early depletion of a prescription will result in no further controlled substances being dispensed to that patient from our unit. The need does not necessarily result, however, in cessation of the therapeutic relationship with our unit, or in our ceasing to prescribe non-controlled substances.
7. There are to be no prescription refills if a patient arrives without an appointment prior to the time of his or her next scheduled refill. Even when a medical follow-up visit is not necessary, the patient must still inform the center at least the day before picking up a prescription. Failure to do so disrupts the center's schedule and needlessly inconveniences those working in it or waiting to be seen.
8. Options for physician therapy, behavioral medicine treatment, or other consultations (e.g., psychiatry, orthopedics), as appropriate, should be offered to patients who are being tapered from chronic opioid use. These options may be offered through an inpatient rehabilitation program, providing insurance is available to cover it, or, if not, through MGH outpatient departments (e.g., Addictions Service).

9. No longer than 2 months should elapse between scheduled follow-up appointments during the long-term follow-up of any patient receiving controlled substances in the absence of malignant disease.

Apart from the regulatory dimension, our first role is to treat the patient. Thus it is essential that our notes document the history, physical and laboratory findings, diagnosis, and plans for medical and other therapies (including specifics and timing of schedules for tapering opioids). Initiation or tapering controlled substances in the absence of a documented medical rationale is not acceptable.

Appendix VI

Guidelines for the Prescription of Controlled Substances Issued by the Drug Enforcement Agency

1. A prescription for a controlled substance is lawful only if issued for a legitimate medical purpose by an individual practitioner acting in the usual course of professional practice. Prescriptions under the law may not be issued for narcotic drugs for the purpose of detoxification or maintenance of narcotic addicts.
2. All prescriptions for controlled substances must bear the following information:
   a. Name of patient
   b. Home address of patient
   c. Name of practitioner
   d. Address of practitioner
   e. Registration number of practitioner
   f. Name of the drug, strength, and quantity of the medicine to be dispensed
   g. Directions for use
3. All prescriptions must be dated with the day when issued to the patient and must be signed manually on that day by the practitioner.
4. It is illegal under both federal and state law to issue a prescription for other than a legitimate bona fide medical need or to date a prescription other than the date when it is issued to the patient and signed by the practitioner.
5. Schedule II controlled substances require written prescriptions prior to dispensing. They may not be refilled. A Schedule II drug may be dispensed in an emergency by a pharmacist upon oral prescription of a practitioner if the quantity is limited to the emergency period, if the prescription is reduced immediately to writing by the pharmacist and contains all the information required of written prescription except the signature of the prescriber, if the pharmacist knows the prescriber, or makes a reasonable effort to verify the order's validity, and if the prescriber issues to the pharmacist a written prescription within 48 hours of the oral order. If the pharmacist does not receive a written prescription from the prescriber within 72 hours, he or she must by law notify the DEA regional office.
6. A controlled substance prescription must be for no more than 30 days of medicine.

Appendix VII

Food and Drug Administration State Drug Schedules

There are five established schedules of controlled substances, known as schedules I, II, III, IV, and V. These schedules currently consist of the substances listed in Table 1.

Table 1. Schedules for controlled substances prescribed for patients in pain

Schedule 1

The drug or other substance has a high potential for abuse.

The drug or other substance has no currently accepted medical use in treatment in the United States.

There is a lack of accepted safety for use of the drug or other substance under medical supervision.

None

Schedule 2

The drug or other substance has a high potential for abuse.

The drug or other substance has a currently accepted medical use in treatment in the United States or a currently accepted medical use with severe restrictions.

Abuse of the drug or other substances may lead to severe psychological or physical dependence.

Opioids: morphine, codeine, fentanyl, hydromorphone, meperidine, levorphanol, oxycodone.

Stimulants: amphetamine, methylphenidate

Marijuana: dronabinol

Schedule 3

The drug or other substance has a potential for abuse less than the drugs or other substances in schedules I and II.

The drug or other substance has a currently accepted medical use in treatment in the United States.

Abuse of the drug or other substance may lead to moderate or low physical dependence or high psychological dependence.

Opioids: nalorphine; mixtures of limited specified quantities of codeine, dihydrocodeine, hydrocodone, morphine, or opioid with noncontrolled medicinal ingredients

Schedule 4

The drug or other substance has a low potential for abuse relative to the drugs or other substances in schedule III.

The drug or other substance has a currently accepted medical use in treatment in the United States.

Abuse of the drug or other substance may lead to limited physical dependence or psychological dependence relative to the drugs or other substances in schedule III.

Opioids: pentazocine

Benzodiazepines: valium, clonazepam, flurazepam, midazolam, triazolam

continued

Table 1.   *Continued*

Schedule 5

The drug or other substance has a low potential for abuse relative to the drugs or other substances in schedule IV.

The drug or other substance has a currently accepted medical use in treatment in the United States.

Abuse of the drug or other substance may lead to limited physical dependence or psychological dependence relative to the drugs or other substances in schedule IV.

Opioids: cough suppressant preparations

Drugs Commonly Used in Pain Practice

Salahadin Abdi and Jatinder S. Gill

NOTE: This table provides a ready reference to the drugs frequently used in pain practice. The information provided is not comprehensive and the reader is encouraged to refer to the Physicians Desk Reference (PDR) or other source for a complete description of these drugs.

Acetaminophen (Tylenol)

Description:	Analgesic, antipyretic.
Indications:	Used to relieve mild to moderate pain and has minimal anti-inflammatory effects.
Dosage:	325–1000 mg PO every 4–6 hours not to exceed 4,000 mg/day.
Side Effects:	Overdoses of acetaminophen can cause severe, even fatal, hepatic dysfunction. Allergies to this drug can also occur.
Precautions:	Use with caution in presence of alcoholism or liver disease. Daily use of alcohol, especially when combined with phenobarbital, may enhance acetaminophen's hepatotoxicity. It may produce a slight increase in prothrombin time in patients receiving oral anticoagulants, but the clinical significance of this effect is not clear.

Acetylsalicylic acid (see NSAIDs)
Amitriptyline (see TCAs)
Amoxapine (see TCAs)
Anafranil (see TCAs)
Anaprox (see NSAIDs)
Ansaid (see NSAIDs)
Asendin (see TCAs)
Aspirin (see NSAIDs)
Atarax (see hydroxyzine)
Ativan (see lorazepam)
Baclofen (see Lioresal)
Benadryl (see diphenhydramine)
Benylin (see dextromethorphan)

Bretylium (Bretylol)

Description:	Anti-arrhythmic.
Indications:	Bier block for neuropathic (sympathetically maintained) chronic pain. Releases norepinephrine from adrenergic nerve terminals, prevents reuptake and decreases release of norepinephrine in response to sympathetic stimulation.
Dosage:	50 mg or 1 mg/kg IV
Side Effects:	Hypotension, arrhythmias (bradycardia), vertigo, dizziness, and light-headedness.

Precautions: Use with caution under ECG and blood pressure monitoring and additional intravenous access.

Bretylol (see bretylium)

Butalbital-caffeine-Tylenol/ASA (Fioricet/Fiorinal)
Description: Barbiturate, caffeine, and analgesic mixture.
Indications: Tension (or muscle contraction) headache and conditions where a simultaneous sedative and analgesic action is required, such as mixed migraine headaches, postdural puncture headache, and menstrual and postpartum tension and pain.
Dosage: Two tablets or capsules at once, followed if necessary, by one tablet or capsule every 3 to 4 hours; up to six capsules or tablets daily.
Side Effects: Bloating; dizziness or lightheadedness; drowsiness; nausea, vomiting, or stomach pain.
Precautions: Caution in patients with history of alcohol abuse, heart disease, mental depression, kidney and liver disease, diabetes mellitus, porphyria.

Butazolidin (see NSAIDs)

Capsaicin (Zostrix, topical)
Description: Topical analgesic, antipruritic, antineuralgic.
Indications: Arthritis, shingles, diabetic neuropathy.
Dosage: Apply to affected areas (rub well) three to four times a day.
Side Effects: Warm, burning feeling, stinging, redness.
Precautions: Avoid contact with eyes or on other sensitive areas of the body.

Carbamazepine (Tegretol)
Description: Anticonvulsant, antineuralgic.
Indications: Neuropathic pain medication especially useful for trigeminal neuralgia.
Dosage: Usually initiated at 100 mg PO BID with escalation by 100 mg every 12 hours as tolerated. Effective dose for pain may range from 200 mg to 1,200 mg/day.
Side Effects: Dizziness, drowsiness, blurred vision, pruritus and rash, hematologic and hepatic complications.
Precautions: Obtain baseline hematologic function test and subsequent monitoring on the basis of clinical indication. Liver function tests prior to initiating therapy and periodically thereafter. Caution in patients with history of bone marrow depression and liver dysfunction.

Celebrex (see celecoxib)

Celecoxib (Celebrex)
Description: NSAID, selective COX-2 inhibitor.
Indications: Pain with peripheral inflammatory component.
Dosage: 100 mg PO BID or 200 mg PO QD.
Side Effects: Lower incidence of GI complications than traditional NSAIDs. Usual doses do not appear to af-

fect platelet aggregation. Renal toxicity similar to traditional NSAIDs.

Precautions: Caution with history of GI bleed, fluid retention, or renal impairment.

Chlorpromazine (Thorazine)

Description: Phenothiazine, dopamine antagonist, antipsychotic, antiemetic, sedative.

Indications: Psychoses, hiccups, anxiety, and nausea and vomiting.

Dosage: 10–50 mg PO/IM two to four times daily.

Side Effects: Constipation, drowsiness, vision changes or dry mouth, extrapyramidal symptoms, occasional tardive dyskinesia.

Precautions: Caution with extreme hypertension or hypotension, liver or heart disease, alcohol or drug dependencies, history of neuroleptic syndrome.

Choline magnesium trisalicylate (see NSAIDs)
Clinoril (see NSAIDs)
Clomipramine (see TCAs)

Clonazepam (Klonopin)

Description: Benzodiazepine, sedative–hypnotic, anxiolytic, amnestic, anticonvulsant, skeletal muscle relaxant.

Indications: Patients with chronic neuropathic pain exhibiting sleep disturbances, anxiety and restlessness, skeletal muscle spasm.

Dosage: Start at 0.5 mg PO at bedtime. May be given as a TID dose for patients with daytime anxiety/panic attack, usually not exceeding 3–4 mg/day with largest dose given at bedtime.

Side Effects: Sedation, drowsiness, increased salivation, constipation.

Precautions: Avoid alcohol, caution with hepatic impairment, periodic blood counts, and positive liver function tests.

Clonidine (Catapres)

Description: Centrally acting alpha-2 agonist, antihypertensive, suppresses manifestations of opioid withdrawal syndrome, adjunct analgesic.

Indications: Neuropathic pain with sympathetic dependency; opioid withdrawal.

Dosage: Clonidine has been used orally, topically, and neuraxially for pain. Start at 0.1 mg PO BID or TID and gradually escalate by 0.1–0.2 mg/day every few days until side effects, or maximum dose of 2.4 mg/day. Use 0.2–0.4 mg/day for opioid withdrawal.

Transdermal: 0.1–0.3 mg once every 7 days.

Epidural: 2–10 µg/kg (about 150–800 µg for a normal adult) bolus, and 10–40 µg/hour continuous infusion.

Spinal: 10–30-µg bolus.
Side Effects: Bradycardia, hypotension, sedation, xerostomia, constipation, urinary retention, impotence, pruritus, and insomnia.
Precautions: Patients should be warned about the risk of rebound hypertension with abrupt discontinuation. Caution in patients with coronary artery disease, cerebrovascular disease, Raynaud's disease, and depression.

Codeine (see opioids)
Compazine (see prochlorperazine)

Cyclobenzaprine (Flexeril)
Description: Skeletal muscle relaxant; structurally and pharmacologically related to TCAs.
Indications: Myofascial pain in conjunction with physical therapy, usually short term.
Dosage: Usually 10 mg PO TID with gradual increase to maximum of 60mg/day.
Side Effects: Drowsiness, dry mouth, fatigue, tiredness, blurred vision, constipation, flatulence.
Precautions: Follow the guidelines for tricyclic antidepressants.

Demerol (see opioids)
Desipramine (see TCAs)

Dexamphetamine (Dexedrine)
Description: Central stimulant. CNS and respiratory stimulant with weak sympathetic activity.
Indications: Excessive sedation due to opioids, especially in cancer patients.
Dosage: 5–10 mg PO is administered in the morning after a 2.5-mg test dose. Maximum daily dose is 20 mg/day.
Side Effects: Nervousness, insomnia, anorexia, angina, tachycardia, thrombocytopenia, leukopenia.
Precautions: Tolerance and psychological dependence may occur. Use with caution in seizure disorder, psychiatric symptoms. Contraindicated in presence of uncontrolled hypertension, significant coronary artery disease, and in patients exhibiting anxiety, agitation.

Dexedrine (see dexamphetamine)

Dextromethorphan (Benylin)
Description: Antitussive, weak analgesic with some N-methyl-D-aspartate (NMDA) receptor antagonism.
Indications: Combined with opioids to decrease the development of tolerance, second-line medication for neuropathic pain.
Dosage: 30 mg PO every 6–8 hours. Dosage can be titrated high (typically up to 90 mg PO TID) as tolerated.

Side Effects: Dizziness, drowsiness, nausea and vomiting.
Precautions: Asthma, chronic bronchitis, emphysema, diabetes, liver disease.

Diazepam (Valium)
Description: Benzodiazepine, sedative-hypnotic, anxiolytic, amnestic, anticonvulsant, skeletal muscle relaxant.
Indications: Patients with chronic neuropathic pain exhibiting sleep disturbances, anxiety and restlessness, skeletal muscle spasm.
Dosage: Start at 5 mg PO at bedtime. May be given as a TID dose for patients with daytime anxiety/panic attack, usually not exceeding 3–4 mg/day with largest dose given at bedtime.
Side Effects: Sedation, drowsiness, increased salivation, constipation.
Precautions: Not recommended for use in depressive neurosis or in psychotic reactions; avoid alcohol; careful when given to elderly or seriously ill patients with limited pulmonary function, those with hepatic or renal disease, debilitated patients, or those with organic brain syndrome.

Dibenzyline (see phenoxybenzamine)
Diclofenac sodium (see NSAIDs)
Diflunisal (see NSAIDs)

Dihydroergotamine (D.H.E. 45, Ergomar, Ergostat)
Description: Antihypotensive, vascular headache suppressant, ergot alkaloid.
Indications: Severe throbbing headaches, such as migraine and cluster headaches.
Dosage: For the abortion of migraine with aura (also called classic migraine) or migraine without aura (also called common migraine), intranasal dose of dihydroergotamine mesylate is 0.5 mg (one spray) administered in each nostril (1 mg total) initially, followed by 1 mg [one spray (0.5 mg) in each nostril] 15 minutes later for a total dose of 2 mg. For rapid response, dihydroergotamine mesylate may be administered IV. (Total IV dose should not exceed 2 mg; and total weekly IM or IV dosage should not exceed 6 mg.) For the prevention or abortion of vascular headaches, the usual adult IM dose of dihydroergotamine mesylate is 1–2 mg initially, followed by 1 mg at 1-hour intervals until the attack has abated or until a total of 3 mg has been given in 24 hours.
Side Effects: Dizziness, drowsiness, stomach upset (nausea and vomiting), anxiety, tremor.
Precautions: Liver, kidney or vascular disease; hypertension, poor circulation; arterial vasospasm when given with heparin; ischemic heart disease (e.g., angina pectoris, Prinzmetal angina, myocardial infarc-

tion, documented silent myocardial ischemia); peripheral vascular disease, coronary artery disease, uncontrolled hypertension.

Dilaudid (see opioids)

Diphenhydramine (Benadryl)

Description:	Antihistamine, antiemetic, sedative–hypnotic.
Indications:	Nausea, vomiting, and itching.
Dosage:	For PO, use 25–50 mg every 4–6 hours. For IV/IM, use 10–50 mg every 4–6 hours (not to exceed 400 mg/day).
Side Effects:	Antihistaminic effect such as drowsiness, sedation, dry mouth, vertigo, urinary retention.
Precautions:	Caution in patients with GI obstruction, seizure, increased intraocular pressure.

Disalcid (see NSAIDs)
Dolobid (see NSAIDs)
Dolophine (see opioids)
Doxepin (see TCAs)

Droperidol (Inapsine)

Description:	Butyrophenone, dopamine antagonist, antipsychotic, antiemetic.
Indications:	Nausea/vomiting, and anxiety.
Dosage:	0.625–2.5 mg IV every 4–6 hours; higher doses for anxiolysis.
Side Effects:	Shares toxic potential of phenothiazines: dysphoria, hypotension, sedation, and respiratory depression, especially in combination with opioids.
Precautions:	Contraindicated in patients with Parkinson's disease and a history of neuroleptic syndrome.

Elavil (see TCAs)
Etodolic acid (see NSAIDs)
Feldene (see NSAIDs)
Fenoprofen (see NSAIDs)
Fioricet (see butalbital)
Flexeril (see cyclobenzaprine)

Fluoxetine

Description:	Selective serotonin reuptake inhibitor (SSRI), first-line antidepressant.
Indications:	Depression, panic disorder, obsessive-compulsive disorder.
Dosage:	10–80 mg/day PO.
Side Effects:	These are rare but include headaches, stimulation or sedation, fine tremor, tinnitus, rare extrapyramidal symptoms, palpitations, nausea and vomiting, bloating, and diarrhea.
Precautions:	Known sensitivity, interactions with monoamine oxidase inhibitors (MAOIs).

Flurbiprofen (see NSAIDs)

Gabapentin (Neurontin)

Description:	Anticonvulsant, adjunct antineuralgic.
Indications:	Commonly used neuropathic pain medication marketed as anticonvulsant.
Dosage:	Start at 300 mg PO QHS or lower (100 mg) in elderly patients. Gradual escalation in dose every 3–5 days to the range of 1,200 mg TID as tolerated. Maximum dose varies depending on efficacy and patient's tolerance of side effects. Beneficial effects expected in 1–3 weeks of therapy.
Side Effects:	Usually well tolerated with self-limiting mild to moderate side effects. Somnolence, dizziness or fatigue, ataxia (CNS), mild dyspepsia (GI), and diplopia and amblyopia.
Precautions:	Do not discontinue abruptly; reduce dose in renal dysfunction.

Haldol (see haloperidol)

Haloperidol (Haldol)

Description:	Butyrophenone, antipsychotic, antiemetic.
Indications:	Nervous, mental, and emotional conditions (e.g., agitation, confusion); Tourette's syndrome.
Dosage:	0.5–5 mg PO 2–3 times daily.
Side Effects:	Drowsiness, dizziness, or blurred vision, stomach upset, loss of appetite, headache, drooling, dry mouth, sweating, sleep disturbances or restlessness.
Precautions:	Difficulty urinating, Parkinson's disease, glaucoma, lung disease, heart or blood vessel disease, seizure disorder, or disease of the thyroid, kidney, liver, or prostate.

Hydromorphone (see opioids)
Hydrocodone (see opioids)

Hydroxyzine (Atarax, Vistaril)

Description:	Antihistamine, antiemetic, sedative–hypnotic.
Indications:	Itching, emesis, anxiety.
Dosage:	For PO and IM use 25–100 mg Q6 hours. Adjust dose to patient response.
Side Effect:	Drowsiness, dry mouth, dizziness, discomfort at site of injection.
Precautions:	Epilepsy, prostatic hypertrophy, glaucoma, hepatic disease.

Ibuprofen (see NSAIDs)
Imipramine (see TCAs)
Imitrex (see sumatriptan)
Inapsine (see droperidol)
Indocin (see NSAIDs)
Indomethacin (see NSAIDs)
Kenalog (see triamcinolone)

Ketoprofen (see NSAIDs)

Ketorolac (Toradol)

Description:	Potent, injectable NSAID
Indications:	Acute postoperative pain, acute inflammatory pain, available for intravenous, intramuscular and oral use. Recommended for short-term use only. Superior adjunct drug for patients with inadequately controlled postoperative pain.
Dosage:	15–30 mg IV or IM every 6 hours; 10 mg PO every 6 hours. It is used preferably as a fixed regimen; lower dose for elderly, low-weight patients, and renal impairment. Total usage not to exceed 5 days.
Side Effects:	Dizziness, nausea, vomiting, pain/redness at the injection site may occur. Enhanced risk of bleeding, adverse GI effects, renal function impairment and some concerns about bone remodeling in acute fractures and bone fusion procedures.
Precautions:	Caution in presence of hematologic, GI, and renal dysfunction. Use minimum effective doses and adjust for low weight, age, and renal impairment.

Klonopin (see clonazepam)

Lactulose

Description:	Laxative.
Indication:	Constipation.
Dosage:	10–40 g daily or two divided doses.
Side Effects:	Skin rash, abdominal cramping, potassium loss.
Precautions:	Caution in presence of kidney disease, heart disease, high blood pressure, intestinal blockage (ileostomy/colostomy), inflamed bowel.

Lamictal (see lamotrigine)

Lamotrigine (Lamictal)

Description:	Anticonvulsant, adjunct antineuralgic.
Indications:	Used as a neuropathic pain medication when first-line medications fail. Neuronal membrane stabilizing drug blocking voltage sensitive sodium channels and inhibiting release of excitatory amino acid neurotransmitters. Beneficial effects may be slow to occur, as dose escalations are gradual.
Dosage:	Start at 25 mg PO QHS with dose escalations every 2 weeks as tolerated up to the maximum of 200 mg BID.
Side Effects:	Dizziness, ataxia, somnolence, headache, diplopia, blurred vision, maculopapular rash, nausea and vomiting.
Precautions:	Do not discontinue abruptly. Rapid dose escalations increase the risk of rash.

Levo-Dromoran (see opioids)
Levorphanol (see opioids)

Lidocaine (Xylocaine) patch, ointment, oral gel, infusion, eutectic mixture

Description:	Local anesthetic, antiarrhythmic.
Indications:	Itching and pain of various disorders [postherpetic neuralgia (PHN), peripheral diabetic neuropathy (PDN), burns]; irritation and inflammation in the mouth and throat; as an infusion, this is a diagnostic test for neuropathic pain.
Dosage:	As a diagnostic test for neuropathic pain, prepare an IV infusion of 1–5 mg/kg in 20–100 mL of normal saline and infuse for 20–60 min; for PHN, Lidoderm patch 12 hrs on and 12 hrs off; for PDN, lidocaine cream/ointment apply to affected areas one to four times a day.
Side Effects:	Stinging, burning, redness, tenderness, swelling, or rash.
Precautions:	Heart disease, serious illness, infections, or allergies.

Lioresal (Baclofen)

Description:	Antispastic analgesic.
Indications:	Myofascial pain in conjunction with physical therapy, spasticity. May also be used for the treatment of facial pain (trigeminal neuralgia).
Dosage:	Usually started at 5 mg PO TID. Dose escalations of 15 mg every 3 days as tolerated to a maximum of 40–80 mg daily. Intrathecal administration is often beneficial for cases of severe spasticity.
Side Effects:	Drowsiness, fatigue, nausea, vertigo, hypotonia, muscle weakness, mental depression, and headache may occur.
Precautions:	Seizure disorder, peptic ulcer disease, and psychotic disorders.

Lodine (see NSAIDs)

Lorazepam (Ativan)

Description:	Benzodiazepine, sedative–hypnotic, anxiolytic, amnestic, anticonvulsant, skeletal muscle relaxant.
Indications:	Patients with chronic neuropathic pain exhibiting sleep disturbances, anxiety and restlessness, skeletal muscle spasm.
Dosage:	Initial adult daily oral dosage is 2 mg in divided doses of 0.5 mg, 0.5 mg, and 1 mg, or of 1 mg and 1 mg. The daily dosage should be carefully increased or decreased by 0.5 mg depending on tolerance and response.
Side Effects:	Drowsiness, dizziness, weakness, fatigue and lethargy, disorientation, ataxia, anterograde amnesia, nausea, change in appetite, change in

weight, depression, blurred vision and diplopia, psychomotor agitation, sleep disturbance, vomiting, sexual disturbance, headache, skin rashes, and GI, ear, nose, and throat, musculoskeletal, and respiratory disturbances.

Precautions: Not recommended for use in depressive neurosis or in psychotic reactions; avoid alcohol; caution in elderly or seriously ill patients with limited pulmonary function; hepatic or renal disease; and debilitated patients, and those with organic brain syndrome.

Lorcet (see opioids)
Meclofenamate (see NSAIDs)
Meclomen (see NSAIDs)
Meperidine (see opioids)
Methadone (see opioids)

Methylphenidate (Ritalin)

Description: Central stimulant. CNS and respiratory stimulant with weak sympathetic activity, similar to amphetamines.

Indications: For excessive sedation due to opioids, especially in cancer patients.

Dosage: Start at 5–10 mg PO in the morning. Avoid late evening or night dose. Maximum dose 40 mg/day.

Side Effects: Nervousness, insomnia, anorexia, angina, tachycardia, thrombocytopenia, leukopenia.

Precautions: Periodic blood counts (use clinical judgment), tolerance and psychological dependence may occur. Caution in seizure disorder, psychiatric symptoms. Contraindicated in presence of uncontrolled hypertension, significant coronary artery disease, and in patient exhibiting anxiety, agitation.

Methylprednisolone (Medrol, Solu-Medrol, Depo-Medrol)

Description: Corticosteroid, anti-inflammatory.

Indications: Swelling, arthritis, skin diseases (psoriasis, hives), asthma, chronic obstructive pulmonary disease, pain.

Dosage: Epidural 20–80 mg.

Side Effects: Dizziness, nausea, indigestion, increased appetite, weight gain, weakness, or sleep disturbances.

Precautions: Extreme hypertension or hypotension, liver or heart disease, Reye's syndrome, alcohol or drug dependencies, neurologic disease.

Metoclopramide (Reglan)

Description: Dopamine antagonist, antiemetic, peristaltic stimulant.

Indications: Nausea and emesis.

Dosage: Oral, IM, IV, 10 mg up to four times daily.

Side Effects: Restlessness, drowsiness, anxiety, headache, extrapyramidal symptoms.

Precautions: Contraindicated in obstructive GI pathology, neuroleptic syndrome. Caution in presence of seizure disorder and depression.

Mexiletine (Mexitil)
Description: Sodium channel blocker, antiarrhythmic, antineuralgia adjunct.
Indication: Adjunct medication for neuropathic pain.
Dosage: Starting dose is 150 mg PO QHS, gradually titrated as tolerated up to 900 mg/day in three divided doses.
Side Effects: Nausea, vomiting, heartburn, dizziness, tremor, changes in vision, nervousness, confusion, headache, fatigue, depression, rapid heartbeat, general weakness.
Precautions: Caution in patients with cardiac disease, especially congestive cardiac failure, hypotension, liver disease, a history of seizures or allergies, especially allergies to amide-type anesthetics (e.g., lidocaine, tocainide).

Mexitil (see mexiletine)
Morphine (see opioids)
Motrin (see NSAIDs)
MS Contin (see opioids)
Nalfon (see NSAIDs)

Naloxone (Narcan)
Description: Mu opioid receptor antagonist.
Indication: Reversal of opioid effects.
Dosage: 0.02–0.04 mg IV every 2–3 minutes, titrated to effect. Avoid high doses to prevent complete reversal of opiate effects. Use higher doses 0.4–2 mg every 2–3 minutes to a maximum of 10 mg in emergency situations only. Infusions may be required to prevent renarcotization. Used orally 1.2–2.4 mg every 4–6 hours until the first bowel movement or to a maximum of 5 mg for reversing opiate-induced constipation.
Side Effects: Acute cardiovascular and CNS excitability caused by rapid reversal of opiate effects, acute withdrawal symptoms.
Precautions: Use low doses and titrate to effect. Care in the presence of history of opioid dependency.

Naproxen (see NSAIDs)
Naproxen sodium (see NSAIDs)
Narcan (see naloxone)
Neurontin (see gabapentin)
Norpramin (see TCAs)
Nortriptyline (see TCAs)

NSAIDs (nonsteroidal anti-inflammatory drugs)
Description: Nonsteroidal anti-inflammatory agents, prostaglandin inhibition secondary to cyclooxygenase (COX) inhibition.

Indications: First-line medications in mild to moderate pain, especially of musculoskeletal origin. Valuable adjuncts in severe pain by attacking the peripheral inflammatory cascade; opioid sparing. CNS effects not clearly elucidated but under investigation.

Dosage: See Table 1.

Side Effects: Prostaglandin inhibition leading to decreased platelet adhesion, gastric mucosal damage with or without GI bleeding, and renal function impairment.

Table 1.   Commonly used oral NSAIDs

Generic Name	Trade Name	Adult Dosage
Acetaminophen	Tylenol	500–1000 mg q4h
Acetylsalicylic Acid	Aspirin	325–650 mg q4h
Celecoxib	Celebrex	100 mg BID or 200 mg qd
Choline Magnesium Trisalicylate	Trilisate	500–750 mg q8–12h
Diclofenal sodium	Voltaren	25–75 mg q8–12h
Diflunisal	Dolobid	250–500 mg q8–12h
Etodolic Acid	Lodine	200–400 mg q6–8h
Fenoprofen calcium	Nalfon	200 mg q4–6h
Flurbiprofen	Ansaid	100 mg q8–12h
Ibuprofen	Motrin	400–800 mg q6–8h
Indomethacin	Indocin	25–50 mg q8–12h
Ketoprofen	Orudis	25–75 mg q6–8h
Ketorolac	Toradol	10 mg q6–8h
Meclofenamate sodium	Meclomen	50 mg q4–6h
Naproxen	Naprosyn	275–500 mg q8–12h
Naproxen Sodium	Anaprox	275–550 mg q6–8h
Phenylbutazone	Butazolidin	100 mg q6–8h
Piroxicam	Feldene	10–20 mg qD
Rofecoxib	Vioxx	12.5–50 mg qD
Salsalate	Disalcid	500 mg q4h
Sulindac	Clinoril	150–200 mg q12h
Tolmetin	Tolectin	200–600 mg q8h

NSAID, nonsteroidal anti-inflammatory drugs; q, every; BID, twice a day.

Precautions: Caution in elderly and in the presence of coagu-
                  lopathy, renal impairment, and peptic ulcer dis-
                  ease. Use lowest effective doses.

Ondansetron (Zofran)
Description: $5HT_3$ receptor antagonist, antiemetic.
Indications: Nausea and emesis.
Dosage: Oral or IV (4 mg IV every 6 hours), higher doses
                  used for patients undergoing chemotherapy and/
                  or radiation treatment.
Side Effects: Headache, blurring vision, diarrhea, unspecified
                  chest pain, pruritus, fever.
Precautions: Rapid intravenous injections may increase the
                  risk for headache.

Opioids
Description: Ligands at endogenous opioid receptors, opium
                  constituents (morphine, codeine) or their deriv-
                  atives (hydromorphone, hydrocodone, buprenor-
                  phine, oxycodone) or synthetic (levorphanol,
                  methadone, meperidine, fentanyl).
Indications: Potent analgesics for severe pain including post-
                  operative pain, cancer pain; gaining acceptabil-
                  ity in chronic nonmalignant pain (CNMP).
Dosage: See Table 2.
Routes: PO, IM, SC, transdermal, IV, nasal, sublingual,
                  epidural, intrathecal.
                     Start at lowest dose and gradually titrate to
                  effect. Dose depends on effect versus side effects.
                  There is no ceiling effect.
                     Add adjuncts for opioid-sparing effects.
                     Approximate conversion ratio for intrathecal:
                  epidural: IV: PO is 1: 10: 100: 300.
                     Tolerance to analgesic effects as well as to side
                  effects is common. Rotate opioid if excessive tol-
                  erance develops. New opioid can be started at $\frac{1}{2}$
                  to $\frac{1}{4}$ the calculated equivalent dose of the new
                  opioid because of incomplete cross-tolerance.
                     Use short-acting opioids for breakthrough or
                  incidental pain, and long-acting opioids for
                  background analgesia.
                     Avoid rapid or frequent dose escalations in
                  CNMP.
Side Effects: Respiratory depression, sedation, euphoria, dys-
                  phoria, weakness, agitation, seizure, nausea,
                  vomiting, constipation, biliary spasm, urinary
                  retention, sweating, flushing, bradycardia, toler-
                  ance, physical dependence, and addiction.
Precautions: Caution in elderly, opioid naive, respiratory dis-
                  ease, infants, hepatic or liver disease, and pa-
                  tients with history of drug abuse and chemical
                  dependence, and patients performing tasks re-
                  quiring high mental alertness.

Orudis (see NSAIDs)
Oxycodone (see opioids)

Table 2. Commonly used opioids

Generic name	Trade name	Equianalgesic dosage Oral	Equianalgesic dosage Parenteral	Average adult dosage Oral	Average adult dosage Parenteral
Codeine		30 mg q 3–4h	10 mg q 3–4h	30 mg q 3–4h	10 mg q 3–4 h
Fentanyl Patch	Duragesic	N/A	N/A	25micg/hr patch q72h	N/A
Hydrocodone	Vicodin, Lorcet	N/A	N/A	10 mg q3–4h	N/A
Hydromorphone	Dilaudid	7.5mg q3–4h	1.5mg q 3–4 h	6mg q 3–4h	1.5 mg q 3–4h
Levorphanol	Levo-Dromoran	4mg q 6–8 h	2 mg q6–8 h	4mg q 6–8 g	2 mg q 6–8 h
Meperidine	Demerol	300 mg q 2–3h	100 mg q3h	100 mg q 3h	100 mg q 3h
Methadone	Dolophine	20 mg q 6–8h	10 mg q 6–8 h	10 mg q 8–12h	5mg q8–12 h
Morphine		30 mg q 3–4h	10 mg q 3–4 h	30 mg q 3–4h	10 mg q 3–4 h
Morphine SR	MSContin	N/A	N/A	15mg q 12h	N/A
Oxycodone	Percocet, Percodan	N/A	N/A	5 mg q 3–4h	N/A
OxyContin		N/A	N/A	10 mg q 8–12h	N/A

OxyContin (see opioids)
Pamelor (see TCAs)
Percocet (see opioids)
Percodan (see opioids)

Perphenazine
Description:	Phenothiazine, dopamine antagonist, antipsychotic, antiemetic, sedative.
Indications:	Psychoses, anxiety, nausea and vomiting.
Dosage:	PO or IM 4 mg two to four times daily.
Side Effects:	Constipation, sedation, vision changes or dry mouth, extrapyramidal symptoms, occasional tardive dyskinesia.
Precautions:	Extreme hypertension or hypotension, liver or heart disease, alcohol or drug dependencies, history of neuroleptic syndrome. Avoid in children.

Phenergan (see promethazine)

Phenoxybenzamine (Dibenzyline)
Description:	Alpha-adrenergic blocker.
Indications:	Sympathetically mediated/maintained pain.
Dosage:	Start at 10 mg PO TID and increase by 10 mg every 2 days, titrating to effect and as tolerated. Maximum dose (as an antihypertensive agent) 90–120 mg/day.
Side Effects:	Orthostatic hypotension, reflex tachycardia, meiosis, lethargy, nausea, vomiting, nasal congestion and headaches.
Precautions:	Extreme caution in the elderly and in presence of cardiovascular disease.

Phentolamine (Regitine)
Description:	Alpha-adrenergic antagonist.
Indications:	Diagnostic IV injection in suspected sympathetically mediated/maintained pain.
Dosage:	Infuse 35–70 mg in 250 mL normal saline over 20 minutes.
Side Effects:	Hypotension, dizziness, reflex tachycardia, syncope.
Precautions:	Monitor heart rate and blood pressure; patent IV access. Preload with 500 mL normal saline or lactated Ringer's solution prior to infusion; propranolol pretreatment (2 mg) for preventing reflex tachycardia recommended; have resuscitation equipment available.

Phenylbutazone (see NSAIDs)

Phenytoin (Dilantin)
Description:	First-generation sodium channel blocking anticonvulsant, adjunct antineuralgic.
Indications:	Seizures, epilepsy, and neuropathic pain.
Dosage:	PO 100 mg TID.
Side Effects:	Constipation, dizziness and drowsiness, blurred

vision, unsteadiness, nausea, mood changes or confusion, slurred speech, rash, insomnia, or headache.

Precautions: Porphyria, liver disease, myocardial insufficiency, cardiac arrhythmias, hypotension. Measure therapeutic levels.

Piroxicam (see NSAIDs)

Prednisolone
Description: Corticosteroid, anti-inflammatory.
Indications: Suppression of inflammatory and allergic disorders including asthma, chronic obstructive pulmonary disease, rheumatic disease, pain due to inflammation.
Dosage: Usual starting dose is 10–30 mg PO per day.
Side Effects: Dizziness, nausea, indigestion, increased appetite, weight gain, weakness, or sleep disturbances.
Precautions: Extreme hypertension or hypotension, liver or heart disease, Reye's syndrome, alcohol or drug dependencies, neurologic disease.

Prilocaine (see lidocaine–eutectic mixture)

Prochlorperazine (Compazine)
Description: Antiemetic.
Indications: Nausea and vomiting.
Dosage: Oral 5–10 mg three to four times daily, usually not exceeding 40 mg; rectal, 25 mg twice daily; IM, 5–10 mg every 3–4 hours, not to exceed 40 mg/day; IV, 2.5–10 mg every 3–4 hours, not to exceed 40 mg/day.
Side Effects: Extra pyramidal syndrome, neuroleptic malignant syndrome, drowsiness, postural hypotension, leukopenia, anorexia, dyspepsia, hyperpyrexia.
Precautions: Caution in elderly patients and patients with seizure disorder, glaucoma, and prostate hypertrophy.

Promethazine (Phenergan)
Description: Phenothiazine, dopamine antagonist, antipsychotic, antiemetic, sedative, antihistamine.
Indications: Nausea and vomiting.
Dosage: Can be used PO, IV, or IM for antiemesis, 12.5 to 25 mg every 4 hours, not to exceed 100 mg/day.
Side Effects: Shares the side effects of antihistamines, anticholinergic effects (dry mouth, blurring vision), phenothiazines (extrapyramidal symptoms), leukopenia, obstructive jaundice.
Precautions: Caution with cardiovascular or hepatic disease, and in the presence of other CNS depressants.

Protriptyline (see TCAs)
Prozac (see fluoxetine)

Regitine (see phentolamine)
Reglan (see metoclopramide)
Ritalin (see methylphenidate)

Rofecoxib (Vioxx)
Description: NSAID, selective COX-2 inhibitor.
Indications: Pain with peripheral inflammatory component.
Dosage: 12.5–50 mg PO once daily.
Side Effects: Lower incidence of GI complications than tradi-
                 tional NSAIDs. Usual doses do not appear to af-
                 fect platelet aggregation. Renal toxicity similar
                 to that of traditional NSAIDs.
Precautions: History of GI bleed, fluid retention, or renal im-
                 pairment.

Salsalate (see NSAIDs)
Senna (Senokot)
Description: Laxative.
Indication: Constipation.
Dosage: One to two tablets PO once or twice per day.
Side Effects: Diarrhea, nausea, vomiting, rectal irritation,
                 stomach cramps, or bloating.
Precautions: Kidney disease, heart disease, high blood pres-
                 sure, edema, or allergies, especially to tartrazine.

Sertraline (Zoloft)
Description: Selective serotonin reuptake inhibitor (SSRI),
                 first-line antidepressant.
Indications: Depression, panic disorder, obsessive-compulsive
                 disorder.
Dosage: PO 50–200 mg/day.
Side Effects: These are rare but include headaches, stimulation
                 or sedation, fine tremor, tinnitus, rare extrapyra-
                 midal symptoms, palpitations, nausea and vom-
                 iting, bloating, and diarrhea.
Precautions: Known sensitivity, interactions with MAOIs.

Sinequan (see TCAs)
Sodium valproate (see valproic acid)
Sulindac (see NSAIDs)

Sumatriptan (Imitrex)
Description: "Triptan," selective $5HT_{1B}$ agonist, antimigraine
                 agent.
Indication: Migraine headache attacks.
Dosage: For *nasal* dosage form (nasal solution), 5 or 10 mg
                 (one or two sprays into each nostril) or 20 mg (one
                 spray into one nostril). Do not use more than
                 40 mg in a 24-hour period. For *oral* dosage form
                 (tablets), 25 to 100 mg as a single dose. If the mi-
                 graine comes back after being relieved, another
                 dose may be taken 2 hours after the last dose. Do
                 not take more than 300 mg in any 24-hour period.
                 For *parenteral* dosage form (injection), One 6-mg

injection. One more 6-mg dose may be injected, if necessary, if the migraine comes back after being relieved. However, the second injection should not be given any sooner than 1 hour after the first one. Do not use more than two 6-mg injections in a 24-hour period.

Side Effects: Tingling sensations, feelings of warmth or heaviness, dizziness, flushing, drowsiness.

Precautions: Cardiovascular disease, high blood pressure, kidney disease, liver disease stroke.

TCAs (tricyclic antidepressants)

Description: Norepinephrine and serotonin reuptake inhibitors.

Indications: Depression, neuropathic pain, evening dose may improve overnight sleep.

Dosage: Usually given once daily at bedtime. Start at 25 mg (10 mg for elderly patients) and gradually escalate dose in small increments every 3–5 days as tolerated to a maximum of 75–150 mg at bedtime (see Table 3 for range of doses). Beneficial effects may be noticed in 1–3 weeks or sometimes earlier.

Side Effects: Dry mouth, blurred vision, urinary retention, constipation, reflux (anticholinergic), weakness, lethargy, fatigue, paradoxical excitement, exacerbation of psychiatric symptoms (CNS), postural hypotension, cardiac arrhythmias.

Precautions: Benign prostatic hypertrophy, urinary retention, closed-angle glaucoma, severe respiratory disease, seizure disorder, cardiac dysrhythmias, other cardiac disease.

Tegretol (see carbamazepine)
Thorazine (see chlorpromazine)

Tizanidine (Zanaflex)

Description: Antispasmodic.

Indications: Myofascial pain (muscle spasms).

Table 3. Commonly used tricyclic antidepressants (TCAs)

Generic name	Trade name	Adult dosage range (mg/day)
Amitriptyline[a]	Elavil	10–300
Amoxapine	Asendin	50–400
Clomipramine[a]	Anafranil	25–300
Desipramine[a]	Norpramin	10–300
Doxepin	Sinequan	10–300
Imipramine[a]	Tofranil	10–300
Nortriptyline[a]	Pamelor	10–200
Protriptyline	Vivactil	10–60

[a]Commonly used for neuropathic pain.

Dosage: Start with 2–4 mg PO QHS, then gradually
                   increase to maximum of 36 mg/day in divided
                   doses.
Side Effects: Nausea, drowsiness, dizziness, constipation, un-
                   usual weakness, or dry mouth.
Precautions: Caution in patients with hypotension, hepatic,
                   cardiac, renal, or eye diseases.

Tofranil (see TCAs)
Tolectin (see NSAIDs)
Tolmetin (see NSAIDs)
Topamax (see topiramate)

Topiramate (Topamax)
Description: Anticonvulsant, adjunct antineuralgic.
Indications: Second-line medication for neuropathic pain. May
                   act by inhibiting voltage-dependent sodium chan-
                   nels, enhancing activity of inhibitory neurotrans-
                   mitter gamma aminobutyric acid (GABA) and
                   antagonism of NMDA receptor.
Dosage: Usually start at 50 mg QHS and gradually in-
                   crease by 25 mg every week up to a maximum of
                   200 mg BID as tolerated. Gradual improvement
                   may be noticed over weeks, as doses are titrated
                   gradually.
Side Effects: Weakness, tiredness, drowsiness, dizziness, tin-
                   gling sensations, loss of appetite and weight,
                   unsteadiness, slowing or shakiness, speech prob-
                   lems, mental/mood changes, stomach/abdominal
                   pain or vision problems may occur.
Precautions: Caution in patients with renal or hepatic disease.

Toradol (see ketorolac)

Tramadol (Ultram)
Description: Analgesic, weak mu agonist with additional inhi-
                   bition of norepinephrine and serotonin reuptake.
Indications: Mild to moderate pain, adjunct in severe pain.
                   Useful in patients who cannot tolerate opioids.
Dosage: PO 50–100 mg every 4–6 hours as needed. Start
                   at low dose to minimize side effects (not to ex-
                   ceed 400 mg/day).
Side Effects: Dizziness, vertigo, headache, constipation, nau-
                   sea and vomiting, dyspepsia, pruritus, and se-
                   dation.
Precautions: At high doses, seizures may occur, especially if
                   used in combination with TCAs. Respiratory
                   depression, constipation, and dependence are
                   extremely rare. Prolonged international nor-
                   malized ratio (INR) in presence of warfarin; re-
                   duce dose in renal impairment and the elderly.

Triamcinolone (Aristocort, Kenalog)
Description: Corticosteroid, anti-inflammatory.
Indications: Inflammation, swelling, and pain.

Dosage: For epidural or nerve root injection, 10–80 mg as a single dose.

Side Effects: Increased or decreased appetite, insomnia, indigestion, nervousness.

Precautions: Extreme hypertension or hypotension, liver or heart disease, Reye's syndrome, alcohol or drug dependencies, neurologic disease.

Tricyclic antidepressants (see TCAs)
Trilisate (see NSAIDs)
Tylenol (see acetaminophen)
Ultram (see tramadol)
Valium (see diazepam)

Valproic acid (Depakene)
Description: Anticonvulsant, adjunct antineuralgic.

Indications: Seizure disorders, migraine headache prophylaxis, manic phase of bipolar disorder, neuropathic pain.

Dosage: 15 mg/kg per day in two or three divided doses, increasing every week up to maximum dose of 60 mg/kg per day.

Side Effects: Stomach pain, loss of appetite, change in menstrual periods, diarrhea, mild hair loss, unsteadiness, dizziness, drowsiness, rash, or headache.

Precautions: Liver disease, bleeding disorder.

Vicodin (see opioids)
Vioxx (see rofecoxib)
Vistaril (see hydroxyzine)
Vivactil (see TCAs)
Voltaren (see NSAIDs)
Zanaflex (see tizanidine)
Zofran (see ondansetron)
Zoloft (see sertraline)

Subject Index

Note: Page numbers followed by *f* indicate figures; those followed by t indicate tables.